Pharmacology of the
Contraceptive Steroids

Pharmacology of the Contraceptive Steroids

Chief Editor

Joseph W. Goldzieher, M.D.

Department of Obstetrics and Gynecology
Baylor College of Medicine
Houston, Texas

Associate Editor

Kenneth Fotherby, Ph.D.

Royal Postgraduate Medical School
Hammersmith Hospital
London, England

Raven Press   New York

Raven Press, Ltd., 1185 Avenue of the Americas, New York, New York 10036

Made in the United States of America

Library of Congress Cataloging-in-Publication Data

Pharmacology of the contraceptive steroids / chief editor, Joseph W.
  Goldzieher ; associate editor, Kenneth Fotherby.
      p. cm.
    Includes index.
    ISBN 0-7817-0097-3
    1. Contraceptive drugs.   2. Steroid hormones.   I. Goldzieher,
Joseph W. (Joseph William), 1919–   .   II. Fotherby, K. (Kenneth),
1927–   .
    [DNLM: 1. Estrogens—pharmacology.   2. Progestational Hormones—
pharmacology.   QV 177 P5364 1994]
RG137.4.P48   1994
615′.766—dc20
DNLM/DLC
for Library of Congress
                                                          93-38571
                                                             CIP

9 8 7 6 5 4 3 2 1

"There is nothing more difficult to take in hand, more perilous to conduct, or more uncertain in its success, than to take the lead in the introduction of a new order of things."

Niccolo Machiavelli

Contents

Part VI. Drug Interactions

Part VII. Statistical and Epidemiological Issues

Contributors

Michael R. Adams, D.V.M.   *Department of Comparative Medicine, Comparative Medicine Clinical Research Center, Bowman Gray School of Medicine of Wake Forest University, Medical Center Boulevard, Winston-Salem, North Carolina 27157*

Kosin Amatayakul, M.B., Ch.B., FRCOG   *Department of Obstetrics and Gynecology, Faculty of Medicine and Research Institute for Health Sciences, Chiang Mai University, Chiang Mai 50002, Thailand*

David J. Back, Ph.D.   *Department of Pharmacology and Therapeutics, University of Liverpool, P.O. Box 147, Liverpool L69 3BX, United Kingdom*

Fritz K. Beller, M.D., D.Sc.   *W. C. Keettel Professor (Emeritus), Department of Obstetrics and Gynecology, University of Iowa College of Medicine, Iowa City, Iowa 52242*

Giuseppe Benagiano, M.D.   *First Institute of Obstetrics and Gynecology, University la Sapienza, Policlinico Umberto I, Rome 00161, Italy*

Helmut Blode, Ph.D.   *Institue of Pharmacokinetics, Research Laboratories, Schering AG, 13342 Berlin, Germany*

Ivo Brosens, M.D., Ph.D.   *Department of Obstetrics and Gynecology, University Hospital Gasthuisberg, Herestraat 49, B-300 Leuven, Belgium*

James H. Clark, Ph.D.   *Department of Cell Biology, Baylor College of Medicine, One Baylor Plaza, Houston, Texas 77030*

Thomas B. Clarkson, D.V.M.   *Department of Comparative Medicine, Comparative Medicine Research Center, Bowman Gray School of Medicine of Wake Forest University, Medical Center Boulevard, Winston-Salem, North Carolina 27157*

Göran Cullberg, M.D., Ph.D.   *Department of Obstetrics and Gynecology, University of Gothenburg, Hallegårsv. 19, S-43362 Partille, Sweden*

David Edelman, Ph.D.   *Medical Research Consultants, 20 Bedford Court, Madison, New Jersey 07940*

Richard A. Edgren, Ph.D.   *Pharmaceutical Consultant, 50 Oakhaven Way, Woodside, California 94062*

Karen Elkind-Hirsch, Ph.D.   *Internal Medicine Specialty Laboratories, 7550 Fannin, Suite 104, Houston, Texas 77054*

Kenneth Fotherby, Ph.D. *Reader Emeritus, Royal Postgraduate Medical School, Hammersmith Hospital, London W12 0HS, England*

Robert Fraser, M.D. *MRC Blood Pressure Unit, Western Infirmary, Medical Research Council, Glasgow G11 6NT, Scotland*

T. B. P. Geurts, Ph.D. *Organon Scientific Development Group, P.O. Box 20, 5340BH Oss, The Netherlands*

Joseph W. Goldzieher, M.D. *Professor and Director of Endocrine/Metabolic Research (ret.), Department of Obstetrics and Gynecology, Baylor College of Medicine, One Baylor Plaza, Houston, Texas 77030*

E. M. Goorissen, Ph.D. *Organon Scientific Development Group, P.O. Box 20, 5340BH Oss, The Netherlands*

J. M. W. Hazes, M.D., Ph.D. *Department of Rheumatology, University Hospital Leiden, P.O. Box 9600, 2300RC, Leiden, The Netherlands*

Elisabeth Johannisson, M.D., Ph.D. *Laboratory of Analytical and Quantitative Cytology, International Committee for Research in Reproduction, CH-1208 Geneva, Switzerland*

David Keefe, M.D. *Department of Obstetrics and Gynecology, Yale School of Medicine, 333 Cedar Street, New Haven, Connecticut 06510*

Wilhelm Kuhnz, Ph.D. *Institute of Pharmacokinetics, Research Laboratories Schering AG, 13342 Berlin, Germany*

Morris Notelovitz, M.D., Ph.D. *Women's Medical and Diagnostic Center and The Climacteric Clinic, Inc., Gainesville, Florida 32607*

Michael L'E. Orme, M.D., FRCP *Department of Pharmacology and Therapeutics, University of Liverpool, P.O. Box 147, Liverpool L69 3BX United Kingdom*

Nicola Perone, M.D. *Department of Obstetrics, Gynecology and Reproductive Sciences, University of Texas Health Science Center, 1631 North Loop West, Suite 560, Houston, Texas 77008*

Steven M. Petak, M.D. *Department of Pharmacology, University of Texas School of Medicine at Houston, and Texas Institute for Research in Reproductive Medicine and Endocrinology, Houston, Texas 77054*

Malcolm Potts, M.B., B.Chir., Ph.D. *International Family Health, 15, Bateman's Buildings, Soho Square, London WIV 5TW, England*

Francesco M. Primiero, M.D. *First Institute of Obstetrics and Gynecology, University la Sapienza, Policlinico Umberto I, Rome 00161, Italy*

A. H. W. M. Schuurs, Ph.D.   *Organon Scientific Development Group,*
P.O. Box 20, 5340BH, Oss, The Netherlands

M. H. Sillem, Dr. Med.   *Klinikum Aschaffenburg, University of Würsburg, Am*
Hasenkoph I, 8750 Aschaffenburg, Germany

Frank Z. Stanczyk, Ph.D.   *Department of Obstetrics and Gynecology,*
University of Southern California School of Medicine, Los Angeles,
California 90033

Emil Steinberger, M.D.   *Texas Institute for Research in Reproductive Medicine*
and Endocrinology, University of Texas School of Medicine at Houston,
7400 Fannin Suite 850, Houston Texas 77054

A. T. Teichmann, Prof. Dr. Med.   *Klinikum Aschaffenburg, University of*
Würsburg, Am Hasenkoph 1, 8750 Aschaffenburg, Germany

H. A. M. Verheul, Ph.D.   *Organon Scientific Development Group,*
P.O. Box 20, 5340BH, Oss, The Netherlands

Janice D. Wagner, D.V.M., Ph.D.   *Department of Comparative Medicine,*
Comparative Medicine Clinical Research Center, Bowman Gray School of
Medicine of Wake Forest University, Medical Center Boulevard,
Winston-Salem, North Carolina 27157

Scott A. Washburn, M.D.   *Departments of Obstetrics and Gynecology, and*
Comparative Medicine, Comparative Medicine Clinical Research Center,
Bowman Gray School of Medicine of Wake Forest University, Medical Center
Boulevard, Winston-Salem, North Carolina 27157

Ronald J. Weir, M.D.   *MRC Blood Pressure Unit, Medical Research Council,*
Glasgow G11 6NT, Scotland

John C. Wirth, Ph.D.   *Department of Physical Education, Wayne State*
University College of Education, Detroit, Michigan 48202

Preface

Fundamental advances in medical science have usually been met with resistance or outright hostility by the Establishment, and often by the public as well: consider vaccination (Jenner, Pasteur), antisepsis (Semmelweiss), anesthesia (Morton) and, more recently, genetic engineering. When, in addition, a new development impacts on deepseated sociocultural and religious beliefs and traditions, an even more intense reaction can be expected. This has, in fact, turned out to be the case with contraception. Hormonal contraceptives have been more widely studied and intensively researched than any other medicinal agent in history, yet misinformation prevails and controversy continues. This ranges from the ridiculous (one religious group claims that an agent which prevents ovulation is an abortifacient) to sophisticated scientific publications which imperturbably conclude what they set out to prove *a priori*, ignoring "minor" factors such as the known hazards of cigarette smoking in studies of cardiovascular risks. The literature is so vast and the many excellent reviews so closely focused that it is difficult for someone not profoundly involved in this field to gain access to the basic information.

After more than thirty years of evolution, the field of steroid contraception has matured considerably and the intellectual threads are coming together. A great deal has been learned about the ways in which such agents should be developed and tested, and what improvements would yield practical benefit. The overriding importance of factors which improve compliance, whether pharmacological or sociocultural, is clear. It is our prediction (one which we hope will be proved wrong) that this branch of "steroidery" is not going to see revolutionary developments in the near future. Therefore, it now may be the time to collect basic information on various aspects of hormonal contraception in one place, and that is the intent of this book. Hopefully the knowledge garnered and the mistakes committed in the past will expedite future investigation.

Fields of chemical contraception involving substances other than the current class of steroids will bear watching. Immunocontraception, long delayed by lack of funding and bureaucratic and professional obstructionism, may benefit by technical advances such as PCR, which increase enormously our investigative capabilities. Photochemistry, long neglected by a shortsighted pharmaceutical industry as simply not cost-effective, may have been given a critical boost by the impact of environmentalism, especially rain-forest destruction, and by technology which permits mass screening of raw materials. Hopefully, investigators will access anthropological, as well as chemical, skills (perhaps we need another Russell Marker!) to benefit from the centuries of experience of native peoples with the medicinal plants in their surroundings. Exciting times are ahead.

Joseph W. Goldzieher

Introduction

Malcolm Potts

The invention of the Pill was the greatest revolution that has ever occurred, or will ever occur, in family planning. It disassociated contraception from sexual intercourse; it was virtually 100% effective and totally reversible. It was particularly remarkable that this revolution grew out of research in Boston, Massachusetts, because at the time the Pill was tested, birth control was illegal in that state. It was not until 1965 that the US Supreme Court struck down *Griswold v Connecticut*, the last of the 19th century Comstock laws, which treated contraceptives as obscene items.

Revolutions, however, have their limitations, and when Pincus, Rock, and Chang worked on the Pill, the possibility of therapeutic abortion was unthinkable. The normal clinical titration of an effective dose was impossible. To complicate matters, synthetic steroids are less effective orally in rodents than in people, so extrapolation from animal doses led to human overdosing. It took many years to demonstrate that much lower doses of steroids could be equally effective in preventing pregnancy. Unfortunately, oral contraceptives still live under the shadow of the high-dose pills, which had both tiresome short-term side effects and unsolved questions about cancer.

Revolutions, by definition, are controversial. The Pill has been alternately hailed as signifying the ultimate liberation of women and as an evil example of a deliberate effort by the medico-industrial complex to exploit women in an unnatural and highly dangerous fashion. Use of the Pill has gone up and down with the degree of media coverage and current medical opinion. Following first market approval in the USA in 1960, use of the Pill rose rapidly in many developed countries, sometimes reaching a third of all married women of reproductive age. Use then declined when the first reports of associated cardiovascular complications appeared from Europe. For the first time, a great many physicians and the public at large had to make decisions based on large-scale and sometimes difficult-to-interpret epidemiological studies. Epidemiological methodologies were pushed to the limit, but in the process, important discoveries were made about the effect of estrogen dose in oral contraceptives, and the interrelationships between age and the smoking practices of users. By the late 1970s the selection of low-dose pills, combined with the screening of women for smoking, either eliminated the cardiovascular risks of the Pill or reduced them to such a level that they became virtually unmeasurable.

The use of contraceptive steroids also brought about another revolution. The Pill is the first therapy that protects against an important group of malignancies. By the 1980s there was mounting evidence of a consistent, duration-of-use dependent, powerful protective effect of Pill use against ovarian and uterine cancer. It was a revolution practically no one had thought possible. Yet biologically it was perfectly predictable. It is clear from several sources that patterns of human reproduction have been finely tailored by evolution to encompass late puberty and a relatively small number of pregnancies spaced by long intervals of breast feeding. Rather than being "unnatural," as some feminist critics of the Pill suggest, the use of oral contraceptives is in some ways less "unnatural" than long uninterrupted intervals of ovulation and repeated menstruation.

Will it ever be possible to turn a welcome but still accidental protection against neoplasia into a planned defense? Epidemiological study to date shows no overall relationship between oral contraceptive use and the incidence of breast cancer, although breast cancer itself is much more common in women who have an early puberty, late childbearing and fewer pregnancies, and (some studies suggest) who do not breast feed their babies. There is a question about the relationship between the Pill and the rare occurrence of breast cancer in women under 35, but biologically speaking, it is remarkable that a stronger adverse or beneficial effect does not exist. It is possible that new progestins, or new approaches to the formulation of hormonal contraceptives, could eventually create an orally active formulation that would not only allow a woman to control her fertility in a totally reversible way, but if used for a number of years at a critical age, might also end up protecting the user against ovarian, uterine, and breast cancer later in her reproductive life.

One of the many remarkable things about oral contraceptives is that they can be mass produced in high quality at very low cost. When purchasing in bulk for programs of international family planning, the cost of oral contraceptives, in non-inflationary terms, has fallen over the last few decades. In countries where oral contraceptives can be freed from unrealistic medical restrictions and actively promoted, oral contraceptives can be made available at a price that is acceptable to many people in the cash economy. Empirical observations suggest that people will spend about 1% of their disposable income on family planning. However, for some of the poorer regions of the world, such as South Asia and sub-Saharan Africa, even the low cost of the Pill is too high. Fortunately, it is quite within the grasp of international agencies and national governments to subsidize the price of pills and "socially market" them so they do become generally available to all women who need them. Since the 1970s, the International Planned Parenthood Federation and other bodies have endorsed the philosophy that whoever normally provides for the health care of the community can be an appropriate person to distribute oral contraceptives. As low-dose pills are safer than aspirin, there is also a movement in some western countries to reconsider the need for medical prescription. At a global level, it has almost certainly been a combination of muddled medical philosophies and a territorial eagerness among some physicians to control any therapy that has kept the Pill on prescription. Medical barriers, from lack of perspective on risks to the expense and deterrent of prescription and examination, along with the tendency of many doctors to prefer treatment over prevention, have been the primary restraining factors holding back oral contraceptive use.

There may well be genuine sociocultural differences in the acceptability of different methods of family planning in different cultures, although they are often overshadowed by simple lack of availability. Some societies, for example in the Caribbean, appear to prefer to receive steroidal contraceptives through a syringe rather than as a tablet. In other parts of the world, women are in partial (or) total seclusion. In Bangladesh, it is men who purchase packets of pills to take home to their wives. In Iran, among one group of women using oral contraceptives, 78% discontinued use within 6 months of taking the first tablet. Most people would have concluded that the Pill was unacceptable in that community, were it not for an Iranian psychologist. He took the husbands of the same group of women, gave them the Pill, provided them with instructions on its use and side effects, and suggested that they pass it on to their wives; at the end of 6 months, more than 90% of the wives continued taking the Pill. This difference in continuation rates is much greater than has ever been observed between two different pill formulations. Perhaps it is not so much that there are societies for whom the Pill is unacceptable, as that there are societies where the method of distribution needs to be altered to meet the perceptions of the consumers.

One important quantitative difference between developed and developing countries is the lower use-effectiveness of the Pill in many Third World communities. There are interesting differences in the ways in which different ethnic groups or women with different diets metabolize steroids, but large differences in failure rate are almost certainly due to variations in compliance. Field studies show as many as 10% or more women getting pregnant in the first year of use, whereas the theoretical effectiveness should be 99% or better. Over the years, improvements in package design and the use of placebo pills may have been as important as some changes in formulation. There is still a long way to go. A recent study in Egypt showed that more women made the transition between one packet and the next incorrectly than made it correctly. Recent efforts by the US Food and Drug Administration (FDA) to work with manufacturers to produce a common set of instructions, particularly when tablets are forgotten, are to be welcomed. In the future development of oral contraceptives, improvements in compliance are likely to prove more important than improvements in chemistry. After all, the most common "side effect" of the Pill remains unintended pregnancy.

As a result of yesterday's population explosion there will be one-third more women of fertile age in 10 years' time than there are today. The prevalence of contraceptive use in many developing countries rose rapidly in the past 10 or 15 years. Sufficient demand probably exists so that the number of contraceptive users in Third World countries might be doubled in the coming decade. If this is to occur, there can be no doubt that oral contraceptives will play a major role.

Lack of money and medicolegal fears have practically stopped the development of new methods of contraception. The levonorgestrel implant is likely to remain a minority method for reasons of expense and difficulty in use. Incidentally, this implant, with its systemic release of steroid, might have been developed before the Pill; if it had, we can be sure the race would now be on to develop an oral formulation!

The Pill is going to be with us for a long time. We can expect to see further incremental improvements in dose and formulation. A wider variety of progestational agents are likely to be used. Further insight into the relationship between contraceptive steroids and breast cancer will slowly become available. In short, there is every reason to believe that more women will use oral contraceptives in the future than have used them in the past 30 years.

Pharmacology of the Contraceptive Steroids,
edited by Joseph W. Goldzieher.
Raven Press, Ltd., New York © 1994.

1

The Progestins

Nicola Perone

*Clinical Associate Professor, Department of Obstetrics, Gynecology and Reproductive
Sciences, University of Texas Health Science Center at Houston
Houston, Texas 77008*

The introduction of oral contraception in 1960 was not the result of one person's fortuitous discovery, as happened with x-rays or penicillin. It was, rather, the product of small accretions of knowledge resulting from the effort, talent, and determination of many people over a period of years.

THE CHEMICAL HISTORY OF THE PILL

The chemical history of the Pill begins with the isolation of progesterone in May, 1933 by Corner and Allen. With the help of Dr. Hickman from the research laboratory of the Eastman Kodak Company, they used high-vacuum distillation of the oils extracted from corpora lutea to isolate the hormone in a crystalline form, which they named "Progestin." Before the end of that year, Wintersteiner and Allen (1934) determined the structural formula of the hormone ($C_{21}H_{30}O_2$). This admittedly was not difficult, since the structural formula of pregnanediol was known from previous work by Butenandt. As Allen later recalled (Allen, 1974), the correct structural formula of progesterone had originally been sketched on a napkin during a lunch with William Strain, long before the definitive structural proof was furnished!

In the summer of 1934, the isolation of crystalline progesterone was announced also by Butenandt and Westfall (1934) in Danzig, by Slotta et al. (1934) in Breslau, and in Switzerland by Hartman and Wettstein (1934). A short time later, Butenandt and Schmidt (1934) converted the dihydroxy compound pregnandiol to progesterone and Fernholz succeeded in synthesizing progesterone from stigmasterol.[a]

---

[a]This international race for the isolation of the hormone did not proceed without incidents (Allen, 1974). In December of 1934, Wintersteiner received a letter from Slotta in which he was informed that the two had agreed to call the new hormone "luteo-sterone," unaware of the previous name "progestin" given by Allen and Corner in 1933. In his answer Corner suggested as a compromise to name the new hormone progesterone or progestenone. The question of the name for the new hormone was eventually settled in 1935 during a garden party in London given by Sir Henry Dale, and attended by Allen, Butenandt, and Slotta. The conference had been specifically organized to collect standard samples of

A few years later (in 1945), an international legal controversy arose. Percy Julian, a chemist with the Glidden paint company, had been making progesterone from the oils used in the manufacture of paint. The Schering Co. filed suit against Glidden for infringement of the German patent, based on Butenandt's work. When told of the suit by Julian, Allen started to prepare for the trial by diligently reviewing his notes, which clearly indicated his priority in the isolation of the hormone. The contest was eventually settled out of court.

The early production of progesterone was extremely complex and laborious and the resulting product prohibitively expensive. Butenandt required a ton of cholesterol, obtained from the brains and spinal cords of cattle and the grease from sheep's wool, to obtain 20 pounds of starting material from which commercial quantities of progesterone could be produced. Progesterone, when available, was quoted at $1000 per gram.

What opened the door for the development of the Pill were two advances in steroid chemistry: the introduction of a new technique, which changed progesterone from an expensive rarity to the cheapest of all steroid hormones, and the subsequent modification of the progesterone molecule to make it orally effective. The first of these two discoveries was made by a genius chemist by the name of Russel E. Marker who, in addition to a brilliant mind, possessed extraordinary determination in pursuing his ingenious researches.[b] By working at all hours of the day and night at the Pond Laboratory at Penn State, he repeated the experiments of various European chemists to get the feel of steroid chemistry. Then, with some sarsaparilla obtained from Mexico, he was able to determine the configuration of the sarsapogenin side chain, which, as he had suspected, was not the configuration pro-

---

progesterone, estradiol, estradiol benzoate, and androsterone, and to define an international unit for each of these sex steroids. Sir Henry was able to convince Butenandt and Slotta that "progesterone" was, after all, a composite of Allen's "progestin" and their "luteo-sterone," and thus an acceptable compromise.

[b]Marker, the man regarded as the "chemical father of the birth control pill," was born in 1902 near Hagerstown, Maryland, the son of a farmer. He saw early on that education was the only way out of the farm. With considerable effort he finished high school and enrolled at the University of Maryland, where in 1923 he received his BS in organic chemistry, and the following year, his Master's degree in colloidal chemistry. In 2 years, he completed the research required for his PhD. However, when told that he had to take additional formal courses for his doctorate in physical chemistry, he found that idea boring, and simply walked out. His teacher at the University of Maryland predicted that, without a doctorate, he could only hope to become a "urine analyst." Oblivious of the prediction, he married and took a job as a research chemist with the new Ethyl Gasoline Corporation in Yonkers, NY. There he studied hydrocarbons, discovered important characteristics of gasoline, and developed the octane rating system. He was subsequently invited to join the Rockefeller Institute, where he developed the now well-known optical rotatory dispersion technology. He first became involved with methods to produce steroid hormones from plant material while at the Rockefeller Institute. His laboratory was adjacent to that of a colleague (Dr. Walter Jacobs) who had been trying unsuccessfully to derive progesterone from sarsapogenin, obtained from the sarsaparilla rhizome. Marker was aware of the increased demand for steroid hormones and saw in this area a tremendous challenge. He was convinced that he could succeed where Jacobs had failed, and asked the head of the Rockefeller Institute for permission to pursue this area of research. To his disappointment, he was told to continue instead with his current work. He remembered that Dr. Frank Whitmore, the dean at Pennsylvania State University, had told him to call if he ever thought to change employers. He did, and in September 1934 was offered a job at $1800 per year (which represented a 55% pay cut from the Rockefeller Institute), but with complete freedom as to the type of research he did. In 1935, he was given a Professorship at Penn State University in organic chemistry.

posed by the German chemists. He found that it consisted of a keto-spiral-acetal grouping that, under certain conditions, could be easily removed. Meanwhile, T. Tsukamoto, in Japan, had isolated a product called diosgenin from *Dioscorea Tokoro*, which Marker felt was even more suitable for hormone production than sarsapogenin, since it had a 5,6 double bond and one hydroxyl group in the 3-position, having the beta-configuration as in cholesterol. Tsukamoto obtained tigogenin by catalytic reduction, demonstrating that it had the same side chain characteristics as the sapogenins. Thus, Marker concluded that diosgenin was an ideal compound to apply the same reactions that he had applied to sarsapogenin for the removal of the side chain, thus leading to derivatives of the pregnane and androstane series (Marker et al., 1939, 1940). He obtained a small (30 g) sample of diosgenin from Japan and from it was able to derive, with a unique chemical process later called "Marker's degradation," progesterone.[c]

The successful attempt to obtain progesterone from diosgenin led Marker to a search for American plants that stored diosgenin. He found one in North and South Carolina, but the rhizome was "the size of a thumb" and thus not suitable for commercial production. He also went to College Station, Texas, where he contacted V.L. Cory, range ecologist for Texas A & M University. While at Cory's house, he picked up a book and, quite by accident, found the picture of a large dioscorea (*Dioscorea mexicana*), which grew in Vera Cruz, Mexico. He returned to Penn State to unload the plants collected in Texas and decided to go to Mexico (it took 3 days by train in those days) in search of the large dioscorea. He went the first time in November of 1941 and was told he needed a plant collecting permit from the Mexican government, and was advised to return to the US to get typhoid shots while the American embassy would attempt to secure his permit. In January 1942, with a rented truck and a Mexican botanist, he went as far as Tehuacan without, however, getting any plants. He returned to Mexico City, where he reported his failure to the American embassy and was told to forget about his plants and to return to the US. Instead, Marker got on the bus and went to Orizaba with a stop overnight at Puebla. He remembered having read in the book he saw at Cory's house that the dioscorea (known locally as "cabeza de negro," i.e., negro's head, due to the scale-like markings on the rhizome reminiscent of a black man's curls) grew along a stream between Orizaba and Cordoba. He took the bus to Cordoba and, 10 miles out of Orizaba, he found the stream and nearby a small country store manned by an Indian named Alberto Moreno. With some difficulty, since he spoke no Spanish, Marker asked Moreno to get him some cabeza de negro, and the man secured two plants for him. The next morning he loaded the two bags containing cabeza de negro onto the bus and went back to Orizaba, where he found out that the plants had been stolen; however, the local policeman was willing to sell them both back to him for $20.

---

[c]Marker notified Butenandt, among others, of his ability to derive progesterone from plant material and was invited to discuss his new process (Butenandt, along with other European chemists, had demonstrated that sex hormones were all based on a steroid nucleus). Marker eventually crossed the Atlantic on the Queen Mary, but once in Germany, Butenandt refused to receive him, possibly because he had been told that Marker, while in Berlin, had befriended a Jewish couple.

Marker was only willing to part with a $10 bill and salvaged one of the two plants, with which he returned to Penn State. He used half of it to obtain diosgenin and the other half to demonstrate the process to the Parke-Davis chemists, in hopes of convincing Dr. Oliver Kamm, then Director of Research at Parke-Davis, to gather large amounts of dioscorea from Mexico to use as a source for hormone production.[d] Dr. Kamm was unconvinced that anything constructive could be done in Mexico and believed that bull's urine and sarsaparilla were adequate sources. Unable to get the backing of Parke-Davis, Marker took half of his life savings and, at the start of the dry season in October 1942, returned to Vera Cruz. There, with the help of a new Mexican botanist (Dr. Benevides), he gathered various plants he thought might be of interest and shipped them from Laredo to Penn State. He also gathered more "cabeza de negro," which Moreno dried for him. Then he found a man with a small-scale extractor who was able to extract and evaporate the product to a syrup.

While waiting for this to be done, he thought of searching for a Mexican company that could be interested in the production of hormones. While looking through the "yellow pages" in the Mexico City telephone directory, he noticed a company called Laboratorios Hormona, owned by Emeric Somlo, a lawyer who had emigrated to Mexico from Hungary. He called up the company and arranged a meeting with Dr. Federico Lehman, a physician who was the production manager and company co-founder (Somlo being in New York at that time). Dr. Lehman called Somlo, who immediately returned to Mexico, and the three of them agreed to form a Mexican company for the production of hormones, with Laboratorios Hormonas financing the entire project. Marker, with his 5-gallon cans of syrup, returned to Penn State. He arranged with a friend in New York to make progesterone from this syrup, promising him one-third of the yield as compensation, and absolute anonymity. The yield, to his surprise, was 3 kg of progesterone, of which he retained 2 kg; the friend was given the rest. This was more progesterone than had ever been produced before, and Marker's friend established a price of $80 per gram, breaking the international hormone cartel controlled by the European companies.

In 1943, Marker returned to Mexico to get some more plants and to see if Laboratorios Hormona had purchased the necessary equipment and chemicals. As he was leaving, he mentioned to Lehman that he had 2 kg of progesterone in the US, produced from cabeza de negro. As soon as he returned to State College, he received a call from Somlo, who asked if he still had the 2 kg of progesterone, and if so, would he meet with him in New York.

Marker took his progesterone to New York, where Somlo convinced him to turn it over to him and in return he would get 40% of the new company to be established in Mexico, with Somlo retaining 52% and Lehman receiving the remaining 8% for having gotten the two together. Marker agreed and returned to Mexico in December of 1943 to start production of hormones in two small laboratories that belonged to Laboratorios Hormona; he had the help of four young women, none of whom had

---

[d]The reason why Marker had approached Parke-Davis was that the pharmaceutical company had established a few graduate fellowships to study the possibility of extracting estrone and estradiol from urine of pregnant women and mares.

more than a fourth-grade education or spoke English. The following month, Somlo applied for a charter for the new company, which Marker proposed be called Syntex, (from *Synt*hesis and M*e*xico). Syntex was incorporated in March, 1944. Meanwhile, a four room laboratory had been built adjacent to Laboratorios Hormona, to which Marker moved in May of 1944. During the remainder of that year, he was able to produce over 30 kg of progesterone and 10 kg of dehydroepiandrosterone, to be converted later into testosterone.[e]

Marker soon realized the mistake he had made in setting up production in Mexico and tried until May of 1945 to reach some kind of settlement. Since none could be reached, he left Syntex and started a new company of his own in Texcoco, 30 miles from Mexico City, with the financial support of his friend from New York with whom he had produced the first 3 kg of progesterone. The new company, called Botanica-Mex SA, had considerable difficulty getting started. A man collecting dioscorea for him was killed, a guard he had was shot, and one of the women working for him was choked and beaten (Marker, 1987). The starting material he used was a different dioscorea (*Dioscorea barbasco*), which, although more difficult to collect, gave a much higher yield of diosgenin. Marker knew that *Dioscorea barbasco* was a better source of diosgenin than cabeza de negro, since he had tested its rhizome at Penn State along with several other specimens brought back from one of his early trips to Mexico. He had opted, however, for cabeza de negro simply because it was easier to collect. His friend and business associate decided to drop the price of progesterone to $10 per gram and later to $5 per gram. Meanwhile, Syntex hired a chemist from a pharmaceutical company in Havana, George Rosencranz, who had trained in Switzerland with Nobel prize winner Leopold Ruzicka. With the help of the women whom Marker had left behind at Syntex and who were familiar with the various steps, he was able to reconstruct the process, enabling Syntex to continue to produce progesterone.[f]

With progesterone readily available, the door was open for its investigational and clinical use. However, it had to be injected, since it had negligible oral potency.

---

[e]During all this time, Syntex paid the expenses for Marker and his family, which had joined him in Mexico, but no salary, with the understanding that at the end of the year, the company profits would be distributed and he would receive 40% of the net. Nor had he received his 40% shares of stock in Syntex. At the end of the year, he did not receive his share of the profits, which had been considerable (since the company had been selling progesterone at $50 per gram). Marker went to Somlo in March, 1945 to discuss this matter. Somlo told Marker that there were no profits and, when questioned further, Somlo stated that he had taken all of the profit for his salary.

[f]A few months after Marker started production at Botanica-Mex, Somlo, the owner of Syntex, had a meeting with Marker's lawyer and demanded that he turn over to him all correspondence between them, especially a letter stating that Marker was to have 40% of the shares of Syntex. If he did not do so, he would have Marker jailed "for stealing Syntex processes" (!) and eventually force him to leave Mexico. Marker's lawyer, who strangely never met with Somlo's lawyer, advised him to comply, which he did, losing his two original 2 kg of progesterone and his shares of Syntex. Because of continued harassment of the workers at Botanica-Mex, production of progesterone and dehydroepiandrosterone was discontinued in March of 1946. The equipment and the unprocessed roots were sold to Gedeon Richter SA, which started production under the name of Hormo-synth SA, later changed to Diosynth SA, and eventually sold to Organon of Holland, which is using it at the present time under the name of Quimica Esteroides SA.

This limitation stimulated steroid chemists to look for an orally active compound with progestational activity. A breakthrough was achieved independently by two chemists: Carl Djerassi[g] and Frank Colton.[h]

In 1949, at the age of 28, Djerassi was asked to head the research team at Syntex in Mexico City. The main objective at the time was to synthesize cortisone and estradiol. To obtain estradiol from diosgenin-derived testosterone, Djerassi had used a chemical procedure known as "aromatization." When he applied the same procedure to progesterone, he came up with a substance that possessed the structural features of both estradiol and progesterone. Such a hybrid, however, proved devoid of any biological activity. Then he "dearomatized" the hybrid compound, using a new procedure developed by the Australian chemist A.J. Birch, to restore its ring properties to those of natural progesterone. The resulting compound had one key difference, however, when compared to progesterone: in position 19, it had a hydrogen atom rather than a methyl group. This new compound, called 19-nor-progesterone, was, surprisingly, 4 to 8 times more potent than its natural counterpart. Next, Djerassi set out to synthesize an orally active compound.

Hans H. Inhoffen of Berlin had found that introducing an acetylene group into one ring of the estradiol molecule altered it in such a way that it was stable in the stomach and could be used orally. Djerassi applied the same process to testosterone and obtained a substance that he called ethisterone, active when taken orally, but with progestational rather than androgenic activity. In the fall of 1951, Djerassi thought to dearomatize ethisterone, as he had his hybrid compound, to increase its progestational activity without disturbing its oral effectiveness. The new substance, with a hydrogen atom in position 19 rather than a methyl group, was called nor-ethisterone and later became known as norethindrone; it proved to be more potent, when taken orally, than any other known compound with progestational activity. A US patent was issued on May 1, 1956, with Djerassi and two associates (L. Miramontes and G. Rosencranz) as assignors.

In 1952, Frank Colton,[h] a chemist at Searle, independently synthesized a closely related 19-nor compound, norethynodrel, which was in fact the first orally active progestational agent to receive a US patent. It was issued on November 29, 1955, with Colton as the sole assignor.

---

[g]Djerassi was born in Vienna, Austria, and immigrated to the US at the age of 16. He earned his undergraduate degree at Kenyon College and at the age of 19 was already working as a chemist at Ciba Pharmaceutical. Subsequently, he completed his doctorate, in only 2 years, at the University of Wisconsin.

[h]Frank Colton was born in Poland in 1923 and arrived in the United States in 1934 at the age of 11. He received his BS and MS degrees in chemistry from Northwestern University in Evanston, Illinois and his PhD from the University of Chicago in 1950. He gained expertise in steroid research while completing work on his PhD as a research fellow at the Mayo Foundation of the Mayo Clinic in Rochester, New York.

THE BIOLOGICAL HISTORY OF THE PILL

The biological history of hormonal birth control began when Ludwig Haberlandt (1885–1932), a physiologist from Innsbruck, Austria, started his animal experiments on the antiovulatory action of the corpus luteum (Haberlandt, 1921). In 1919, he transplanted the ovaries of a pregnant rabbit under the skin of an adult nonpregnant rabbit. Despite frequent coitus, the recipient of the graft became infertile for about 2½ months. Haberlandt reported his findings in a paper titled "On Hormonal Sterilization of the Female Animal Organism" and advanced for the first time the idea that such a method of contraception, if tried in women, could provide an effective means of temporary sterilization. Following his initial transplantation experiment, he reported, at the 1923 meeting of the German Physiological Society, that injection of extracts of corpora lutea from pregnant cows rendered rabbits infertile (Haberlandt, 1923). In 1927, he reported the first successful attempt at oral contraception. Six mice had been given ovarian extracts and five were given placental extracts, resulting in sterility for 1–2½ months in some of the animals (Haberlandt, 1927).

Haberlandt was clearly influenced in his animal studies by a hypothesis (advanced in the late 19th century) and by experimental evidence (accumulated in the early 20th century) on the suppressive action of the corpus luteum on ovulation. The corpus luteum had been the object of attention since its description by Reinier De Graff (1641–1673) (De Graff, 1672) and Marcello Malpighius (1628–1694) (Malpighius, 1648) who coined the name "the yellow body." Both De Graff and Malpighius, however, assumed that the whole content of the follicle was the ovum and thus incorrectly hypothesized that the function of the corpus luteum was its expulsion.

Their "mechanical" hypothesis of the function of the corpus luteum prevailed for over two centuries until 1898, when the French histologist Louis-Auguste Prenant (1861–1927) suggested that the corpus luteum was an organ of internal secretion (Prenant, 1898). At about the same time, this conclusion was reached by an embryologist from Breslau, Gustav Born (1851–1900) (Born, 1901). In both cases the suggestion of endocrine function was based on the histological similarity between the corpus luteum and other endocrine glands. Prenant hypothesized the suppressive action of the corpus luteum upon ovulation during pregnancy and postulated that it secreted a substance or substances. Born, on the other hand, suggested that the specific endocrine function of the corpus luteum consisted in preparing and supporting the uterus after ovulation and implantation.

The task of putting Born's idea to experimental test fell to one of his students, Ludwig Fraenkel (1870–1953) (Fraenkel, 1903). In 1901, Fraenkel mated rabbits and during the following week excised or cauterized the corpora lutea. The result was interruption of pregnancy (Fraenkel, 1910).

About the same time, the French embryologist Paul Ancel and the histologist Paul Bouin discovered (Bouin et al., 1910), in the rabbit, the endometrial changes that occur during pregnancy, and correctly inferred that such changes were produced by the endocrine activity of the corpus luteum. They were able to test this supposition by mating female rabbits with vasectomized males: no pregnancy ensued although progestational changes developed in the endometrium. These experiments provided a method of bioassay, which eventually made possible the identification of progesterone.

In 1909, Leo Loeb (1869–1959), then working at the Laboratory of Experimental Biology of the University of Pennsylvania, had provided the first experimental evidence for ovulation suppression by the corpus luteum (Loeb, 1909a). He reached this conclusion after having observed in guinea pigs that ovulation almost always occurred earlier than normal when corpora lutea were removed. He brought his findings to the attention of other investigators (presumably including Haberlandt) through reports in the English and German literature (Loeb, 1909b, 1910, 1911).

Haberlandt knew about Prenant's writings, and he was also aware of most of the attempts to demonstrate the influence of the corpus luteum upon ovulation. It is also likely that he knew of the common veterinary practice, used as early as the middle of the 19th century, of restoring fertility in cows with persistent corpora lutea by squeezing the cysts manually *per rectum*. Although Haberlandt had been guided not just by his own reasoning but by previous concepts and experiments, it was to his great credit that he assimilated the isolated studies and observations on the inhibitory action of the corpus luteum on ovulation and understood their implications for hormonal contraception in the human. While the objective for many of the investigations conducted prior to and during Haberlandt's lifetime had been to gain a better understanding of reproductive physiology, Haberlandt's aim was clearly the possible application of hormonal sterilization to women. Thus he should be regarded as the direct forerunner of birth control by progestins. He even formulated, with the pharmaceutical company of G. Richter in Budapest, an oral preparation under the name of "Infecundin" (Von Brucke, 1932), to be used for clinical experimentation. Haberlandt, not being a clinician, approached several physicians in an attempt to induce them to apply hormonal contraception to women. However, no record exists of any systematic trial before his untimely death in 1932, at the age of 47, of a heart attack. Haberlandt, who had coined the phrase "hormonal sterilization," was indeed a lonely crusader for hormonal contraception in the human.

In the next 2 decades, extensive biological work led to the discovery of progesterone, its isolation and, finally, its synthesis.[i]

With the pure hormone of the corpus luteum available, Makepeace et al. (1937) reported from the University of Pennsylvania that mated female rabbits did not ovulate when treated with progesterone. The final step was the demonstration that

---

[i]In 1929, Corner and Allen (1929) announced that alcoholic extracts of the corpus luteum contained a substance that, when injected into castrated adult female rabbits, induced a characteristic progestational proliferation of the endometrium identical to that shown by Ancel and Bouin to be due to the presence of corpora lutea. They thus concluded that extracts of the corpora lutea contained a special hormone that had for one of its functions the preparation of the uterus to the reception of the embryos. This important discovery was soon followed by the isolation and synthesis of progesterone.

progesterone was also an effective inhibitor of ovulation in the human. This was accomplished by a biologist, Gregory Pincus.[j]

In 1945, Hoagland and Pincus recruited M.C. Chang, who had worked at Cambridge University on methods of preservation of mammalian sperm and other problems concerning the improvement of fertility in domestic animals. His assignment was perfusion of cow ovaries, induction of superovulation, the recovery of eggs, their fertilization *in vitro*, and subsequent transfer to another cow for the production of genetically superior calves. Pincus and Chang often discussed various possible methods of contraception—particularly after the "population explosion" made the headlines at the end of World War II—without, however, arriving at any specific research plan.

In 1950, Pincus was contacted by Margaret Sanger, (who pioneered the US family planning movement and founded the International Planned Parenthood Federation) and by her wealthy friend Katherine Dexter McCormick, who was willing to provide resources for the development of a safe and effective contraceptive. Soon Pincus and Chang decided to begin their research by repeating Makepeace's experiment (Makepeace et al., 1937). Before starting, however, Pincus became concerned about the availability of progesterone and in 1950, during a trip to Mexico City, he contacted Russel Marker, who assured him that large amounts of progesterone could be produced easily. As the reclusive Marker later recalled, Pincus succeeded in getting in touch with him at the Hotel Genève only because the regular hotel operator, who had been given orders not to forward any calls to Marker, had been temporarily replaced!

Chang started his first study (Pincus & Chang, 1953) on female rabbits in April 1951 and confirmed that high doses of progesterone indeed inhibited ovulation. A second experiment followed using rats, whose physiology is more similar to humans, since the female rat ovulates regularly whether mated or not. The same conclusions were reached. A third series of experiments followed in 1953, in which the newly synthesized 19-norsteroid compounds were tested and found the most effective for the prevention of ovulation (Pincus et al., 1956).

Meanwhile, Pincus enlisted Dr. John Rock as collaborator for human testing. Rock, a friend for many years, was Professor of gynecology at Harvard and director of a busy fertility clinic at the Free Hospital For Women. Rock's main interest at the time was not contraception, but rather the treatment of idiopathic infertility. He postulated that hypoplastic reproductive organs were often the cause of infertility.

---

[j]The son of a Russian Jewish immigrant, Pincus was born in 1903 in a farming community in Woodbine, New Jersey. He enrolled in agriculture at Cornell University, where he received his BS, and in 1928 he received his doctorate in mammalian genetics from Harvard University. He then spent a year and half in Cambridge (England) on a National Research Council Fellowship, becoming for the first time interested in reproductive physiology. In the fall of 1930, he became instructor in general physiology at Harvard and 2 years later was appointed Assistant Professor. Before the end of his term, Pincus was told that he would not be promoted to Associate Professor, a decision which by the administrative rules of the time terminated his faculty appointment. Hudson Hoagland, chairman of the biology department at Clark University, found Pincus' dismissal from Harvard unfair and in 1938 offered him a position as a Visiting Professor. Then in 1944, they together established the Worcester Foundation for Experimental Biology.

Knowing that in pregnancy the uterus and the tubes underwent a marked increase in size, Rock theorized that the same could be accomplished with the administration of estrogen and progesterone. He tested his theory in 1952 on 80 volunteer patients who for 3 months orally took diethylstilbestrol in doses that increased from 5 mg/day during the first week to 30 mg/day during the eleventh week. In addition they were given progesterone, also orally, in doses of 50 mg/day, increasing to 300 mg/day. Thirteen of the 80 women became pregnant within 4 months of treatment (Rock et al., 1957). He referred to the prompt resumption of ovulation after the treatment with hormones as a "rebound reaction." The large doses of diethylstilbestrol and natural progesterone, however, caused considerable side effects. Particularly disturbing was the suppression of menstruation, which some of the infertile couples, although they had been warned, found disquieting and confusing. Rock discussed these disadvantages with Pincus and expressed concern about the known relationship between large doses of estrogen and various kinds of cancer in laboratory animals.

Pincus suggested to try progesterone alone, from the 5th to the 25th day of the menstrual cycle, in order to prevent any suppression of menstruation. In 1953, following such a regimen, 4 pregnancies occurred in 27 patients (Rock et al., 1957). Rock and Pincus also noted that suppression of ovulation occurred in at least 85% of the first cycles of administration. Pincus felt that the elimination of breakthrough bleeding and an even more complete suppression of ovulation could be achieved with a more potent form of progesterone and, following Chang's encouraging animal tests with 19-norprogestins, suggested their use instead of the natural progesterone. Pincus reported the results of their clinical trial with progesterone at the Fifth International Conference on Planned Parenthood in Tokyo in October of 1955 and publicly stated for the first time the possibility of using progestational compounds for oral contraception, attracting world press attention.

Subsequently, Rock, aided by Pincus and Celso-Ramon Garcia (Garcia et al., 1958), began his third clinical trial in 50 women to test the biological activity of three new products: norethisterone (Norlutin), norethynodrel (Enovid), and norethylsterone (Nilevar), in doses between 5 and 50 mg/day, from the 5th day of the menstrual cycle. Within 5 months following the treatment, 7 conceptions occurred after total inhibition of ovulation, and with fewer and milder side effects. Rock used, as indices of the occurrence of ovulation, daily basal temperature and vaginal smears, and from the 19th to the 22nd day of the menstrual cycle, an endometrial biopsy. Furthermore, a number of laparotomies were done, which documented the absence of corpora lutea.

During these early trials it became clear that the norethynodrel was contaminated by estrogen. Some patients complained of severe nausea and vomiting, as previously observed in patients treated with stilbestrol. The manufacturers discovered that the original samples were contaminated with as much as 4–7% of mestranol. They promptly removed the contaminant while the clinical testing was still in progress. With the pure product, inhibition of ovulation became inconsistent and breakthrough bleeding increased. Both problems were corrected by reverting to the use of "partially contaminated" progestin, i.e., containing only 1.5% of mestranol. The finding that the estrogen allowed better cycle control and, as discovered much later, that it had a synergistic action with the progestin in ovulation inhibition, was responsible for the eventual combined use of estrogen and progestin in the formulation of the Pill. The above trials demonstrated to Rock that the 19-norsteroids were very useful in the treatment of "inexplicable childlessness" and more importantly, to Pincus, that they were very effective in inhibiting ovulation in the human, with relatively rare and mild side effects.

The next step for Pincus was to generate clinical investigations with these products, specifically to see how reliable they were as contraceptives. Pincus had worked as a paid consultant for the G.D. Searle Company, and approached the management on this matter. Despite their initial reluctance (due to the known opposition of the Catholic church), he was able to convince them of the need to proceed with a field trial. Eventually, in April of 1956, Puerto Rico was selected because it had a tremendous population problem, the population was relatively immobile, there was a willingness on the part of the local government to cooperate, and, also, there were already family planning clinics in place. At the beginning of 1956, Pincus approached Dr. Edris Rice-Wray, medical director of the Public Health Training Center in Rio Piedras, Puerto Rico; she was immediately receptive to the idea of a study of the contraceptive effects of norethynodrel in volunteer subjects from San Juan. They selected a government housing development where people had been relocated from El Fanguito, one of the worst slums (thus, they were unlikely to move away).

In 1958, a population of 125 women was given 20 tablets containing 10 mg of norethynodrel plus 0.15 to 0.23 mg of mestranol to be taken from the 5th to the 24th day of the menstrual cycle. Data from this initial experience showed that if the regimen was followed faithfully, unfailing contraception occurred. These results were subsequently confirmed by projects in Humacao, Puerto Rico and Port-Au-Prince, Haiti, with a total of 830 subjects for a total of 8,133 cycles, or 635 woman-years (Pincus et al., 1959). Further clinical trials were conducted by J. W. Gold-zieher in San Antonio, E. Rice-Wray in Mexico City, and by E.T. Tyler in Los Angeles. The combination tested by Pincus was immediately patented by Searle as Enovid-10, becoming its exclusive property. In 1960, the US Food and Drug Administration (FDA) approved Enovid-10 as a contraceptive agent and "the Pill" was officially born.

EPILOGUE

After Marker sold Botanica-Mex, he remained as a consultant to Hormosynth for 3 years; then in 1949, at the age of 47, he retired completely from chemistry and moved back to Pennsylvania. After having worked for the US government on a secret project, Marker's interest shifted completely from steroid chemistry to ro-coco-style silver made in the mid-18th century; he would search through the antique shops and museums of Europe and make commissioned replicas. In 1969, he was finally honored by the Mexican Chemical Society. In 1970, the Mexican government offered him the Order of the Aztec Eagle for his important contribution to the establishment of the Mexican chemical industry; he declined. In 1979, Marker was featured on TV's "Nova." His Mexican experience, furthermore, was made the subject of a German TV movie ("Die Spur Führt Nach Mexico"). Pennsylvania State University established, in 1984, the annual Marker Lectures in Science and, in 1987, the Russell and Mildred Marker Professorship of Natural Product Chemistry. In December of 1987 Marker, a spry octogenarian, traveled back to College Park, Maryland, to receive the honorary Doctorate in Science from the University of Maryland, which he had failed to receive in 1926!

In 1952, Carl Djerassi joined the faculty of Wayne State University, where he remained until 1959, when he accepted his current position of Professor of chemistry at Stanford University. He authored a book *The Politics of Contraception*, which has been the subject of controversy. Dr. Djerassi won the highest scientific honors, including the National Medal of Science. In 1978, he was inducted into the National Inventors Hall of Fame. In 1979–1980 he became a member of the President's Committee on the National Medal of Science. He was the invited speaker at the first Russell Marker Lecture in Chemical Sciences at Penn State University.

Dr. Frank Colton retired from Searle in 1986. Among the awards and honors he received are the Professional Achievement Award (in 1978) from his alma mater, the University of Chicago, and more recently the Inventors Hall of Fame Award from the United States Patent Office.

In 1960, Gregory Pincus received the Albert D. Lasker award in Planned Parenthood. In 1964, he received the Modern Medicine Award for distinguished achievement "for his contribution to understanding the physiology of human reproduction, the factors that influence fertility and practical methods for the hormonal control of ovulation." He died at age 67 in Boston, Massachusetts.

Min C. Chang was nominated as Professor of reproductive biology at Boston University in 1961. At the age of 83 he was Principal Scientist Emeritus at the Worcester Foundation for Experimental Biology in Shrewsbury, Massachusetts. In 1987, Dr. Chang was presented the award of Scientific Merit during the Fifth World Congress on IVF-ET, held in Norfolk, Virginia, "in recognition of his valuable scientific contribution to the field of reproductive physiology." In addition to having participated in the development of oral contraceptives, Chang is credited with the discovery of capacitation of sperm in the female tract (Chang, 1951), also discovered independently by Austin (1951). In addition, in 1959, he reported the birth of young rabbits following the transfer of rabbit eggs fertilized *in vitro* by capacitated sperm from the uterus (Chang, 1959). Virtually all the advances made in assisted reproduction are believed to derive directly or indirectly from the publication of his landmark paper. In his reminiscences, Chang recalls joining the Worcester Foundation precisely to learn the technique of *in vitro* fertilization from Pincus, who first reported *in vitro* fertilization of rabbit eggs in 1934 (Pincus et al., 1934). Chang admits, however, doing his early *in vitro* experiments with the idea that such studies might be useful for animal breeding but not for human sterility. He passed away in 1991.

After the Pill was approved by the FDA, John Rock concentrated his efforts on "his mission to convert the Catholic church on birth control." He had been a proponent of birth control, despite being a practicing Catholic, long before he started his studies with steroid hormones. However, his predominant interest at the time was in the "rebound reaction" and he was well aware that birth control was illegal in the Commonwealth of Massachusetts. His close friend and professional associate, Arthur T. Hertig, recalls being lectured, as a medical student, by Rock on birth control in the early 1930s (Hertig, 1989). Celso-Ramon Garcia confirms this fact by adding that, the subject being illegal, he would indicate to the students that the law did not permit him to provide birth control information; then he proceeded to indicate what the law did not permit him to say. In 1963, he published the book *The Time Has Come: A Catholic Doctor's Proposal To End The Battle Over Birth Control*, and, although 73 at the time, embarked on a strenuous promotional tour advocating the use of oral contraception. Rock sincerely felt that the pill was "an adjunct to nature." His argument was that by preventing the release of the egg, the Pill stretched out the infertile period, used as the theological basis of the rhythm method, approved by the Church.

Of course, Rock did not succeed in changing the Catholic church's anti-Pill stance and, although saddened, he used to observe optimistically "when Galileo declared that the earth revolved around the sun, the church delayed application of his scientific insight for human benefit. But the delay was slight, really,[k] and the truth eventually triumphed" (Hendin, 1976).

In 1985, the American Fertility Society published a memorial in its newsletter, in which, in addition to Rock's contribution to the development of the Pill, his less-known pioneering efforts in the recovery of human eggs and embryos from patients undergoing gynecologic procedures (leading to the fertilization *in vitro* of human ova) (Rock & Menkin, 1944) were acknowledged. As a true visionary, Rock had published an editorial in the *New England Journal of Medicine* as early as 1937, in which he mentioned the possibility of using *in vitro* fertilization and embryo transfer for the treatment of patients with tubal disease (Rock, 1937). Dr. Rock passed away in 1984.

Dr. Edris Rice-Wray, after the field trials in Puerto Rico were completed, moved to Mexico City where, in 1959, she founded and directed the Asociacion Mexicana Pro Bienestar De La Familia (Mexican Family Welfare Association), whose stated purpose was to prevent the necessity of abortion. After her retirement, she moved from Mexico City to Puebla, where she lived to the age of 86.

Dr. Goldzieher, whose early studies on synthetic progestational compounds actually predated those of Pincus (Goldzieher, 1957; Goldzieher et al., 1958), conducted extensive clinical trials with norethindrone. He then went on to re-examine the role of estrogen in oral contraceptives and showed, in small-scale clinical trials conducted in Mexico together with Dr. Rice-Wray (Goldzieher et al., 1963), that 80 μg/day of mestranol, without the concomitant administration of a progestin, consis-

---

[k]400 years (Ed.).

tently inhibited ovulation. This finding paved the road for the introduction in 1965 of sequential oral contraceptives. However, these were withdrawn in 1970 from the US market by the FDA, concerned about their alleged lower contraceptive effectiveness and reports of endometrial pathology associated with certain sequential preparations, particularly one marketed under the name Oracon. Goldzieher felt that the perceived differences in effectiveness were the result of biases in clinical trials, while the worrisome endometrial pattern associated with sequential Oracon might have been due to the poor balance of the steroids (Goldzieher, 1982).

The synergism between estrogen and progestins (which Dr. Goldzieher was among the first to point out and which the manufacturers of the Pill pointedly ignored for some time), once widely recognized, permitted dosage reductions leading eventually to the current, widely used low-dose oral contraceptives.

In 1966, he published the first report (Zanartu et al., 1966) in the medical literature on the use of long-acting injectable steroids for fertility control. Although only recently approved in the United States, long-acting injectable contraceptives, using medroxyprogesterone acetate or norethindrone enanthate, have been available, for quite sometime, in more than 90 countries.

Edward T. Tyler, whose reputation on the West Coast as an infertility specialist was similar to that of Rock's on the East Coast, served as the first president of Planned Parenthood of America; he continued his work in several family planning centers that he opened in the Los Angeles area. Dr. Tyler died in Los Angeles at 62 years of age in 1975. From 1977 on, Edward Tyler Symposia on Infertility were held in Hawaii to honor his memory.

Acknowledgment

The Author wishes to thank R. E. Marker, C. Djerassi, F. Colton, M. C. Chang, C. Ramon-Garcia, E. Rice-Wray, and J. W. Goldzieher for their helpful comments.

REFERENCES

Allen WM. Recollection of my life with progesterone. *Gynecol Invest* 1974;5:142.
Austin CR. Observation on the penetration of the sperm into the mammalian eggs. *Aust J Sci Res* 1951;B4:581.
Born G (as quoted by Fraenkel L, Cohn F). Experimentelle Untersuchungen über den Einfluss des Corpus luteum auf die Insertion des Eies (Theorie von Born). *Anat Anz* 1901;20:294.
Bouin P, Ancel P. Sur le determinisme de la preparation de l'uterus a la fixation de l'oeuf. *J Physiol Path Gen* 1910;12:1.
Butenandt A, Westphal O. Zur: Isolierung und Charakterisierung des Corpus-luteum-Hormons. *Ber Deutsch Chem Gesellsch* 1934;67:1440.
Butenandt A, Schmidt J. Uberführung des Pregnandiols im Corpus-luteum Hormon, *Ber Chem Ges* 1934;67:1901.
Chang MC. Fertilizing capacity of spermatozoa deposited into the fallopian tubes. *Nature* 1951;168:697.
Chang MC. Fertilization of rabbit ova in-vitro. *Nature* 1959;184:466.
Corner GW, Allen WM. Production of a special uterine reaction (progestational proliferation) by extracts of the corpus luteum. *Am J Physiol* 1929;88:326.

De Graaf R. De mulierum organis generationi inservantibus. Lugduni Batavorum. Ex. Off. Hackiana (1672).

Fraenkel L. Die Funktion des Corpus luteum. *Arch Gynak* 1903;67:438.

Fraenkel L. Neue Experimente zur Funktion des Corpus luteum. *Arch Gynak* 1910;91:705.

Garcia CR, Pincus G, Rock J. Effects of three 19-Nor steroids on human ovulation and menstruation. *Am J Obstet Gynecol* 1958;75:82.

Goldzieher JW. Lack of androgenicity of 17-hydroxyprogesterone or its 17-caproate ester. *J Clin Endocrinol Metab* 1957;17:323.

Goldzieher JW, Peterson WF, Gilbert RA. Comparison of the endometrial activities in man of anhydrohydroxyprogesterone and 17-acetoxyprogesterone, a new oral progestational compound. *Ann NY Acad Sci* 1958;71:722.

Goldzieher JW, Martinez-Manautou J, Moses LE, et al. The use of sequential estrogen and progestin to inhibit fertility. A preliminary report. *West J Surg Obstet Gynecol* 1963;71:187.

Goldzieher JW. Estrogen in oral contraceptives: Historical perspectives. *Johns Hopkins Med J* 1982;150:165.

Haberlandt L. Ueber hormonale Sterilisierung des weiblichen Tierkörpers. *Münch Med Wochenschr* 1921;68:1577.

Haberlandt L. Ueber hormonale Sterilisierung weiblicher Tiere. *Klin Wochenschr* 1923;2:1938.

Haberlandt L. Ueber hormonale Sterilisierung weiblicher Tiere (Fütterungsversuche mit Ovarial-und Plazenta-Opton). *Münch Med Wochenschr* 1927;74:49.

Hartmann M, Wettstein A. Ein krystallisiertes Hormon aus Corpus luteum. *Helv Chim Acta* 1934;17:878.

Hendin D. *The Life Givers.* W. Narrow and Co; 1976:225.

Hertig AT. A fifteen-year search for first-stage human ova. *JAMA* 1989;261:434.

Loeb L. Ueber die Bedeutung des Corpus luteum. *Zentralbl Physiol* 1909a;23:73.

Loeb L. The experimental production of the maternal placenta and the function of the corpus luteum. *JAMA* 1909b;53:1471.

Loeb L. The function of the corpus luteum, the experimental production of the maternal placenta, and the mechanism of the sexual cycle in the female organism. *Med Rec* 1910;77:1083.

Loeb L. Uber die Bedeutung des Corpus luteum für die Periodizitat des sexuellen Zyklus beim weiblichen Saugetierorganismus. *Deutsch Med Wochenschr* 1911;37:17.

Makepeace SW, Winstein GL, Friedman NW. The effect of progestin and progesterone on ovulation in the rabbit. *Am J Physiol* 1937;119:512.

Malpighius M. Praeclarissimo & Eruditissimo Viro D. Jacobo Sponio Medicinae Doctori & Lugdunens Anatomico Accuratissimo. *Philosoph Transact Royal Soc Lond* 1648;15:630. (see pp. 639–640).

Marker RE, Rohrman E. Sterols. LXXXI. Conversion of Sarsapogenin To Pregnanediol-3 (α), 20 (α). *JACS* 1939;61:3592.

Marker RE, Tsukamoto T, Turner DL. Sterols. C. Diosgenin *JACS* 1940;62:2525.

Marker RE. The early production of steroidal hormones. *CHOC News*, Summer 1987, pp. 3–6.

Pincus G, Chang MC. The effects of progesterone and related compounds on ovulation and early development in the rabbit. *Acta Physiol Lat Am* 1953;3:177.

Pincus G, Chang MC, Hafez ESE, et al. Effects of certain 19-NOR steroids on reproductive processes in animals. *Science* 1956;124:890.

Pincus G, Garcia CR, Rock J, et al: Effectiveness of an oral contraceptive. *Science* 1959;130:81.

Pincus G, Enzmann EV. Can mammalian eggs undergo normal development in vitro? *Proc Nat Acad Sci* 1934;20:121.

Prenant LA. La valeur morphologique du corps jaune. *Rev Gen Sci* 1898;9:646.

Rock J, Garcia CR, Pincus G. Synthetic progestins in the normal human menstrual cycle. *Recent Prog Horm Res* 1957;13:323.

Rock J, Menkin MF. In vitro fertilization and cleavage of human ovarian eggs. *Science* 1944;100:105.

Rock J. Conception in a watch glass. *N Engl J Med* 1937;217:678.

Slotta W, Ruschig H, Fels W. Reindarstellung der Hormone aus dem Corpus luteum. *Ber Deutsch Chem Gesellsch* 1934;67:1270.

Von Brucke ET. Ludwig Haberlandt. *Forsch Forschr* 1932;8:327.

Wintersteiner O, Allen WM. Crystalline progestin. *J Biol Chem* 1934;107:321.

Zanartu J, Rice-Wray E, Goldzieher JW. Fertility control with long-acting injectable steroids. A preliminary report. *Obstet Gynecol* 1966;28:513.

Pharmacology of the Contraceptive Steroids,
edited by Joseph W. Goldzieher.
Raven Press, Ltd., New York © 1994.

2

The Estrogens

Joseph W. Goldzieher

*Department of Obstetrics and Gynecology, Baylor College of Medicine
Houston, Texas 77030*

While one group of veterinarians and biologists was exploring the endocrinology of the corpus luteum, others were looking at the biological activity of ovarian tissue itself. As early as 1912, Adler (1912) and Fellner (1912), in Vienna, and Iscovesco (1912), in Paris, obtained ovarian extracts that gave evidence of estrogenic activity. By 1921, Fellner reported that lipid extracts of pregnant cows' ovaries had potent estrogenic effects. Haberlandt (1921), aware of these findings, concluded that ovarian interstitial tissue also functions in pregnancy to inhibit ovulation. He was, of course, unaware that he was dealing with a hormone different from that found in his extracts of corpus luteum tissue. Some years later, Fellner published additional experiments (1921) in which injectable extracts and an orally active material (he named it "Feminin") produced sterility in rabbits and mice. By 1927 he concluded that these extracts had different effects at different doses (now a known property of estrogens) and that they prevented pregnancy by destruction of ova and by inhibition of corpus luteum formation.

The breakthrough in the study of estrogenic substances came when Aschheim and Zondek (1927) discovered the assay based on an estrus reaction in the immature mouse or rat. With this assay it became apparent that urine was a better starting material than tissue extract. Both Butenandt and Westphal (1934) and the Allen/Doisy team (1923) started work in late 1927, and strove neck and neck for nearly 2 years. Then, in the Fall of 1929 the latter team announced the isolation of crystalline estrone. By 1933 estrone had been converted to estradiol, and 2 years later Doisy showed that this too was a physiological substance; experiments with defined materials became possible. By 1930, Reiprich, in Breslau, suggested that the antifertility action of the estrogens might be brought about by pituitary inhibition. *Thus, by this early date, the concept of contraception with sex steroids had not only been explicitly enunciated, but a mechanism of action had been correctly inferred.*

As soon as estrogenic materials became clinically available, they were tested in a wide variety of gynecological disorders. None of these clinicians gave any evidence of being aware of the work of Adler or Fellner, whose estrogenic extracts inhibited ovulation in rodents. However, at the Conference on Contraceptive Research and

Clinical Practice, held in New York in December 1936, Kurzrok presented a paper entitled "The Prospects for Hormonal Sterilization" (1937). He was apparently unaware of Haberlandt's work and of information on the antiovulatory activity of the corpus luteum and its hormone. He did mention that estrone, by inhibiting ovulation, was a possible modality for hormonal sterilization, and concluded with the opinion that "the potentialities of hormonal sterilization are tremendous." Like Haberlandt, he was ignored. In 1938, Wilson and Kurzrok observed that the complaint of (functional) dysmenorrhea signified ovulation, for it occurred only in patients with a functioning corpus luteum. This led other gynecologists to explore ovulation inhibition as a treatment for dysmenorrhea and, in 1940, Sturgis and Albright, in Boston, reported that frequent injections of estradiol benzoate prevented dysmenorrhea when ovulation was successfully inhibited. Of 65 patients treated for this complaint, 63 were relieved. In the same year, Karnaky (1940), in Houston, "produced a physiologic sterility" with a continuous regimen of 10 to 25 mg stilbestrol daily.

In 1941, Gillman, in Johannesburg, was also making observations on the inhibition of ovulation with estradiol in baboons.

Although many possible applications of these findings were considered, contraception was not among them. Nor was this possibility mentioned in two subsequent communications by Sturgis in 1942. He did, however, confirm Hartman's original observations of the importance of initiating estrogen therapy early in the cycle if ovulation was to be inhibited. Other reports on estrogen treatment for dysmenorrhea—by Hamblen, Goldzieher, and associates in 1943 and 1947 (Hamblen et al., 1943; Haus et al., 1947), and by Lyon (who used ethinyl estradiol) in 1943, also made no mention of contraception, a subject that was simply not discussed in proper academic circles.

However, in 1945, Albright, who had worked with Sturgis, clearly identified the potential of ovulation-inhibiting doses of estrogen as a contraceptive method. The comment, unfortunately, was buried in a section within a chapter in a large textbook on internal medicine. Thus, the suggestion of Albright joined the oblivion of Haberlandt, Fellner, and Kurzrok. In retrospect, none of the treatments used at that time would have had the required efficacy, for most of the estrogens, used in the conventional dosage, were not consistent in their ovulation-inhibiting effect. A clinical trial of the suggestions of Kurzrok or Albright might have proved disastrous to the future of "hormonal sterilization."

Nothing further happened on the estrogen front until 1960, when a meeting about the design of clinical contraceptive trials with the newly available 19-norprogestins took place in Mexico City. J. M. Maas of the Eli Lilly company, Harry Rudel of Syntex, J. Martinez-Manautou and Edris Rice-Wray of Mexico City, and J. W. Goldzieher of Texas reviewed the question of the "contaminant" mestranol in the oral contraceptives then being formulated. Although the earlier treatments for dysmenorrhea with various estrogens had shown inconsistent ovulation inhibition, there was no reason to assume a priori that mestranol, an ethynyl estrogen, would show the same behavior. Small-scale studies (Goldzieher, et al., 1975a) promptly revealed that 20 μg of mestranol per day was not sufficient, but 50 μg seemed to be a consistently effective dose. This immediately raised the question of which substance was responsible for the contraceptive action of the commercial norethindrone or norethynodrel formulations, which contained from 60 to 150 μg of mestranol per tablet. Further investigations (Goldzieher, et al., 1975b) with mestranol led to recognition of the special role of the ethynyl group in potentiating the gonadotropin-suppressing action in relation to the other estrogenic activities, a concept still not fully appreciated by investigators seeking to develop contraceptive formulations containing a "natural" estrogen.

These observations formed the basis for the development of a class of oral contraceptive formulations that became known as "sequentials." Ethynyl estrogens were given for 21 consecutive days at doses of 75 μg or more, and 19-nor or C_{21}-acetoxyprogestins such as medroxyprogesterone or chlormadinone acetate were given concurrently for 7 days or more toward the end of the estrogen treatment cycle to produce adequate progestational changes of the endometrium and ensure clinically satisfactory menstrual bleeding patterns. Eventually, as dosage reduction became the goal of pharmaceutical development, the sequentials became noncompetitive with combined monophasic formulations, which were effective at far lower estrogen dosage. Additionally, there was some question of lowered contraceptive efficacy of the sequentials in actual use and, as a final blow, a worrisome histological appearance of the endometrium of women using a mestranol/dimethisterone sequential formulation led the FDA to require withdrawal of *all* sequentials. They are, however, available in other countries.

From the beginning, pharmaceutical companies experimented with permutations and combinations of estrogen/progestin, attempting to alleviate side effects by dosage reduction while maintaining contraceptive efficacy and good cycle control. Studies of urinary pregnandiol excretion or plasma progesterone levels, as indicators of corpus luteum formation, quickly showed that the initial formulations of Enovid and Ortho-Novum were far higher than necessary; the studies of Goldzieher and his group (1975a, b) indicated that the gonadotropin-suppressing activities of the 19-norprogestin and the ethynyl estrogen were synergistic, permitting consistent ovulation inhibition with quantities of the two substances that were far lower than would have been expected from their individual potencies. This phenomenon made possible the modern generation of oral contraceptive formulations, which differ from the original combination products in dosage by an order of magnitude.

The estrogenic contaminant in the original preparations of norethindrone or noethynodrel was mestranol, the 3-methyl ether of ethynyl estradiol. Subsequent pharmaceutical preparations utilized this estrogen or ethynyl estradiol itself. It has been shown that mestranol must be demethylated to become biologically active. At one time, this led to some confusion, because the ability of rodents to demethylate differs from that of humans; as a consequence, relative potency estimates of mestranol/ethynyl estradiol derived from rodents gave misleading information. Recent pharmacokinetic studies (Brody, et al., 1989) have shown that plasma ethynyl estradiol levels from a single oral dose of 50 μg mestranol are comparable to those produced by a 35 µg dose of ethynyl estradiol itself. This has become an important point in the debate over clinical benefits of lowering the estrogen dose: the rubric "50 µg pills" used in epidemiological studies does not differentiate the two estrogens, hence the interpretation of "high dose" (i.e., 50 µg or more) versus "low dose" (35 µg or less) becomes confounded. However, newer contraceptive formulations tend more and more to use ethynyl estradiol, so this problem is likely to disappear with time.

In the 1980s, another ethynyl estrogen, 11β-methoxy ethynyl estradiol, became available for clinical testing in Germany. This compound turned out to be approximately ten times as potent as ethynyl estradiol itself, a feature that might be of pharmaceutical interest. However, it turned out to have some highly unusual metabolic features: the 11β-methoxy group interferes with enzymatic oxidation of the A-ring, preventing the formation of catechols and epoxides (Purdy et al., 1983). Since certain classes of organic compounds with these structures have mutagenic properties, Purdy et al. (1983) examined this compound and other estrogens in an *in vitro* cell culture system. All the other estrogens formed oxidative metabolites, and the cultured cells showed evidence of mutagenesis as well as tumor formation when injected into nude mice. The 11β-methoxy compound, which did not form oxidative metabolites, did not cause cell transformation, and the transplanted cells did not produce tumors. Whether these observations have any relevance to the clinical question of estrogens and tumorigenesis remains a matter for future research.

REFERENCES

Adler L. Zur Physiologie u. Pathologie der Ovarialfunktion. *Arch Gynak* 1912;95:349–424.

Albright F. In: Musser JH (ed). *Internal Medicine*. Philadelphia: Lea & Febiger; 1945;966.

Allen E, Doisy EA. An ovarian hormone: preliminary report on its localization, extraction, partial purification and action in test animals. *JAMA* 1923;81:819–21.

Aschheim S, Zondek B. *Klin Wschr* 1927;6:1322–4.

Brody SA, Turkes A, Goldzieher JW. Pharmacokinetics of three bioequivalent norethindrone/mestranol-50 mcg and three norethindrone/ethynyl estradiol-35 mcg OC formulations: Are low-dose pills really lower? *Contraception* 1989;40:269–84.

Butenandt A, Westphal O. Zur Isolierung und Characterisierung des Corpus-Luteums-hormons. *Ber Deutsch Chem Gesellsch* 1934;67:1440–2.

Fellner O. Experimentell erzeugte Wachstumsveränderungen am weiblichen Genitale der Kaninchen. *Centralbl Allg Path Anat* 1912;23:673–6.

Fellner O. Über die Tätigkeit des ovarium in der Schwangerschaft (interstitielle Zellen). *Monatschr Geburts Gynakol* 1921;54:88–94.

Fellner O. Die Wirkung des Feminin auf das Ei. *Med Klin* 1927;23:1527–9.

Gillman J. A quantitative study of the inhibition of the ovary and of the turgescent perineum of the normal baboon produced by a single injection of estradiol benzoate. *Endocrinology* 1941;29:633–8.

Goldzieher JW, de la Pena A, Chenault CB, Cervantes A. Comparative studies of the ethynyl estrogens used in oral contraceptives. Potency. *Am J Obstet Gynecol* 1975a,b;122:619–36.

Haberlandt L. Über hormonale sterilizierung des weiblishen Tierkorpers. *Munch Med Wschr* 1921;68:1577–8.

Hamblen EC, Hirst DV, Cuyler WK. Effects of estrogenic therapy upon ovarian function. *Am J Obstet Gynecol* 1943;45:268–77.

Haus LW, Goldzieher JW, Hamblen EC. Dysmenorrhea and ovulation: correlation of the effect of estrogen therapy on pain, the endometrium and the basal body temperature. *Am J Obstet Gynecol* 1947;54:820–8.

Iscovesco H. Les lipoides de l'ovaire. *Compt Rend Soc Biol* 1912;73:16–8.

Karnaky KJ. Endocrines in gynecology and obstetrics with special reference to stilbestrol in the treatment of uterine bleeding—original research on menstruation. *Texas State J Med* 1940;36:379–85.

Kurzrok R. The prospects for hormonal sterilization. *J Contracept* 1937;2:27–9.

Lyon R. Relief of essential dysmenorrhea with ethinyl estradiol. *Surg Gynecol Obstet* 1943;77:657–60.

Purdy RH, Goldzieher JW. Toward a safer estrogen in aging. In: *Intervention in the aging process*, Part A. Quantitation, Epidemiology and Clinical Research. New York: Alan R. Liss; 1983;247–266.

Purdy RH, Goldzieher JW, LeQuesne PW, et al. Active intermediates and carcinogenesis. In: Merriam GR, Lipsett MB (eds). *Catechol Estrogens*. New York: Raven Press; 1983;123–140.

Reiprich W. Experimenteller Hyperfeminismus. Seine Bedeutung for weibliche Generationsorgane und Gestation. *Arch Gynak* 1930;141:27–46.

Sturgis S, Albright F. The mechanism of estrin therapy in the relief of dysmenorrhea. *Endocrinology* 1940;46:68–72.

Wilson L, Kurzrok R. Studies on the motility of the human uterus in vivo—a functional myometrial cycle. *Endocrinology* 1938;23:79.

Pharmacology of the Contraceptive Steroids,
edited by Joseph W. Goldzieher.
Raven Press, Ltd., New York © 1994.

3

Mechanism of Action of Steroid Hormones and Antagonists

James H. Clark

Department of Cell Biology
Baylor College of Medicine, Houston, Texas 77030

Steroid hormones have effects at all levels of biological organization; however, it is clear that most of their actions are mediated by interactions at the gene level via hormone receptors. Therefore, a generalized model of steroid hormone action that gives an overview of these actions at the cellular and molecular level will be presented.

Steroid hormones enter most cells by diffusion, although in some cases active uptake may be involved. In target cells (i.e., cells sensitive to hormone) the steroid binds to macromolecules called receptors. These molecules are relatively large proteins that have specific binding sites for the hormone and are found in both the cytoplasm and nuclear fractions of the cell. Binding of the steroid to its receptor molecule results in ill-defined conformational (allosteric) changes in structure, which convert the receptor from an inactive to an active conformation. These changes result in the formation of an "activated or transformed" receptor–steroid complex that has a high affinity for various nuclear binding sites. Receptor–steroid complexes bind to regulatory DNA sequences in the 5′-end of a responsive gene. In the past it was thought that the activation or transformation step occurred in the cytoplasm; however, recent evidence indicates that this process may also occur in the nuclear compartment. The binding of the receptor hormone complex to regulatory elements usually results in gene activation, i.e., transcription of the gene by RNA polymerase to produce messenger RNA. The mRNA is translated on cytoplasmic ribosomes to produce the appropriate protein, which alters cell function, growth, or differentiation.

In some cases receptor–gene interaction causes gene activity to be decreased rather than increased. Once the receptor–hormone complex has interacted with a gene, the protein undergoes reactions that are not well understood; these result in the reestablishment of unoccupied receptor (recycling) and elimination of the steroid from the cell. These steps may involve dissociation of the steroid from the receptor and conversion of the receptor to a form that can subsequently re-bind hormone again and recycle. The steroid may be metabolized to forms that do not bind tightly to the receptor and hence diffuse out of the cell.

BIOCHEMISTRY AND MOLECULAR BIOLOGY OF STEROID RECEPTORS

Steroid receptors represent a class of ligand-activated transcription factors including, for instance, the thyroid hormone and vitamin D receptors. Many of the known steroid receptors have been cloned, and as a result, we now know a great deal about steroid receptor structure (Evans, 1988; Green & Chambon, 1986; O'Malley, 1989).

Structural Organization of Receptor Proteins

Sequence comparisons of the cloned receptors reveal three regions of consensus homology. The first region of homology, Consensus 1 (C1), is the most highly conserved, and is a cysteine-rich DNA binding domain. C2 and C3 are less highly conserved, yet still have significant homology. The carboxyl terminal region has been associated with ligand binding, transcriptional activation, and potential protein–protein interactions with other steroid receptors as well as potential inhibitory factors. These structural observations suggest that the steroid receptor supergene family represents an old family of transcription factors. One can speculate that the early forms of these receptors were regulated by intracellular metabolic ligands, in an intracrine fashion (O'Malley, 1989). Some of the receptors may have lost the ligand binding domain, and hence became constitutive transcription factors, such as v-erb-A (Debuire et al., 1984). Other receptors may have acquired the ligand specificity for steroids, thyroid hormones, retinoic acid, and perhaps even other unidentified ligands. Low-stringency southern blot hybridization analysis with the DNA binding domain of the glucocorticoid receptor has suggested an abundance of related receptor proteins (Giguere et al., 1988). Some of these receptor proteins have been cloned, but the ligands are yet to be identified. These "orphan receptors" or receptor variants, may represent the earliest forms of the steroid receptor gene family.

The Steroid Receptor Gene Family

Steroid receptor proteins have molecular weights of about 80,000–100,000. Each monomeric unit binds a single steroid molecule, but the receptors are known to dimerize when bound to the genes they regulate. They are acidic, asymmetric, and present in low abundance in cells. With the exception of phosphate, no other covalent posttranslational modifications are known. There is no evidence for either lipid, carbohydrate, or nucleic acid in their structures, and no confirmed evidence that any receptor possesses an intrinsic enzymatic activity. Rather, the proteins are thought to function primarily by virtue of their DNA-binding activity.

Most steroid-regulated genes share one important structural feature, the presence of steroid receptor binding sites referred to as steroid response elements (SREs). SREs have all of the characteristics of a classical enhancer element (Maniatis et al., 1987). They are position and orientation independent, and their presence has a profound effect on transcriptional activity when stimulated by hormone (Chandler et al., 1983; Ponta et al., 1985).

Binding to the SRE DNA sequence involves receptor dimerization on the DNA, concentration of activated steroid receptors. Transcriptional response to steroids in different tissues and cells is additionally controlled by limiting the tissue-specific expression and concentration of the various different steroid receptors.

HORMONAL CONTROL OF GENE EXPRESSION

Hormone-dependent transcription of the vitellogenin gene in crude extracts of Xenopus nuclei has been observed (Corthesy et al., 1988), and it has been demonstrated that bacterially expressed, truncated glucocorticoid receptor fragment (Freedman et al., 1989) and native progesterone receptor (Klein-Hitpass et al., 1990) are capable of enhancing RNA synthesis in an *in vitro* transcription assay. These findings suggest that enhancer binding proteins may interact with one or a subset of general transcription factors to recruit and stabilize the formation of preinitiation complexes at distal proximal promoters and thus enhance the initiation of transcription. Preliminary investigations using other steroid receptors (e.g., glucocorticoid and estrogen) indicate that this may be a general mechanism by which all receptors act to regulate the expression of their respective target genes.

Steroid hormone response elements are often found in multiple copies in the 5'-flanking regions of hormone-responsive genes (Glass et al., 1988; Jantzen et al., 1987). Transient transfection studies demonstrate that deletion or mutation of one of two SREs leads to a dramatic decrease in the inducibility of a target gene, suggesting that the SREs cooperate with one another to confer synergistic induction. Cooperative binding of receptors to PREs appears to contribute to the hormone induced synergism in gene expression observed *in vivo*. Taken together, these results demonstrate that complex regulation of eukaryotic gene expression can be achieved by assembling unique subsets of cis elements. Through either cooperative binding or cooperative interactions of specific activation domains with other transcription factors at target genes, expression of a given gene can be regulated over a wide range.

It is well documented that steroid receptor-mediated induction of target gene expression *in vivo* is dependent on the presence and concentration of steroid hormone (Beato, 1989; O'Malley et al., 1979; Yamamoto, 1985). Consistent with this model, specific hypersensitive sites, which correlate well with the state of expression of hormone responsive genes, are detected in and around the SREs in the presence of the cognate hormone (Fritton et al., 1984). A nuclear genomic footprint, demonstrating receptor binding to the PRE/GRE element of the tyrosine amino-transferase gene, is only observed in the presence of hormone (Becker et al., 1986). Furthermore, estrogen or progesterone (Bagchi et al., 1988) receptors in crude nuclear extracts bind to their respective SRE DNAs only when the extracts are prepared from hormone-treated cells. Recent results of *in vitro* transcription experiments have revealed that highly purified progesterone receptors bind and function to enhance the expression of PRE-containing target genes in a hormone-independent manner. In contrast, less pure nuclear extracts isolated from T47D cells contain ligand-free progesterone receptors that do not bind to PRE sites; these receptors also fail to enhance transcription of PRE-containing test genes. Upon treatment with progesterone ligand, either *in vitro* or *in vivo*, the receptors in such extracts now bind specifically to their respective PREs and enhance transcription of PRE-containing test genes. This transcriptional stimulation is specific for progestins and is inhibited by 70% when the anti-progestin RU 486 is added to the reaction.

Such evidence indicates that hormone is needed to effect an additional structural alteration(s) in the receptor molecule, an event not induced completely by anti-hormones or steroid antagonists. *In situ*, this event could be represented by dissociation of additional inhibitory proteins, by inducing a specific conformation change in the receptor via covalent modifications such as phosphorylation, or likely by a combination of these parameters. Following such an alteration, the receptor gains the capacity to bind and activate hormone responsive genes. Steroid antagonists are inefficient in affecting this process. In highly purified forms of receptor, this "active" conformation may be achieved via the purification process itself.

In summary, steroid-activated receptor dimers bind to SRE elements and further stabilize crucial transcription factors bound at the distal and proximal promoter elements. Receptor tetramers, bound to two SREs, are most efficient in this process. When these transcription factors are bound stably, they are able to recruit RNA polymerase repeatedly to that gene and a high rate of transcription is achieved.

STEROID HORMONE ANTAGONISM

Compounds that block the action of a given steroid hormone are called antagonists or anti-hormones. Most of these are thought to act by binding to receptors and interfering with their normal function. However, this generalization requires qualification depending on the specific hormone. Therefore, the steroid hormone antagonists have been divided according to the class of hormone that they inhibit.

Anti-Estrogens

Anti-estrogens can be divided into the following three groups: (1) short-acting antagonists, such as estriol; (2) long-acting antagonists, such as tamoxifen and clomiphene; and (3) physiological antagonists, such as progesterone, androgens, and glucocorticoids. Each of these will be discussed separately.

Short-Acting Antagonists

Short-acting estrogens such as estriol and 17α-estradiol are actually time-dependent, mixed agonist–antagonists. They have the ability to stimulate early uterotropic responses while having little effect on true uterine hypertrophy and hyperplasia when they are injected in saline (Clark & Guthrie, 1981; Clark & Peck, 1979).

Short-acting agonists cause binding of the receptor hormone complex in the nucleus for short periods of time and thus they are able to stimulate early uterotropic events. However, they are unable to maintain the receptor in the nucleus for a sufficient period of time to cause true uterine growth. The antagonistic action of these compounds results from the competition between receptor estradiol and receptor estriol complexes for functional nuclear sites. This competition reduces the number of effective receptor estrogen complexes retained in the nuclear compartment, and thus reduces the long-term uterotropic stimulation. When short-acting estrogens are administered by pellet implant, which results in a continuous release of hormones and continuous occupancy of the receptor, no antagonism is observed. Thus the biological response obtained with short-acting estrogens is dependent on the conditions of administration and are the consequence of receptor occupancy.

The reasons why short-acting estrogens occupy nuclear bound receptors for short periods of time following an injection are complex and not clear. The dissociation rate of estriol from the receptor is more rapid than that of estradiol (Brecher & Wotiz, 1968), leading to the suggestion that this difference in dissociation rate accounts for short-term nuclear retention (Bouton & Raynaud, 1979). Estriol is also cleared from the body more rapidly than estradiol (Jensen et al., 1966). Therefore, the equilibrium between tissue and blood levels would result in more rapid dissociation of nuclear bound receptor–estriol complexes. It is also possible that receptor–estriol complexes dissociate from their nuclear binding sites more rapidly than receptor–estradiol complexes. This could result in a more rapid turnover or processing of receptor and loss of hormone from the tissues.

Long-Acting Antagonists

Triphenylethylene derivatives, such as tamoxifen or clomiphene, are mixed agonist–antagonists of estrogen action (Clark & Markaverich, 1982). Mixed agonism/ antagonism is very common among the anti-steroid hormones; therefore, an explanation of this term will be offered here as a general example. An agonist is a compound that stimulates a response while an antagonist will completely inhibit the action of an agonist. A mixed agonist–antagonist will partially inhibit the action of an agonist but, because it has inherent agonistic properties, it will partially mimic the response of the agonist. The degree of agonist or antagonist activity observed depends on the species, organ, tissue, or cell type that is being examined and upon the end-point assay chosen. Clomiphene and tamoxifen stimulate the rat uterus to grow when administered alone, but they inhibit the growth-promoting effects of estradiol when both substances are given simultaneously. These stimulatory and inhibitory functions are the result of the ability of these drugs to stimulate cellular hypertrophy of the epithelial cells of the endometrium while having little effect on the stromal or myometrial compartments. Estradiol, on the other hand, stimulates cellular hypertrophy and hyperplasia in all three tissue layers and hence produces a uterus that is considerably larger than that seen with clomiphene use alone. The elevation in uterine weight caused by clomiphene or tamoxifen use alone is due primarily to the hypertrophy of epithelial cells and some slight, but significant, stimulation of the stroma and myometrium. The inhibition of estradiol action on uterine growth results from the antagonism of cellular growth in the stromal and myometrial compartments. Therefore, triphenylethylene drugs act like partial estrogen agonists in the epithelial cells and as estrogen antagonists in other uterine cells.

The mechanisms by which long-acting estrogen antagonists act to block estrogen action in some cell types, yet stimulate estrogen responses in others, are not fully understood. However, it is known that these drugs bind to the estrogen receptor and cause nuclear accumulation of receptor antagonist complexes. This accumulation is accompanied by long-term depletion of cytosol receptors and altered nuclear processing of the receptor antagonist complex. It is possible that all of these altered receptor functions are involved in the mechanism by which these antagonists block estrogen action.

Some investigators have reported specific but subtle differences in the physicochemical characteristics of receptor anti-estrogen and receptor estradiol complexes (Tate & Jordan, 1984; Tate et al., 1984). However, it is not clear how such differences relate to hormone antagonism. No difference between receptor–anti-estrogen and receptor–estradiol complexes has been found with respect to their recognition by monoclonal antibodies to the receptor, or binding to their DNA or polynucleotides (Murphy & Sutherland, 1983; Tate et al., 1983). Evans et al. (1982) did show that estradiol receptor complexes bind more tightly to calf thymus DNA than receptor–anti-estrogen complexes. Perhaps this observation relates to the finding that nuclear bound receptor–anti-estrogen complexes can be readily extracted by high salt, whereas a portion of estrogen–receptor complexes cannot (Ruh & Baudendistel, 1977). These salt-extracted forms of the receptor do not differ significantly from those of the estradiol-receptor complex (Ruh & Ruh, 1983). Differential extraction of estrogen and tamoxifen receptors has also been observed with the nonionic detergent Nonidet P40 (Ikeda et al., 1984). All of the nuclear tamoxifen–receptor complex from MCF-7 cells is extracted with this detergent and sediments as 7 and 5S peaks on sucrose density gradients. In contrast, nuclear estradiol complexes resist extraction. These results suggest that the interactions of these two receptor complex forms with chromatin differ in some way.

The interpretation of the mechanism of action of long-acting agonist–antagonists is complicated further by interspecies variation. In contrast to the mixed agonistic-antagonistic function of nonsteroidal anti-estrogens in the rat, in the adult mouse these compounds are estrogenic with little if any anti-estrogenic activity (Terenius, 1971). In the chick oviduct and liver, however, these compounds are estrogen antagonists with virtually no detectable agonist activity under most circumstances (Binart et al., 1979). In primates, clomiphene and tamoxifen are primarily anti-estrogenic; however, estrogenicity has been noted depending on the species and endpoint used (Clark & Guthrie, 1981; Natrajan & Greenblatt, 1979). Other species manifest a broad spectrum of agonistic-antagonistic responses to nonsteroidal anti-estrogens, discussion of which goes beyond the scope of this chapter (for review see Clark & Markaverich, 1982; Furr & Jordan, 1984).

These species' differences in response to nonsteroidal anti-estrogens essentially disappear when these compounds are tested in cell culture. Tamoxifen and 4-hydroxytamoxifen block the estrogen-stimulated increases in several specific proteins in MCF-7 cells and have no agonistic activity (Westley & Rochefor, 1979). Tamoxifen and nafoxidine inhibit [^{3}H]thymidine incorporation and DNA polymerase activity, and reduce cell number in MCF-7 cell cultures (Coezy et al., 1982). Estrogen-stimulated prolactin synthesis is inhibited by tamoxifen and no agonist effect is seen with the drug alone (Klein-Hitpass et al., 1990).

It is also possible that these drugs act via indirect mechanisms that do not involve the estrogen receptor at all. Estrogen target tissues, as well as other nontarget tissues, contain triphenylethylene anti-estrogen binding sites (TABS). These TABS bind anti-estrogens, such as tamoxifen and clomiphene, with high affinity ($K_d \approx 1$ nM), and are present in estrogen target and nontarget tissues (Sutherland et al., 1980; Sutherland, 1981). In addition, somewhat similar sites with lower affinity ($K_d \approx 10$ nM) are associated with low-density lipoprotein in rat serum (Winneker & Clark, 1983).

The physiological function of TABS has not been defined, and although it is tempting to suggest that these sites are anti-estrogen receptors; in general, the data do not support this hypothesis. The estrogenic and anti-estrogenic properties of nonsteroidal anti-estrogens correlate with their relative binding affinities for the estrogen receptor and not for TABS (Miller & Katzenellenbogen, 1983). The cis and trans isomers of clomiphene bind to TABS with similar affinities, yet they have dissimilar agonist–antagonist profiles. Tamoxifen resistance has been described in a cell line of MCF-7 breast cancer cells that contained very low levels of TABS and normal levels of estrogen receptor. However, it has not been possible to relate the levels of TABS to tamoxifen sensitivity (Miller & Katzenellenbogen, 1983).

Pure Anti-Estrogens

All of the compounds discussed previously have been mixed estrogen agonist–antagonists. Recently a new class of drugs have been introduced which appear to be pure antagonists (Wiseman et al., 1989). ICI 164,384 is a 7α-alkyl amide analogue of estradiol that lacks agonist activity for uterine growth in both rats and mice and is unable to induce the progesterone receptor in the immature rat. ICI 164,384 binds to the estrogen receptor with an affinity similar to estradiol; however, its ability to inhibit estrogen induced mRNA synthesis is 50 to 150 fold less than predicted (Wiseman et al., 1989). Similar discrepancies have been noted for tamoxifen and hydroxytamoxifen (May & Westley, 1987), and may result from a differential ability of these compounds to enter cells, or their binding interactions with nonreceptor proteins.

Physiological Estrogen Antagonists

The blood levels of estrogen fluctuate according to the stage of the reproductive cycle, and this is accompanied by changing levels of estrogen receptor binding. Thus the effects of estrogen wax and wane as a result of these changes in ovarian secretion of estrogens. In addition to these influences of estrogen alone, other hormones act to alter the actions of estrogen at the cellular level and modify estrogen-directed functions.

Progesterone

Progesterone acts on the estrogen-primed uterus to alter cell function and reproductive competence. Often this ability of progesterone is considered to be antagonistic to estrogen; however, it probably should be referred to as a modifier of estrogen action rather than an antagonist. Nevertheless, progesterone will reduce the ability of estrogens to cause uterine growth and vaginal cornification. This ability of progesterone to modify or antagonize estrogen action is generally considered to involve receptor mechanisms that have been previously discussed. These effects of progesterone involve decreasing the number of cytosol and nuclear bound estrogen receptor complexes. Such reductions in receptor number have been correlated with a reduced sensitivity of the uterus to estradiol (Clark et al., 1977).

Most of the studies concerned with progesterone effects on estrogen receptor levels have been done under nonphysiological circumstances. However, in the elegant studies of Brenner et al. (1974), physiological conditions were maintained by creating artificial menstrual cycles in ovariectomized rhesus monkeys. Under these conditions, estradiol blood levels were maintained at a constant level throughout the cycle and progesterone was elevated during the second half of the cycle. Cytosol estrogen receptor levels were elevated during the first half of the cycle and dramatically decreased during the second half. These data suggest that progesterone does lower cytosol estrogen receptor even when estradiol is present. Although nuclear estrogen receptors were not examined in this study, progesterone does decrease their level in the hamster uterus under physiological circumstances. In the pig endometrium, progesterone induces estrogen sulfotransferase, an enzyme that inactivates estradiol, which interferes with the estrogen-dependent replenishment of the estrogen receptor (Saunders et al., 1989). Therefore, there are several different mechanisms that exist whereby progesterone can decrease the level of estrogen receptor and reduce the ability of a tissue to respond to estrogen.

Modulated estrogen receptor levels are correlated with striking changes in the morphology of the uterine luminal epithelium (Clark & Peck, 1979). When nuclear receptor levels are elevated, the epithelium is hypertrophied and mitotic, whereas when receptor levels are suppressed, the epithelium is atrophied and shows degenerative changes. Such changes in morphology and functional state of uterine cells probably reflect the normal cyclic interaction of estrogen and progesterone on the reproductive tract.

In addition to these effects on the estrogen receptor, progesterone also inhibits the stimulation of nuclear type II estrogen binding sites. This inhibition of nuclear type II sites is correlated with reduced uterotropic response to estrogen, and does not appear to be related to any effects of progesterone on estrogen receptor levels. The inhibitory effects of progesterone do appear to be mediated by the progesterone receptor, since estrogen priming is necessary in order to observe the inhibitory effects of progesterone.

Androgens

Androgenic steroids are known to inhibit the actions of estrogen on the growth of estrogen target tissues (Rochefort & Garcia, 1984). Indeed, androgen therapy has been used in the treatment of estrogen-dependent breast cancer. This treatment is based on the rationale that androgens should block or antagonize the estrogen-stimulated growth of breast cancer cells. The mechanisms by which androgens antagonize estrogenic functions are not known; however, it is known that androgen receptors are present in estrogen target tissues (Garcia & Rochefort, 1979). Physiological concentrations of androgens do not cause growth or stimulate other known functions of MCF-7 breast cancer cells, even though nuclear binding of the receptor–androgen complex is readily observed (Rochefort & Garcia, 1984). Likewise, in the rat uterus there appears to be no biological response to nuclear binding of the receptor–androgen complex. However, chronic exposure to physiological levels of androgens in the rat does depress uterine weight, an indication that androgens are antiestrogenic by some mechanism.

In contrast, high doses of androgens stimulate growth of the rat uterus, mammary tumors, and MCF-7 cells (Garcia & Rochefort, 1978). Thus, androgens appear to have the capacity both to inhibit and stimulate estrogen target tissues depending on the dose used. The low-dose inhibition may be mediated directly by the androgen receptor or it may operate indirectly via interactions at the hypothalamic–pituitary level or some other pathway. The high-dose stimulation effect is mediated by the estrogen receptor, since it is known that high concentrations of androgens will bind to the estrogen receptor, cause nuclear accumulation, and produce an estrogen-like response (Rochefort et al., 1972).

Type II Estrogen Binding Sites and Estrogen Antagonism

One of the pleiotropic events stimulated by exposure to estrogen is an elevation of type II estrogen binding sites. These sites are present in the cytosol and nuclei and are different from the estrogen receptor (type I). Nuclear type II sites are occupied by an endogenous ligand that appears to be an inhibitor of cell proliferation, and as such, may constitute a new class of anti-estrogen (Maniatis et al., 1987). Since estrogen-induced uterine cell proliferation is observed only when nuclear type II sites are elevated, this may mean that the inhibitory ligand has dissociated from these sites. Such dissociation would open up sites that are measured by the binding of labeled estradiol. Nuclear type II sites are tightly associated with the nuclear matrix and may be coupled to the regulatory components involved with DNA synthesis. Therefore, the dissociation of an inhibitory ligand from these sites may act as a positive regulation signal that initiates DNA synthesis and cell proliferation.

Glucocorticoids

Glucocorticoids inhibit several of the early uterotropic responses induced by estrogen. These include water imbibition, histamine mobilization, eosinophil infiltration, and vasodilation, which are all components of the support pathway facilitating uterine growth. When these estrogen-induced responses are blocked by glucocorticoid administration, the biosynthetic ability of estrogen is not blocked; however, the total effect of estrogen on uterine growth is somewhat reduced. This reduction is probably due to the reduced availability of substrates to the growing uterus. The mechanisms involved in the antagonism of early uterotropic responses are not known, however, since they involve such uterine components as the vasculature, mast cells (histamine release) and eosinophil infiltration. They undoubtedly are quite complex. Uterine cells do contain glucocorticoid receptors but their functional relationships to estrogen antagonism is not known.

Anti-Progestins

Although there are several exogenous and endogenous anti-estrogens, anti-progestational compounds are rare. RU 486 (mifepristone), which was synthesized by Roussel UCLAF, has been shown to interrupt the luteal phase of the menstrual cycle and terminate pregnancy in women (Herrmann et al., 1982). RU 486 induces early onset of vaginal bleeding when administered during the luteal phase of cycling monkeys (Asch & Rojas, 1985; Healy et al., 1983). Such actions are considered to be due to a direct antagonistic effect of RU 486 at the receptor level in the uterine endometrium. This compound binds to progesterone receptors in the rabbit uterus and glucocorticoid receptors in the thymus where it acts as an anti-glucocorticoid (Herrmann et al., 1982). In T47D cells, RU 486 binds to the progesterone receptor and inhibits cellular proliferation, as does R5020, a synthetic progesterone (Horwitz, 1985). Thus, RU 486 is an agonist by this criterion; however, it does antagonize the stimulation of insulin receptors by R5020. These agonistic properties have also been observed in T47D cells, which grow in response to RU 486 (Bowden et al., 1989). Therefore, in T47D cells, RU 486 manifests mixed agonist–antagonist properties.

RU 486 binds well to all mammalian progesterone receptors except those of the hamster (Glass et al., 1988). In this species, the drug also has no anti-progestational effects. Progesterone receptors from the chick oviduct also do not bind this compound. Such loss of affinity in the hamster and chicken indicate some important structural differences exist in the receptor in these animals.

The mechanism by which RU 486 exerts its antagonistic activity does not involve any differences in activation and transformation of the drug-receptor complex (Bagchi et al., 1992; ElAshry et al., 1989). Both progesterone and RU 486 form complexes that bind to hormone response elements in a qualitative and quantitatively similar manner. This binding even involves the same G nucleotides. The only difference appears to be in the sedimentation properties and the gel retardation characteristics of the two receptor–hormone–response element complexes. Thus it seem likely that the binding of the receptor–RU 486 complex to hormone response elements results in a conformation that is different from that of the receptor–progesterone complex. This different conformation does not permit the protein–protein interaction's necessary induction of gene transcription.

As pointed out earlier for anti-estrogens, the actions of anti-steroid hormone drugs *in vitro* are not necessarily identical to their actions *in vivo*. Obviously more work *in vivo* is needed on this important class of anti-progestins before definitive statements can be made regarding their mechanism of action and their true pharmacologic and physiologic actions.

An inhibitor of progesterone-receptor binding has been described in the cytosol from rat placenta (Olge, 1981). This inhibitor is a macromolecule that decreases the affinity of the receptor for progesterone but has no effect on the number of receptor sites. The function of this inhibitor is not known; however, inhibitory activity in trophoblast cytosol is greatest on days 9 and 12 of pregnancy and declines thereafter. By day 18 inhibitory activity is no longer detectable and this coincides with a sharp decrease in progesterone receptor concentration. The presence of such inhibitors in other systems has not been described; however, their potential physiological significance in the regulation of progesterone action is considerable.

REFERENCES

Asch RH, Rojas FJ. The effects of RU 486 on the luteal phase of the rhesus monkey. *J Steroid Biochem* 1985;22:227–30.

Bagchi MK, Elliston JF, Tsai SY, et al. Steroid hormone-dependent interaction of human progesterone with its target enhancer element. *Mol Endo* 1988;2:1221–9.

Bagchi MK, Tsai SY, Tsai MJ, et al. Progesterone-dependent cell free transcription: identification of a functional intermediate in receptor activation. *Nature* (in press).

Bagchi MK, Tsai SY, Weigel NL, et al. Regulation of *in vitro* transcription by progesterone receptor-characterization and kinetic studies. *J Biol Chem* 1990;265:5129–34.

Beato M. Gene regulation by steroid hormones. *Cell* 1989;56:335–44.

Becker PB, Gloss B, Schmid W, et al. *In vivo* protein DNA interactions in a glucocorticoid response element require the presence of the hormone. *Nature* 1986;324:686–8.

Binart N, Catelli MH, Geynet G, et al. Monohydroxytamoxifen: an antiestrogen with high affinity for the chick oviduct oestrogen receptor. *Biochem Biophys Res Commun* 1979;91:812–8.

Bouton M, Raynaud JP. The relevance of interaction kinetics in determining biological responses to estrogens. *Endocrinology* 1979;105:509–15.

Bowden RT, Hissom JR, Moore MR. Growth stimulation of T47D human breast cancer cells by the antiprogestin RU 486. *Endocrinology* 1989;124:2642–4.

Brecher PI, Wotiz HH. Nuclear binding and an assay for the estrogen receptor. *Proc Soc Exp Biol Med* 1968;128:470–2.

Brenner RM, Resko JA, West NB. Cyclic changes in oviductal morphology and residual cytoplasmic estradiol binding capacity induced by sequential estradiolprogesterone treatment of spayed rhesus monkeys. *Endocrinology* 1974;95:1094–1104.

Chandler VL, Maler BA, Yamamoto KR. DNA sequences bound specifically by glucocorticoid receptor *in vitro* render a heterologous promoter hormone responsive *in vivo*. *Cell* 1983;33:489–99.

Clark JH, Markaverich BM. Agonist and antagonist properties of clomiphene: a review. *Pharmacol Ther* 1982;15:467–519.

Clark, JH, Markaverich BM. The agonistic and antagonistic effects of short acting estrogens: a review. *Pharmacol Ther* 1982;21:429–53.

Clark JH, Guthrie SC. The agonistic and antagonistic effects of clomiphene and its isomers. *Biol Reprod* 1981;25:667–72.

Clark JH, Paszko Z, Peck EJ Jr. Nuclear binding and retention of the receptor estrogen complex: relation to the agonistic and antagonistic properties of estriol. *Endocrinology* 1977;100:91–6.

Clark JH, Peck EJ Jr. Female sex steroids: receptors and function. *Monog Endocrinol* 1979;14:4–36.

Coezy E, Borgna JL, Rochefort H. Tamoxifen and metabolites in MCF7 cells: correlations between binding to estrogen and cell growth inhibition. *Cancer Res* 1982;42:317–23.

Corthesy B, Hispking R, Theulaz I, Wahli W. Estrogen-dependent *in vitro* transcription from the vitellogenin promoter in liver nuclear extracts. *Science* 1988;239:1137–9.

Debuire B, Henry C, Banaissa M, et al. Sequencing the erbA gene of avian erythroblastosis virus reveals a new type of oncogene. *Science* 1984;224:1456–9.

ElAshry D, Onate SA, Nordeen SK, Edwards DP. Human progesterone receptor complexed with the antagonist RU 486 binds to hormone response elements in a structurally altered form. *Mol Endo* 1989;3:1545–58.

Evans E, Baskevitch PP, Rochefort H. Estrogen receptor DNA interactions: difference between activation by estrogen and antiestrogen. *Eur J Biochem* 1982;128:185–91.

Evans RE. The steroid and thyroid hormone receptor superfamily. *Science* 1988;240:889–95.

Freedman L, Yoshinaga S, Vanderbilt J, Yamamoto K. *In vitro* transcription enhancement by purified derivatives of the glucocorticoid receptor. *Science* 1989;245:298–300.

Fritton HP, Igo-Kemenes TI, Nowock J, et al. Alternative sets of DNaseI-hypersensitive sites characterize the various functional states of the chicken lysozyme gene. *Nature* 1984;311:163–5.

Furr BJA, Jordon VC. The pharmacology and clinical uses of tamoxifen. *Pharmacol Ther* 1984;25:127–205.

Garcia M, Rochefort H. Androgen effects mediated by estrogen receptor in 7,12dimethylbenz(a)anthraceneinduced rat mammary tumors. *Cancer Res* 1978;38:3922–9.

Garcia M, Rochefort H. Evidence and characterization of the binding of two 3H androgens to the estrogen receptor. *Endocrinology* 1979;104:1797–804.

Giguere V, Yang N, Segui P, Evans RM. Identification of a new class of steroid hormone receptors. *Nature* 1988;331:91–4.

Glass CK, Holloway JM, Devary OV, Rosenfeld MG. The thyroid hormone receptor binds with opposite transcriptional effects to a common sequence motif in thyroid hormone and estrogen response elements. *Cell* 1988;54:313–23.

Gray OG, Leavitt WW. RU 486 is not an antiprogestin in the hamster. *J Steroid Biochem* 1987;28:493–7.

Green S, Chambon P. A superfamily of potentially oncogenic hormone receptors. *Nature* 1986;324:615–7.

Healy DL, Baulieu EE, Hodgen GD. Induction of menstruation by an antiprogesterone steroid (RU 486) in primates: site of action, dose-response relationships, and hormonal effects. *Fertil Steril* 1983; 40:253–7.

Herrmann W, Wyss R, Riondel A, et al. The effects of an antiprogesterone steroid in women: interruption of the menstrual cycle and of early pregnancy. *CR Sciences Acad Sci (III)* 1982;294:933–8.

Horwitz KB. The antiprogestin RU 38486: receptor-mediated progestin versus antiprogestin actions screened in estrogen-insensitive T47D human breast cancer cells. *Endocrinology* 1985;116:2236–45.

Ikeda M, Omukai Y, Hosokawa, K, Senoo T. Differences in extractability of estradiol and tamoxifen receptor complex in the nuclei from MCF7 cells with Nonidet P40. *Steroids* 1984;43:481–9.

Jantzen K, Fritton HP, Igo-Kemenes T, et al. Partial overlapping of binding sequences for steroid hormone receptors and DNase I hypersensitive sites in the rabbit uteroglobin gene region. *Nucl Acid Res* 1987;15:4535–52.

Jensen EV, Jacobson HI, Flesher JW, et al. Estrogen receptors in target issues. In: Pincus G, T. Nakao T, Tait JF (eds) *Steroid Dynamics*. New York: Academic Press; 1966;133–57.

Klein-Hitpass L, Tsai SY, Weigel NL, et al. The progesterone receptor stimulates cell-free transcription by enhancing the formation of a stable preinitiation complex. *Cell* 1990;60:247–57.

Maniatis T, Goodbourn S, Fischer JA. Regulation of inducible and tissue-specific gene expression. *Science* 1987;236:1237–44.

May FEB, Westley BR. Effects of tamoxifen and 4hydroxytamoxifen on the pNR1 and pNR2 estrogenregulated RNAs in human breast cancer cells. *J Biol Chem* 1987;262:15894–9.

Miller MA, Katzenellenbogen BS. Characterization and quantitation of antiestrogen binding sites in estrogen receptor-positive and negative human breast cancer cell lines. *Cancer Res* 1983;43:3094–100.

Murphy LC, Sutherland RL. Antitumor activity of clomiphene analogs *in vitro*: relationship to affinity for the estrogen receptor and another high affinity antiestrogenbinding site. *J Clin Endocrinol Metab* 1983;57:373–9.

Natrajan PK, Greenblatt RB. *Clomiphene Citrate: Induction of Ovulation*. Philadelphia: Lea and Febiger; 1979;35–76.

O'Malley BW, Roop DR, Lai EC, et al. The ovalbumin gene: organization, structure, transcription and regulation. *Rec Prog Hormone Res* 1979;35:1–46.

O'Malley BW. Did eucaryotic steroid receptors evolve from intracrine gene regulators? *Endocrinology* 1989;125:1119–20.

Olge FF. Kinetic and physiochemical characteristics of an endogenous inhibitor to progesterone receptor binding in rat placental cytosol. *Biochem J* 1981;199:371–81.

Ponta H, Kennedy N, Skroch P, et al. Hormonal response region of the mouse mammary tumor virus long terminal repeat can be dissociated from the proviral promoter and has enhancer properties. *Proc Natl Acad Sci USA* 1985;84:1020–4.

Rochefort H, Garcia G. The estrogenic and antiestrogenic activities of androgens in female target tissues. *Pharmacol Ther* 1984;23:193–216.

Rochefort H, Lignon F, Capony F. Formation of estrogen nuclear receptor in uterus: effects of androgen, estrone and nafoxidine. *Biochem Biophys Res Commun* 1972;47:662–70.

Ruh TS, Baudendistel LJ. Different nuclear binding sites for antiestrogen and estrogen receptor complexes. *Endocrinology* 1977;100:420–6.

Ruh TS, Ruh MF. The agonistic and antagonistic properties of the high affinity antiestrogen H1285. *Pharmacol Ther* 1983;21:247–64.

Saunders DE, Lozon MM, Corombos JD, Brooks SC. Role of porcine endometrial estrogen sulfotransferase in progesterone mediated down regulation of estrogen receptors. *J Steroid Biochem* 1989;32:749–57.

Sutherland RL, Murphy LC, Foo MS, et al. High affinity antioestrogen binding site distinct from the oestrogen receptor. *Nature* 1980;288:273–5.

Sutherland RL. Estrogen antagonists in chick oviduct: antagonist activity of eight synthetic triphenylethylene derivatives and their interactions with cytoplasmic and nuclear estrogen receptors. *Endocrinology* 1981;09:2061–8.

Tate AC, Jordan VC. Nuclear [³H]4hydroxytamoxifen (40HTAM) and [³H]estradiol (E2) estrogen receptor complexes in the MCF7 breast cancer and GH3 pituitary tumor cell lines. *Mol Cell Endocrinol* 1984;36:211–9.

Tate AC, DeSombre ER, Greene GL, et al. Interaction of [³H]monohydroxytamoxifen-estrogen receptor complexes with a monoclonal antibody. *Breast Cancer Res Treat* 1983;3:267–77.

Tate AC, Greene GL, DeSombre ER, et al. Differences between estrogen and antiestrogenestrogen receptor complexes from human breast tumors identified with an antibody raised against the estrogen receptor. *Cancer Res* 1984;44:1012–8.

Terenius L. Structure activity relationships of antioestrogens with regard to interaction with 17boe-stradiol in the mouse uterus and vagina. *Acta Endocrinol* 1971;66:431–47.

Westley BR, Rochefort H. Estradiolinduced proteins in the MCF7 human breast cancer cell line. *Biochem Biophys Res Commun* 1979;90:410–6.

Winneker RC, Clark JH. Estrogen stimulation of the antiestrogen specific binding site in rat uterus and liver. *Endocrinology* 1983;112:1910–5.

Wiseman LR, Wakeling AE, May FE, Westley BR. Effects of the antioestrogen, ICI 164,384 on oestrogen induced RNAs in MCF-7 cells. *J Steroid Biochem* 1989;33:1–6.

Yamamoto KR. Steroid receptor-regulated transcription of specific genes and gene networks. *Annu Rev Genet* 1985;19:209–52.

Pharmacology of the Contraceptive Steroids,
edited by Joseph W. Goldzieher.
Raven Press, Ltd., New York © 1994.

4

Pharmacokinetics of Selected Contraceptive Steroids in Various Animal Species

Wilhelm Kuhnz and Hartmut Blode

Institute of Pharmacokinetics, Research Laboratories, Schering AG
13342 Berlin, Germany

During drug development, the pharmacological profile of a new compound is assessed in several suitable animal models which try to adequately describe the different individual agonistic or antagonistic properties of the drug. Having selected an animal species, the pharmacologist then needs to interpret the measured effects in relation to the dose administered. At this point of data evaluation, a knowledge of the basic pharmacokinetic parameters of the drug in this particular species is a prerequisite for a meaningful correlation of the drug level/time curves measured in body fluids and the time course and duration of the pharmacodynamic effects observed. Similarly, when toxicological studies have to be evaluated, a detailed knowledge on the pharmacokinetics of the drug, such as bioavailability, clearance, and half-life is mandatory for an interpretation of the absence or presence of toxicological effects and for the decision about whether a particular species can serve as a model for risk assessment in the human.

This will be an overview over the pharmacokinetics of certain contraceptive steroids in commonly used laboratory animals such as rat, mouse, rabbit, dog, and monkey. The steroids included are ethinylestradiol (EE) as the most important estrogen, and several progestins either of the 19-nortestosterone series (norethindrone, levonorgestrel, and gestodene) or derived from 17-hydroxy progesterone, such as medroxyprogesterone and cyproterone acetate. For desogestrel or chlormadinone acetate, there were no studies available that were within the scope of this review.

METHODS

The literature was screened over for the period 1970 to 1991. In addition, unpublished data produced during preclinical drug development at Schering were also included in this review. Reports were considered only if drug analysis had been performed by a specific analytical method, such as radioimmunoassay, HPLC, or gas chromatography–mass spectrometry; data based on nonspecific measurements, such as total radioactivity, were not included. Also excluded were papers dealing with biotransformation, protein binding, or other *in vitro* studies.

In one instance, drug concentration data were published, but no or only limited pharmacokinetic data were given in the original paper. In this case (which is marked in the respective tables), we used the original data for further pharmacokinetic calculations based on either an open three- or open two-compartment model, using the computer program TOPFIT (Goedecke, Schering, Thomae). The pharmacokinetic parameters selected from the available literature are oral bioavailability, AUC, half-lives, total plasma clearance, and volume of distribution. The doses administered orally in the various studies were in the range of 0.03 to 6.7 mg/kg. For a better comparison, we decided to present only the AUC-values measured after intragastric (IG) administration of doses between 0.5 and 1.5 mg/kg, normalized to a dose of 1 mg/kg with the assumption of dose-linear pharmacokinetics. All values presented in the tables are mean values without SD or ranges. The number of animals used for the calculation of each time point in the drug concentration–time curves was between 3 and 7, and typically between 3 and 4 for all species.

Ethynyl Estradiol

A summary of the pharmacokinetic parameters of EE, determined after parenteral (IV) and IG administration to different animal species is presented in Table 1. Doses of 0.1 mg/kg (IV) and 1.0 mg/kg (IG) were administered to female Wistar rats and a bioavailability of 3% was calculated. Since EE is completely absorbed following IG

TABLE 1. *Pharmacokinetic parameters of HEE in selected animal species*

Species	f (%)	AUC[a] (ng·h/ml)	$t_{1/2}\lambda_1$ (h)	$t_{1/2}$ (h)	CL (ml/min/kg)	V_z (L/kg)	Reference
Rat	3	7.6	0.3[b]	2.5[b]	64	73	Düsterberg et al., 1986
Rabbit	4	—	0.2[b] 0.3[c]	1.4[b] 1.1[c]	52.5	7.5	Back et al., 1980
	0.3	1.3	0.5[b]	3.0[b]	37	31.7	Düsterberg et al., 1986
Dog	9	75	0.4[b]	2.3[b]	25	16.8	Düsterberg et al., 1986
Monkey							
Rhesus	0.6	11.3	0.3[b]	2.7[b]	17	6	Düsterberg et al., 1986
Baboon	2	11.3	0.4[b]	2.5[b]	22	6.9	Düsterberg et al., 1986
Baboon	64	—	1.8[b] 7.0[c]	10[b] 7.2[c]	—	—	Newberger et al., 1983
	61	—	0.4[b] 0.2[c]	2.2[b] 7.8[c]	47.5	9	Recalculated from Newburger et al., 1983

[a]AUC values are corrected for an IG dose of 1 mg/kg. [b]IV administration. [c]IG administration.

administration, this indicates an extensive presystemic elimination during the absorption process and the first liver passage. From the IV administration of the drug, a total plasma clearance of 64 ml/min/kg, which exceeds total plasma liver flow, and an apparent volume of distribution (V_z) of 73 L/kg were obtained. Total plasma clearance rates almost exclusively represent metabolic clearance since practically no unchanged parent drug is excreted in the urine. Post-maximum drug levels in plasma declined biphasically with half-lives of 0.3 hr and 2.5 hr, respectively. An AUC of 7.6 ng·h/ml was observed following an oral dose of 1 mg/kg (Düsterberg et al., 1986).

The pharmacokinetics of EE in the rabbit (New Zealand White strain) was investigated at doses of 0.1 mg/kg administered both intravenously and intragastrically (Back et al., 1980). A bioavailability of 4% was found and clearance and volume of distribution were determined to be 52.5 ml/min/kg and 7.5 L/kg, respectively. As already seen in the rat, the metabolic clearance exceeded the hepatic plasma flow in the rabbit, indicating an additional contribution of extrahepatic metabolism. The biphasic pattern of drug disposition in the plasma was characterized by half-lives in the range of 0.2 to 0.3 hr and 1.1 to 1.4 hr, respectively. In another study, very similar results were obtained, although bioavailability was less and volume of distribution was found to be larger as compared to the previous study (Düsterberg et al., 1986).

In the beagle dog a slightly higher bioavailability of about 9% was found. A total clearance of 25 ml/min/kg, being close to the hepatic plasma flow, and a mean volume of distribution of 16.8 L/kg were derived from the intravenous administration of the drug. Intragastric administration of a dose of 1 mg/kg gave an AUC of 75 ng·h/ml (Düsterberg et al., 1986).

Studies in monkeys were performed in rhesus monkey and the baboon (Düsterberg et al., 1986; Newburger et al., 1983). Oral bioavailability of EE was 0.6% and 2% in rhesus monkey and the baboon, respectively. Both the clearance and volume of distribution were similar in the two species. They were 17 ml/min/kg and 6 L/kg in the rhesus monkey and 22 ml/min/kg and 6.9 L/kg in the baboon, respectively. As already seen in the other species, a high first pass was also observed in the monkey, which is in accordance with the high clearance values. Somewhat contradictory to these findings are the high bioavailability of about 64% and the long terminal half-lives of about 10 hr (after IV administration) in castrate female baboons, which have been reported in one study (Newburger et al., 1983). A reevaluation of these data based on an open two-compartment model, however, gave similar half-lives as those found in the other study (Düsterberg et al., 1986), where drug levels in the plasma declined in both species in two disposition phases, characterized by half-lives of 0.3 to 0.4 hr and 2.5 to 2.7 hr, respectively.

Norethindrone

A summary of the pharmacokinetic parameters of norethindrone (NET), determined after IV and IG administration to different animal species is given in Table 2.

TABLE 2. *Pharmacokinetic parameters of NET in selected animal species*

Species	f (%)	AUC[a] (ng·h/ml)	$t_{1/2}\lambda_1$ (h)	$t_{1/2}$ (h)	CL (ml/min/kg)	V_z (L/kg)	Reference
Rat	16	41.9	0.09[b]	0.8[b] 1.8[c]	70.8	5.2	Back et al., 1980
	18	—	—	3.7[b] 5.5[c]	63.1	19.9	Düsterberg et al., 1981; unpublished results
	14	—	0.28[b] 0.09[c]	0.7[b] 1.1[c]	80.1	5.2	Back et al., 1978
Rabbit	54	—	0.4[b] 0.7[c]	7.4[b] 10.4[c]	35.5 31.2	28.3 20	Back et al., 1980 Back et al., 1978
Dog	43	809	—	5.7[b,c]	26	12.7	Düsterberg et al., 1981; unpublished results
Monkey							
Rhesus	38	—	—	6[b] 15.1[c]	—	—	Barkfeldt et al., 1983
Rhesus	16	306	—	2.0[b] 4.1[c]	16	2.8	Düsterberg et al., 1981; unpublished results

[a]AUC values are corrected for an IG dose of 1 mg/kg. [b]IV administration. [c]IG administration.

Following the administration of oral doses of 0.5 mg/kg to Wistar rats in one study (Back et al., 1980) and 6.7 mg/kg in another study (Düsterberg et al., 1981), the bioavailability of NET was determined to be 16% and 18%, respectively. Parenteral administration of NET allowed the calculation of total clearance and volume of distribution. Clearance values between 70.8 and 63.1 ml/min/kg exceeded plasma liver blood flow and thus indicated a contribution of extrahepatic metabolism. The volume of distribution was 5.2 L/kg in one study (Back et al., 1980); a somewhat higher value of 19.9 L/kg was reported by others (Düsterberg et al., 1981). The disposition of NET from plasma followed a biphasic or triphasic pattern, depending on the route of administration (IG or IV). The terminal half life was in the range of 0.8 to 1.8 hr in one study (Back et al., 1980), while in another study (Düsterberg et al., 1981) mean values of 3.7 hr and 5.5 hr were observed following IV and IG administration, respectively. These differences are probably due to the different periods of time post-administration during which the drug was measured in the plasma. An AUC of about 42 ng·h/ml was calculated after the oral administration of a dose of 1 mg/kg.

In the rabbit (New Zealand White), NET showed a bioavailability of about 54%. Clearances of 35.5 ml/min/kg and 31.2 ml/min/kg and apparent volumes of distribution of about 28.3 L/kg and 20 L/kg were derived from parenteral administration of the drug. Two disposition phases of NET levels in the plasma were seen both following IV and IG administration, with half-lives in the range of 0.4 to 0.7 hr and 7.4 to 10.4 hr, respectively (Back et al., 1978, 1980).

In the beagle dog, NET showed a bioavailability of about 43% following an oral dose of 0.8 mg/kg. The mean metabolic clearance rate was 26 ml/min/kg, which is close to the plasma liver flow rate; and a terminal half-life of about 5.7 hr was observed, both following IV and IG administration (Düsterberg et al., 1981; unpublished results).

Bioavailability in the rhesus monkey was found to be in the range of 38% to 16% following the administration of oral doses of 0.6 to 1.5 mg/kg and the dose-normalized AUC was 306 ng·h/ml. A clearance rate of 16 ml/min/kg and a volume of distribution of 2.8 L/kg were observed, and drug disposition in plasma followed a triphasic pattern both after IV and IG administration. The corresponding half-lives obtained after both routes were in the range of 1.7 to 2.7 hr ($t_{1/2}\lambda_1$), 2.5 to 4.3 hr ($t_{1/2}\lambda_2$) and 6 to 15.1 hr ($t_{1/2}$), respectively (Barkfeldt et al., 1983). Somewhat shorter terminal half-lives of 2.0 hr and 4.1 hr following parenteral and enteral drug administration were reported in another study (Düsterberg et al., 1981).

Levonorgestrel

Table 3 summarizes the pharmacokinetic parameters of levonorgestrel (LNG) in various animal species. In the Wistar rat, bioavailability was 6%. The terminal half-lives were 0.5 hr and 5.9 hr after IV and IG administration, respectively (Düsterberg et al., 1981). In another study, oral bioavailability was about 44%, and following IV administration, a clearance rate of 1.3 ml/min/kg and a volume of distribution of 0.74 L/kg were found (Gomaa et al., 1984). The terminal half-life of

TABLE 3. *Pharmacokinetic parameters of LNG in selected animal species*

Species	f (%)	AUC[a] (ng·h/ml)	$t_{1/2}\lambda_1$ (h)	$t_{1/2}$ (h)	CL (ml/min/kg)	V_z (L/kg)	Reference
Rat							
Wistar	6	—	—	0.5[b] 5.9[c]	—	—	Düsterberg et al., 1981; unpublished results
Wistar	44.3	—	0.3	6.7	1.3	0.74	Gomaa et al., 1984
Sprague-D.	—	—	—	23	32.5[d]	1.3[d]	Naqvi et al., 1984
Mouse	67	—	0.5	9.3	1.7	1.4	Gomaa et al., 1983
Rabbit	63	—	—	17	27	—	Hümpel, 1987
Dog	20	455	—	1.2[b] 10.0[c]	—	—	Düsterberg and Beier, 1981; unpublished results
	—	—	—	1.1	8.9	1.7	Düsterberg et al., 1984
Monkey	10	1073	—	4.5[b] 9.4[c]	1.5	0.6	Düsterberg et al., 1981; unpublished results

[a]AUC values are corrected for an IG dose of 1 mg/kg. [b]IV administration. [c]IG administration.
[d]These values were calculated subsequently from the original publication.

LNG was 6.7 hr in that study. In a third study, where female Sprague-Dawley rats received an IV administration of 0.03 mg/kg, the decline of drug levels in plasma followed a triphasic pattern, with half-lives of about 0.2 hr, 0.7 hr, and 23 hr, respectively. However, since drug levels were only measured for 48 hr, a reliable estimate of the terminal half-life was not obtained (Naqvi et al., 1984). Based on these data, a metabolic clearance rate of 32.5 ml/min/kg, which is equal to the hepatic plasma flow, and a volume of distribution of 1.3 L/kg were calculated using a three-compartment model.

A relatively high bioavailability of 67% was found for LNG after IG administration to the mouse. Total plasma clearance was 1.7 ml/min/kg and the volume of distribution was about 1.4 L/kg. Following IV administration, drug levels declined in a biphasic pattern, with half-lives of about 0.5 hr and 9.3 hr, respectively (Gomaa et al., 1983).

In the rabbit, a bioavailability of 63% was found, along with a total clearance of 27 ml/min/kg, which is equivalent to the hepatic plasma flow, and mean terminal half-life of 17 hr (Hümpel, 1987).

In the beagle dog, the bioavailability of LNG was 20% and the AUC amounted to 455 ng·h/ml. A metabolic clearance rate of 8.9 ml/min/kg and a volume of distribution of 1.7 L/kg were obtained. The mean terminal half-life was in the range of 1.1 to 1.2 hr after IV administration, while a mean value of 10 hr was observed after IG administration when drug levels were measured over a comparatively longer time period (Düsterberg et al., 1981; Düsterberg & Beier, 1984).

The bioavailability of LNG in the rhesus monkey was about 10%. A metabolic clearance rate of about 1.5 ml/min/kg, a volume of distribution of 0.6 L/kg, and mean terminal half-lives of 4.5 hr (IV), and 9.4 hr (IG) were reported (Düsterberg et al., 1981; unpublished results).

Gestodene

Pharmacokinetic parameters of gestodene (GSD) in various animal species are presented in Table 4. The bioavailability of GSD in Wistar rats was found to be 10% following an oral dose of 6.7 mg/kg. Following IV administration, a biphasic decline in drug plasma levels was seen, with a mean terminal half-life of 0.4 hr (Düsterberg et al., 1981). The total plasma clearance was about 81 ml/min/kg and the volume of distribution was 2.8 L/kg. Following an oral dose, the mean terminal half-life was 7.3 hr; however, it was measured over a longer period of time compared to the IV administration (Düsterberg et al., 1981; unpublished results).

In the rabbit, the bioavailability of GSD was about 29% and the plasma clearance was determined to be 28 ml/min/kg with a corresponding volume of distribution of 5.2 L/kg. A biphasic decline was observed for the drug levels in plasma, with mean half-lives of 0.3 and 1.2 hr $^1(t_{1/2}, \lambda_1)$ and 2.2 and 9.1 hr $^2(t_{1/2})$, after IV and IG administration, respectively (unpublished results).

In the beagle dog, GSD bioavailability was about 36% to 42% and AUC values

TABLE 4. *Pharmacokinetic parameters of GJD in selected animal species*

Species	f (%)	AUC^a (ng·h/ml)	$t_{1/2}\lambda_1$ (h)	$t_{1/2}$ (h)	CL (ml/min/kg)	V_z (L/kg)	Reference
Rat	10	—	—	0.4^b 7.3^c	81	2.8	Düsterberg et al., 1981; unpublished results
Rabbit	29	—	0.3^b 1.2^c	2.2^b 9.1^c	28	5.2	unpublished results
Dog	36	1160	—	5.2^b 17.4^c	14.9	6.7	Düsterberg et al., 1981; unpublished results
	42	927	1.3^b 5.1^c	4.5^b 20.7^c	7.6	2.9	unpublished results
Monkey	9	1193	—	5^b 12.5^c	1.7	0.8	Düsterberg et al., 1981; unpublished results

^{a}AUC-values are corrected for an IG dose of 1 mg/kg. ^{b}IV administration. ^{c}IG administration.

between 927 and 1160 ng·h/ml were observed. Clearance was calculated to be between 7.6 and 14.9 ml/min/kg, and the mean terminal half-life, measured after IV administration, was between 4.5 and 5.2 hr, while values of 17.4 and 20.7 hr were observed after IG administration. The apparent volume of distribution was between 2.9 and 6.7 L/kg (Düsterberg et al., 1981; unpublished results).

In the rhesus monkey, the bioavailability of GSD was about 9%. A clearance of 1.7 ml/min/kg was calculated, and a biphasic pattern was seen for the decline in drug plasma levels following IV administration of the drug with a mean terminal half-life of 5 hr. Following an oral dose, the mean terminal half-life was 12.5 hr (Düsterberg et al., 1981). As already pointed out, the difference in half-lives determined after IV and IG administration of the drug is mainly due to differences in the length of the observation period.

Medroxyprogesterone Acetate

The pharmacokinetic parameters of medroxyprogesterone acetate (MPA) determined in the rabbit (New Zealand White) are presented in Table 5. Corresponding data from other animal species were not available. Clearance was determined following IV administration of solutions of the drug in DMSO in doses of 0.1 mg/kg, 0.5 mg/kg, and 1 mg/kg. The corresponding clearance rates were 6.6, 11.2, and 15.7 ml/min/kg, respectively, indicating dose-dependence over this dose range. The

TABLE 5. *Pharmacokinetic parameters of MPA in the rabbit, determined after IV administration*

Species	$t_{1/2}\lambda_1$ (h)	$t_{1/2}\lambda_2$ (h)	$t_{1/2}$ (h)	MRT (h)	CL (ml/min/kg)	V_{ss} (L/kg)	Reference
Rabbit							
0.1 mg/kg	0.04	1.1	13.3	16.2	6.6	6.9	Pannuti et al., 1987
0.5 mg/kg	0.06	0.62	12.8	11.8	11.2	8.5	
1.0 mg/kg	0.04	0.42	12.4	11.1	15.7	11.3	

corresponding values for the volume of distribution were 6.9, 8.5, and 11.3 L/kg. Since no IG administration was included in this study, data on the oral bio-availability are not available. Following parenteral administration, triphasically de-clining plasma drug levels were seen, with half-lives of 0.04 to 0.06 hr ($t_{1/2} \lambda_1$) 0.4 to 1.1 hr ($t_{1/2} \lambda_2$) and 12.4 to 13.3 hr ($t_{1/2}$), respectively (Pannuti et al., 1987).

Cyproterone Acetate

A summary of the pharmacokinetics of cyproterone acetate (CPA) is presented in Table 6. In the Wistar rat, CPA was completely bioavailable following an IG dose of 6.7 mg/kg. From parenteral administration, a mean clearance value of 6.6 mL/min/kg, which is very low compared to hepatic plasma flow, and a volume of distribution of 15 L/kg were calculated. Drug disposition from plasma followed a biphasic pattern, with mean terminal half-lives of about 26 hr and 10 hr after IV and IG administration, respectively. In this case, the observation period was the same for both routes of administration (Düsterberg et al., 1981).

In the rabbit, a bioavailability of 57% was seen after IG administration of CPA. The metabolic clearance rate was calculated to be 2.9 ml/min/kg and the mean terminal half-life was 41 hr (Hümpel, 1987).

In the beagle dog, CPA bioavailability was about 73% and the plasma clearance was calculated to be 0.9 ml/min/kg. The mean terminal half-life of CPA following IV administration was reported to be 95 hr; however, since drug levels were mea-sured only up to 96 hr, the actual terminal half-life might be even longer. Following the administration of an oral dose of CPA, a terminal half-life of 202 hr was ob-served (Düsterberg et al., 1981).

In rhesus monkeys, CPA was almost completely bioavailable (88%); the volume of distribution was 11.6 L/kg and total clearance was 4.6 ml/min/kg. The mean terminal half-life of disposition was about 29 hr following IV administration and 33 hr following IG administration (Düsterberg et al., 1981).

TABLE 6. *Pharmacokinetic parameters of CPA in selected animal species*

Species	f (%)	AUC^a (ng·h/ml)	$t_{1/2}\lambda_1$ (h)	$t_{1/2}$ (h)	CL (ml/min/kg)	V_z (L/kg)	Reference
Rat	100	—	—	26.3^b 10^c	6.6	15	Düsterberg et al., 1981; unpublished results
Rabbit	57	—	—	41	2.9	—	Hümpel, 1987
Dog	73	24 000	—	95^b 202^c	0.9	7.3	Düsterberg et al., 1981; unpublished results
Monkey	88	3327	—	29^b 33^c	4.6	11.6	Düsterberg et al., 1981; unpublished results

[a]AUC values are corrected for an IG dose of 1 mg/kg. [b]IV administration. [c]IG administration.

DISCUSSION

Once the basic pharmacokinetic parameters of each contraceptive steroid are known in several animal species, it is of interest to try to identify certain trends. Looking at one particular steroid, one could take each of its pharmacokinetic parameters and compare them between species. On the other hand, looking at a particular pharmacokinetic parameter, one could try to find differences or similarities by a comparison of the three groups of contraceptive steroids (EE, 19-nortestosterone derivatives, and 17-hydroxy progesterone derivatives).

The absolute bioavailability of EE reveals no striking difference between species. A range of 0.3% to 9% (64% in the baboon) was observed, and the lowest values were found for the rat, the rabbit, and the rhesus monkey, while the highest value was seen in the dog. Terminal half-lives following an IV dose were also much the same in the species investigated. They ranged from about 1 to 3 hr, and in only one study, a half-life of 10 hr was reported for the baboon. Total plasma clearance on the other hand, was about twice as high in the rat and rabbit as compared to the dog and monkey (except for the baboon) and thus there seems to be no clear trend.

The bioavailability of NET was in the range of 16% to 54%. The lowest values were seen in the rat and rhesus monkey and the highest values in the rabbit and dog. The terminal half-lives ranged from about 1 to 15 hr, with the rat at the lower end and the rabbit and monkey at the higher end of the range. A clear trend was only seen with clearance, which was low in the monkey, intermediate in the dog and the rabbit, and high in the rat.

There was no such trend in any of the pharmacokinetic parameters of LNG. The bioavailability of LNG was in the range of 6% to 67%. The rat and monkey represented the lower end, while the highest values were seen in the rabbit and mouse. The terminal half-lives were relatively short in the rat and dog, intermediate in the mouse and monkey, and the highest in rats. The highest clearance values of 33 and 27 ml/min/kg were reported for the rat and rabbit, respectively, while values between 1.7 and 1.5 ml/min/kg were observed in the mouse and rhesus monkey. For the dog, both high and intermediate values were reported. In contrast to NET, there was no clear decrease in the metabolic clearance rate of LNG from rodent to primates.

For GSD, the lowest bioavailability was seen in the monkey and rat, an intermediate value for the rabbit, and the highest values were observed in the dog. The longest terminal half-life was seen in the dog, which was twice as high as the values observed in the rabbit and monkey. The plasma clearance showed a clear trend with markedly decreasing values from rodents to dog and monkey.

For MPA, only data from one species were available, but for CPA, the other progestin of the 17-hydroxy progesterone group, an interspecies comparison was possible. CPA was almost completely bioavailable in the rat and monkey and to a lesser extent in the dog and rabbit. The longest half-life was seen in the dog and the shortest half-lives were seen in the monkey and rat, with the rabbit taking an intermediate position. Clearance values were highest in the rat and monkey and somewhat lower in the rabbit and dog.

Obviously, there is no clear trend in the bioavailability of these steroids when compared among the animal species. There is, however, a difference between the three different groups of contraceptive steroids. For each species, the lowest bioavailability was seen with EE, markedly higher values were observed for the 19-nor testosterone derivatives, and generally the highest values were obtained with CPA. EE is subject to conjugation reactions in the gastrointestinal tract, which may largely contribute to the high first pass effect observed in all animal species investigated. Direct conjugation plays no important role in the biotransformation of the progestins, which instead are characterized by a number of oxidation and hydroxylation reactions. Thus the first pass effect observed for the progestins is basically due to metabolic reactions in the liver. In the case of CPA, enzymic attack is impeded by the presence of additional functional groups like the methylene bridge in ring A, the chlorine atom in ring B, and the esterified 17-hydroxyl group in ring D. This could account for the almost complete oral bioavailability of CPA in all animal species.

There are fairly large interspecies differences in the terminal half-lives of a particular steroid and no clear trend can be recognized. That was even true if one compared representatives that belonged to the same group of compounds, such as NET, LNG, and GSD. A comparison between the three groups of contraceptive steroids, however, revealed in most cases very short half-lives for EE, slightly longer half-lives for the 19-nortestosterone derivatives, and markedly longer half-lives for CPA.

The clearances of NET and GSD showed a clear trend from high values in the rodent species to comparatively lower values in the monkey. However, this was not true for EE, LNG, and CPA. In the rat and rabbit, the clearance rates of all steroids, except for CPA, exceeded the plasma liver flow, which points to the contribution of extrahepatic metabolism in these two species. In the other species, the metabolic clearance rates of all steroids were less than or close to the respective plasma liver flow rates, and the liver was obviously the major site of biotransformation. There was no obvious distinction in the clearance values when the three groups of steroids were compared.

The pharmacokinetic parameters of a particular steroid showed large interspecies variabilities. This can partly be attributed to similarly large differences in physiological and biochemical parameters between the species. These differences include, for example, specific binding proteins, which are present in one species and absent in another; or, variabilities may be due to different amino acid compositions of these proteins, which may result in different binding characteristics in the various species. Further examples are the capacity and the distribution pattern of cytochrome P-450 isozymes, which can both be very different among species, leading to differences in metabolic pathways and rates of elimination of a particular steroid. These and other factors make it nearly impossible to extrapolate the pharmacokinetic characteristics of a particular steroid in one species to any other species. Even within a group of closely related compounds of similar chemical structure, corresponding pharmacokinetic parameters do not necessarily show the same trends in different species.

In order to make the best use of the potential of pharmacokinetics in the design and interpretation of pharmacological and toxicological studies, it is therefore necessary to assess the pharmacokinetic parameters of each particular compound in the selected species. Both in the pharmacokinetic and the pharmacodynamic study to be evaluated, the same route of administration and, if possible, the same doses should be chosen, unless linearity of pharmacokinetics over a dose range could be demonstrated. With this basic information, one can then interpret drug level time courses measured in pharmacological or toxicological studies.

REFERENCES

Back DJ, Breckenridge AM, Crawford FE, et al. Phenobarbitone interaction with oral contraceptive steroids in the rabbit and rat. *Br J Pharmacol* 1980;69:441–52.

Back DJ, Breckenridge AM, Crawford FE, et al. First pass effect of norethindrone in rabbits and rats. *J Pharmacol Exp Therap* 1978;207:555–65.

Barkfeldt JOA, Odlind V, Victor A. Interaction between phenytoin and norethisterone in the rhesus monkey. *Contraception* 1983;27:423–9.

Düsterberg B, Hümpel M, Speck U. Terminal half-lives in plasma and bioavailability of norethisterone, levonorgestrel, cyproterone acetate and gestodene in rats, beagles and rhesus monkeys. *Contraception* 1981;24:673–83.

Düsterberg B. Plasma levels of levonorgestrel, gestodene, norethisterone and cyproterone acetate on single dose subcutaneous administration in oily solution in the rat, beagle and rhesus monkey. *Steroids* 1984;43:43–56.

Düsterberg B, Beier S. Plasma levels and progestational activity of levonorgestrel after repeated intravenous and subcutaneous administration in the beagle bitch. *Contraception* 1984;29:345–57.

Düsterberg B, Kühne G, Täuber U. Half-lives in plasma and bioavailability of ethinylestradiol in laboratory animals. *Drug Res* 1986;36:1187–90.

Gomaa AA, Osman FH. Influence of acetaminophen-induced hepatic necrosis on the pharmacokinetics of levonorgestrel. *Contraception* 1983;28:149–57.

Gomaa AA, Osman FH, Salem HT, Abdel Wareth AA. A study of interaction between levonorgestrel and ethanol. *Contraception* 1984;29:535–42.

Hümpel M. Comparative pharmacokinetics of selected contraceptive steroids in animal species and man. In: Safety requirements for contraceptive steroids. Proceedings of a symposium on improving safety requirements for contraceptive steroids convened by the WHO Special Programme of Research, Development and Research Training in Human Reproduction. 1987:193–210.

Naqvi RH, Mitra SB, Saksena IF, Lindberg MC. Pharmacokinetics of levonorgestrel in the rat. *Contraception* 1984;30:81–8.

Newburger J, Castracane VD, Moore PH, et al. The pharmacokinetics and metabolism of ethinyl estradiol and its three sulfates in the baboon. *Am J Obstet Gynecol* 1983;146:80–7.

Pannuti F, Camaggi CM, Strocchi E, Comparsi R. Medroxyprogesterone acetate plasma pharmacokinetics after intravenous administration in rabbits. *Cancer Chemother Pharmacol* 1987;19:311–4.

Pharmacology of the Contraceptive Steroids,
edited by Joseph W. Goldzieher.
Raven Press, Ltd., New York © 1994.

5

Metabolism of Contraceptive Steroids in Animals

Frank Z. Stanczyk

*Department of Obstetrics and Gynecology, University of Southern California
School of Medicine, Los Angeles, California 90033*

To select a relevant pharmacological animal model, it is essential to have sufficient knowledge about contraceptive steroid metabolism in various species so that a valid comparison can be made to humans. A review of species differences in the metabolism of contraceptive steroids by Fotherby (1986) showed that very little is known about this subject. The present chapter aims to update information about how different animal species transform contraceptive progestins and estrogens. An additional goal is to look critically at the methodology used to identify steroid metabolites in order to gain a better understanding of the reliability of the accumulated information.

Both *in vivo* and *in vitro* studies of the metabolism of contraceptive progestins and estrogens have been performed in a variety of animal species. They relate chiefly to the older 19-nor C_{19} derivatives—i.e., norethindrone, norethynodrel, and levonorgestrel—and to the C_{21}-acetoxy steroids medroxyprogesterone acetate, megestrol acetate, and chlormadinone acetate. However, virtually nothing is known about the metabolism of the new progestins (norgestimate, desogestrel, and gestodene) in animals. Of the two synthetic estrogens that have been used in contraceptive preparations, ethinylestradiol and mestranol, there is more information about the metabolism of the former compound.

C-19 DERIVATIVE PROGESTINS

Norethindrone

Dog

Cook et al. (1974) studied the *in vitro* metabolism of norethindrone by the beagle dog and identified two novel oxygenated metabolites of this precursor. Following the incubation of norethindrone with the $10,000 \times g$ fraction from the liver of phenobarbital-treated beagles, the amount of norethindrone and its metabolites of intermediate polarity decreased with time, with a concomitant increase in the amount of highly polar metabolites. The major metabolites of intermediate polarity were nor-ethindrone-4β,5β-epoxide and 6-keto-5α-dihydronorethindrone. These metabolites were identified using rigorous analytical methods including nuclear magnetic resonance (NMR), gas chromatography-mass spectrometry, and circular dichroism.

Rabbit

The *in vivo* metabolism of ^{14}C-norethindrone in female rabbits was investigated by Kamyab et al. (1967), using the experimental design as described for the metabolism of norgestrel (q.v.). The results of both studies were presented in the same publication, and were similar. Following the injection of ^{14}C-norethindrone into the rabbits (n = 6; 1 pregnant), there was a rapid decline in the radioactivity, and after 24 hours, less than 0.5% of the injected dose was found in plasma. Large amounts of the radioactivity were present in the liver, intestine, and bile even though the precursor was intravenously administered. Insignificant amounts of norethindrone were found in the tissues and most of the radioactive material was present in a conjugated form within 3 hours post-injection. Approximately 40% of the administered dose was excreted in urine within 2 days post-treatment. The estimated amount of radioactivity excreted by the fecal route was less than 10%. As in the study of norgestrel metabolism, fractionation of urine yielded an unconjugated and conjugated fraction. These fractions were subjected to paper partition chromatography. On the basis of chromatographic mobilities of the peaks of radioactive material relative to the mobilities of authentic norethindrone derivatives, Kamyab et al. (1967) concluded that the metabolites of norethindrone were mainly polar compounds and suggested that norethindrone underwent extensive hydroxylation. However, no rigorous identification of the metabolites was carried out in this study and no quantification of the hydroxylated metabolites was given.

There is evidence of deethynylation of norethindrone based on data from an *in vitro* study. Palmer et al. (1969a) incubated a $10,000 \times g$ supernatant fraction of rabbit (New Zealand White) liver homogenate with ^{3}H-norethindrone, and found that 19-nortestosterone was the principal metabolite (>25% yield).

Rodent

Urinary, fecal, and biliary excretion of norethindrone and characterization of its metabolites has been studied by Hanasono and Fischer (1974) in female rats (Sprague-Dawley). In the urinary and fecal collection experiments, three rats (240–300 g) were infused with ^{3}H-norethindrone intraperitoneally at a dosage of 48 μg/kg. Urine and feces were collected at various intervals during a 7-day period. The results showed that the mean half-life for the appearance of radioactive material in urine was 16.8 hours, and urinary excretion of radioactive material was essentially completed by 48 hours post-treatment. The mean percentage of the radioactive dose excreted in urine during the 7-day period was 25%. In contrast, the radioactivity in the feces continued to increase until the end of the 7-day experimental period, at which time the mean recovery was approximately 80% of the administered dose.

Fractionation of the urinary radioactive material showed that only about 10% of the total radioactivity was present in an unconjugated (9%) and β-glucuronidase hydrolyzable (2%) form. The rest of the radioactive material (90%) consisted of nonhydrolyzable metabolites. There was no evidence for the presence of any significant amounts of the sulfate metabolites of norethindrone.

Only part (76%) of the radiolabeled compounds present in the fecal samples could be extracted with methanol. Analysis of the radiolabeled compounds showed that only unconjugated and polar nonhydrolyzable metabolites were present. However, it was not possible to rule out the presence of glucuronide metabolites of norethindrone because of the partial recovery of radioactive material from feces.

Hanasono and Fischer (1974) used a different experimental design to study biliary excretion of radiolabeled norethindrone and its metabolites. Prior to precursor administration, the femoral vein and common bile duct of the rats (n = 3) were cannulated, and then ^{3}H-norethindrone was infused via the femoral vein using the same dose as for the urinary and fecal excretion experiments. Collection of bile samples was carried out at various time intervals during an 8-hour period. The results showed that the biliary excretion of radioactive material was rapid. The mean half-lives for the appearance of steroid-related radioactivity in the bile during the initial rapid phase of excretion and during the subsequent slower phase of excretion were 0.45 and 1.2 hours, respectively. The latter value is 14 times less than the corresponding half-life of the urinary excretion of radioactive material following dosing with ^{3}H-norethindrone, and emphasizes the relative slowness of urinary excretion of norethindrone metabolites.

Characterization of the biliary radioactive material was carried out after pooling the 0 to 2-hour fractions from each of the three rats. These fractions contained most of the biliary radioactivity. The majority of the radioactive material consisted of β-glucuronidase-hydrolyzable metabolites (60%), and the remainder was present as nonhydrolyzable metabolites (33%) and unconjugated steroids (6%). Little or no sulfate conjugates of norethindrone and its metabolites were found. Only the unconjugated fraction was processed further. Thin-layer chromatography showed the absence of untransformed precursor and the presence of polar norethindrone metabolites.

The enterohepatic circulation of biliary metabolites of norethindrone was also studied by Hanasono and Fischer (1974). Female rats (n = 3) were prepared with bile fistulas and were administered single intravenous injections of ^{3}H-norethindrone. The bile that was excreted during the first 2 hours in each animal was collected and infused, via the duodenum, into a recipient rat previously prepared with a bile fistula. Bile collection from the recipient rats was then made at appropriate time intervals during a 24-hour period. The percentage of the administered radioactivity that appeared in the bile of the recipients was utilized as an index of the degree of enterohepatic circulation of radioactive steroid metabolites. The results showed that 59% of the intraduodenally infused bile-containing radioactive material underwent enterohepatic circulation and emerged in the bile of the recipient rats during a 24-hour period. It was also shown that the β-glucuronidase-liberated biliary metabolites of norethindrone underwent enterohepatic circulation more rapidly and extensively than did the nonhydrolyzable biliary metabolites.

The metabolism of norethindrone has also been studied *in vitro*. In the study by Peter et al. (1981), in which it was shown that ^{3}H-levonorgestrel is converted to its 4β,5-epoxide by rat (male Wistar) liver microsomes, a similar conversion of ^{3}H-norethindrone to ^{3}H-norethindrone-4β,5-epoxide, was demonstrated. Both the epoxide of levonorgestrel and of norethindrone were quantitatively the most important metabolites found. Another similarity to the data obtained when ^{3}H-levonorgestrel was used as substrate was suggestive evidence, based on chromatographic data, for the transformation of ^{3}H-norethindrone to hydroxylated and ring A-reduced metabolites.

A considerable amount of attention was focused on the epoxides of both norethindrone and levonorgestrel when the tumorigenic effect of synthetic sex steroids on liver was being evaluated. This evaluation became necessary after the first report of seven cases of hepatic tumors in women taking oral contraceptives (Baum et al., 1973). Subsequently, the number of anecdotal cases reported increased rapidly (Klatskin, 1978; Sherlock, 1978). During that time it was shown that some progestational compounds, such as norethindrone and norethynodrel, fed to rodents in very large doses for a prolonged time, produced hepatocellular adenomas (Schuppler & Gunzel, 1978). However, no mutagenic effect of norethindrone and other synthetic progestins in a bacterial system was found (Kappus et al., 1976; Lang & Redmann, 1979). Furthermore, no irreversible binding of either norethindrone, norgestrel, or their epoxides to DNA was observed (Kappus & Bolt, 1976; Bolt, 1977). Nevertheless, the epoxides of these progestogens drew attention as potential tumorigenic agents due to their reactivity and capability of irreversible binding (covalently) to sulfhydryl groups of proteins (Kappus & Remmer, 1975).

The study by Peter et al. (1981) showed that norethindrone-4β,5-epoxide inhibits two enzyme systems that are involved in the deactivation of carcinogenic epoxides originating from environmental polycyclic hydrocarbons. These enzymes include microsomal epoxide hydrolase and cytoplasmic glutathione-5-transferases. In the same study, the investigators also showed that levonorgestrel inhibits the latter enzyme system but not the former one. The Ki of norethindrone epoxide with epoxide hydrolase was shown to be 1.6×10^{-4} M, indicating that relatively high concentrations of this epoxide are required to produce an effective inhibition. The inhibitory potency of norethindrone-4β,5-epoxide is consistent with data obtained by White (1980), who also showed that norethindrone-4,5-dihydrodiol may be formed by incubating norethindrone-4β,5-epoxide with rat liver microsomes. Similar information was not obtained with glutathione-S-transferases since distinct isoenzymes purified to homogeneity were not available for kinetic studies. On the basis of their findings, Peter et al. (1981) proposed that formation of liver tumors may be explained, in part, by the extent of interaction of norethindrone-4β,5-oxide with metabolic steps involved in the deactivation of environmental carcinogens. They argued that relatively large amounts of norethindrone epoxides are required for effective inhibition of the epoxide hydrolyase, and that such amounts are administered to rats in toxicological long-term experiments in which liver tumors have been observed (Schuppler & Gunzel, 1978). The authors also pointed out that high levels of norethindrone epoxide are never attained in women during the use of oral contraceptives containing norethindrone.

Comparison of the Metabolism of Norethindrone Among Animals and Man

It is difficult to compare the metabolism of norethindrone with that of man since so few metabolites have been identified in animals. Most of the available data in animals are concerned with the formation of norethindrone-4β,5-epoxide. As mentioned earlier, this metabolite drew attention as a potential tumorigenic agent due to its reactivity and capability of irreversible binding (covalently) to sulfhydryl groups of proteins. It was also pointed out earlier that high levels of norethindrone epoxide are never attained in women during the use of oral contraceptives containing norethindrone.

In the human, it has been shown that norethindrone undergoes extensive reduction of the α,β-unsaturated ketone in ring A forming the corresponding dihydro and tetrahydro reduced products. Whether or not norethindrone is hydroxylated remains to be established. The metabolites of norethindrone circulate primarily as sulfates, whereas in urine norethindrone metabolites are present in approximately equal amounts as sulfates and glucuronides. Sizeable amounts of norethindrone are found in an unconjugated form in the circulation.

NORETHYNODREL

Rabbit

The metabolic fate of norethynodrel in the female rabbit (New Zealand White) was studied both *in vivo* and *in vitro* by Arai et al. (1962). Distribution of radioactivity in urine, bile, or feces following oral administration of randomly tritiated norethynodrel (4 μCi plus 20 mg of unlabeled norethynodrel) was measured in five rabbits with bile drainage cannulae, and in a control group of three normal and two sham-operated rabbits during 7 days. In the five experimental animals, 33%, 21%, and 17% of the administered radioactivity was excreted in the bile, urine, and feces, respectively. In contrast, 52% and 16% of the radioactivity was found in urine and feces of the control group, respectively. The results indicate that there was considerable reabsorption of biliary metabolites from the intestine of the rabbits and that these metabolites are ultimately excreted in urine. In addition, the data showed that

TABLE 1. *Percentage of radioactivity accounted for as either recovered substrate or specific metabolites in pooled glucuronide extracts of bile and urine and in the unconjugated fraction of feces, following oral administration of ^{3}H-norethynodrel to rabbits (cannulated and control groups)*

Compound	Bile	Urine		Feces	
		Cannulated	Control	Cannulated	Controls
Norethynodrel				57.3[a]	27.3[a]
3β-Dihydronorethynodrel	90.5[a]	21.8	37.3		15.3
Norethindrone				17.5	19.0
10β-Hydroxynorethindrone				6.3	1.8
10β-Hydroxy-3ε-dihydronorethindrone[b]	} 8.0	29.0	19.8	2.8	12.7
10β-Hydroxy-3ε,5ε-tetrahydronorethindrone[b]					
Unidentified ketone				10.7	2.3
Unidentified alcohol		12.1	15.6		
TOTAL	98.5	62.9	72.7	94.6	74.4

[a]Metabolite was identified by infrared spectroscopy and melting point mixture.
[b]Compounds were identified tentatively since the corresponding standards were not available.

there were two definite peaks of radioactivity in the urines of the control group, suggesting the existence of considerable enterohepatic circulation.

Fractionation of the excreta was carried out by subjecting pooled bile, urine, and feces (from three cannulated rabbits or two controls) to chloroform extraction (unconjugated fraction), and subsequently subjecting the extracted bile and urine to hydrolysis. β-Glucuronidase was used to cleave the glucuronides, whereas a chemical solvolysis procedure presumably hydrolyzed the sulfates. Individual metabolites were identified by thin-layer chromatography of the various extracts. In a few instances, it was possible to confirm identification of the metabolites by use of infrared spectroscopy and the effect of admixture with isolated material on the melting point of a reference standard.

The pattern of metabolites differed among the three forms of excreta. The isolated metabolites and their quantities, reported as percentage of recovered radioactivity, are shown in Table 1.

In bile, most of the radioactive material was in a conjugated form, predominantly as the glucuronide (81%); the remainder was in a sulfurylated form. Less than 1% of the radioactive material was unconjugated. Most of the glucuronide fraction consisted of 3β-dihydronorethynodrel. In the same fraction, 10β-hydroxy-3ε-dihydronorethindrone and 10β-hydroxy-3ε,5ε-tetrahydronorethindrone were tentatively identified; together they comprised 8% of the recovered radioactivity.

In urine, only 1–2% of the radioactive material was unconjugated, whereas 35–40% and 10–15% of the radioactive material was present in glucuronide and sulfate forms, respectively. As shown in Table 1, the 3β-reduced metabolite of norethynodrel (3β-dihydronorethynodrel) accounted for 22% of the radioactivity in the glucuronide fraction from the cannulated rabbits, and for a somewhat larger proportion (37%) in the control group. Also, 20–29% of the radioactivity in the glucuronide fraction from both the cannulated and control groups was attributed to tentatively identified 10β-hydroxy-3ε-dihydronorethindrone and 10β-hydroxy-3ε,5ε-tetrahydronorethindrone, and 12–16% of the same radioactivity was in the form of an unidentified alcohol.

In feces from the cannulated animals, 57% of the unconjugated radioactive material was identified as norethynodrel and 17% was norethindrone; the corresponding values for the feces from control rabbits were 27% and 19%, respectively. The remainder of the unconjugated radioactive material was attributed to an unidentified ketone, to 10β-hydroxynorethindrone, and to tentatively identified 10β-hydroxy-3ε-dihydronorethindrone plus 10β-hydroxy-3ε,5ε-tetrahydronorethindrone. These metabolites accounted for 2–11%, 2–6%, and 3–13% of the unconjugated radioactivity in the feces of both groups of animals, respectively. In addition, 3β-dihydronorethynodrel accounted for 15% of the unconjugated radioactive material in the control group.

In the same study by Arai et al. (1962), ^{3}H-norethynodrel was separately incubated *in vitro* with gastric juice, blood, or liver from adult female rabbits. The same methods were used to isolate and identify the products and recovered precursor as in the *in vivo* experiments. When gastric juice or blood was used, 34–55% of the substrate was still unaltered after 2.5 hours of incubation at 37°C, an additional 26–42% was in the form of norethindrone, 4–5% was present hydroxylated at carbon-10, and an unidentified ketone accounted for 7–14% of the recovered radioactivity (Table 2). Surprisingly, the same products were found following incubation of ^{3}H-norethynodrel in aqueous medium at pH 1, but not in phosphate buffer at pH 7.8, at 37°C.

When homogenates of liver were used in the incubation, the pattern of isolated metabolites differed from that found with gastric juice, blood, or buffer. The major products isolated were 3β-dihydronorethynodrel (33%) and the tentatively identified metabolites found in the *in vivo* experiments, namely, 10β-hydroxy-3ε-dihydronorethindrone and 10β-hydroxy-3ε,5ε-tetrahydronorethindrone (19.7%). Small

TABLE 2. *Percentage of radioactivity accounted for as either recovered precursor or specific metabolites, following in vitro incubation of ^{3}H-norethynodrel with rabbit tissues*

Compound	Gastric Juice	Blood	Liver
Norethynodrel	55.4[a]	34.2[a]	
3β-Dihydronorethynodrel			33.4[a]
Norethindrone	26.2[a]	41.9[a]	5.7[a]
10β-Hydroxynorethindrone	4.3	5.2[a]	3.2[a]
10β-Hydroxy-3ε-dihydronorethindrone[b]		}	19.7
10β-Hydroxy-3ε,5ε-tetrahydronorethindrone[b]			
Unidentified ketone	7.1	14.2	
TOTAL	93.0	95.5	62.0

[a]Metabolite was identified by infrared spectroscopy and melting point mixture.
[b]Compounds were identified tentatively since the corresponding standards were not available.

amounts of norethindrone (6%) and 10β-hydroxynorethindrone (3%) were also found.

The *in vitro* metabolism of norethynodrel in the rabbit has also been studied by Palmer et al. (1969b). These investigators incubated unlabeled norethynodrel (115 mg) with the $100,000 \times g$ supernatant fraction of rabbit liver homogenates. Two main metabolites, 3α-dihydronorethynodrel and 3β-dihydronorethynodrel, were isolated in pure form and their identification was established unequivocally by nuclear magnetic resonance. The 3β-epimer was present in greater amount; the 3α/3β-epimer ratio was 1:1.8. A third metabolite, norethindrone, was also identified using rigorous methodology.

Rodent

Urinary, fecal, and biliary excretion of norethynodrel and its metabolites was investigated in rats in the same study by Hanasono and Fischer (1974), in which the excretion of radioactive material following administration of ^{3}H-norethindrone to rats was assessed. To study the excretion of norethynodrel, the investigators administered ^{3}H-norethynodrel to rats (n = 3) in the same manner as described for ^{3}H-norethindrone. The results showed that both the urinary and fecal excretion of radioactive material was similar to that found for norethindrone. The data also showed that the mean half-lives (slow and rapid phases) for the appearance of radioactive material in bile were similar to those obtained for norethindrone; however, the percentage of biliary radioactive material present as glucuronide conjugates (21%) was approximately three-fold less than the corresponding value for norethindrone (60%). This finding is surprising in view of the fact that the two progestins differ in chemical structure only in the positions of their double bonds [Δ 5(10) vs Δ 4(5)]. Only 3% of the biliary radioactive material was present in an unconjugated form and as much as 76% was found as nonhydrolyzable metabolites.

In vitro studies of norethynodrel metabolism by rat liver have been reported. Unlabeled norethynodrel (115 mg) was incubated with the $10,000 \times g$ supernatant of female and male rat liver (as well as guinea pig) homogenates, using the same methodology described above for the rabbit (Palmer et al., 1969b). Quantification of two of the identified metabolites, 3α-dihydronorethynodrel and 3β-dihydronorethynodrel, showed that the 3α-epimer was the predominant product in the rat but not in the guinea pig. The 3α/3β-epimer ratio was 24:1 in the male rat and 9:1 in the female rat, whereas the ratio in the guinea pig was 1:10.1.

A follow-up to this study was carried out by Freundenthal et al. (1971), who used time-sequence incubation procedures with tritiated norethynodrel and the postmitochondrial supernatant from rat liver homogenates. The investigators identified the same three metabolites (3α- and 3β-dihydronorethynodrel and norethindrone) as in the study by Palmer et al. (1969b), and also showed that these steroids are further converted to more polar metabolites, which they thought were unconjugated polyhydroxylated end-products.

Comparison of the Metabolism of Norethynodrel Among Animals and Man

Very few studies have been carried out on the metabolism of norethynodrel in animals. The most elaborate study was carried out in the rabbit (Arai et al., 1962). It showed that, in urine, the glucuronide metabolites were predominant; however, a sizeable sulfate fraction was present as well. 3β-dihydronorethynodrel was the major urinary metabolite identified, but tentative identification of 10β-hydroxy-3ε-dihydronorethindrone and 10β-hydroxy-3ε,5ε-tetrahydronorethindrone was also made. In feces, there was a large amount of untransformed norethynodrel and sizeable amounts of norethindrone and 3β-dihydronorethynodrel as well.

In the human, norethynodrel undergoes conversion to ring A reduction products (3α-dihydronorethynodrel, 3β-dihydronorethynodrel, 3β,5α-tetrahydronorethynodrel, and 3α,5β-tetrahydronorethynodrel), which can be considered either as norethynodrel or norethindrone metabolites (Stanczyk & Roy, 1990). Despite reports to the contrary, there is no convincing evidence that norethynodrel is converted to norethindrone in the human.

LYNESTRENOL

Rabbit

The metabolism of lynestrenol has been studied *in vitro* by Yasuda et al. (1984). These investigators incubated a combination of 0.5 mg of unlabeled lynestrenol and 0.8 μCi of ^{14}C-lynestrenol with the 105,000 g microsomal pellet from rabbit liver for varying times. Three products, norethindrone, 3α-hydroxylynestrenol, and 3β-hydroxylynestrenol were isolated by gas-liquid chromatography and identified by mass spectrometric analysis. The concentration of 3α-hydroxylynestrenol during the course of incubation was always considerably higher than that of 3β-hydroxylynestrenol. On this basis, the investigators concluded that the metabolic conversion of lynestrenol to norethindrone probably proceeds primarily via 3α-hydroxylynestrenol.

Comparison of the Metabolism of Lynestrenol Among Animals and Man

Since the metabolism of lynestrenol has apparently not been studied *in vivo* in animals, no comparisons can be made. In the human no classical metabolic study has been performed to substantiate the view that lynestrenol is converted to norethindrone. However, support for this conversion was obtained by Odlind et al. (1979), following oral administration of different doses of lynestrenol to women and subsequent measurement of norethindrone levels in plasma by radioimmunoassay. In a subsequent study, Yasuda et al. (1981) measured norethindrone in serum by HPLC, following the administration of lynestrenol to women. On the basis of their data, they suggested that the transformation of lynestrenol to norethindrone is rapid and almost complete.

NORGESTREL

Monkeys

African Green Monkey. With the exception of the human, the most extensive studies of the metabolism of levonorgestrel have been carried out by Sisenwine et al. (1974, 1979) in two different species of monkeys, namely, the African green monkey (*Cercopithecus aethiops*) and the rhesus monkey (*Macaca mulatta*). In those studies, radiolabeled norgestrel and one or both of its enantiomers were administered individually to the animals in separate experiments.

In the study with African green monkeys, two female and two male animals, weighing between 3.0 and 5.0 kg, were given a single dose (1 mg/kg) of ^{14}C-norgestrel (approximately 16–26 μCi) via a nasal tube. The same monkeys were dosed in a similar manner with ^{14}C-levonorgestrel and then with ^{14}C-dextronorgestrel at 5-month intervals. Total urine and feces were collected daily for 7 days after each dosing. Approximately 1 year later, the same amounts of the same steroids were administered once again in the same manner, but only to the female monkeys. Thus, a total of six animals were dosed with each radioactive precursor.

Most of the radioactivity was excreted during the first 3 days following administration. The mean percentage ($\pm$ standard deviation) of the radioactive dose excreted in urine and feces after administration of ^{14}C-norgestrel, ^{14}C-levonorgestrel, and ^{14}C-dextronorgestrel was 51.4 ± 5.0 and 41.3 ± 6.7; 37.5 ± 5.4 and 54.3 ± 19.4; 44.2 ± 8.9 and 55.1 ± 15.6, respectively. Analysis of the urines showed that the majority of the radioactive material was present in an unconjugated form (48–62%), whereas an additional 13–27% was released by β-glucuronidase preparations, regardless of which ^{14}C-labeled precursor was administered.

Aliquots (¼ volume) from each of the first 4 days of urine collection were pooled and used for isolation and identification of metabolites. Fractionation of the pooled urine was carried out by chromatography on DEAE-Sephadex A-25, solvent extraction and enzymatic cleavage. After combining corresponding fractions from the animals in each study group, metabolites were identified in unconjugated and glucuronide fractions of urine. No urinary sulfate conjugates were found in any of the experiments.

It is important to note that the metabolites of norgestrel and its enantiomers will be named as derivatives of the parent compound administered. We assume that the optical rotation of an isolated metabolite is the same as that of the administered compound, since no attempt was made to characterize the optical rotatory properties of the identified metabolites in this study. This assumption may not be valid since additional asymmetric carbons may be formed following enzymatic transformation of the administered compound.

Table 3 shows the approximate quantities of the compounds that were identified in the urines of African green monkeys dosed with either ^{14}C-norgestrel, ^{14}C-levonorgestrel, or ^{14}C-dextronorgestrel. The quantity of each isolated metabolite was reported in terms of a range of the percent of urinary radioactivity within which

TABLE 3. *Conversion of the racemic mixture of norgestrel or its separate enantiomers to urinary metabolites, following intranasal administration of ^{14}C-norgestrel, ^{14}C-levonorgestrel and ^{14}C-dextronorgestrel to African Green monkeys[a]*

	% of urinary radioactivity					
	^{14}C-Norgestrel		^{14}C-Levonorgestrel		^{14}C-Dextronorgestrel	
Compound[b]	Unconjugated	Glucuronide	Unconjugated	Glucuronide	Unconjugated	Glucuronide
Norgestrel	0.1–1	0.1–1	0.1–1	0.1–1	0.1–1	0.1–1
3α,5β-Tetra-hydro-norgestrel	5–20	1–5	50–60	< 0.1	1–5	< 0.1
2α-Hydroxy-norgestrel	1–5	5–20	0.1–1	0.1–1	0.1–1	5–20
16α-Hy-droxynor-gestrel	0.1–1	0.1–1	—	—	0.1–1	0.1–1
16β-Hydroxy-norgestrel	5–20	1–5	—	—	50–60	< 0.1
16-Hydroxy-tetra-hydronor-gestrel	1–5	0.1–1	1–5	< 0.1	—	—
17β-De-hydro-homonor-gestrel	0.1–1	0.1–1	< 0.1	< 0.1	0.1–1	< 0.1

[a]Data are taken from a study by Sisenwine et al. (1974). Each animal (two females and two males) was given a single dose (1 mg/kg; 16–26 μCi) of ^{14}C-norgestrel, ^{14}C-levonorgestrel, or ^{14}C-dextronorgestrel at 5-month intervals. The same labeled compounds were administered once again to the female animals in the same manner. Total urine was collected daily for 7 days after each dosing.

[b]The appropriate prefix (levo- or dextro-) should be added to the name, norgestrel, when reference is made to the compounds isolated after administration of ^{14}C-levonorgestrel, or ^{14}C-dextronorgestrel.

each value was found. There was extensive metabolism, as judged by the low amount (0.1–1%) of each precursor found unaltered in urine. Similar amounts of each precursor were also found as the glucuronide.

Following administration of the radiolabeled racemic mixture of norgestrel, the most abundant urinary metabolites isolated were 3α,5β-tetrahydronorgestrel (5–20%) and 16β-hydroxynorgestrel (5–20%) in the unconjugated fraction, and 2α-hydroxynorgestrel (5–20%) in the glucuronide fraction. The former compounds were also isolated in the glucuronide fraction, but in smaller amounts (1–5%). Similarly, a lesser amount (1–5%) of 2α-hydroxynorgestrel was found in the unconjugated fraction as compared to the conjugated one. 16-Hydroxytetrahydronorgestrel (orientation of the hydroxyl at carbon-3 and the hydrogen at carbon-5 is unknown) was present in higher amounts in the unconjugated fraction (1–5%) compared to the glucuronide fraction (0.1–1%). Two other urinary metabolites, 16α-hydroxynorgestrel and 17β-dehydrohomonorgestrel ([±]-13-ethyl-D-homogon-4-ene-3,17-dione), were present in approximately equal amounts (0.1–1%) in both the unconjugated and conjugated fractions. There is evidence that the latter compound is an artifact that results from decomposition of the methylester of (±)-13-ethyl-D-homogon-4-ene-3,17-dione-17-carboxylic acid during the isolation procedure. The formation of this interesting compound is discussed in the section on the metabolism of norgestrel in the rhesus monkey.

Evidence for stereoselective biotransformations was found in monkeys dosed with the ^{14}C-labeled enantiomers of norgestrel. The most notable stereoselective conversions were ring A reduction of levonorgestrel and 16β-hydroxylation of dextronorgestrel, yielding 3α,5β-tetrahydrolevonorgestrel and 16β-hydroxydextronorgestrel, respectively. Both metabolites were present in very high amounts (50–60%) relative to the other isolated metabolites. No 16β-hydroxynorgestrel was found in either the unconjugated or glucuronide fractions of urine after the monkeys were dosed with ^{14}C-levonorgestrel. However, after treatment with ^{14}C-dextronorgestrel, 3α,5β-tetrahydrodextronorgestrel in amounts of 1–5% and <0.1% was found in the unconjugated and glucuronide fractions of urine, respectively. These amounts are relatively small compared to the amount (50–60%) of 3α,5β-tetrahydrolevonorgestrel found after ^{14}C-levonorgestrel dosing. The pattern of metabolites for the racemate (^{14}C-norgestrel), showed an approximate composite of the metabolite pattern of each enantiomer.

When ^{14}C-levonorgestrel was used as precursor, a smaller number of metabolites were identified in comparison to treatment of the monkeys with ^{14}C-norgestrel. In addition to 3α,5β-tetrahydrolevonorgestrel, only small amounts (0.1–1%) of 2α-hydroxylevonorgestrel and 2α-hydroxylevonorgestrel glucuronide, as well as trace amounts (<0.1%) of 3α,5β-tetrahydrolevonorgestrel glucuronide, 17β-dehydrohomolevonorgestrel, and 17β-dehydrohomolevonorgestrel glucuronide were found.

In contrast to the relatively small number of metabolites isolated following treatment with ^{14}C-levonorgestrel, the number of metabolites found following ^{14}C-dextronorgestrel dosing was the same as that obtained with ^{14}C-norgestrel as precursor. In addition to 16β-hydroxydextronorgestrel, a sizeable amount (5–20%) of 2α-hydroxydextronorgestrel glucuronide, smaller amounts (1–5%) of 3α,5β-tetrahydrodextronorgestrel, and very small amounts (0.1–1%) of 2α-hydroxydextronorgestrel, 16α-hydroxydextronorgestrel, 16α-hydroxydextronorgestrel glucuronide, and 17β-dehydrohomodextronorgestrel were found. Also, trace amounts (<0.1%) of 3α,5β-tetrahydrodextronorgestrel glucuronide, 16β-hydroxydextronorgestrel glucuronide, and 17β-dehydrohomodextronorgestrel glucuronide were isolated.

Different methods were utilized to identify the compounds isolated from urine. Following treatment with ^{14}C-norgestrel, the identification of three metabolites, namely, 16β-hydroxynorgestrel, 3α,5β-tetrahydronorgestrel, and 16-hydroxytetrahydronorgestrel was confirmed by mass spectrometric analysis or gas chromatography. Corresponding metabolites obtained after dosing with the ^{14}C-labeled enantiomers were identified in the same manner. Other metabolites were identified by analytical thin-layer chromatography. In addition to the metabolites reported in Table 3, there were as many as 17–20, 16–19, and 10–12 unidentified compounds in the unconjugated and glucuronide fractions of urine, following dosing with ^{14}C-norgestrel, ^{14}C-levonorgestrel, and ^{14}C-dextronorgestrel, respectively.

Rhesus Monkey. Sisenwine et al. (1979) studied the metabolism of norgestrel and its levorotatory enantiomer using an experimental design that was similar to that just described for the study with the African green monkey. ^{14}C-norgestrel (0.5 mg/kg; 40.0–65.1 μCi) was administered intranasally to three female rhesus monkeys weighing between 4.3 and 7.0 kg. Similarly, a group of three other female rhesus monkeys (4.7–5.1 kg) received ^{14}C-levonorgestrel (37.7–40.9 μCi). Total urine and feces were collected daily for 7 days. In addition, blood samples were drawn at variable times after dosing. On the average, 86.7–90.1% of the administered radioactivity was recovered in urine and feces. Urinary and fecal excretion accounted for 52.6 ± 5.4% (mean ± standard error) and 37.2 ± 4.4%, and for 29.5 ± 2.0% and 57.1 ± 4.0% following dosing with ^{14}C-norgestrel and ^{14}C-levonorgestrel, respectively. Measurement of radioactivity in plasma showed that 10.0–11.6% of the dose was found at 2–3 hours after dosing. These values declined with time, falling to 3.2–3.8% of the dose at 24 hours.

Isolation and identification of unaltered precursor and of metabolites in urine were carried out as described for the study with African green monkeys, except that the compounds were not quantified. At least 20 metabolites were detected in the unconjugated and glucuronide fractions of urine, however, only a small number of them were identified. Following administration of ^{14}C-norgestrel, the following metabolites were found in minor amounts in each fraction: 3α,5β-tetrahydronorgestrel, 2-hydroxynorgestrel, 16α-hydroxynorgestrel, 16β-hydroxynorgestrel, and 16β-hydroxy-3α,5β-tetrahydronorgestrel. In addition, a relatively large amount of 17β-dehydrohomonorgestrel was found unconjugated. The levorotatory form of these metabolites was also detected following administration of ^{14}C-levonorgestrel to the second group of monkeys. All the metabolites, including 17β-dehydrolevonorgestrel, were present in minor amounts. No sulfurylated metabolites were detected in any of the urines analyzed.

In the same study the investigators obtained convincing evidence for the occurrence of D-homoannulation (expansion of the D ring by one carbon). They isolated and identified the methyl ester of 13-ethyl-D-homogon-4-ene-3,17-dione-17-carboxylic acid in pooled urine from two monkeys treated daily with single 10 mg/kg intragastric doses of unlabeled norgestrel for 7 days, and postulated that D-homoannulation occurs by an initial oxidation of the triple bond in the ethinyl group of norgestrel to an activated oxygen complex. This complex undergoes rearrangement to form a transient β-ketoaldehyde, which is oxidized further to the β-keto acid. The instability of the free β-keto acid prevented its isolation, however, the methyl ester derivative was isolated and identified by mass spectrometry. Furthermore, the degradation product of the acid, 17-dehydrohomonorgestrel, was identified.

Separate experiments, in which ^{14}C-norgestrel was administered to two rhesus monkeys, were carried out to measure urinary phenolic metabolites. Negligible amounts of 18-homoethynylestradiol (13-ethyl-18,19-dinor-17α-pregn-1,3,5(10)-triene-20-yne-3,17-diol) and other phenolic metabolites (<0.2% of the dose) were found.

Fractionation of pooled plasma specimens from rhesus monkeys yielded two major and one minor fractions following dosing with either ^{14}C-norgestrel or ^{14}C-levonorgestrel. The radioactivity in one of the major fractions was associated with unconjugated compounds. The major radioactive component in that fraction was the administered precursor (norgestrel or levonorgestrel). It was detected up to 8 hours after dosing and accounted for as much as 25% of the total plasma radioactivity. At 24 hours after dosing, each isolated precursor accounted for <6% of the total plasma radioactivity. 17β-dehydrohomonorgestrel was detected in plasma between 2 and 8 hours after dosing with ^{14}C-norgestrel, but not with ^{14}C-levonorgestrel. In addition, numerous polar metabolites were detected in the 24-hour plasma samples following dosing with ^{14}C-levonorgestrel. The other major plasma fraction contained approximately 50% of the total plasma radioactivity. This radioactivity was associated primarily with glucuronides, of which the major component was 3α,5β-tetrahydronorgestrel glucuronide, when ^{14}C-norgestrel was the administered precursor. The identification of the main compounds in plasma is based on chromatographic (thin-layer) data. In addition to these compounds, the presence of numerous minor metabolites was also indicated chromatographically.

Rabbit

The *in vivo* metabolism of ^{14}C-labeled norgestrel was studied in female rabbits (type of rabbit not stated) (n = 6; 1 pregnant) by Kamyab et al. (1967). Following injection into the animals, the radioactivity in the circulation declined rapidly, and less than 0.5% of the dose remained after 24 hours. Up to 5 hours post-injection, large amounts of radioactivity were present in the liver and intestine. Paper chromatography of tissue extracts showed that extensive metabolism of the substrate had occurred within 3 hours post-injection. At least half of the radioactive material was found in a conjugated form, and there were insignificant amounts of substrate present in the tissues. More than half of the administered dose was excreted in urine (56.7 ± 15%), mostly within 2 days. The investigators estimated that less than 10% of the radioactivity was excreted via the fecal route. Fractionation of urine yielded unconjugated and conjugated extracts. Although the nature of the conjugated extracts was not well defined, the data suggested the possibility that sulfurylated metabolites of norgestrel were present in the urine. The unconjugated and conjugated fractions were chromatographed on paper, and on the basis of the mobility of the peaks of radioactive material relative to that of norgestrel, Kamyab et al. (1967) found that norgestrel metabolites were similar to the compounds produced by partial or complete reduction of the α,β-unsaturated ketone group in ring A of norgestrel. However, no rigorous identification of the metabolites was performed and no estimate of the quantities of reduced metabolites was reported.

The *in vitro* metabolism of ^{14}C-labeled norgestrel and its enantiomers by female New Zealand white rabbit liver microsomes was studied by Khan and Fotherby (1983). Unchanged precursor and products were isolated and identified by use of thin-layer and gas-liquid chromatography. The results showed that levonorgestrel was metabolized rapidly: more than 50% was transformed within 10 minutes and more than 80% within 30 minutes. In contrast, only 50% of dextronorgestrel and

60% of norgestrel were metabolized after 30 minutes of incubation. When levonorgestrel was used as precursor, two types of metabolic transformations were found after 30 minutes: hydroxylations (at C-6α, C-16α, and C-16β) and ring A reductions (3α,5β- and 3β,5β-tetrahydro). These conversions accounted for 41% and 32% of the radioactivity added, respectively. However, when either dextronorgestrel or norgestrel were utilized as precursor, ring A reduction was a relatively minor process (11–13% of the radioactivity) compared to the hydroxylations that collectively accounted for 37–38% of the added radioactivity.

Rodent

In a study by Peter et al. (1981) in which ^{3}H-levonorgestrel was incubated with NADPH and liver microsomes from rats pretreated with phenobarbital or 3-methylcholanthrene, there was suggestive evidence for the transformation of the precursor to hydroxylated metabolites, reduced metabolites, and to its epoxide, levonorgestrel-4β,5-epoxide. The evidence was based on the mobility on thin-layer chromatograms of peaks of radioactive material relative to that of authentic derivatives of levonorgestrel. There was no indication as to which individual metabolites of levonorgestrel were chromatographically detected. Under the conditions used, the epoxide was quantitatively the most important metabolite found. The significance of this metabolite, as well as other progestin epoxides, is discussed in the section on the metabolism of norethindrone in rats.

Comparison of the Metabolism of Norgestrel and Its Enantiomers Among Animals and Man

Metabolic pathways of norgestrel and levonorgestrel that are operative in man and the African green monkey occur only to a minor extent in the rhesus monkey. This conclusion is derived from results of the studies by Sisenwine et al. (1974, 1979), described earlier, as well as similar studies in three women by the same investigators (Sisenwine et al., 1975). In the human study, fractions of pooled urine obtained following oral administration of either ^{14}C-norgestrel, ^{14}C-levonorgestrel, or ^{14}C-dextronorgestrel showed different profiles from those observed in the two species of monkeys. The most important difference was that a major urinary sulfate fraction was found after administration of ^{14}C-norgestrel and ^{14}C-dextronorgestrel to the women (17.5% and 32.1% of the dose, respectively). The sulfate fraction following ^{14}C-levonorgestrel treatment was relatively small (5.4% of the dose). In contrast to these findings, the sulfate fraction contained an insignificant amount of the administered ^{14}C-norgestrel, ^{14}C-levonorgestrel, or ^{14}C-dextronorgestrel radioactivity in the monkey experiments.

Similar to the findings in the African green monkey study, evidence for stereoselective biotransformations of the norgestrel enantiomers was also found in the pattern of urinary metabolites of each drug following dosing of the women (Table

TABLE 4. *Urinary metabolites of ^{14}C-norgestrel and ^{14}C-levonorgestrel in women*

Compound[b]	% of urinary radioactivity[a]					
	^{14}C-Norgestrel			^{14}C-Levonorgestrel		
	Unconjugated	Glucuronide	Sulfate	Unconjugated	Glucuronide	Sulfate
Norgestrel	0.2	0.4	—[c]	0.1	0.5	<0.1
3α,5β-Tetra-hydronorgestrel	0.1	4.1	1.2	0.1	9.5	1.5
2α-Hydroxynorgestrel	0.1	0.2	—	<0.1	0.2	—
16α-Hydroxynor-gestrel	—	—	—	—	—	<0.1
16β-Hydroxynorgestrel	0.2	1.2	11.9	—	0.5	0.1
16β-Hydroxy-3α,5β-tetra-hydronorgestrel	<0.1	0.6	0.5[d]	<0.1	1.3	0.5
17β-Dehydrohomonor-gestrel	0.1	—	—	<0.1	0.1	—

[a]Data are taken from a study by Sisenwine et al. (1975) in which women received oral doses of ^{14}C-norgestrel (n = 5) and ^{14}C-levonorgestrel (n = 5). Urine was collected from three selected study subjects in each group during the first 4 days after dosing and was pooled; the pools were used to identify metabolites of each administered drug.

[b]The prefix levo- should be added to the compound name when reference is made to the compounds isolated after ^{14}C-levonorgestrel administration.

[c]The dash indicates that the compound was not isolated.

[d]The value was estimated from Figure 2 in the publication by Sisenwine et al.

4). The most notable stereoselective conversions were ring A reduction of levon-orgestrel and 16β-hydroxylation of dextronorgestrel. Both products were excreted primarily in the glucuronide form. The pattern of identified metabolites for the racemate was an approximate composite of the identified metabolite patterns of each enantiomer. The stereoselective conversions in the women were similar to those found in the African green monkey, with the exception that the urinary ring A-reduced and 16β-hydroxylated metabolites were present in an unconjugated form, instead of a glucuronide form.

With the exception of the sulfurylated metabolites that were absent in both species of monkeys, the urinary metabolites found in the monkeys and women were, in general, qualitatively but not quantitatively similar, following the dosing with either ^{14}C-norgestrel, ^{14}C-levonorgestrel, or ^{14}C-dextronorgestrel. This is evident when comparing the data between Tables 3 and 4. Note that Sinsenwine et al. (1974, 1975) reported the conversions differently in the two studies. The reactions that were common to all three studies (Sisenwine et al., 1974, 1975, 1979) include the following: ring A reduction, 2α-hydroxylation, 16α-hydroxylation, 16β-hydroxylation, and D-homoannulation. It is important to realize that, in addition to the identified metabolites, there were numerous unidentified products in all three studies.

Although there is only a limited amount of data on the metabolism of norgestrel and its enantiomers in the rabbit, it suggests that additional *in vivo* metabolic studies with this progestin are warranted in this species to determine whether or not it could serve as a useful model for the human. Support for this proposal can be found in the *in vitro* study with rabbit liver microsomes reported by Khan and

Fotherby (1983), in which stereoselective biotransformations of levonorgestrel and dextronorgestrel were observed. As discussed earlier, similar stereoselective conversions have been reported in women. Additional support originates from the report by Kamyab et al. (1967) on the *in vivo* metabolism of norgestrel in the rabbit, in which there was a suggestion that sulfurylated norgestrel and/or its metabolite(s) was present in urine. The importance of this finding lies in the fact that in the human there is a sizeable urinary sulfate fraction, but not in the African green or rhesus monkeys, following the administration of norgestrel, levonorgestrel, or dextronorgestrel as discussed earlier.

C-21 PROGESTINS

Megestrol Acetate

Baboon. There is sketchy information about the metabolism of megestrol acetate in the baboon. Goldzieher and Kraemer (1972) reported preliminary data on the transformation of this progestin. After oral administration of 500 mg of radiolabeled (radiolabel not stated) megestrol acetate, there was a gradual, continuous increase in the concentration of plasma radioactivity that reached a plateau at about 24 hours. In urine, 6–36% of the administered dose was excreted during the first 24 hours, and 33–43% was excreted after 5 days; only 0.4–2.8% was found in the feces.

Monkey. A study similar to the one described above with the baboon was also carried out with the rhesus macaque (*Macaca mulatta*) (Goldzieher & Kraemer, 1972). Plasma levels of radioactivity reached a maximum within an hour and these levels were maintained during the next 24 hours. In urine, 22% of the dose was excreted after 24 hours, and 14–33% was excreted after 6 days. There was a relatively high fecal excretion of radioactivity in this species (36–44% of the dose).

Dog. The metabolism of megestrol acetate has been investigated in the beagle dog. Chainey et al. (1970) found that 79–92% of administered tritiated megestrol acetate was excreted in feces, but only 6–10.5% of the dose was found in urine. These data indicate that the main route of megestrol acetate excretion in the beagle is the biliary–fecal axis. Although no data were given, these findings are apparently supported by the study of Martin and Adlercreutz (1977), who investigated megestrol acetate metabolism in a female and male beagle dog, following oral administration (100 mg) for 10 days. Gas chromatography–mass spectrometry was used to identify metabolites. No untransformed megestrol acetate or any of its metabolites were detected in either plasma or urine. However, the investigators found evidence for the presence of 6-hydroxymethylmegestrol acetate and an unidentified metabolite in the unconjugated fraction from female beagle liver.

Rabbit. The *in vivo* metabolism of megestrol acetate in the rabbit has been studied by Cooper et al. (1965). These investigators administered ^{3}H-megestrol acetate to one group of rabbits (n = 4) and the ^{14}C-labeled form of the same progestin to another group of rabbits (n = 4). Both substrates were administered by stomach cannulas. Two of the rabbits in each group received a dose of radiolabeled megestrol acetate that had a high specific activity, whereas the precursor administered to the other two animals in each group had low specific activity. No significant difference was observed between the rates of excretion of the precursor with high and low-specific activity. However, the combined recovery of tritium (40.9%) in urine and feces during the first 7 days after dosing was considerably less than the recovery of carbon-14 (70.4%). On the average, 32.3% of the administered tritium was found in urine and the rest (8.6%) in feces. Following extraction of the urine, it was shown that the unconjugated and conjugated fractions contained 10.8% and 20.9% of the administered dose, respectively. β-Glucuronidase hydrolysis and solvolysis of the conjugated fraction showed that most of this fraction consisted of glucuronide metabolites, and virtually no metabolites in the sulfurylated form. The combined tritium of the two subfractions accounted for virtually all of the tritium in the conjugated extract. When a similar comparison was made with recovered carbon-14, there was lack of agreement between the total radioactivity in the conjugated extract and the combined radioactivity of the glucuronide and sulfate subfractions.

For identification of megestrol acetate metabolites, urinary glucuronide extracts from two rabbits were processed. Infrared and ultraviolet spectroscopy, as well as chemical transformations were used to identify two metabolites of megestrol acetate; these were 2α-hydroxymegestrol acetate and 6-hydroxymethyl megestrol acetate.

Numerous other homogeneous radioactive components were found in both the glucuronide and unconjugated fractions of urine but were not identified. However, evidence was obtained for the inhibition of reduction of the α,β-unsaturated 3-ketone group of megestrol acetate. Furthermore, no hydroxylation at C-21 of this molecule was observed. The investigators concluded, "This difficulty in hydroxylation of megestrol acetate as a step prior to conjugation is reflected in the relatively high biological half-life of the compound and may be a reason for the high biological activity of this progestogen."

The metabolism of megestrol acetate by the rabbit has also been studied *in vitro*. Cooke and Vallance (1965) investigated the structural features of megestrol acetate that prevent its rapid metabolism by measuring the rates of metabolism of progesterone, 6α-methylprogesterone, 17α-acetoxyprogesterone, 17α-acetoxy-6α-methylprogesterone and megestrol acetate, using microsome-supernatant fractions of liver from female New Zealand White rabbits. The different products were isolated by paper partition chromatography and were quantified by their extinction coefficients. The results show that megestrol acetate (100 μg) was metabolized very slowly at a tissue:substrate ratio of 1000:1. Additional metabolism occurred when the tissue:substrate (20 μg) ratio was increased to 15,000:1. In addition, when both the 6α-methyl and 17-acetoxy groups were introduced into the progesterone molecule, there was a marked decrease in the rate of metabolism of the new substrate. Additional resistance to metabolism was obtained when the $\Delta^{6(7)}$-bond was incorporated into that precursor. The investigators concluded that the enhanced progestational activity of megestrol acetate may be explained, in part or totally, by the substituents which were added to the progesterone molecule.

Rat. In the study by Cooke and Vallance (1965) described above in the section on the rabbit, the *in vitro* metabolism of megestrol acetate by rat liver preparation was also studied in the rat. Megestrol acetate was metabolized very slowly at a tissue:steroid (100 μg) ratio of 250:1. Although additional metabolism occurred at a higher ratio (15,000:1), the substrate (20 μg) was not completely metabolized even after 4 hours of incubation. In contrast, both 17-acetoxyprogesterone and 6α-methylprogesterone were rapidly metabolized at this high tissue:steroid ratio.

Cook and Vallance (1968) carried out another study on the metabolism of megestrol acetate. This time they incubated 100 μg of megestrol acetate with rat (mature female Sprague-Dawley) adrenal glands. They tentatively identified 3 metabolites, 11β-hydroxymegestrol acetate, 17,18-dihydroxy-6-methylpregna-4,6-diene-3,20-dione and the α-ketol form of the latter compound, resulting from ring closure between the hydroxyl group at carbon-18 and the ketone group at carbon-20. In order to characterize these products, the investigators utilized paper chromatography, ultraviolet and infrared spectroscopy, as well as chemical methods.

Comparison of the Metabolism of Megestrol Acetate Among Animals and Man

Species differences in the urinary and fecal excretion of radioactive material following the administration of radiolabeled megestrol acetate have been reported (Goldzieher & Kraemer, 1972). After the first 24 hours post-ingestion of the progestin (500 mg), the percentage of urinary radioactivity excreted was 6–36% in the baboon, 22% in the rhesus, and 8–15% in man. Also, there was a relatively high fecal excretion of radioactive material in the rhesus (36–44% of the dose) compared to the baboon (0.4–2.8% of the dose).

Goldzieher and Kraemer pointed out that reports in the literature on the presence of urinary unconjugated metabolites in subhuman primates are difficult to interpret because of technical problems related to urine collection. For example, they found negligible amounts of unconjugated steroids in urine compared to those of other investigators by preventing bacterial hydrolysis.

Although the metabolism of megestrol acetate has been studied in a variety of animal species, the most extensive studies were carried out in the rabbit. Both the *in vivo* and *in vitro* studies in the rabbit suggest that certain structural features of the megestrol acetate molecule, the 6α-methyl and 17-acetoxy groups, may prevent its rapid metabolism. A similar conclusion may be drawn about the metabolism of megestrol acetate in the rat, based on scanty *in vitro* data.

An extensive study of megestrol acetate metabolism was carried out in women by Cooper and Kellie (1968). Following oral dosing with ^{14}C-megestrol acetate (60–91 mg in four women; 4 mg in one woman), a mean recovery of 66.4% and 19.8% of the dose was obtained in the urine and feces, respectively, within 7 days. Three major metabolites were identified in the glucuronide fraction of urine pooled from the five study subjects: 2α-hydroxymegestrol acetate, 17α-acetoxy-6-hydroxymeth-ylpregn-4,6-diene-3,20-dione, and 17α-acetoxy-2α-hydroxy-6-hydroxymethylpregn-4, 6-diene-3,20-dione. They were identified by paper chromatography, ultraviolet and infrared spectroscopy, as well as chemical reactions.

Chlormadinone Acetate

Monkey. There are only sketchy data from an *in vivo* study on the metabolism of chlormadinone acetate in the rhesus monkey (*Macaca mulatta*) Goldzieher & Kraemer (1972). The overall urinary and fecal excretion was reported to be 35–36% and 26–28% respectively, following the administration of 5 mg of chlormadinone acetate.

Dog. Chlormadinone acetate metabolism was also studied *in vivo* in the dog (species not reported) as reported by Goldzieher and Kraemer (1972). The fecal excretion was 33–46%, whereas the urinary excretion was only 8–9% of the admin-istered dose (5 mg).

Rabbit. In comparison to other *in vivo* studies of progestin metabolism, a rela-tively high number of urinary and biliary metabolites of chlormadinone acetate have been identified in the rabbit (type of rabbit not stated) in a study carried out by Abe and Kambegawa (1974). In the study of urinary metabolites, two experiments were carried out. In the first experiment, three male rabbits (2.3–3.1 kg) received an oral dose of 150 mg of 1,2-^{3}H-chlormadinone acetate (specific activity, 3.4 μCi/mmol; amount of radioactivity given is unspecified) twice daily for 4 days, and urine was collected daily for 7 days after dosing. In the second experiment, three male rabbits (3.3–3.5 kg) were given 200 mg of 1-^{3}H-chlormadinone acetate (amount of radio-activity given is unspecified) orally twice a day for 7 days, and urine collection was carried out for 9 days post-treatment. Although hydrolysis of urinary conjugated metabolites was carried out in the two experiments, the authors did not report the relative quantities of either the sulfurylated, glucuronidated, or unconjugated radio-active urinary fractions.

The latter experiment utilizing 1-^{3}H-chlormadinone acetate as the precursor was required because the investigators found that 42% of the urinary radioactivity was excluded in the wash step during extraction of urinary metabolites with XAD-2 resin, when 1,2-^{3}H-chlormadinone acetate was used as substrate. This loss did not occur with 1-^{3}H-chlormadinone acetate. The discrepancy in the recovery of radioac-tive material was attributed to loss of tritium at carbon-2 from the dual radiolabeled substrate, resulting either from enolization of the 3-ketone group or hydroxylation at carbon-2 of chlormadinone acetate.

Unconjugated and conjugated metabolites were combined and subjected to puri-fication and identification. Rigorous methods, including nuclear magnetic reso-nance, mass spectrometry, infrared spectroscopy, and ultraviolet spectroscopy, as well as reverse isotope dilution, were utilized to identify untransformed chlor-madinone acetate (17α-acetoxy-6-chloro-4,6-pregnadiene-3,20-dione) and its me-tabolites. The following metabolites were found: 17α-acetoxy-6-chloro-2α-hydroxy-

4,6-pregnadiene-3,20-dione, 17α-acetoxy-6-chloro-2α-hydroxy-1,4,6-pregnatriene-3,20-dione, 17α-acetoxy-6-chloro-2α,3β-dihydroxy-4,6-pregnadien-20-one, 6-chloro-17α, 20E, 21 = trihydroxy-4, 6-pregnadiene-3-one, 17α-acetoxy-4-pregnene-3, 20-dione, 17α-acetoxy-2α-hydroxy-4-pregnene-3,20-dione, and 17α-acetoxy-2ε,3ε-dihydroxy-5ε-pregnan-20-one and its isomers, and the enol derivative of 17α-acetoxypregnane-2,3,20-trione. Although no quantities of these urinary products were reported, the investigators did state that, of the ten metabolites identified in urine, the main metabolite was 17α-acetoxy-2ε,3ε-dihydroxy-5ε-pregnan-20-one. Fifteen additional urinary metabolites were isolated, but remain unidentified.

Two different experiments were also carried out by Abe and Kambegawa (1974) to characterize biliary metabolites of chlormadinone acetate in the rabbit. In the first experiment, a single oral dose of 200 mg of 1-³H-chlormadinone acetate (amount of radioactivity not stated) was administered to two male rabbits (2.1 and 3.4 kg), which had cannulated bile ducts. Bile was collected continuously for 16 hours after dosing. In the second experiment, two other male rabbits (4.1 and 3.5 kg) with cannulated bile ducts were infused with 130 and 80 mg of 1,2-3H-chlormadinone acetate (amount of radioactivity not stated), and their bile was collected for 19 hours after dosing. Following hydrolysis of the conjugates, the same metabolites of chlormadinone acetate that were identified in urine were also identified in the bile. However, in contrast to the urine, the main biliary metabolite was 17α-acetoxy-6-chloro-2ε,3ε-dihydroxy-4,6-pregnadiene-20-one.

Abe and Kambegawa concluded that chlormadinone acetate is metabolized by two major routes: one includes oxidation at carbon-2 and the other involves dechlorination at carbon-6. Although oxidation of steroids at carbon-2 is a common *in vivo* biochemical reaction, there is little information about dechlorination of steroid metabolites in the literature.

Rodent. The excretion of chlormadinone acetate in urine, feces, and bile by the rat has been investigated in the study by Hanasono and Fischer (1974). Following the administration of ³H-chlormadinone acetate to the rats, the mean percentage of the radioactive dose excreted in urine and feces during the 7-day post-treatment period was 17% and approximately 85%, respectively.

After fractionation of the urinary radioactive material it was shown that as much as 64% of the total urinary radioactivity was present in an unconjugated form, and that the β-glucuronidase hydrolyzable and nonhydrolyzable metabolites (10% and 26%, respectively) accounted for the rest of the radioactivity.

The mean half-life for the appearance of radioactive material in bile during the initial rapid phase and subsequent slower phase was 0.45 and 2.7 hours, respectively. Fractionation of the bile showed that 20% of the biliary radioactive material was present in an unconjugated form, whereas the rest of the material was found as β-glucuronidase hydrolyzable metabolites (26%) and nonhydrolyzable metabolites (54%). It was also shown that 34% of the biliary radioactive material which was infused into recipient rats, underwent enterohepatic circulation and appeared in the bile during a 24-hour period. The β-glucuronidase-liberated metabolites underwent enterohepatic circulation more rapidly and extensively than the other metabolites.

Comparison of the Metabolism of Chlormadinone Acetate Among Animals and Man

A comparison of the data obtained on the metabolism of chlormadinone acetate in the human, rhesus and dog (Goldzieher & Kraemer, 1972) shows that the excretion pattern in man and the rhesus was quite similar, but significantly different from that of the dog. However, the administered doses of chlormadinone acetate differed among the animals, since the rhesus and dog received a 5 mg dose where human subjects were dosed with only 0.4 mg of the drug.

The study carried out by Abe and Kambegawa (1974), in which they identified urinary and biliary metabolites of chlormadinone acetate in the rabbit, is impressive. Not only did these investigators use rigorous methodology, including nuclear magnetic resonance and mass spectrometry, to characterize metabolites but also showed proof of radiochemical homogeneity of isolated metabolites. Unfortunately, similar data in the human are lacking.

In the rat, chlormadinone acetate showed a different pattern of metabolism compared to norethindrone and norethynodrel. The most apparent difference was the relatively large amount of unconjugated radioactive material excreted in urine (64% for chlormadinone acetate compared to 9% and 10% for norethindrone and norethynodrel, respectively). Other differences include a lower excretion of administered radioactive chlormadinone acetate in urine and an approximate 2-fold higher slow phase of excretion of the same substrate in bile, compared to the other two progestins.

Medroxyprogesterone Acetate

There is virtually nothing known about the metabolism of medroxyprogesterone acetate in animals. The metabolism of this progestin by rabbit and rat liver was investigated *in vitro* by Cooke and Vallance (1965) in the same study in which the structural features of megestrol acetate that prevent its rapid metabolism were investigated. Medroxyprogesterone acetate was metabolized very slowly at a tissue: steroid ratio of 250:1 and 1000:1 by rat and rabbit liver, respectively. More metabolism occurred at a higher ratio (15,000:1) but the steroid was not completely metabolized by rat liver even after 4 hours of incubation. Medroxyprogesterone acetate was metabolized more rapidly than megestrol acetate by rabbit liver and possibly also by rat liver (insufficient data available for comparison).

The available information in the human indicates that medroxyprogesterone acetate undergoes ring A reduction, hydroxylation (primarily at carbons 6 and 21), and conjugation (primarily glucuronidation (Castegnaro & Sala, 1962; Fukushima et al., 1979; Helmreich & Huseby, 1962; Mathrubutham & Fotherby, 1981).

ESTROGENS

Ethynyl Estradiol

Baboon. There is a sizeable amount of information about the metabolism of ethinylestradiol in the baboon. Kulkarni (1970) determined the amounts of radioactivity in the plasma and urine of two normally cycling baboons (*Papio* sp.), following intravenous administration of ^{14}C-ethynylestradiol (250 μg) labeled in the ethynyl side-chain. Blood sampling was carried out at frequent intervals during the first 7½ hours and at 24 and 48 hours after dosing. There was no attempt to recover the precursor from plasma or to identify specific plasma metabolites. Urine was collected for 6 continuous days posttreatment. An experiment in which ^{14}C-estradiol (6 μg) was administered to a single baboon was carried out simultaneously in the same manner as the experiments with ^{14}C-ethynylestradiol.

Disappearance of radioactivity from plasma differed between the animals receiving the two different substrates. The plasma radioactivity was calculated to be 8.5–14.4% of the ^{14}C-ethynylestradiol dose during the first hour and then it dropped progressively. In contrast, the plasma radioactivity in the baboon that received ^{14}C-estradiol was found to be 26–27% of the dose per liter of plasma during the first hour, and then it dropped dramatically to 9.5% in 2 hours, and decreased further to less than 1% within 7½ hours. No radioactivity was found in the blood of that baboon after 24 hours, whereas in the other two baboons that received ^{14}C-ethynylestradiol, there was still radioactivity in their circulation after 48 hours.

Following dosing with ^{14}C-ethynylestradiol, 76.9–83.3% of the administered dose was recovered in urine within the 6 days of collection, however, approximately one-half of that radioactivity was excreted in the first 24 hours. In contrast, the animal that received ^{14}C-estradiol excreted only 61% of the dose within 6 days.

Fractionation of the urines from each of the two baboons injected with the labeled synthetic estrogen showed that less than 1% of the total urinary radioactivity was present in an unconjugated form, whereas 57.2–70% and 14% of the radioactivity was liberated by enzymic hydrolysis and solvolysis, respectively. Paper chromatographic analysis of the β-glucuronidase-hydrolyzed fraction containing compounds with an ethynyl group gave suggestive evidence for the presence of at least 11 metabolites, most of which may have been hydroxylated as judged by their polarities.

Newburger et al. (1983) have reported data from a study of the metabolism of ethynylestradiol and its three sulfates, namely, ethynylestradiol-3-sulfate, ethynylestradiol-17β-sulfate, and ethynylestradiol-3,17β-disulfate. In their study, oral and/or intravenous doses of ethinylestradiol or each of its three sulfates were administered to castrate female baboons (*Papio* sp.), and plasma levels of ethynylestradiol and its sulfate forms were quantified by radioimmunoassay or radioisotope counting. The results show that following intravenous administration of ethynylestradiol, the 3-sulfate and the 3,17-disulfate forms of this estrogen are the major circulating metabolites. In contrast, after oral administration, the 3-glucuronide and, in some instances, the 3,17-diglucuronide also become important. The data also suggest that hydrolysis at the carbon-17 position of ethynylestradiol occurs when ethynylestradiol-17-sulfate is administered orally but not intravenously.

Comparison of the Metabolism of Ethinylestradiol Among Animals and Man

Urinary excretion of ^{14}C-ethynylestradiol in the baboon can be compared with that in the human since the excretion study in the baboon (Kulkarni, 1970), described earlier, was carried out in the same manner as an excretion study by Kulkarni and Goldzieher (1970) in women. The comparison shows that the overall urinary excretion of radioactive material (74.5–80.4% of the dose) over a period of 5 days in the baboon was substantially higher than that (36.5–54.7%) obtained in two women over the same time period.

The metabolism of ethynylestradiol is similar to that of the natural estrogens. Thus, ethynylestradiol undergoes extensive hydroxylation at the C-2, C-6, and C-16 positions of the molecule. The 2- and 3-methyl ethers of ethynylestradiol have also been identified as major metabolites. Both ethynylestradiol and its metabolites undergo extensive conjugation. Most of the conjugates in plasma and urine exist as glucuronides. The principal circulating form of ethynylestradiol appears to be ethynylestradiol sulfate; the ratio of these compounds in plasma was found to be 1:6.5 following the administration of ^{3}H-ethynylestradiol in women.

Mestranol

Rabbit. The metabolism of mestranol in rabbits has been studied *in vivo* by Abdel-Aziz and Williams (1969). In that study, a mixture of approximately 5 μCi of ^{3}H-mestranol, 0.5 μCi of the ^{14}C-methyl ether of ethynylestradiol, and 25 mg of unlabeled mestranol was administered to four virgin New Zealand does daily for 5 days by gavage. Urine was collected for 9 days. After hydrolysis of the steroid conjugates, three products were identified by rigorous analytical methods (mass spectrometry, nuclear magnetic resonance, and infrared spectroscopy). The major isolated urinary metabolite of mestranol was ethynylestradiol; the other metabolites were estradiol-17α, and D-homoestradiol-17α.

Rat. The urinary, fecal, and biliary excretion of mestranol in the rat was examined by Hanasono and Fischer (1974) in the study described earlier, dealing with the excretion of administered norethindrone, norethynodrel, and chlormadinone acetate. Following treatment of the rats (n = 3) with ^{3}H-mestranol, the mean percentage of the radioactive dose excreted during the 7-day period posttreatment was only 5%. The urinary elimination of the steroid was essentially complete by 48 hours after dosing. Fractionation of the radioactive material excreted in the 0 to 24-hour samples showed that 26%, 18%, and 56% of the total urinary radioactivity constituted of unconjugated steroids, β-glucuronidase-hydrolyzable, and nonhydrolyzable metabolites, respectively.

Fecal excretion of radioactive compounds was also low (5% of dose). Only 30% of the radioactive material was extracted in methanol.

Mean half-lives for the appearance of radioactive material in bile during the initial rapid and succeeding slower phases of excretion were 0.29 and 2.3 hours, respectively. The percentage of total biliary radioactivity excreted as unconjugated steroids was only 7%, whereas that excreted as glucuronides and as nonhydrolyzable metabolites was approximately equal (48% and 45%, respectively). It was also shown that 59% of infused biliary metabolites underwent enterohepatic circulation and emerged in the bile of recipient rats during a 24-hour period.

In vitro studies with rat liver have been carried out to demonstrate demethylation of mestranol to ethynylestradiol. Lee and Chen (1971) showed this conversion by incubating microsomes from male and female rat (Charles River) liver microsomes with mestranol (1 mM) and a NADPH-generating system. The product was identified by measuring formaldehyde production and by chromatography (thin-layer and gas-liquid). In the following year, Kappus et al. (1972) performed a similar study with male rat (Wistar) liver microsomes, except that they used ^{3}H-mestranol as precursor and identified the transformation product, ethynylestradiol, by addition of carrier steroid and recrystallization of the mixture to constant specific activity. The same investigators also demonstrated a minimum rate of demethylation of mestranol using *in vivo* conditions. This was shown by measuring the amount of tritiated water exhaled by phenobarbital-treated (n = 4) and control (n = 3) female rats after they were injected with ^{3}H-mestranol.

Comparison of the Metabolism of Mestranol Among Animals and Man

Although only a limited number of studies of mestranol metabolism have been carried out in animals (rabbit, rat), it appears that demethylation of mestranol may be a reaction common to both animals and man. In the human, it is well established that the liver can demethylate mestranol to ethynylestradiol. On the basis of the urinary pattern of mestranol metabolites, it appears that mestranol is largely transformed to ethynylestradiol, which undergoes further metabolism (Helton & Goldzieher, 1977).

CONCLUSIONS

The goal of this chapter has been to update the available information about the metabolism of contraceptive steroids in animals and to look critically at the experimental methods used in the studies on this subject. Unlike other reviews, we have purposely provided a considerable amount of detail about the methodology, so that the reader can realize that we know very little about the qualitative and quantitative aspects of contraceptive steroid metabolites. Many of the studies utilized pharmacological doses of precursor and an insufficient number of animals, and lacked rigorous analytical techniques for identifying metabolites. Inadequate attention has been paid to preventing hydrolysis of steroid conjugates during collection of excreta. Although some studies did use sophisticated methods such as mass spectrometry and nuclear magnetic resonance to characterize the chemical structure of isolated steroids, very few investigators demonstrated proof of radiochemical homogeneity of isolated metabolites. In addition, in many studies urine or plasma from individual animals was pooled prior to isolation and identification of metabolites, so that we know virtually nothing about interanimal variability of the compounds.

Because of the limitations just discussed and the paucity of studies carried out in animals, it is difficult to compare the metabolism of contraceptive steroids among different animal species and between animals and man. Nevertheless, some generalizations can be made. One pertains to the metabolism of norgestrel and its enantiomers in two species of monkeys (African green and rhesus). The urinary metabolites found in these monkeys were qualitatively but not quantitatively similar to those in women, with the exception that sulfurylated metabolites were absent in the monkeys.

A suitable animal model for studying toxicological effects of contraceptive steroids would be of great value. Data on the metabolism of norgestrel and its enantiomers in the rabbit suggest that additional studies with levonorgestrel as well as other progestins in this species may be warranted to detemine if it could serve as a useful model for the human. Nair et al (1981) have published data showing that the rabbit may be a useful animal model for comparing the pharmacokinetics of levonorgestrel in women. Obviously, many more studies are required to understand the metabolism of contraceptive steroids in animals so that a suitable model for the human can be found.

REFERENCES

Abdel-Aziz MT, Williams KIH. Metabolism of 17α-ethynylestradiol and its 3-methyl ether by the rabbit; an in vivo D-homoannulation. *Steroids* 1969;13:809.

Abe T, Kambegawa A. Urinary and biliary metabolites of 17α-acetoxy-6-chloro-4,6-pregnadiene-3,20-dione in the rabbit. *Chem Pharm Bull* 1974;22:2824.

Arai K, Golab T, Layne DS, Pincus G. Metabolic fate of orally administered ^{3}H-norethynodrel in rabbits. *Endocrinology* 1962;71:639.

Baum JK, Holtz F, Bookstein JJ, Klein EW. Possible association between benign hepatomas and oral contraceptives. *Lancet* 1973;2:626.

Bolt HM. Structural modifications in contraceptive steroids altering their metabolism and toxicity. *Arch Toxicol* 1977;39:13.

Castegnaro E, Sala G. Isolation and identification of 6β,17α,21-trihydroxy-6α-methyl-Δ^4pregnene-3,20-dione (21-acetate) from the urine of human subjects treated with 6α-methyl-17α-acetoxyprogesterone. *J Endocrinol* 1962;24:445.

Chainey D, McCoubrey A, Evans JM. The excretion of megestrol acetate by beagle bitches. *Vet Rec* 1970;86:287.

Cook BA, Vallance DK. Metabolism of megestrol acetate and related progesterone analogues by liver preparations in vitro. *Biochem J* 1965;97:672.

Cook BA, Vallance DK. Metabolism of megestrol acetate by rat adrenal glands in vitro. *Biochem J* 1968;109:121.

Cook CE, Dickey MC, Christansen HD. Oxygenated norethindrone derivatives from incubation with beagle liver. Structure, synthesis and biological activity. *Drug Metab Disp* 1974;2:58.

Cooper JM, Jones HEH, Kellie AE. The metabolism of megestrol acetate (17α-acetoxy-6-methyl-pregna-4,6-diene-3,20-dione) in the rabbit. *Steroids* 1965;6:255.

Cooper JM, Kellie AE. The metabolism of megestrol acetate (17α-acetoxy-6-methylpregna-4,6-diene-3,20-dione) in women. *Steroids* 1968;11:133.

Fotherby K. Species differences in metabolism of contraceptive steroids. In: Gregoire AT, Blye RT (eds) *Contraceptive Steroids: Pharmacology and Safety*. New York: Plenum Press; 1986;113.

Freundenthal RI, Cook CE, Rosenfeld R, Wall ME. The effect of different incubation systems on the in vitro metabolism of norethynodrel. *J Steroid Biochem* 1971;2:77.

Fukushima DK, Levin J, Liang JS, Smulowitz M. Isolation and partial synthesis of a new metabolite of medroxyprogesterone acetate. *Steroids* 1979;34:57.

Goldzieher JW, Kraemer DC. The metabolism and effects of contraceptive steroids in primates. *Acta Endocrinol (KBH) Suppl* 1972;166:389.

Hanasono GK, Fischer LJ. The excretion of tritium-labeled chlormadinone acetate, mestranol, norethindrone and norethynodrel in rats and the enterohepatic circulation of metabolites. *Drug Metab Disp* 1974;2:159.

Helmreich ML, Huseby RA. Isolation of a 6,21-dihydroxylated metabolite of medroxyprogesterone acetate in human urine. *J Clin Endocrinol Metab* 1962;22:1018.

Helton E, Goldzieher JW. Metabolism of ethynyl estrogens. *J Toxicol Env H* 1977;3:231.

Kamyab S, Littleton P, Fotherby K. Metabolism and tissue distribution of norethindrone and norgestrel in rabbits. *J Endocrinol* 1967;39:423.

Kappus H, Bolt HM, Remmer H. Demethylation of mestranol to ethinylestradiol in vitro and in vivo. *Acta Endocrinol* 1972;71:374.

Kappus H, Bolt HM. Irreversible protein binding of norethisterone (norethindrone) epoxide. *Steroids* 1976;27:29.

Kappus H, Greim H, Bolt HM. Formation of reactive metabolites from ethynylestradiol and norethisterone by rat liver microsomes. 5th International Congress of Endocrinology. Hamburg 1976, abstract 766.

Kappus H, Remmer H. Metabolic activation of norethisterone (norethindrone) to an irreversibly protein-bound derivative by rat liver microsomes. *Drug Metab Disp* 1975;3:338.

Khan FS, Fotherby K. In vitro hydroxylation of the synthetic gestagen, norgestrel. *J Steroid Biochem* 1983;19:1169.

Klatskin G. Possible relationship between oral contraceptives and hepatic tumors. In: *Advances in Pharmacology and Therapeutics*, 7th Internat Congr Pharmacol Paris, 1978. Vol 8, Oxford: Pergamon Press; 1978;169.

Kulkarni BD. Metabolism of [14C] ethinyloestradiol in the baboon. *J Endocrinol* 1970;48:91.

Kulkarni BD, Goldzieher JW. A preliminary report on urinary excretion pattern and method of isolation of 14C-ethinylestradiol metabolites in women. *Contraception* 1970;1:47.

Lang R, Redmann U. Non-mutagenicity of some sex hormones in the Ames salmonella/microsome mutagenicity test. *Mutation Res* 1979;67:361.

Lee S, Chen C. Liver microsomes demethylation of mestranol and some of its effects on drug metabolism. *Steroids* 1971;18:565.

Martin F, Adlercreutz H. Aspects of megestrol acetate and medroxyprogesterone acetate metabolism. In: Garattini S, Berendes HW (eds) *Pharmacology of Steroid Contraceptive Drugs*. New York: Raven Press; 1977;99.

Mathrubutham M, Fotherby K. Medroxyprogesterone acetate in human serum. *J Steroid Biochem* 1981;14:783.

Nair KM, Sivakumar B, Rao BSN. The rabbit as an animal model to study pharmacokinetics of levonorgestrel in women. *Contraception* 1981;23:89.

Newburger J, Castracane VO, Moore PH, Williams MC, Goldzieher JW. The pharmacokinetics and metabolism of ethinyl estradiol and its three sulfates in the baboon. *Am J Obstet Gynecol* 1983;146:80.

Odlind V, Weiner E, Victor A, Johansson EDB. Plasma levels of norethindrone after single oral dose administration of norethindrone and lynestrenol. *Clin Endocrinol* 1979;10:29.

Palmer KH, Fierabend JF, Baggett B. Metabolic removal of a 17α-ethinyl group from the antifertility steroid, norethindrone. *J Pharmacol Exp Ther* 1969a;167:217.

Palmer KH, Ross FT, Rhodes S, Baggett B, Wall ME. Metabolism of antifertility steroids. I. Norethynodrel. *J Pharmacol Exp Ther* 1969b;167:207.

Peter H, Jung R, Bolt HM, Oesch F. Norethisterone 4β,5-oxide and levonorgestrel-4β,5-oxide: formation in rat liver microsomal incubations and interference with microsomal epoxide hydrolase and cytoplasmic glutathione-S-transferase. *J Steroid Biochem* 1981;14:83.

Schuppler J, Gunzel P. Synthetic steroid sex hormones and liver tumors in experimental animals. In: *Advances in Pharmacology and Therapeutics*, 7th Internat Congr Pharmacol Paris, 1978, Vol. 8. Oxford: Pergamon Press; 1978;159.

Sherlock S. Hepatic tumors and sex hormones. In: Remmer H, Bolt HM, Bannasch P, Popper H (eds) *Primary Liver Tumors*. Lancaster, UK: MTP Press; 1978;201.

Sisenwine SF, Kimmel HB, Liu AL, Ruelius HW. Stereoselective biotransformations of dl-norgestrel and its enantiomers in the African green monkey. *Drug Metab Disp* 1974;2:65.

Sisenwine SF, Kimmel HB, Liu AL, Ruelius HW. Excretion and stereoselective biotransformations of *dl,-d-* and *l*-norgestrel in women. *Drug Metab Disp* 1975;3:180.

Sisenwine SF, Kimmel HB, Liu AL, Ruelius HW. The metabolic disposition of norgestrel in female Rhesus monkeys. *Drug Metab Disp* 1979;7:1.

Stanczyk FZ, Roy S. Metabolism of levonorgestrel, norethindrone, and structurally related contraceptive steroids. *Contraception* 1990;42:67.

White INH. Chemical reactivity and metabolism of norethisterone 4β,5β-epoxide by rat liver microsomes in vitro. *Chem Biol Interact* 1980;29:103.

Yasuda J, Fujii M, Tsukamoto T, Honjo H, Okada H. Pharmacokinetics of norethindrone and lynestrenol studied by HPLC. *Folia Endocr Jap* 1981;57:1159.

Yasuda J, Honjo H, Okada H. Metabolism of lynestrenol: Characterization of 3-hydroxylation using rabbit liver microsomes in vitro. *J Steroid Biochem* 1984;21:777.

Pharmacology of the Contraceptive Steroids,
edited by Joseph W. Goldzieher.
Raven Press, Ltd., New York © 1994.

6

Issues in Animal Pharmacology

Richard A. Edgren

Pharmaceutical Consultant, Woodside, California 94062

The oral contraceptives (OCs) create a major, if not unique and unprecedented problem for the endocrine pharmacologist. Predicting clinical effects from laboratory animal research is particularly difficult. OCs are compound and complex drugs. With the exception of the few progestin-only preparations, OCs are compound, i.e., combinations of an estrogen and a progestational agent. OCs are complex in that one of the two estrogens employed is a pro-hormone (mestranol) that must be converted to the other, ethynyl estradiol, before it becomes biologically active; similarly, several of the commonly employed progestins, e.g., ethynodiol diacetate, lynestrenol, and perhaps norethindrone acetate, must be converted to norethindrone before they become physiologically active. Among the newer preparations, desogestrel is oxidized to the biologically active 3-keto-desogestrel (11-methylene-levonorgestrel). As a result, although the endocrine pharmacology of the estrogens and progestins has been well studied and is well documented in the literature, application of this knowledge to the clinical effects of combined preparations must be carried out with more caution than it normally receives. Components of OCs have altered with time. The early preparations contained mestranol, the 3-methyl ether of ethynyl estradiol, while over the last decade or so ethynyl estradiol (EE) itself has become the most commonly used estrogen (Gerstman et al., 1991). Even more recently estradiol-17β and its esters have received closer attention when alternate routes of administration have been explored.

The progestins have involved a broader range of compounds. Among orally effective agents, those related to 19-nortestosterone have proved the most successful. Despite very high levels of potency in laboratory animal assays, such progesterone derivatives as the acetoxyprogesterones have not proved particularly satisfactory as components of oral preparations. On the other hand, medroxyprogesterone acetate (MPA) has provided a basis for a satisfactory injectable product. The utility of norethindrone enanthate for injectable contraception and levonorgestrel in subdermal implants suggests that 19-nor compound, if explored as extensively as MPA, could provide acceptable parenteral drugs.

The estrogenic agents have a relatively narrow range of pharmacological properties that do not differ markedly from those of the natural estrogens. Vaginal cornification, uterine growth, and pituitary blockage are among the critical physiological effects of estrogens that have been adapted to pharmacological assay procedures; the first of these responses was utilized by Allen and Doisy during the late 1920s in the original extraction, purification, and identification of estrone. All of these assay procedures are dependent upon the binding of the steroid to the estrogen receptor, which does not seem to differ significantly from tissue to tissue.

The progestins, on the other hand, have a wide range of endocrine–pharmacological properties (Edgren, 1980b). Again, each of these appears to result from receptor binding, effects on receptor biosynthesis, or both. The progestins that are components of contraceptive preparations or their metabolites variously exhibit binding to receptors that normally bind progesterone, testosterone, the estrogens, and the corticoids. Subsequent to this binding are characteristic target organ responses defined as progestational, androgenic, estrogenic, and gluco- or mineralocorticoid.

In addition, the estrogenic and progestational components of combination contraceptives interact to modify each other's actions and even to produce responses not otherwise apparent. For example, both the estrogen and the progesterone receptor are estrogen-dependent, i.e., the receptors are synthesized in appropriate target cells under stimulation by the estrogens, while progesterone will interfere with the biosynthesis of the estrogen receptor and act as an anti-estrogen. Synthetic progestins also act as anti-estrogens variously by preventing receptor formation and by competing for binding sites. Estrogens function as anti-progestins.

Finally the acetoxyprogesterones particularly show a substantial degree of corticoid activity, which does not seem to complicate clinical use of the 19-nortestosterones. Among this latter class of progestins, desogestrel has been shown to bind to the corticoid receptor, but whether this has clinical significance remains to be determined.

This review will focus on the most clinically relevant endocrine pharmacology that characterizes the steroidal components of contraceptives, despite the fact that these well-defined properties cannot be employed to predict the entire spectrum of activities of the final combination products.

BIOASSAY AND POTENCY

The administration of a physiologically active material to animals, whether they are conventional laboratory species or not, is normally associated with biochemical or morphological differences between the treated animals and controls. When those differences can be assessed with precision and quantitatively, the induced changes may be adapted for bioassay purposes. For example, growth of the uterus and cornification of the vaginal epithelium have provided satisfactory assay systems for estrogens; changes in the glandular characteristics of the estrogen-primed rabbit uterus and maintenance of pregnancy in rats spayed during pregnancy are suitable assays for progestins; growth of the prostate of castrated male rats may be used to measure androgenicity; alterations in concentration of urinary sodium and potassium are measures of the mineralocorticoid effects of steroids. Measures of binding of the steroids to appropriate cytosolic receptors have had considerable currency in recent years. However, the bulk of the pharmacological work with contraceptive steroids was completed before the receptors were identified and binding assays were developed. Furthermore, the biological effects of various progestins often depend upon metabolites while the parent compound is not bound to the receptor.

Protocols for these bioassays, which have been defined by Dorfman (1962, 1965, 1966) and others, vary slightly from laboratory to laboratory—for example, the estrogen used to prime rabbits for progestational assays varies in kind (estrone or estradiol-17β) and in dose. Route of administration has varied from laboratory to laboratory, with many workers orally dosing the rabbits to simulate human use. Since such natural steroids as estradiol-17β, progesterone, and testosterone are largely inactive orally, such approaches necessitate selection of synthetic rather than natural agents as standards. In addition animal "strain" has varied as have statistical interpretations of the data generated. Finally, a degree of subjectivity creeps into most procedures: An obvious example is in evaluation of the degree of endometrial glandular proliferation in rabbits; a less obvious problem involves the trimming of tissues and expulsion of fluid from the uteri of rats or mice before weighing. Presumably as a result of these divergencies in technique, published results of assay data have differed markedly over the years and from laboratory to laboratory (Tausk, 1972). These differences largely affect quantitative evaluations, while qualitative assessments have been reasonably consistent. In an effort to limit this broad variability, I have attempted in the past to restrict my own evaluations to assays carried out in my own laboratory (Edgren et al., 1967a; Edgren et al., 1968), but it is not currently possible to so limit interpretations concerning the newer progestins, which will be considered in a separate section below.

The purpose of pharmacological assays is to predict clinical effects of a drug, both efficacy and side effects, and to provide rough estimates of likely human doses. In general, qualitative prediction has been satisfactory in the past (Table 1), although, as discussed below, data on certain of the newer progestins may not fit the mold established in the 1950s and 1960s.

Perhaps the most difficult problem to address is that of potency, in part because the term is used in a series of overlapping popular connotations, as well as in imprecise ways by various investigators. The qualitative concept of activity and the quantitative concept of potency are frequently used interchangeably. Defined from a strict pharmacological point of view, potency refers to the amount of a drug necessary to produce a specified effect (Edgren, 1980a). Thus, a material that produces an effect at low doses is more potent than one that requires a large dose to produce the same effect.

In most situations, pharmacologists define a standard for comparison and define "relative potencies" based on this standard. Such a procedure creates a number of problems. The first problem is the selection of a standard. I have always selected a

TABLE 1. *Comparative biological effects of progestational agents in laboratory animals and humans*

Compound	Effect Progestational		Estrogenic		Androgenic		Anti-estrogenic		Glucocorticoid	
	Lab Animal	Human	Lab Animal	Human	Lab Animal	Human	Lab Animal	Human	Lab Animal	Human
Progesterone	+	+	−	−	−	−	+	+	?	?
Norethindrone	+	+	+[a]	−	+	+	+	+	−	−
Norethindrone acetate	+	+	+	+	+	+	+			
Ethynodiol diacetate	+	+	+	+	+	+	+	+		
Norgestrel	+	+	−	−	+	+	+	+		
Norethynodrel	+	+	+	+	+	+	−	−		
Medroxyprogesterone acetate	+	+	−	−	−[b]	−	+	−	+	+
Chlormadinone acetate	+	+	−	−	−	−	+	+	+	−
Cyproterone acetate	+	+	−	−	−	−	+			

[a]Long-term studies only
[b]Fetal masculinization only
From Edgren, 1986.

natural hormone, estrone or estradiol-17β, progesterone, testosterone, cortisone or cortisol, or aldosterone. However, since these substances are largely inactive by the oral route or have very low oral potency, I have tended to quantify on the basis of parenteral administration and later determined the ratio of oral to parenteral potencies. Others have chosen to select orally effective structural modifications of the natural hormones or orally active materials as standards such as ethynyl estradiol, methyl testosterone, or norethindrone. Either approach has proved satisfactory in the hands of various investigators. However, a caveat must be interjected at this point: In general, when estrogenic or progestational steroids are administered orally to laboratory rodents or rabbits at the human dose, based upon milligrams per kilogram body weight, they are ineffective. Few publications have explored this problem in detail, but toxicological studies based on multiples of the clinical dose are probably not meaningful at the lower dose range. Some years ago, my associates and I (Edgren et al., 1968) studied norgestrel (the racemate) and ethynyl estradiol by the oral route in a series of assays at 1-, 5-, and 25-fold multiples of the 0.5/0.05 preparation (Ovral, Wyeth). Only uterine growth effects were evident in the clinical range; there was no evidence of gonadotropin blockade, vaginal smear effects, or androgenic or myotrophic effects until the higher doses were administered. No dose in this entire range supported pregnancy, induced significant changes in glandular proliferation, or had gluco- or mineralocorticoid activities.

These data suggest caution in application of quantitative laboratory results to clinical situations, since norgestrel-containing contraceptives have proved satisfactory at even lower doses than the 0.5 mg employed as a base in this study, not to mention the activity of minipill preparations containing only 0.075 mg of the racemate or 0.030 mg of the levorotatory enantiomer. Furthermore, this progestin is androgenic at this dose in women (i.e., there is a decrease in HDL-cholesterol) despite the lack of an effect on the ventral prostate, seminal vesicles, or levator ani muscles of rats treated with 25 times the basic dose.

The second problem created by defining a standard for comparison and then defining relative potencies based on that standard is that there are a number of strictures that must be observed for relative potencies to be valid even when presumably identical experimental protocols are employed. In essence, the dose–effect curves for the standard and the compound under study must be congruent, i.e., they must have parallel slopes, and maximum responses must be the same (Edgren, 1980a). Both concepts are regularly ignored, leading to broad variations in potency estimates. Furthermore, there are some obvious statistical problems that must be considered. In quantal assays the use of the ED_{100}, which is common practice in evaluation of various anti-ovulatory assays, is unsatisfactory. Most dose–effect curves are sigmoid in shape, approaching an upper limit asymptotically. Selection of an ED_{100} in such circumstances is unlikely to be precise; use of the minimum effective dose is equally subject to variability in estimate. A midrange point is far more satisfactory. This is also true for quantitative assays. Both minimally and maximally effective doses are subject to error in estimate, and one at the middle of the effect dispersion is more satisfactory.

The third problem created is that pharmacological protocols must be identical for relative potencies to be meaningful. Animal species and often strain, route of administration, and temporal relations between drug administration and reading of the end point must all be the same.

These variations from laboratory to laboratory preclude precise comparisons of relative potencies, and their direct application from one assay system to another is questionable. Some years ago 18-homologated "derivatives" of estradiol-17β were compared with the parent compound across a range of bioassays for estrogenic potency in my laboratory (Edgren et al., 1967b). The broadly discrepant results from assay to assay reinforce the contention that quantitative comparisons based upon published data are futile. In short, one can only determine whether a given compound has an activity and whether the laboratory data suggest a relative potency that is likely to be clinically meaningful. Such potency estimates are valuable in suggesting dose ranges for initial clinical evaluation, but utilizing data of this type to project differential safety of various compounds is probably invalid (Edgren & Sturtevant, 1976). Only data based on specific preparations and specific end points are likely to be meaningful.

Even less likely to provide useful information is the frequent effort to relate the incidence of one or another adverse experience to the dose of estrogen. Few such studies discriminate between mestranol or EE. They ignore the fact that most OCs with estrogen doses above 50 μg were formulated with mestranol while those with doses less than 50 μg contained EE. The OCs that contain 50 μg of estrogen may be made up with either EE or mestranol. The fact that these two estrogens may be equipotent with respect to pituitary blockade does not justify pooling the data without demonstration that they are indeed identical with respect to whatever end point may be under study.

This problem is more than a simple theoretical difficulty. Recently Brody et al. (1989) showed that in the conversion of mestranol, which does not bind to the estrogen receptor, demethylation was associated with a loss of material such that human blood levels of EE, which does bind, were essentially identical after administration of 50 μg of mestranol and 35 μg of EE. Assuming linear kinetics—an assumption by no means supported by adequate data—80 μg of mestranol is likely to convert to and provide roughly the same circulating levels as 50 μg of EE. The so-called high-dose estrogen OCs, those containing 75 to 80 μg of mestranol, should probably be included with middose preparations containing 50 μg of EE, while middose 50-μg mestranol preparations are clearly the equivalent of low-dose 35-μg EE formulations. Thus, much that has been written about the relationship of estrogen dose to side effects is pharmacologically unacceptable. Application of these concepts to individual subjects is characteristically fraught with difficulties since ability to demethylate mestranol is likely to vary from subject to subject, suggesting the possibility of greater variability of blood levels of EE with mestranol-containing preparations than with EE-containing OCs. However, I know of no acceptable evidence in support of this concept.

PHARMACOLOGICAL ASSAYS

Detailed discussion of assay systems for progestational and estrogenic steroids seems unwarranted at this late date. Standard bioassay techniques have been defined in detail in volumes by Emmens (1950) and Dorfman (1962, 1964, 1965, 1966), and systems I have found useful have been defined by Edgren et al. (1968). I shall, therefore, confine myself to some general remarks.

Estrogen Assays

The primary sites of action of estrogenic hormones are the uterus and vagina, and a range of measures of activity at both targets has been applied to assays. I have preferred assays based on vaginal effects since they appear to be more specific than uterine systems.

Vaginal Smear Assays. Both EE and MEE are effective in inducing keratinization of the vaginal epithelium of spayed female rodents, and at least some of the progestins related to 19-nortestosterone are effective in standard, short-term protocols. A high degree of subjectivity intrudes on reading the vaginal smears. Biggers and Claringbold (1954) evaluated this problem several decades ago and concluded that the presence or absence of leucocytes in the smear provided the most satisfactory end point, although even here a degree of subjectivity intrudes since occasional leucocytes occur in cornified smears. Modifications of the Allen–Doisy assay are particularly satisfactory, since a colony of spayed rats or mice may be maintained and the animals reused repeatedly for rather extended periods of time. In my hands rats were employed every second week for assay of miscellaneous compounds; the animals were "primed" on alternate weeks with a standard dose of estrone and only those responding were used for assay purposes. Since the estrogen receptor is estrogen dependent, this procedure probably increases sensitivity of the assay.

In addition to acute effects of progestins like norethynodrel and ethynodiol diacetate, longer-term oral administration of norethindrone produces a characteristic estrogenic effect on the vaginal mucosa (Jones & Edgren, 1973). This activity presumably results from hepatic conversion of the norethindrone to 5,10-dihydronorethindrone (Reel et al., 1979). The possibility of simple A-ring aromatization seems unlikely.

Uterine Growth Assays. The progestational 19-nortestosterone derivatives and, to a lesser degree, progesterone derivatives induce growth of the uterus that is marked in assay systems employing spayed female rats, but less so in intact prepubertal mice. The nature of this effect is not entirely clear; it would not seem to be based upon an estrogenic metabolite of the progestin since norgestrel, which has no folliculoid activity at the level of the vagina, has a clear uterine growth effect. Androgens like testosterone and, of course, estrogenic agents induce growth of both the mouse and the rat uterus, although testosterone has minimal activity in mice. In addition to simple weight of the uterus, increases in uterine imbibition of water and various other chemical end points have been employed to assay estrogens. There seems little reason to believe that these approaches provide more predictable data than uterine weight.

Estrogen-receptor binding assays are based on the displacement of a radio-labelled ligand (perhaps estradiol itself) from the receptor, which is usually extracted from the estrogen-treated uterus. Ethynyl estradiol binds to the estrogen receptor, as do some progestins (norethynodrel, ethynodiol diacetate, and, to a lesser degree, norethindrone), but mestranol does not.

Progestational Assays

For bioassay purposes these procedures primarily focus on glandular proliferation of the uterine epithelium of rabbits or the maintenance of pregnancy in rodents spayed during pregnancy.

Endometrial Glandular Proliferation. McPhail (1934) illustrated a graded series of changes in arborization of the endometrial glands of progesterone-treated, estrogen-primed rabbits. This study has provided the basis for a series of assay procedures that have been employed successfully in various laboratories. Intact immature rabbits (the Clauberg test) have been used in many laboratories with the progestin either injected or administered orally. Spayed adults may also be employed for assay by systemic routes, or at laparotomy, the progestin may be administered locally into an isolated segment of the uterine horn (the McGinty test). In the latter case, the contralateral horn may be used as a control, both for the assay drug itself and to determine whether the administered material is passing into the systemic circulation.

As a correlate to the glandular proliferation, carbonic anhydrase levels may be evaluated in rabbit uteri.

Interpretation and especially quantification of the Clauberg test is complicated by the fact that the dose–response curves for commonly employed products are not parallel and the maximum response varies (Edgren, 1980b). In general, progesterone, the acetoxyprogesterones, and norgestrel (both the racemate and levonorgestrel) have dose–response curves with steep parallel slopes, validating the use of simple potency estimates. Norethindrone and norethynodrel, in contrast, have curves with shallow slopes. The compounds with steep slopes tend to produce maximal McPhail readings that average $+3$ to $+3.5$ (maximum response $+4$) in my laboratory, while norethindrone has a maximum response of about $+2$ and norethynodrel about $+1.3$. Various statistical manipulations of Clauberg data are helpful (log–log transformations proved especially useful), but entirely precise results are unlikely to emerge from the Clauberg test.

Some years ago Elton (1962) showed that a variety of the progestins under study at the time behaved like mixtures of estrogen and progesterone in their impact on the cytology of the uterine epithelium. When estrogen is given simultaneously with progesterone, the epithelial cells progressively increase in height from low to tall columnar, and subnuclear vacuoles are developed at higher dose levels. Progesterone derivatives and norgestrel produce low columnar epithelia while norethynodrel, norethindrone, and ethynodiol diacetate are associated with tall columnar epithelia; subnuclear vacuoles are seen in norethynodrel-treated rabbits.

The clinical relevance of these changes remains obscure at this time; however, they correspond to other characteristics that tend to define synthetic progestins in terms of progesterone itself (Edgren et al., 1967a).

The carbonic anhydrase content of uteri provides a dose-related index of the progesterone effect (Pincus & Bialy, 1963). This enzyme is largely restricted to the epithelium, so various workers have improved precision of the assay by separating the endometrium from the underlying myometrium before chemical evaluation. Although carbonic anhydrase provides an objective measure of progesterone effect on the uterus, there is an ambiguity involved since the carbonic anhydrase inhibitor Diamox (acetazolamide) will prevent the progesterone-induced rise in enzyme, while glandular proliferation remains unaltered (Knudsen et al., 1969).

The progestational response in the Clauberg test is inhibited by graded doses of estrogen in a dose-related fashion (norgestrel *vs* ethynyl estradiol) (Edgren et al., 1967c).

Administration directly into an isolated segment of the estrogen-primed rabbit uterus was followed by distinct glandular arborization when the progestin was an acetoxyprogesterone or norgestrel, while norethindrone, norethynodrel, and ethynodiol diacetate (Elton & Nutting, 1961) were ineffective.

Pregnancy Support. In rats and various other species, early pregnancy following implantation is dependent upon ovarian progesterone. In other species, including humans, placental progesterone is more critical, particularly in later stages of gestation. A convenient assay employs pregnant rats, spayed on about day 8 of pregnancy and maintained with daily progestin administration until autopsy at about term. Norethynodrel and norethindrone are inactive in this protocol, while the acetoxyprogesterones are effective. Norgestrel is effective at low, but not high, doses. Various studies that have suggested activity for norethindrone are apparently based upon the presence of implantation sites at the time of sacrifice.

Estrogens are ineffective in this assay and will inhibit the effects of active progestins when administered at sufficient dose levels.

Inhibition of Parturition. Progesterone, when administered late in pregnancy, will delay delivery to the point of maternal and fetal death. This observation was adapted for assay of progestins by Edgren and Peterson (1966). Norethindrone, norgestrel, chloroethynyl norgestrel, and medroxyprogesterone acetate were active. This bioassay apparently fails to distinguish among the various progestins.

Receptor Binding Assays. A detailed protocol for this assay, employing estrogen-primed rabbit uteri, has been published by Reel et al. (1979), and an extensive series of compounds was assayed. Briggs (1975) reported on binding of a series of progestins to human endometrial and myometrial receptors. Briggs' data suggest that progesterone, norethindrone, norgestrel (and levonorgestrel), and the acetoxyprogesterones bind to the receptor, whereas norethindrone acetate, norethynodrel, ethynodiol diacetate, lynestrenol, and EE and MEE do not. Other studies (Reel et al., 1979; Kuhl, 1987) suggest that norethindrone acetate will bind to the progesterone receptor. The obvious clinical and systemic progestational effects of the latter group of nortestosterones must result from metabolites, probably norethindrone itself.

Androgenic/Anabolic Assays

Some of the main problems encountered with clinical use of oral contraceptives appear to be related to the androgenic and anabolic effects of the progestins that are chemically related to testosterone. Early studies of the OCs focused on such clinical problems as hirsutism, acne, and deepening voice as measures of androgenicity. As pointed out by Tausk (1966) we had no objective, reliable method for measuring clinical androgenic effects at the time. More recently the impact of these drugs on circulating levels of HDL-cholesterol has proved a sensitive measure of androgenic effects in humans. Furthermore, increase in weight has been a common problem for many women using OCs. In experimental animals, several assays have been employed with success in various laboratories.

Growth of the comb in newly hatched domestic fowl may be stimulated by injection of the progestin or by inunction directly onto the developing comb, which is removed and weighed at autopsy.

More commonly, weights of the ventral prostate and seminal vesicles of rats are employed as measures of androgenicity, while weight of the levator ani muscle, the myotrophic response, is considered by many investigators to be an index of the anabolic effect. Eisenberg and Gordan (1950) proposed use of these end points in adult, castrated rats, while Hershberger et al. (1963) codified an assay based upon castrated immature male rats; this is probably the most commonly used system. Either assay is satisfactory and provides a reliable measure of androgenicity by oral or parenteral routes, while the applicability of the myotrophic response to human anabolic effects remains controversial. Assayed in these systems, most of the norsteroidal progestins show both androgenic and anabolic effects; progesterone itself, the acetoxyprogesterones, and norethynodrel (and of course, EE and MEE) are essentially inactive when evaluated on the basis of growth of the ventral prostate. Seminal vesicle weight is not specific for androgenic effects since it shows a positive response to estrogen administration.

Of the androgenically active progestins, norgestrel and levonorgestrel are unequivocally the most potent materials, and this high level of effect certainly carries over to clinical use as reflected in suppression of HDL-cholesterol levels. The long-term clinical meaning of this effect remains obscure.

A side issue of androgenic impact is the masculinization of female fetuses following administration of androgenic progestins during late pregnancy in rats. This effect appears to carry over to humans since virilization has been reported by Wilkins (1960) in newborn young of women who received androgenic progestins in an effort to salvage pregnancies in habitual aborters. Little has been heard of this problem since this use of progestins has gone out of style. The clinical data, however, are confused by the report of virilization in the child of a norethynodrel-treated woman —norethynodrel is not androgenic, nor does it masculinize rat fetuses. Medroxy-progesterone acetate will masculinize female rate fetuses, but it apparently has little or no effect in humans.*

Anti-Estrogenic Effects

Progesterone and many progestational agents will reverse the effects of various estrogens on the uterine growth or vaginal smear of laboratory rodents. Possible interactions at the level of the hypothalamic–pituitary system are not so clearly defined. Vaginal smear techniques employing either spayed rats or mice are suitable, as are mouse uterine growth effects. I have not found rat uterine growth satisfactory, since there are substantial synergistic relationships between estrogens and progestins in such assays. In general, the administration of an estrogen is followed by vaginal keratinization or increase in uterine weight. In both cases the change is dose-related so a high dose that produces a slightly sub-maximal response may be chosen as a basis; increasing doses of antagonists reverse this effect and reduce the proportion of animals with positive vaginal responses or the uterine weights toward control levels.

Most of the nortestosterone progestins and the acetoxyprogesterones are active antiestrogens; norethynodrel is ineffective.

This property is important in that the use of progestins alone in the so-called minipills may reflect their antiestrogenic effect in reversing the mid-cycle liquefaction of cervical mucus necessary for sperm migration from the vagina to the upper reproductive tract. Furthermore, combination contraceptives appear to have a similar effect, which is important in the event of a failure of ovulatory block.

Pituitary Blockade

A range of bioassay procedures has been employed to estimate the inhibiting effects of contraceptive steroids on the hypothalamic–pituitary system in the belief that this is the primary mode-of-action of these drugs. Such assays have involved suppression of gonadal growth, measurement of circulating gonadotropin, evaluation of ovulation by egg counts, or examination of the ovary for corpora lutea or corpora hemorrhagica.

Gonadal Growth Methods. The administration of gonadal steroids to laboratory rodents leads to failure of growth of both the ovary and testes. The toxicological

---

*At the time these observations were made (and one was a report of masculinization by an estrogen), the frequency of genetic, masculinizing congenital adrenal hyperplasia was unrecognized, and indeed untestable; it is entirely possible that this disorder was the underlying cause of all these reports.

literature presents a large number of studies in which gonadal growth/size is suppressed by estrogen or progestin administration. Early controlled studies were based upon parobiotic unions in which two animals, usually rats, were surgically joined side by side. In such pairs, the gonadotropic hormones passed readily across the union while the gonadal steroids did not. As a result, suppression of secretion of the gonadotropins can be measured by administration of the steroid to one of the pair and evaluation of gonadal size in the other individual. This technique is labor-intensive and unions can only be carried out successfully in immature animals, prior to development of immunological capacity. These studies supported the contention that estrogens and progestins suppressed gonadotropin secretion.

In an effort to overcome the difficulties of the parabiotic system, an assay based upon compensatory ovarian hypertrophy in hemicastrated rats was developed in my laboratory (Peterson et al., 1964). In this technique, the compensatory hypertrophy caused by unilateral ovariectomy is evaluated by dual controls, one intact and one hemicastrated. This effect is suppressed by the administration of steroids. The progestins produce simple linear curves that project below the baseline level of the intact controls, while estrogen suppression proceeds linearly to about the 100% suppression level and then reverses to a growth phase associated with the formation of very large corpora lutea.

Gonadotropin Methods. The extensive work on control of the estrous cycle in rats has demonstrated that in females with regular 4-day cycles, gonadotropins rise to a peak on the afternoon of proestrus. This increase, which induces ovulation early the next morning, can be inhibited by the administration of steroids. However, since much of the pharmacological work that led to the development of the OCs was completed prior to the establishment of radioimmunoassay methods for gonadotropins, such methods have seldom been carried out for comparative purposes.

Ovulatory Methods. During the 1950s and 1960s, coitus-induced ovulation in rabbits was extensively employed as an assay procedure. Progesterone and other progestational agents are certainly active when administered prior to pairing with males. However, these agents suppress mating behavior in a significant proportion of the does, thus compromising efforts to quantify the data. This antiovulatory effect appears to result from an inhibition of release of gonadotropins from the pituitary, since administration of exogenous gonadotropins to steroid-treated rabbit does is followed by normal ovulatory responses (Edgren & Carter, 1962).

Duration of Effect

It has been apparent for some years that long-acting, parenteral preparations of a contraceptive steroid would be desirable in a number of circumstances. This led to an extensive synthetic program sponsored by WHO (Crabbè et al., 1983). The compounds produced were assayed by studying the duration of estrus suppression following administration of these agents. The results of such a test are, of course, ambiguous since it is not possible to determine whether the estrus suppression results from a pituitary blockade or from a direct antiestrogenic effect at the level of the vagina. In the event, however, it probably was not important since such distinctions may be made following identification of a long-acting agent.

Several of the assay systems discussed above may be adapted to studying duration of action. R. C. Jones and I (unpublished) have employed a variant of the Clauberg test where rabbits were sacrificed at extended intervals following injection of the progestin to estrogen-primed rabbits. In this test norgestrel and medroxyprogesterone were long-acting.

Corticoid Effects

The discovery, some years ago, that medroxyprogesterone acetate produced adrenal suppression, both physical and physiological, in treated rats (Edgren et al., 1959) led to a number of studies assessing the corticoid activities of progestins. In general, the acetoxyprogesterone derivatives and to a lesser degree progesterone itself, show marked glucocorticoid activity, while the relatives of 19-nortestosterone demonstrated little effect, although they did show a degree of binding to the corticoid receptor. Similarly, progesterone and the acetoxyprogestins bind to the mineralocorticoid receptor, retain sodium, and have a degree of anti-aldosterone potency. The nortestosterones, with the possible exception of gestodene (see below) seem largely devoid of such activity.

These activities are usually assayed on the basis of measures of sodium retention in adrenalectomized rats (Kagawa, 1964).

THE MAMMARY TUMOR PROBLEM

Steroidal hormones, particularly estrogens, have been associated with mammary tumors in rodents since the 1940s (Burrows, 1949). These mammary tumors are not simple results of estrogen administration, since estrogen-induced prolactin release is involved in both rats and mice and the mouse situation is confused by tumor viruses. This laboratory animal information plus the apparent, if obscure, relationship of human mammary cancer to ovarian function led to concerns over the possibility that oral contraceptive use might predispose women to an increased incidence of breast cancer. At the human level this problem has yet to be resolved (Mann, 1990). In laboratory animals, extensive work has been required by regulatory agencies, and a mass of material was summarized by the British Committee on Safety of Medicines in 1972. Although certain studies showed increased mammary tumor incidence, this appeared to be restricted to susceptible rodent strains that received high doses of steroids for most of the animals' life span. The effects are not generally considered of significance to humans.

An even greater impact resulted from the appearance, some 25 years ago, of mammary tumors in the beagle bitches used for routine toxicity studies. This observation led to regulatory requirements for extensive carcinogenesis studies in dogs

TABLE 2. *Biological effects of newer progestagens*

	Progestational		Estrogenic		Androgenic		
	Clauberg	Receptor Binding	Vaginal Smear	Receptor Binding	Prostate Growth	Receptor Binding	Anti-estrogenic
3-Ketodeso-gestrel (11-methy-lene-levo-norgestrel)	+		−		+		
Gestodene	+	+		−	+	+	+
Norgestimate	+	+	−	−	+	+	+

and monkeys. The US FDA demanded 7 years of continuous administration to dogs and 10 years to monkeys. The results of these studies are proprietary and only a few of the monkey studies have been published—no basis for concern seems to have emerged. In dogs, however, various progestins, particularly the acetoxyproges-terone derivatives, have been associated with high incidences of mammary nodules and a few cases of frank carcinoma. Recently, Larsson and Mackin (1989) collected data from the pharmaceutical industry through the US Freedom of Information Act and summarized the situation. Characteristically, the results of the tumor studies are as widely scattered as their provenances. However, it seems clear from that review that the beagle data are not applicable to human breast cancer risk, a view shared by a special Toxicology Review Panel of the World Health Organisation.

Cyproterone Acetate

This compound is the 1,2-cyclopropal derivative of chlormadinone acetate. Like other progesterone derivatives, it has anti-androgenic effects and was developed primarily as an androgen antagonist. It is currently employed at a dose of 2 mg in combination with EE at 50 or 35 μg as an oral contraceptive that is marketed world-wide (except for the United States) as appropriate for women with acne, seborrhea, or hirsutism.

Cyproterone acetate appears to have a biological spectrum of activities that is similar to that of other acetoxyprogesterone derivatives (Table 1). It would appear to be the only progesterone derivative still marketed as a component of a combina-tion oral contraceptive. The anti-androgenic activity appears to result from competi-tive interactions with androgens at the target organ sites (Neumann, 1977).

NEWER PROGESTINS

Over the past several years, three new progestins have emerged as components of oral contraceptives in Europe. These compounds—norgestimate, gestodene, and desogestrel—are all homologated at carbon 18, i.e., they are derivatives of le-vonorgestrel. Gestodene is simply Δ^{15}-levonorgestrel; norgestimate is the 3-oxime of levonorgestrel acetate, and desogestrel is 11-methylene, 3-desoxolevonorgestrel. All three are purported to share the high potency of levonorgestrel, but they lack the clinical androgenicity of the parent compound. This latter point needs confirmation since all show androgenic effects in rat prostate assays. The biological effects of these compounds are summarized in Table 2.

According to Hahn et al. (1977) norgestimate is a "moderately potent progestin, as judged by the classic Clauberg assay, . . . which binds to the progesterone receptor; is less androgenic than levonorgestrel; is not estrogenic; is markedly anti-estrogenic; and is a more potent uterotrophic agent than levonorgestrel." Binding of norgestimate itself to the progesterone receptor is surprising since, in my experience, an intact ketone at carbon 3 is necessary for such binding. A later paper (Phillips et al., 1990) confirmed binding to the progesterone receptor, but showed that the 3-ketone was appreciably better bound. They also showed substantial binding to the testosterone receptor.

Düsterberg et al. (1988) have summarized the pharmacology of gestodene. This progestin appears to be more potent in its progestational, antiovulatory, and anti-estrogenic effects, but slightly less androgenic than levonorgestrel. Pollow et al. (1989) later showed expected binding to the progesterone and androgen receptors and perhaps unexpectedly to both gluco- and mineralocorticoid receptors; binding to the estradiol receptor was not seen.

Desogestrel functions as a pro-hormone; it is biologically active only after oxygenation at carbon 3 to form 3-ketodesogestrel (11-methylene-levonorgestrel). This material is reported to have progestational, antiovulatory, and weak androgenic/anabolic activities and no estrogenic effects (de Visser et al., 1975).

As was true of the earlier studies on progestins, evaluations of these compounds were not carried out in comparable situations, so quantitative comparisons are not possible. However, based on the consistency of binding to the testosterone receptor and growth effects at the level of the prostate in rats, one would expect clinical evidence of an androgenic activity such as is reported with norgestrel (levonorgestrel or the racemate) or with norethindrone at high doses. Such problems have apparently not been reported, and contraceptive preparations containing these progestins with EE are reported to increase circulating levels of HDL-cholesterol, an estrogenic effect.

REFERENCES

Biggers JD, Claringbold PJ: Criteria of the vaginal response to oestrogens. *J Endocrinol* 1954;11:277.

Briggs M: Contraceptive steroid binding to the human uterine progesterone-receptor. *Cur Med Res Opinion* 1975;3:95.

Brody SA, Turkes A, Goldzieher JW: Pharmacokinetics of three bioequivalent norethindrone/mestranol-50 μg and three norethindrone/ethinyl estradiol-35 μg OC formulations: are "low-dose" pills really lower? *Contraception* 1989;40:269.

Burrows H: *Biological Actions of Sex Hormones*, 2nd ed. Oxford: Cambridge University Press, 1949.

Carcinogenicity tests of oral contraceptives. A report by the Committee on Safety of Medicines. Her Majesty's Stationery Office, London, 1972.

Crabbè P, Archer S, Benagiano G et al.: Long-acting contraceptive agents: design of the WHO chemical synthesis programme. *Steroids* 1983;41:243.

de Visser J, de Jager E, de Jongh HP et al.: Pharmacological profile of a new orally active progestational steroid: Org 2969. *Acta Endocrinol (Suppl)* 1975;199:405.

Dorfman RI (ed): *Methods in Hormone Research, Vol. II: Bioassay.* New York: Academic Press, 1962.

Dorfman RI (ed): *Methods in Hormone Research, Vol. III: Steroidal Activity in Experimental Animals and Mice, Part A.* New York: Academic Press, 1964.

Dorfman RI (ed): *Methods in Hormone Research, Vol. IV: Steroidal Activity in Experimental Animals and Mice, Part B.* New York: Academic Press, 1965.

Dorfman RI (ed): *Methods in Hormone Research, Vol. V: Steroidal Activity in Experimental Animals and Mice, Part C.* New York: Academic Press, 1966.

Düsterberg B, Beier S, Schneider WHF, Spona J: Pharmacological features of gestodene in laboratory animals and man. In: Breckwoldt M, Düsterberg B (eds): *Gestodene: A New Direction in Oral Contraception.* Carnforth, England: Parthenon Publishing Group, 1988, p. 13.

Edgren RA: Relative potencies of oral contraceptives. In: Moghissi KS (ed): *Controversies in Contraception.* Baltimore: Williams and Wilkins, 1980a.

Edgren RA: Progestagens. In: Givens JR, Andersen RN, Cohen BM, Wendt AC (eds): *Clinical Use of Sex Steroids.* Chicago: Year Book Medical Publishers, 1980b.

Edgren RA: Endocrine effects of systemic, steroidal contraceptives. In: Gregoire AT, Blye RT (eds): *Contraceptive Steroids.* New York: Plenum Press, 1986, p. 163.

Edgren RA, Carter DL: Failure of various steroids to block gonadotrophin-induced ovulation in rabbits. *J Endocrinol* 1962;24:525.

Edgren RA, Hanbarrger WE, Calhoun DW: Production of adrenalatrophyly 6-moryl-17-acetoxyprogesterone, with remarks on the adrenal affects of other progestational agents. *Endocrinology* 1959; 65:505.

Edgren RA, Jones RC, Clancy DP, Nagra CL: The biological effects of norgestrel alone and in combination with ethinyl oestradiol. *J Reprod Fert (Suppl)* 1968;5:13.

Edgren RA, Jones RC, Peterson DL: A biological classification of progestational agents. *Fertil Steril* 1967a;18:238.

Edgren RA, Jones RC, Peterson DL: The estrogenic effects of a series of 13β-substituted compounds related to estradiol-17β. *Eur J Steroids* 1967b;2:19.

Edgren RA, Jones RC, Peterson DL, Gillen AL: Studies on the interactions of ethynyl oestradiol and norgestrel. *Acta Endocrinol (Suppl)* 1967c;115:1.

Edgren RA, Peterson DL: Delay of parturition in rats by various progestational steroids. *Proc Soc Exp Biol Med* 1966;123:867.

Edgren RA, Sturtevant FM: Potencies of oral contraceptives. *Am J Obstet Gynecol* 1976;125:1029.

Eisenberg E, Gordan GS: The levator ani muscle of the rat as an index of myotrophic activity of steroidal hormones. *J Pharmacol Exp Ther* 1950;99:38.

Elton RL: Morphological changes in the glandular epithelium of rabbit endometrium due to hormonal treatment. *Anat Rec* 1962;142:469.

Elton RL, Nutting EF: 17-ethynyl-4-estren-3,17-diol diacetate: a unique steroidal "progestin." *Proc Soc Exp Biol Med* 1961;107:991.

Emmens CW: *Hormone Assay.* New York: Academic Press, 1950.

Gerstman BB, Gross TP, Kennedy DL et al.: Trends in the content and use of oral contraceptives in the United States, 1964–88. *Am J Pub Health* 1991;81:90–96.

Hahn DW, Allen GO, McGuire JL: The pharmacological profile of norgestimate, a new orally active progestin. *Contraception* 1977;16:541.

Hershberger LG, Shipley EG, Meyer RK: Myotrophic activity of 19-nortestosterone and other steroids determined by modified levator ani muscle method. *Proc Soc Exp Biol Med* 1963;83:175.

Jones RC, Edgren RA: The effects of various steroids on the vaginal histology of the rat. *Fertil Steril* 1973;24:284.

Kagawa CM: Anti-aldosterones. In: Dorfman RI (ed): *Methods in Hormone Res,* Vol III. New York: Academic Press, 1964, p. 351.

Knudsen KA, Jones RC, Edgren RA: Effect of a carbonic anhydrase inhibitor (Diamox) on the progesterone-stimulated rabbit uterus. *Endocrinology* 1969;85:1204.

Kuhl H: Prostagene zur Empfängnisverhütung. *Wiener Med Woch* 1987:18/19:453.

Larsson RS, Mackin D: Predictability of the safety of hormonal contraceptives from canine toxicological studies. In: Michael D (ed): *Safety Requirements for Contraceptive Steroids,* Oxford: Cambridge University Press, 1989, pp. 230–269.

Mann RD (ed): *Oral Contraceptives and Breast Cancer*. Carnforth England, Park Ridge, NJ: Parthenon Publishing Group, 1990.

McPhail MK: The assay of progestin. *J Physiol* 1934;83:145.

Neumann F: Pharmacology and potential use of cyproterone acetate. *Hormone Metab Res* 1977;9:1.

Peterson DL, Edgren RA, Jones RC: Steroid-induced block of ovarian compensatory hypertrophy in hemicastrated female rats. *J Endocrinol* 1964;29:255.

Phillips A, Demarest K, Hahn DW et al.: Progestational and androgenic receptor binding affinities and in vivo activities of norgestimate and other progestins. *Contraception* 1990;41:399–410.

Pincus G, Bialy G: Carbonic anhydrase in steroid-responsive tissues. *Recent Prog Hormone Res* 1963;19:701.

Pollow K, Juchem M, Grill H-J et al.: Gestodene: a novel synthetic progestin-characterization of binding to receptor and serum proteins. *Contraception* 1989;40:325–341.

Reel JR, Humphrey RR, Shin Y-H et al.: Competitive progesterone antagonists: receptor binding and biologic activity of testosterone and 19-nortestosterone derivatives. *Fertil Steril* 1979;31:552.

Reel JR, Thomas BH, Hartwell BS: 5α-dihydronorethindrone (5α-DNE): a competitive progesterone antagonist with contragestive activity. *The Endocrine Society (Abstract)* 1979;727:754.

Tausk M: Discussion (pp. 334–335). In: Edgren RA, Peterson DL, Jones RL et al.: Biological effects of synthetic gonanes. *Recent Prog Hormone Res* 1966;22:305.

Tausk M: Pharmacology of orally active progestational compounds: animal studies. In: Tausk M (ed): *Pharmacology of the Endocrine System and Related Drugs: Progesterone, Progestational Drugs and Antifertility Agents*. Oxford: Pergamon Press, 1972, p. 35.

Wilkins L: Masculinization of female fetus due to use of orally given progestins. *JAMA* 1960;172:1028.

Pharmacology of the Contraceptive Steroids,
edited by Joseph W. Goldzieher.
Raven Press, Ltd., New York © 1994.

7

Pharmacokinetics and Metabolism of Progestins in Humans

Kenneth Fotherby

*Royal Postgraduate Medical School, Hammersmith Hospital
London W12 0HS, England*

Following a comprehensive review of the pharmacokinetics and metabolism of sex steroids up to 1972 (Fotherby & James, 1972), many reviews have appeared (Fotherby, 1974a, 1984, 1986, 1988, 1990a, 1991b; Breuer, 1977; Ranney, 1977; Hammerstein et al., 1979; Orme et al., 1983; Goebelsmann, 1986; Stanczyk & Roy, 1990; Shenfield & Griffin, 1991), and recently two symposia have been published covering selected aspects of this subject (Skouby & Jespersen, 1990; Kuhl, 1990).

The two major advances in the past 20 years have been the development of (1) sensitive methods, mainly radioimmunoassay (RIA), for estimation of the serum concentrations of the progestins and (2) new, more potent progestins with different spectra of biological activities. The formulae of these compounds are given in the Appendix.

NORETHINDRONE (NET)

Pharmacokinetics

The pharmacokinetic parameters reported in various publications are summarized in Table 1. There are marked variations that arise from a number of causes: (1) mathematical procedure used to calculate the parameters; (2) mode of administration of NET; (3) formulation of NET used, whether progestin-alone or with estrogen, and the NET/estrogen ratio; (4) whether single-dose or steady-state kinetics were examined; (5) small number of subjects studied in most investigations: of the 20 studies summarized, only 6 involved more than 12 subjects; and (6) inter- and intra-subject variation.

Regarding the values in Table 1, the "peak" concentrations are the mean, or range of, the highest NET concentrations recorded in that particular study and therefore not be the true peak concentrations. Even after low doses of NET such as those

TABLE 1. Pharmacokinetic parameters for NET (values derived from published studies are mean ± SD or range, EE denotes ethynylestradiol, ME mestranol)

NET dose (mg)	No. of subjects	'Peak' conc. (ng/ml)	24 h conc. (ng/ml)	Absorption time (h)	Td (h)	Tel (h)	Vd (l)	Cl (l/h)	AUC (ng/ml/h)	Ref.
0.3	5	2-7	0-0.3			7.9				1
0.3	3	3-5	0.5							2
0.35	5	2.1-5.1	0.2-0.9							3
0.35	3	4.3	0.3-0.4		4.4					4
0.35	16	4.7-14.8	0-1.6	1-2	1-1.5	6-13.4				5
0.5	5	4-9	0-0.6			7.9				1
0.5	6	0.7-5	0-0.3	1-3		6				6
0.5	3	6.5	0.2	1						7
1.0	4	6	0.1	1						8
1.05	6				0.4-2.6	7.7 ± 1	264 ± 36	24 ± 1	29.9 + 1	9
1.05	8				0.4	7.9				10
2.5	8				3	9				2
3	3	7-28	1	1-2						3
3	10	18 ± 5	2 + 0.8	1.8 ± 0.8	1.7 ± 1	8.0 ± 1.2	228 ± 60	19.8	132 ± 40	11
5	10	28 ± 6.5	3 ± 1.2	1.9 ± 0.6	1.7 ± 0.5	8.0 ± 0.9	260 + 76	22.5	198 ± 60	11
5	5	30-50	0.5-4			7.7				1
25	2	100-140	5-25							2
0.5 + 35µg EE	3	7.5	0.7-0.8	0.5-4	3.9	11.5 ± 2.4			48.5 ± 9.7	12
0.5 + 35µg EE	5					6.6 ± 1.6			62.6 ± 22	13
1.0 + 35µg EE	24	15.3 ± 4.5				6.4 ± 3.0			72.8 ± 40	14
1.0 + 35µg EE	24	14.0 ± 5.4		1.2 ± 0.6						15
1.0 + 50µg EE	6	4.5	0.1	2						18
1.0 + 50µg EE	6	10.3	0.7 ± 1.5	0.5-4	2.3-3.4	5.4 ± 0.4			36.4 ± 8	12
1.0 + 50µg EE	112	1.8-6.5	0.1-0.7	1-2		7.6 ± 1.9	236 ± 60	22.6 ± 7	53.6 ± 42	16
1.0 + 50µg EE	83	4.3	0.6	1-4		4.1 ± 4.0			87.9 ± 50	17
1.0 + 50µg ME	27	17.1 ± 7.7		1.4 ± 0.8		3.4	217	43.9		15
1.0 + 50µg EE	12	5.3		1.2 ± 0.1		8.1 ± 0.4			84 ± 6	18
1.0 + 120µg EE	24	15.7 ± 1.3	0.7 ± 0.08	0.5 ± 3	0.6	6.3			118	19
2.0 + 70µg EE	18	14.6								20

References: 1, Odlind et al. (1979); 2, Nygren et al. (1974); 3, Saxena et al. (1977); 4, Stanczyk et al. (1978); 5, Prasad et al. (1979); 6, Pasqualini et al., (1975); 7, Warren and Fotherby (1974); 8, Fotherby and Warren (1976); 9, Back et al. (1978); 10, Mills et al. (1974); 11, Song et al. (1986); 12, Stanczyk et al. (1978); 13, El-Raghy et al. (1986); 14, Saperstein et al. (1989); 15, Brody et al. (1989); 16, Kiriwat and Fotherby (1983); 17, Fotherby et al. (1979); Shi et al. (1987); 18, Prasad et al. (1981); 19, Stanczyk et al. (1983); 20, Saperstein et al. (1986).

(0.35–0.50 mg) used in the progestin-only pill, significant amounts are still present in the circulation in the majority of women 24 hr after administration. Almost all women using a combined OC have detectable levels at 24 hr; this is due partly to the fact that the combined oral contraceptives (OCs) contain a higher dose of NET and partly to the increased protein binding of NET in estrogen-treated subjects. However, Back et al. (1978) found no difference in the kinetics of NET when the same dose was administered with or without 50 μg of ethynyl estradiol (EE), although in these two situations there would be a marked difference in the binding of NET.

Absorption of NET is rapid in most subjects, although there are variations: in large-scale studies (Fotherby et al., 1978; Shi et al., 1987) peak serum NET in plasma occurred within 1 hr in 10 of 83 women, in 47 from 1 to 2 hr, and the remaining 26 between 2 and 4 hr. The cause of this variability in absorption has not been determined; it appears not to be connected to food intake or time of day when the dose is taken (Kiriwat & Fotherby, 1983). NET is subject to a first-pass effect (Back et al., 1978a), which reduces the bioavailability by 27 to 53% (mean = 36%). The half-life of distribution is short—usually less than 3 hr—but more information is available for the half-life of elimination ($t_{1/2}\beta$). The mean value derived from the studies listed in Table 1 is about 8 hr but there is at least a threefold variation between the lowest (4 hr) and the highest (11 hr) values (Shi et al., 1987). It is interesting that, from the values in Table 1, the mean elimination half-life for NET administered alone (8.0 hr) was higher than the mean value from the administration of 1 mg NET + EE (6.3 hr). Only a few studies have calculated the volume of distribution, clearance, and bioavailability, but the inter-subject variability of these parameters seems equally large. In a large-scale study (Shi et al., 1987) the variation in bioavailability was almost fivefold—from 20 to 90 ng/ml/hr. Clearance appeared to be the important determinant. In one study (Prasad et al., 1981) a small value for the elimination half-life led to the calculated clearance being significantly higher than that reported in other studies.

Considering the limited data available for peak concentration with NET administered alone, there does not appear to be a linear relation between these values and dose. Since the half-life appears to remain constant irrespective of dose, the lack of correlation between dose and peak concentration is presumably due to a decrease in the proportion absorbed as the dose increases. The peak concentrations for NET given alone appear to be lower than when the same dose is given in conjunction with EE, and this is supported by the limited amount of data on bioavailability and 24-hr plasma levels.

Mean serum concentrations of NET after a 1 mg dose with 50 μg EE, calculated from published reports, are shown in Figure 1. These data relate to single-dose administration; only limited data are available for "steady-state" conditions.

Metabolism

The first studies of the metabolism of NET were performed using the ^{3}H or ^{14}C labelled compounds (Layne et al., 1963; Kamyab et al., 1968; Gerhards et al.,

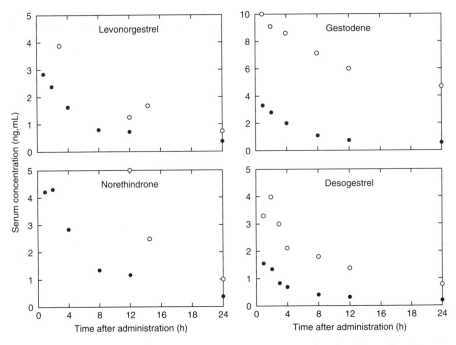

FIG. 1. Serum concentrations of gestagens after administration of oral contraceptives; ● concentrations after a single dose; ○ steady-state concentrations after multiple dosing. (From Fotherby, 1990a, with permission).

1971). These studies showed many of the important aspects of NET metabolism that were confirmed by later studies: (1) rapid absorption from the gastrointestinal tract; (2) rapid excretion of a major portion of the dose (37 to 80%) in the urine mainly within 24 hr of dosing; (3) urinary metabolites mainly conjugated with glucuronic acid (about 40%) with smaller amounts as sulfates (about 15%) and very small amounts (<3%) in a freely extractable form; (4) considerable excretion in the feces (up to 40%); (5) high concentrations in blood (about 10% of the dose during the first 4 hr after administration, decreasing only slowly with time, and with considerable levels (about 5%) still present at 24 hr; (6) most of the radioactivity in blood present in a freely extractable form; and (7) little if any metabolism of the ethynyl group.

Recent investigations have confirmed these findings (Reed et al., 1973; Mills et al., 1974, 1976; Braselton et al., 1977, 1979). Most studies have used radiolabelled NET, although some have used gas chromatography/mass spectrometry (GCMS) and unlabelled compounds. After administration of ^{3}H-NET, the half-life of elimination (T_{el}) of ^{3}H in blood had a mean value of 67 hr (range 43–84 hr). This value is a composite of T_{el} of a number of metabolites; since that of NET itself is much lower (Table 1), it does indicate that some metabolites are eliminated very slowly.

This suggests that, on long-term usage of NET, there may be an accumulation of these metabolites. The nature of these compounds has not been elucidated, but it seems likely that most if not all may be sulfate conjugates. About 3% of a dose may still be present in the circulation 4 days after administration of a single dose, suggesting that metabolites are turned over very slowly or retained in tissues. Much of the NET in the circulation is metabolized quickly: within 30 min of administration, most of the radioactivity can be extracted only after hydrolysis of the steroid extract. This may represent conjugates of reduced NET, but on the evidence available it seems that much of it represents NET sulfate.

Sulfate conjugates appear to predominate in blood and are present in much larger quantities than glucuronides (Reed et al., 1973). NET can be readily sulfated *in vitro* (Khan & Fotherby 1983b); both *in vitro* and *in vivo* sulfation occurred at the C-17β hydroxyl. Sulfate conjugates are also known to be turned over slowly. During the first 24 hr after administration, the proportion of sulfate conjugates in plasma remains constant at about 40 to 50% and the decrease in the free fraction is accompanied by a corresponding increase in the glucuronide fraction (Reed et al., 1973). Compounds other than NET are also present in the freely extractable fraction of plasma. The tetrahydro-reduced metabolites of NET (5β, 3α, the major isomer; 5β, 3β; 5α, 3β, and 5α, 3α) as well as the 5β-dihydrosteroids are present in plasma and urine, but in both fluids metabolites more polar than the tetrahydro steroids are present in larger quantities. These metabolites have not so far been identified. Surprisingly, some unchanged NET is present as sulfate or glucuronide conjugate in the urine.

The four tetrahydro metabolites are found in both blood and urine, the 3α isomers predominating over the 3β ones. After a 2 mg dose of NET, the concentration of 3α, 5β-TH NET was reported to be 22.8–33.9 ng/ml (Watanabe et al., 1983) and the tetrahydro metabolites are present in serum at a concentration about one tenth that of NET (Warren & Fotherby, 1975). In addition to unconjugated NET, both the sulfate and glucuronide are found in serum, but only small amounts of the dihydro metabolites, suggesting that these intermediates are rapidly reduced at C-3. The presence of the 17α-ethynyl group does not prevent sulfation of the 17β-hydroxyl, and sulfation of NET and other ethynyl steroids occurs at C-17 (Khan & Fotherby, 1983b). The mono- and disulfates of all four tetrahydro metabolites are found in blood, with the major ones being the disulfate of the 5α, 3α isomer and the monosulfate of the 5β, 3α isomer. The quantitative and dynamic relationship between NET and its metabolites and the sulfate conjugates requires further study. Whether or not any of the metabolites have biological activity or modify the activity of NET remains to be determined; preliminary reports suggest that they may have some activity (Cerbon et al., 1990; Garza-Flores et al., 1991).

Because of its importance pharmacologically and clinically, there has been considerable interest in the possibility that some NET may be metabolized to EE. Early investigations suggested that such a conversion occurred to an extent that could be important. However, later studies as well as analogous studies of the aromatization of norgestrel (Fotherby, 1974b) suggested that the earlier reports were erroneous and that any aromatization that did occur in humans was so small that it was of no clinical importance. More recently, the aromatization of NET to EE by human placental microsomes (Barbieri et al., 1983), by human liver homogenates (Yamamoto et al., 1988; Urabe et al., 1987), by human ovarian tissue (Yoshiji et al., 1987), and by human hepatocytes (Yamamoto et al., 1988) was demonstrated using methodology that did not result in any artefactual formation of the estrogen. In a preliminary study (Reed et al., 1990) the *in vivo* conversion of NET to EE in two postmenopausal women was demonstrated, to an extent of 0.4 to 2.27%. The higher conversion would result in a significant production of EE (20 μg) in women using a daily oral contraceptive containing 1 mg NET. Obviously, studies are required on a large number of premenopausal women to ascertain the range of conversion and to determine the possible clinical significance.

Assay

The most significant advance in our knowledge of NET pharmacokinetics was the development of RIA (Warren & Fotherby, 1974; Nygren et al., 1974). Many modifications of these original methods have been described (Garza-Flores et al., 1983), competitive protein binding (Okerholm et al., 1978), direct RIA (Pala & Benagiano, 1976), enzyme immunoassay (Turkes et al., 1980, 1982), RIA after HPLC separation (Watanabe et al., 1983; Saperstein et al., 1986; Lee et al., 1987). The RIA originally described used an iodine-labelled ligand, but later, with the availability of ^{3}H-NET of sufficiently high specific activity, the ^{3}H label was found to be more convenient and gave similar values when tested against the iodine label. The iodine label has the advantage that it reacts with some of the NET metabolites (Warren & Fotherby, 1975b; Morris & Cameron, 1975) and hence the RIA can be modified to estimate these metabolites. In a direct comparison, values for serum NET concentrations determined by RIA showed good agreement with those using a specific GC/MS method (Fotherby et al., 1979; Siekmann et al., 1980). Although it was reported (Bedolla-Tovar et al., 1978) that values obtained for NET levels in the same serum samples varied according to the source of the antiserum, this was not found in another study (Sankolli et al., 1979). A serious defect in the first of these studies and to a lesser extent in the second is that the antisera were not compared under the optimum conditions established for each antiserum.

Methods for measuring serum NET levels employing GC/MS have been described (Stillwell et al., 1974; Cook et al., 1975; Siekmann et al., 1980) and although these methods may be more specific than RIA, their cost, sensitivity, and general inconvenience render them less suitable than RIA for widespread use.

Serum Binding

Binding of the progestins in serum occurs mainly to albumin and SHBG. Binding to albumin is relatively weak, so that dissociation of the progestin occurs readily; the binding to SHBG is much stronger and variable, depending on the structure of the progestin, and dissociation occurs much less readily. *In vitro* determinations for NET suggest a concentration of binding sites of 1.53 nmol/mg albumin and an equilibrium dissociation constant (K_d) of 4.8 μmol/L. For SHBG, the binding site concentration was 0.22 nmol/mg protein and a K_d of 0.45 μmol/L (Jenkins & Fotherby, 1980; Li & Hümpel, 1990). The relative binding activity of NET to SHBG compared to 5α-dihydrotestosterone was 2.6%. Using ultracentrifugation-filtration of serum from women not taking OCs, about 61% of NET bound to albumin, 35.5% to SHBG, and 3.5% was unbound (Hammond et al., 1987). However, these values are likely to change in women using OCs containing EE, since the estrogen will increase the serum SHBG concentration. The magnitude of the increase in SHBG will depend on the relative dose of NET and EE, but for the two most widely-used formulations (NET 1 mg + EE 50 μg and NET 0.5 mg + EE 35 μg) the increase is of the order of 80 to 100% (Fotherby, 1988), and presumably under these conditions the proportion of NET bound to SHBG will increase at the expense of that bound o albumin. Changes in women using the NET-only pill will be insignificant since administration of much larger doses (3 and 5 mg) throughout a complete cycle led to only small decreases (approximately 30 and 40% respectively) in SHBG (Song Si et al., 1986).

NORETHINDRONE ENANTHATE (NET-EN)

This compound is used together with estrogen as a 1-month or 2-month injectable contraceptive or alone in a dose of 200 mg administered two or three monthly (see Chapter 9). Most of the NET-EN is hydrolysed to free NET by esterases in liver and other tissues, but not by muscle (Howard et al., 1975a; Bellman et al., 1976; Back et al., 1981). Plasma levels of NET after injection of NET-EN were reported by Howard et al. (1975b) and Weiner and Johansson (1975), and a detailed study of the kinetics and metabolism of NET-EN labelled with ^{3}H at C-7 was performed in two women by Gerhards et al (1976). Maximum levels of radioactivity occurred in plasma at 8 to 14 days after injection, and corresponded to NET concentrations of 0.7–1.0 μg/ml. NET-EN was also detected. The radioactivity was excreted in about equal proportions in urine and feces, but the majority of the dose could not be accounted for. Interestingly, only a minute proportion of the radioactivity in plasma could be accounted for as NET or NET-EN.

A large number of studies have measured serum concentrations of NET after injection of NET-EN (Howard et al., 1975b; Weiner & Johansson, 1975; Fotherby et al., 1978a,b; Goebelsmann et al., 1979; Fotherby et al., 1980; Fotherby, 1980; Werawatgoompa et al., 1980; Prasad et al., 1981; Fotherby & Koetsawang, 1982). The most comprehensive and detailed study was that of Sang et al. (1981). Uptake from the injection site was rapid, and peak concentrations of NET were reached within 8 days. The peak levels varied sixfold—from 4 to 26 ng/ml—with a mean of 11 ng/ml. The length of time that NET was detectable varied from 54 to 120 days (mean 74 days) and the elimination half-life varied from 7.5 to 22.5 days (mean

11.6 days). Much of the variability between subjects' plasma levels probably reflects variability in the dispersion of NET-EN.

Saxena et al. (1977) have described a direct RIA for the specific estimation of NET-EN. Peak concentrations of NET-EN were reached within 8 days and had a mean value of 5.2 ng/ml with a range of 0.8–15 ng/ml. They were always lower than peak values of NET, and showed a greater variability (Sang et al., 1981). NET-EN disappeared from plasma more rapidly than NET, the levels becoming undetectable in 19 to 73 days (mean 43 days), and the elimination half-life was shorter (2.4 to 16 days, mean 8 days). During the first 3 weeks after injection, the ratio of NET/NET-EN decreased, suggesting that NET-EN was absorbed more rapidly than its conversion to NET, and that it might be metabolised by other pathways. The presence of such large concentrations of NET-EN in the circulation over an extended period of time is surprising in view of the wide distribution and activity of tissue esterases. Hydrolysis of NET-EN was not complete even when plasma levels of the ester were low. Calculations suggested that only about 50% of the injected material was converted to NET.

Factors that may affect the pharmacokinetics and duration of action of injectable NET-EN have been examined in detail by Fotherby (1981).

NORETHINDRONE ACETATE

After oral administration, NET acetate is likely to be rapidly and completely hydrolysed to NET, although direct pharmacokinetic studies to support this idea do not appear to have been performed. Esterases capable of hydrolysing the ester are present in many tissues, particularly liver and intestine (Khan & Fotherby, 1980). Most probably, hydrolysis occurs mainly in the gastrointestinal tract, and any ester that escapes would be split by the liver. Studies in Indian women (Sarkar et al., 1983) who took a pill containing 1 mg NET acetate and 50 μg EE showed a peak concentration of 18.3 ± 4.8 ng/ml NET at 2 hr and a concentration of 2.2 ± 0.8 ng/ml at 24 hr. It will be noted that these values are somewhat higher than those shown in Table 1 after administration of an equivalent dose of NET. The values for distribution and elimination half-life were 1.2 ± 0.1 hr and 8.5 ± 1.5 hr respectively. In a previous study, Singh et al. (1979) gave ^{3}H-NET acetate intravenously to six women. Rapid hydrolysis of the ester occurred, although some appeared to escape hydrolysis, since the acetate was still detectable 72 hr after the injection. The mean elimination half-life for NET acetate was 51.5 ± 2.2 hr and that of NET was 34.8 ± 3.5 hr; this latter value is much higher than those shown in Table 1.

LYNESTRENOL (3-DESOXY NET, LYN)

This progestin is now seldom used, and the earlier reports showing its 3-oxidation to NET have been confirmed in more recent *in vivo* studies (Odlind et al., 1979; Shrimanker et al., 1980; Siekmann et al., 1980; Kuhl et al., 1982). All these reports showed the rapid conversion of most of the administered LYN to NET, although the methodology employed does not rule out the possibility that some was metabolised by other pathways. This possibility is supported by a further study with ^{14}C-LYN (Hümpel et al., 1977), which confirms earlier studies; 2.5 mg ^{14}C-LYN was administered orally together with 50 μg EE to six subjects. About 50% of the dose was excreted in urine and 39% in feces. Maximum radioactivity in the total plasma volume occurred at about 4 hr and corresponded to $10.4 \pm 1\%$ of the dose; this declined only slowly to $6.7 \pm 2.4\%$ at 24 hr, and about 3% was still present at 72 hr. The slow absorption was probably due to giving the dose in gelatin capsules. The slow decline in plasma radioactivity may indicate metabolic pathways for LYN other than via NET, although the results could be properly interpreted only if ^{14}C-NET had been similarly given to the subjects.

NORETHYNODREL

This compound was one of the first two 19-nor progestins to be synthesized, and was marketed as an oral contraceptive in 1960, although it had been used for gynecological purposes since 1957. (The same dates apply to norethindrone.) It differs structurally from NET only in having a C_{5-10} instead of a C_{4-5} double bond. After oral administration it disappears essentially completely from the plasma within 30 minutes; the conjugates, chiefly glucuronides, have longer half-lives. The principal free steroids found in plasma are the 3α- and 3β-hydroxy metabolites (Palmer et al., 1969; Cook et al 1972). The C_{5-10} compounds are readily converted to the C_{4-5} analogues norethindrone and ethynodiol, respectively. Although norethynodrel shows a different spectrum of biological activities in animal assays from norethindrone (Colton 1992), in humans it appears to act mainly as a pro-drug for norethindrone (Orme et al, 1983). The possibility that some norethynodrel is metabolised by pathways not involving NET as an intermediate has not been excluded, but there is no evidence in its favor. Norethynodrel was replaced by the more active compound, ethynodiol diacetate.

ETHYNODIOL DIACETATE (EDD)

This progestin also appears to be rapidly and quantitatively converted to NET in humans (Kishimoto et al., 1972; Cook et al., 1973; Walls et al., 1977; Vose et al., 1979; Cooke et al., 1985). Where measured, the peak and 24 hr concentrations of NET and time-to-peak concentration were similar to those after administration of an equivalent dose of NET. Cook et al. (1973) studied the metabolism of ^{3}H-EDD. Within 1 hr, no EDD was found in the plasma; NET was the principal free metabolite and four tetrahydro derivatives of NET were also identified.

LEVONORGESTREL (LNG)

Pharmacokinetics

The pharmacokinetic parameters reported in various papers are summarized in Table 2. The variability among these studies is very apparent, and this is partic-

TABLE 2. Pharmacokinetic parameters for LNG (values derived from published studies are mean ± SD or range; EE denotes ethynylestradiol; *values in l/Kg, + values in ml/h/Kg).

LNG dose (µg)	No. of subjects	'Peak' conc. (ng/ml)	24 h conc. (ng/ml)	Absorption time (h)	Td (h)	Tel (h)	Vd (l)	Cl (l/h)	AUC (ng/ml/h)	Ref.
30	5	0.9-2.0	0.05-0.14			13.7 (8-23)				1
75	3	1.5-1.9	0.2-0.5							2
250	6		0.2-0.7			19.3 (15.1-28.7)			24.3 (15.4-37.7)	3
750	6	9.0-2.2	1.6±0.8	2-4		8.9±1.9	88.6±25.6	7.2±2.7	116±41	4
750	10	11.2±3.4	1.6±0.6	1.9±0.6	1.3±0.6	13.3±3.7	115±41	6.1±1.9	124±43	5
750	10	16.0				14.5 (8.5-18.5)				6
1000	5	14-23	1.8-5.2			12.6 (9-20)				1
75+40µg EE	24	2.5 (1.5-5.3)		0.8 (0.3-3.0)		14(4-38)	1.7 (0.9-3.6)	86	15.5 (4-48)	7
150+30µg EE	3	3.6-4.2	0.6-0.9							2
150+30µg EE	5				1.0+0.2	11.4±1.3	1.9+0.3	105±16	20.4±3.0	9
150+30µg EE	9	3.8±1.2	0.3	2.4±1.0		8.0±3.2			20.2±7.8	10
150+30µg EE	24	3.2 (1.5-6.8)	0.5 (0.4-0.6)			18.0 (8-43)			35 (9-20)	11
150+30µg EE	6	3.2±1	0.36±0.07	1.3 (0.7-3.1)	1.7 (1.4-2.1)	25 (21-35)		5.8 (3.9-15.6)	32.3 (13.7-48.8)	12
150+50µg EE	5	2.6-14.4	0.5-2.3	1-2	5.1	81				8
250+30µg EE	6	4.6-16.2	0.6-1.9	1-2	4.3	62.7				8
250+50µg EE	6	7.1±2	1.2±0.4	2.2±1.3	3.0±0.6	26.4±8				13
250+50µg EE	3	6.3-8.0	1.6-1.9							2
250+50µg EE	5	3.3-5.1	0.3-0.7			12.6 (10-19)				1
250+50µg EE	6		2.8 (1.5-4.7)			30 (18-54)			100 (68-150)	3
250+50µg EE	5	5.1±0.5	0.8	1.2±0.4		11.9±1.7		5.8±2.6	36.2±12.8	14

References: 1, Weiner et al. (1976); 2, Brenner et al. (1977); 3, Dennerstein et al. (1980) and Fotherby (1990); 4, Shi et al. (1988); 5, He et al. (1990); 6, Landgren et al., (1989); 7, Stanczyk et al. (1990); 8, Nair et al. (1979); 9, Back et al. (1981); 10, Back et al. (1987a); 11, Goebelsmann et al. (1986); 12, Humpel et al. (1978); 13, Humpel et al. (1977); 14, Back et al. (1987b).

ularly true for the elimination half-life; excluding the extreme "outlier" values reported by Nair et al. (1979), the means vary from 8 to 30 hr but the variability among individual values is more than tenfold. The overall mean value is 16 hr. All studies agree that absorption is rapid (in most subjects less than 4 hr) but the factors that lead to the variability have not been ascertained. Unlike NET, LNG does not undergo a first-pass effect, a major contributor to inter-individual variability (Hümpel et al., 1978; Back et al., 1981).

There appears to be proportionality between the dose and peak serum concentration when LNG is coadministered with EE. Thus, from Table 2 the mean peak concentration for studies with LNG 150 μg and EE 30 μg was 3.5 ng/ml and that for LNG 250 μg and EE 50 μg was 5.9 ng/ml; however, this does not extend to LNG given without EE, since the mean peak value for LNG 750 μg alone was 12.1 ng/ml. The differences between LNG given alone or with EE are shown more clearly when the two formulations are administered to the same group of women (Dennerstein et al., 1980) and the possible reasons for the differences have been considered in more detail in a recent article (Fotherby, 1990b). Only limited data are available for the other pharmacokinetic parameters.

Mean serum concentrations of LNG after a dose of 150 μg with 30 μg EE, calculated from published reports, are shown in Figure 1; only limited data are available for steady-state concentrations.

Metabolism and Binding

The four tetrahydro metabolites of LNG were identified in urine by DeJongh et al. (1968), with the 3α, 5β-isomer as the major compound; monohydroxylated metabolites were also detected. A more detailed study (Sisenwine et al., 1975a) identified these monohydroxy metabolites as the 2α and 16β-hydroxysteroids. The tetrahydro metabolites are present in serum in concentrations about one-tenth those of LNG itself (Warren & Fotherby, 1975a). There was no evidence for the presence of phenolic metabolites when a procedure eliminating such artefacts was used (Sisenwine et al., 1974). Small amounts of LNG and its metabolites were present in plasma as sulfate and glucuronide conjugates. It is of interest that the metabolism of the biologically inactive L-(d)-norgestrel differs considerably from that of LNG, the biologically active D-(1)-enantiomer (Sisenwine et al., 1975a; Warren & Fotherby, 1975; Khan & Fotherby, 1983a), and LNG is sulfated more rapidly than the inactive isomer (Khan & Fotherby, 1983b).

Like NET, most of the LNG in blood is bound to albumin and SHBG; however, LNG binds to SHBG more avidly than NET and hence there is less to bind to albumin. *In vitro* determinations suggest that the concentration of binding sites in human serum is 1.48 nmol/mg albumin and 0.12 nmol/mg SHBG, with equilibrium dissociation constants of 3.49 μmol/L and 0.11 μmol/L, respectively (Jenkins & Fotherby, 1980; Li & Hümpel, 1990). The relative binding activity of LNG to SHBG compared to 5α-dihydrotestosterone was 14.3%. Using ultracentrifugation-filtration (Hammond et al., 1982) of serum from women not using OCs, about 50% of LNG was bound to albumin, 47.5% to SHBG, and 2.5% was unbound (see Table

6). Due to the strong antiestrogenic activity of LNG, increases in serum SHBG concentrations with OCs containing LNG and EE are less than with OCs containing other progestins. Indeed, the 250 μg LNG + 50 μg EE formulation produces a mean *decrease* of 24% in SHBG concentration; the 150 μg LNG + 30 μg EE formulation produces only a minor increase of about 10%, and the triphasic formulation of LNG and EE a more marked increase (Fotherby, 1990b). Daily administration of 750 μg LNG alone reduces serum SHBG levels by about 33% (He et al., 1990). Thus the proportion of LNG bound to albumin or SHBG or in the free state may vary markedly with different OC formulations. A comparison of binding and other pharmacokinetic parameters after a single dose and long-term treatment with 0.15 LNG and 0.03mg EE has been described by Kuhnz et al. (1992).

Assay

Radioimmunoassay (RIA) has been the preferred method (Warren & Fotherby, 1974; Stanczyk et al., 1975; Victor et al., 1975; Back et al., 1981; Kanluan et al., 1981) although a method based on GC/MS has been described (Tetsuo et al., 1980). As in the case of NET, iodine-labelled ligands were used initially in RIA (Warren & Fotherby, 1974) and a further comparison of tritium-labelled and iodine-labelled ligands for a number of steroids was reported by Stanczyk and Goebelsmann (1981). Standard curves with iodinated ligands were usually more sensitive than with tritium but were less precise. A direct assay that compares well with extraction techniques has been described (Watson & Stewart, 1988). Ten different antisera for LNG were compared by Sankolli et al. (1979).

MEDROXYPROGESTERONE ACETATE (MPA)

Pharmacokinetics

After intravenous injection of ^{3}H-MPA (Utaaker et al., 1988), serum levels of total radioactivity declined only slowly, whereas ether extractable radioactivity declined much more rapidly. From the latter, the MCR was calculated to be about 600 L/day and the volume of distribution 3.4 to 5.9 L. This value for the MCR is much lower than that reported by Gupta et al. (1979)—1668 ± 146—who point out many of the problems that are encountered in trying to determine the pharmacokinetic parameters of steroids with characteristics similar to MPA. Utaaker et al. (1988) showed that all the radioactivity in the ether extract was MPA; its concentration was still 0.07% of the dose per liter of serum 5 days after injection, corresponding to an elimination half-life of 48 to 72 hr. They interpret the findings as showing that MPA is stored in an outer compartment, possibly adipose tissue, from which it is only slowly released. Extracts of the residual water phase after β-glucuronidase hydrolysis contained all the radioactivity as MPA, and they suggest this was originally present as the 3-enol conjugate of MPA, as suggested also by the findings of Mathrubutham and Fotherby (1981) and Pannuti et al. (1984).

After an oral dose of 10 mg to each of five women (Victor & Johansson, 1976), peak concentrations of 1.2 to 5.2 ng/ml were measured within 2 hr. The decline to about 0.25 ng/ml over the next 10 hr was not exponential, making it difficult to calculate the plasma half-life. The elimination half-life for the period 12–48 hr was about 24 hr. Plasma levels at 48 hr were 0.07–0.11 ng/ml and were still detectable at 72–96 hr. These long half-lives and small values for V_d are surprising, considering that no specific binding of MPA occurs in blood (Akpoviroro et al., 1981; Mathrubutham & Fotherby, 1981); over 90% of MPA in blood is bound nonspecifically to albumin, with an apparent association constant of about 2.6×10^{-8} L/mol. The degree of binding was not decreased by the addition of MPA, cortisol, or dihydrotestosterone. The factors that regulate the level of unconjugated MPA in blood are unknown.

A summary of our values for serum MPA concentrations after injection of DepoProvera is shown in Table 3. After injection of 150 mg, MPA is still detectable at the end of the 90-day injection interval in almost all subjects. For all doses of DepoProvera, MPA levels are high, showing a rapid release from the injection site. The factors that regulate the uptake of MPA from the injection site are probably similar to those operative with NET-EN (Fotherby, 1981), except that no hydrolysis

TABLE 3. *Serum concentrations of MPA (ng/ml) after injection of various doses of DepoProvera or of CycloProvera (MPA 25 mg with estradiol cypionate 5 mg). Values are mean for number of subjects (n) indicated, time (days) detectable denotes number of days after injection for which serum MPA concentrations exceeded 100 pg/ml*

Time after injection (weeks)	Depo Provera (mg MPA)				Cyclo Provera (mg MPA)
	150	100	50	25	25
1	7.0	4.5	2.5	1.2	0.65
2	5.2	4.0	1.05	0.95	0.52
3	3.8	3.0	0.8	0.6	0.35
4	2.6	2.5	0.6	(0.5	(0.20
				(0.8[c]	(1.03[d]
5	2.3	2.0	0.5	0.3	1.32[e]
6	1.7	1.5	0.25	0.2	
7	1.2	0.95	0.18	0.15	
8	0.9	0.7	0.11		
9	0.7	0.5			
10	0.6	0.32			
11	0.45	0.2			
12	(0.38	0.14			
	(0.6[a]				
	(0.9[b]				
Time (days) detectable	63-434	76-140	43-68	32-80	28-62
n	25	5	5	5	12
Reference	1, 2, 3	1	1	1	4

[a, b]values relate to 10 subjects after a single injection of DepoProvera and 11 subjects after 8 injections of DepoProvera (ref. 5).

[c]values related to 5 subjects after a single injection of DepoProvera (ref. 5).

[d, e]values relate to 10 subjects after a single injection of CycloProvera and 21 subjects after 31 to 45 injections (ref. 5).

References to Table: 1. Fotherby et al. 1980; 2. Koetsawang et al. 1982; 3. Fotherby and Koetsawang 1982; 4. Fotherby et al. 1982; 5. Koetsawang et al. 1979.

of MPA is necessary for it to become biologically active. It will also be seen from Table 3 that there is little difference between serum concentrations for the 150 and 100 mg doses or the 50 and 25 mg doses; the differences are not statistically significant due to the wide scatter of values. Similarly, there is little difference between the two groups of dose levels when the duration over which MPA was detected in blood was calculated. For the 150 mg dose particularly, there was a wide variation (almost 7-fold) in the duration of detectability. Although the number of studies at doses less than 150 mg is small, similar findings have been reported by Bassol et al. (1984); their serum concentrations are lower than ours (mean peak concentrations of 1000, 1000, 600, and 300 pg/ml for doses of 150, 100, 50, and 25 mg, respectively), and consequently the time over which MPA was detectable in serum was longer (mean durations of 140, 140, 55, and 88 days, respectively).

Other studies (Kirton & Cornette, 1974; Ortiz et al., 1977; Benagiano et al., 1980; Fotherby et al., 1980; Lan et al., 1984) have shown that, in some women, MPA is detectable in serum for 200 days or more after injection of 150 mg. This contrasts with other studies (Jeppsson et al., 1977, 1982) in which plasma MPA levels at the end of the 12-week injection interval were low even in long-term users, and there was no accumulation of MPA. It had been previously suggested (Koetsawang et al., 1979) that subjects who absorb DepoProvera quickly from the injection site show high serum concentrations with the first few days of injection and are the ones who have low levels by the end of the 90-day interval, whereas those in whom the uptake is slow have lower initial serum values that decrease only slowly, and are therefore detectable for an extended duration.

Serum levels of MPA are also very variable after injection of CycloProvera (Table 3) but MPA is still detectable in almost all women at the end of the 28-day injection interval. It seems likely that serum levels of MPA are not different when the progestin is administered with or without estrogen, although no direct comparative study has been reported. Results similar to ours have been reported by Aedo et al. (1985); the mean maximum level was 1.0 ng/ml (range 0.84–1.3 ng/ml); measurable levels were found in all subjects at the end of the injection interval (mean value 0.26 ng/ml), and may remain detectable for up to 90 days.

Metabolism

A recent paper (Utaaker et al., 1988) reported studies in humans of both oral and intravenous ^{3}H-MPA. After oral administration, maximum levels of radioactivity were reached at 2 hr and corresponded to 1% of the dose per liter; total radioactivity remained at these levels for at least 48 hr. MPA and a more polar metabolite were detected by TLC in ether extracts of serum. Hydrolysis of the residual water phase with β-glucuronidase followed by TLC showed that most of the radioactivity was associated with metabolites more polar that MPA. This finding is in agreement with those of Mathrubutham and Fotherby (1981): They found that a mean value of 83% of the assayable MPA in serum extracts could be accounted for as MPA, and the remainder as more polar metabolites. Conjugated MPA was also present in serum and accounted for about 80% of the assayable MPA together with more polar metabolites. There was also evidence for sulfate conjugates. The concentration of conjugated MPA in blood was almost as high as that present in the unconjugated fraction. Chromatographic evidence suggested that the more polar metabolites were ring A-reduced steroids, and this is supported by the work of Utaaker et al. (1988) and Martin et al. (1980). During the first 3 days after oral administration, only 15 to 22% of the dose of ^{3}H-MPA was recovered in the urine (Utaaker et al., 1988) and this agrees with previous findings that excretion in the bile and feces (45 to 80% of the dose is reported to be eliminated in the feces) is more important than urinary excretion. After intravenous injection, 25 to 50% was recovered in urine within 3 days (Utaaker et al., 1988).

Assay

A number of different methods have been used for the assay of MPA: GLC (Kaiser et al., 1974; Pannuti et al., 1978; Rossi et al., 1979); HPLC (Milano et al., 1982; Read et al., 1985; Camaggi et al., 1985); and GC/MS (Phillipou & Frith, 1980; Dikkeschei et al., 1985). Although these methods have a high specificity, they lack sensitivity, so that their use is limited to high-dose studies, but they are unsuitable for the doses of MPA used in contraception. RIA has the required sensitivity and specificity. The first RIA was described by Cornette et al. (1971) but lacked specificity mainly because it was a direct assay—i.e., without extraction. Subsequent methods (Royer et al., 1974; Hiroi et al., 1975; Ortiz et al., 1977; Shrimanker et al., 1978) employed extraction techniques and different antisera. The specificity of the assay described by Shrimanker et al. has been thoroughly assessed (Mathrubutham & Fotherby, 1981) and the results obtained by its use show a good correlation with a GC method (Kozyreff, 1982) and with a method based on GC/MS (Dikkeschei et al., 1985). Many of the possible metabolites do not interfere in this RIA and results obtained after extraction of serum agree with those obtained by a "direct" assay. Utaaker et al. (1988) found, with this RIA, that values obtained from untreated serum or alcohol extracts were more than fourfold those from hexane extracts. These data suggest that any RIA used for MPA measurement need to be thoroughly evaluated for specificity.

NORGESTIMATE (NGM)

Pharmacokinetics and Metabolism

NGM is the 17-acetoxy-3-oxime of LNG, and the extent to which it acts as a prodrug for LNG or LNG-3-oxime has not been studied in detail. The metabolism of NGM labelled with ^{14}C in the ethynyl group was studied after oral administration in four women, and combined with EE in three women. Peak plasma levels of radioactivity were attained within 2 hr, with a rapid decline over the next 6 hr; thereafter, the levels remained fairly constant for 14 hr (Weintraub et al., 1978). The half-life of radioactivity in plasma varied from 45 to 71 hr, although it is not stated to what time period this refers. During the 2 weeks following administration, 35 to 49% was recovered in the urine and 16 to 49% in the feces. Much of the material in feces may have undergone an enterohepatic recirculation. Further examination of urine from subjects receiving NGM alone was reported by Alton et al. (1984). About 12% of the urinary radioactivity was freely extractable, and 57% recovered as conjugates. Almost all the metabolites retained the ethynyl group, although there was presumptive evidence of D-homoannulation.

By GC/MS, the major metabolites were established as LNG, 3α, 5β-tetrahydro-LNG, and trihydroxy compounds; minor metabolites were identified as 16β-hydroxy LNG, 2α-hydroxy LNG, and 3,16-dihydroxy-5α-tetrahydro LNG. Neither intact NGM nor metabolites retaining the oxime group were detected in urine. This extensive metabolism of NGM and the identification of LNG and its metabolites suggests that to some extent NGM is a prodrug for LNG. 17-deacetylated NGM shows a pharmacological profile similar to that of NGM and different from that of LNG and LNG 17-acetate (McGuire et al., 1990).

In vitro, intestinal tissue metabolizes NGM; after 2 hr incubation, 46% of NGM was unchanged and 41% had undergone hydrolysis to LNG-oxime, while only minor amounts were recovered as LNG and LNG acetate. Similar results are obtained on incubating NGM with liver microsomes (Back et al., 1990; Madden & Back, 1991). Steroid oximes are readily hydrolysed under acidic conditions even at 37°C (Khan & Fotherby, 1978) so that considerable hydrolysis may occur in the stomach after oral administration.

A preliminary pharmacokinetic study in women suggests, however, that while hydrolysis of the 17-acetate occurs readily, hydrolysis of the oxime is much slower (McGuire et al., 1990). Doses of 0.18 mg NGM with 35 μg EE were given orally to 10 women and the serum concentrations of NGM and 17-deacetyl NGM were estimated by HPLC and RIA. Mean NGM peak concentrations of about 100 pg/ml were reached within 1 hr, both after single dose and at steady state; there followed a rapid decline and NGM became undetectable at 5 hr. In contrast, peak concentrations of the 17-deacetyl NGM were about 4000 pg/ml at 1 hr, declined rapidly up to 5 hr, and then remained at plateau levels of about 1000 pg/ml up to 36 hr, with an estimated elimination half-life of 16 to 17 hr.

Other studies estimated the fraction of metabolites in the blood as norgestrel oxime, $10.6 \pm 1.8\%$; norgestrel acetate, $9.5 \pm 1.7\%$; and norgestrel, $15.4 \pm 5.4\%$. The blood level of norgestimate itself was less than 0.4% and had completely disappeared within 6 hr. Based on the biological activity of the metabolites, it was believed that the activity of norgestimate is primarily due to norgestrel and norgestrel acetate, with up to 85% of the activity due to the latter compound. Many more pharmacokinetic studies of NGM are required, and the biological activity of the various metabolites needs to be elucidated.

NGM, 17-deacetyl NGM, and the 3-keto metabolites have little affinity for SHBG, and they do not inhibit the EE-induced increase in serum SHBG concentrations (Phillips et al., 1990)

TABLE 4. *Reported pharmacokinetic parameters for DSG after administration of 150 μg DSG + 30 μg EE*

No. of subjects	Peak conc.	24h conc.	Absorption time (L)	Tel (h)	Vd (l)	Cl (l/h)	AUC (ng/ml/h)	Ref
10	6.4 + 1.7	1.0 + 0.8	1.8 + 0.8				45 + 24	1
9	2.0 + 0.7	0.2 + 0.1		11.9 + 4.1		8.7 + 2.9	14.2 + 5.5	2
11								3
25	3.7 + 1.0		1.6 + 1.0	23.8 + 5.3			36 + 8	4
23				22 + 6	88 + 39[a]	5.0 + 1.9		5
13					143 + 61[b]	9.5 + 5.0		6

References: 1 Hassenack et al. 1986; 2 Back et al. 1987; 2 Kuhl et al, 1988; 4 Bergink et al, 1990; 5 Timmer et al. 1990; 6 Back and Orme, 1991.
[a]Values obtained after i.v administration to 4 subjects. [b]Values obtained after single dose i.v. administration.

DESOGESTREL (DSG)

Pharmacokinetics

Reported pharmacokinetic parameters for DSG after its administration with EE are shown in Table 4. All studies except that of Back et al. (1987) were performed under steady-state conditions. It is apparent that serum concentrations, and hence AUC and T_{e1}, are lower under single-dose conditions than under steady state. Kuhl et al. (1988) have performed a detailed study of the serum concentrations of DSG in 11 women; samples were taken on days 1, 10, and 21 of the 1st, 3d, 6th, and 12th cycle of treatment with 150 μg DSG + 30 μg EE. Peak concentrations were usually reached within 2 hr and the mean value after the first dose (equivalent to single-dose administration) was about 1.3 ng/ml compared to 2.5 ng/ml on days 10 and 21 (equivalent to steady-state conditions). Mean $AUC_{0-24\ hr}$ value after the first dose was 14.3 ng/ml hr compared to 30 ng/ml hr at steady state. Serum concentrations of DSG increased from Day 1, reaching a maximum at day 10, and were significantly higher during the 3rd and 6th cycle of treatment than during cycle 1, but thereafter no further increase occurred. There was no correlation between height, weight, and age of the subjects and the serum DSG concentrations. Changes in the serum concentrations of DSG are shown in Fig. 1.

Metabolism

DSG is a prodrug (Viinikka et al., 1976) and in humans is rapidly and almost quantitatively converted to the biologically active metabolite, 3-keto DSG. Values quoted in this chapter refer to the 3-keto compound unless specifically stated otherwise.

The metabolism of ^{3}H-DSG was studied by Viinikka et al. (1979, 1980). The labelled compound was administered with 50 μg EE and the administration was repeated a month later after the subjects had been ingesting this formulation daily for 10 days to achieve steady-state conditions. The amount of radioactivity recovered in urine and feces after a single dose ($48.1 \pm 5.2\%$ and $34.9 \pm 2.7\%$, respec-

TABLE 5. *Reported pharmacokinetic*

GSD dose (μg)	No. of subjects	Peak conc.	24h conc	Absorption time(h)
75 (iv)	6			
25 + 30 μgEE	6	1.0 + 0.4	0.2	1.9 + 1.2
75 + 30 "	6	3.6 + 1.4	0.5	1.7 + 1.2
75 + 30[a] "	1			
75 + 30 "	1			
100 + 30 "	10	7.2 + 3.2		1.3 + 1.1
100 + 30[a] "	10	18.2 + 4.5		0.8 + 0.4
125 + 30 "	6	7.0 + 2.2	1.0	1.4 + 1.2
75 + 30 " (iv)	13			

tively) was slightly but significantly higher than under steady-state conditions $(45.2 \pm 6.5\%$ and $30.9 \pm 1.7\%$, respectively). A high proportion of the urinary radioactivity (14 to 28%) was present in an unconjugated form, with 38 to 61% as glucuronides and 23 to 39% as sulfates. In contrast to urine, levels of total radioactivity in blood were higher under steady-state conditions (peak concentration 4.5 to 5.1% of dose, 24 hr concentration 1.3 to 1.6%) than after a single dose (3.2 to 5.0% and 1.0 to 1.25% for urine and feces, respectively). Almost all the radioactivity in plasma could be accounted for as 3-keto DSG. The half-lives of absorption, distribution, and elimination were computed to be 0.2, 1.5, and 16 hr, respectively.

DSG can be readily converted to 3-keto DSG by human liver reparations (Viinikka, 1979; Madden et al., 1990) and by the intestinal tract (Madden et al., 1989); more polar metabolites, presumably hydroxylated, were also detected. After oral administration of 2.5 mg DSG to one subject (Viinikka, 1978), a peak concentration of 12.7 ng/ml was obtained at 1.5 hr, declining to 1 ng/ml at 12 hr; DSG itself was detected only briefly (up to 3 hr), with a peak concentration of less than 1 ng/ml. Confirmation of the *in vivo* conversion was provided in three studies; Back et al. (1978) reported a mean conversion of $76 \pm 22\%$ (range 40–113%) in 9 women; Hassenack et al. (1986) found similar concentrations of 3-keto DSG in blood after administration of DSG or 3-keto DSG to 10 women; and Timmer et al. (1990) a mean conversion of $81 \pm 27\%$ (range 49–108%) in four women.

Based upon ultrafiltration studies, $66 \pm 12\%$ of DSG was bound to albumin, $31.5 \pm 12\%$ to SHBG, and $2.5 \pm 0.2\%$ was unbound (Kuhnz, 1990); these studies were performed on women on long-term treatment with DSG and EE, and therefore take into account the threefold increase in serum SHBG concentrations that occur with this formulation.

Assay

A number of radioimmunoassays for DSG have been described; antisera raised against 3-keto DSG have been used with an iodinated ligand (Viinikka, 1978) and parmeters for GSD

Td (h)	Tel (h)	Vd (l)	Cl (l/h/kg)	AUC (ng/ml/h)	Ref
1.5 + 1.4	10.0 + 2.3	0.7 + 0.4[b]	0.05 + 0.01	35 + 15	1
1.0 + 0.7	13.9 + 2.9			10.6 + 5	1
0.8 + 0.5	11.8 + 2.3			35 + 16	1
1.5 + 1.0	18.2 + 4.2				2
1.6 + 1.4	10.6 + 6.0				2
	15.8 + 4.9	32 + 19	0.03 + 0.01	74 + 37	3
	22.0 + 4.1			422 + 178	3
1.3 + 1.1	13.9 + 2.7			62 + 21	1
		47 + 24	3.4 + 1.5		4

References: 1. Tauber et al. 1989; 2. Dusterberg et al. 1987; 3. Kuhnz, 1990; 4. Back and Orme, 1991
[a]Steady state studies, all others single dose;
[b]in l/kg.

with tritiated ligands (Kuhl et al., 1988; Berginck et al., 1990). Shaw et al. (1985) used an antiserum raised against LNG with ^{3}H-3-ketoDSG as labelled ligand. HPLC of 3-keto DSG was described by Madden et al. (1989).

GESTODENE (GSD)

Pharmacokinetics and Metabolism

GSD is completely absorbed and appears not to undergo a first-pass effect. After intravenous administration, plasma GSD concentrations decreased in three phases, with mean half-lives of 0.16, 1.5, and 10 hr. After oral administration to the same subjects, the mean value for absolute bioavailability was 99%, although there was a large inter-subject variation (Tauber et al., 1989). When doses of GSD of 25, 75, and 125 μg were given orally with 30 μg EE, there was proportionality between dose and peak serum levels. The bioavailability was also reported to be $87 \pm 19\%$ (Back & Orme, 1991). Reported pharmacokinetic parameters for GSD are summarized in Table 5. Kuhl et al. (1988) have performed a detailed study of the serum concentrations of GSD in 11 women which is similar to but not concurrent with the study described above for DSG. Absorption of GSD appeared to be slower than that of DSG, with values for Tmax up to 4 hr. Serum concentrations of GSD were much higher than for DSG with approximate mean values of 5.7 ng/ml after a single dose and 12.4 ng/ml at steady state. This led to very high values for AUC_{0-24}; approximately 80 ng/ml hr after a single dose and 210 ng/ml hr at steady state. As with DSG, there was no correlation between height, weight, and age of the subjects and the serum concentration. Changes in serum concentrations of GSD are shown in Fig. 1.

With respect to serum binding, more GSD is bound to SHBG than any other progestin. After a single dose of GSD, $47.8 \pm 7.5\%$ was bound to albumin, $50.3 \pm 7.8\%$ to SHBG, and $1.9 \pm 0.3\%$ was unbound, compared to values of $24.1 \pm 0.1\%$, $75.3 \pm 9.1\%$, and $0.6 \pm 0.1\%$ under steady-state conditions (Li & Hümpel, 1990; Tauber et al., 1990).

The metabolism of a single oral dose (500 μg) of GSD, labelled with ^{14}C in the ethynyl group was studied in three women by Düsterberg et al. (1987). Urinary elimination was complete within 7 days and accounted for 50% of the dose. Little if any GSD was excreted unmetabolized, and the metabolites were mainly sulfate (40%) and glucuronide (25%) conjugates and some freely extractable metabolites (25%). A large number of metabolites was produced, based on HPLC analysis of urine extracts. These were mainly hydroxylated metabolites of ring-A reduced (tetrahydro) GSD. Both mono- and dihydroxylated compounds were formed, with hydroxylation occurring at, among others, C-1, C-6, and C-11. D-homoannulation was a minor reaction, but apart from this, no metabolism of the C-15 double bond or ethynyl group occurred, and there was no evidence for conversion to levonorgestrel. About 33% of the dose was recovered from the feces. In plasma, most of the radioactivity was associated with unchanged GSD, but more polar metabolites and also conjugates were detected.

Assay

An RIA for GSD has been described by Nieuweboer et al. (1989) and by Kuhl et al. (1988).

CONCLUSIONS

Despite the numerous studies that have been performed, our knowledge of the pharmacokinetics of the contraceptive steroids is still meager. To take two examples: (1) most of the metabolites of any of the progestins are still inadequately characterized, and (2) the derivation and interpretation of even the simplest pharmacokinetic parameters leaves much to be desired. The second problem arises as a result of study designs, deficiencies in the models used to derive the parameters, especially for compounds with a first-pass effect (see Chapter on ethynyl estrogens), and the many factors that may affect the results. These problems have been discussed elsewhere (Fotherby, 1990a,b,c; 1991).

The progestins are rapidly absorbed, with peak serum concentrations usually being reached within 2 hr, but in some subjects not until 4 hr or more. The effect of diet on absorption needs further study, but is unlikely to be so large as to cause the variation seen in the rate of absorption. NET and DSG undergo a first-pass effect whereas others—for example, LNG and GSD—do not; what determines this difference in a series of closely related compounds is unclear. Enterohepatic recirculation is not important for the progestins, and is unlikely to affect peak serum concentrations.

Although less information is available for the distribution half-life, the values

TABLE 6. *Pharmacokinetic characteristics of gestagens*

	NET	LNG	DSG	GSD
Half-life of elimination (h)	7	16	20	12
Clearance (l/h)	22	6	7	3
Vol. of distribution (l)	240	120	110	32
RBA-SHBG[a]	2.5	12	5	17
Binding in serum %				
albumin	61.0	50.0	64.7	23.3
SHBG	35.5	47.5	31.8	76.0
unbound	3.5	2.5	3.5	0.7

Values are approximate and useful for comparative purposes to show differences among the gestagens. As indicated in text, they will show large variations depending on methodology used and conditions under which they were derived. Insufficient data available for MPA and NGM.
[a]Relative binding affinity compared to 5α-dihydrotestosterone as standard (100).

appear to be more consistent, with mean values varying from 0.8 to 1.6 hr for GSD, to 1.0 to 1.7 hr for LNG and NET, although aberrant values have been reported (Tables 1 and 2). This lack of a distinct difference between the progestins is surprising, in view of the large differences in volume of distribution. The values do suggest, however, that distribution is a rapid process.

Far greater differences are seen in the elimination half-life, both between the progestins and among the values reported for each one. Mean values for GSD reported in 8 investigations varied from 10.0 to 22.0 hr, even though all the studies were performed in the same institution, presumably using the same methodology and in similar subjects. Mean values for LNG also show a similar wide variation (8 to 30 hr), but interstudy mean values are much more consistent. Less information is available for the other pharmacokinetic parameters, which are compared in Table 6.

Marked differences in serum concentrations of the progestins are noted, and these are summarized in Figure 1. The values relate to the doses in the most widely-used OCs. It is clear that the serum concentrations show no correlation with dose: GSD, which is used in the lowest dose (75 μg) produces higher concentrations than 1000 μg NET. For NET, LNG and DSG, the concentrations, even under steady-state conditions, appear to be less than 1 ng/ml 24 hr after administration, whereas those with GSD are much higher. The high values for GSD are undoubtedly due to its low V_d. However, discrepancies exist between the serum concentrations, V_d, and the degree of binding in serum. It should be emphasized that values for the latter are based on very few studies and wide differences are to be expected among subjects since there are not only differences in the rate and extent to which the progestins bind to and dissociate from SHBG (Juchem & Pollow, 1990) but also differences in the extent to which serum SHBG concentrations are raised by the various OCs. Serum SHBG levels show a wide variation in untreated subjects, and are affected by many different factors (Moore & Bulbrook, 1988). The distribution of a progestin between the two proteins and the unbound state will depend on whether the determinations were done on serum from women prior to starting treatment or after a few months of medication, when stable levels of SHBG have been attained. In addition, there will be large intersubject variability in the response of SHBG to the same OC.

The serum concentrations of the progestins, and thus their pharmacokinetic parameters, are likely to be affected by many factors (Fotherby, 1990c), almost all of which have not been adequately investigated. Most of the studies have been single-dose, and the parameters may differ significantly from those pertaining to steady-state conditions, which are more relevant to OC use. It is not widely recognized that the pharmacokinetics of the progestin will be partly determined by the formulation (relative doses of progestin and estrogen).

It has usually been thought that the large intersubject variability is genetic in origin, although evidence to support this is meager. This inference has also been questioned recently on the basis of intrasubject variability that has been demonstrated for the contraceptive steroids (Brody et al., 1989; Fotherby, 1990b, 1991b; Jung-Hoffman & Kuhl, 1990), since this variability may be almost as large as the intersubject variability.

REFERENCES

Aedo AR, Landgren BM, Johannisson E, Diczfalusy E: Pharmacokinetic and pharmacodynamic investigations with monthly injectable contraceptive preparations. *Contraception* 1985;31:453–469.

Akpovororo JO, Mangalam M, Jenkins N, Fotherby K: Binding of MPA and ethynyl oestradiol in blood of various species. *J Steroid Biochem* 1981;14:493–498.

Alton KB, Hetyei NS, Shaw C, Patrick JE: Biotransformation of norgestimate in women. *Contraception* 1984;29:19–29.

Back DJ, Breckenridge AM, Chapman CR et al.: Enzymatic cleavage of NET oenanthate. *Contraception* 1981;23:125–132.

Back DJ, Breckenridge AM, Crawford FE et al.: Kinetics of norethindrone in women. *Clin Pharm Therap* 1978a;24:439–453.

Back DJ, Grimmer SF, Rogers S et al.: Pharmacokinetics of levonorgestrel and ethinyloestradiol after intravenous, oral and vaginal administration. *Contraception* 1978b;36:471–479.

Back DJ, Bates M, Breckenridge AM: Pharmacokinetics of levonorgestrel and ethinyloestradiol in women. *Contraception* 1981;23:229–239.

Back DJ, Killick SR, Stevenson PJ, et al.: Bioavailability of levonorgestrel and ethinyloestradiol from tablets and capsules. *Contraception* 1987a;36:321–326.

Back DJ, Grimmer SFM, Sheppy N, Orme ML: Plasma concentrations of 3-keto desogestrel after oral administration of desogestrel. *Contraception* 1987;35:619–625.

Back DJ, Ward S, Orme M: Recent pharmacokinetic studies of low-dose oral contraceptives. In: Proc Worksh oral contracept and cardiovascular dis. Zatuchni GI, Elstein M (eds). Dordrecht: Kluwer Acad Publ, 1991; vol 7 suppl 3, pp. 164–179.

Barbieri RL, Petro Z, Carmick JA, Ryan DJ: Aromatization of norethindrone by human placental microsomes. *J Clin Endocrinol Metab* 1983;57:299–303.

Bassol S, Garza-Flores J, Cravioto MC et al.: Ovarian function after administration of DMPA at different doses. *Fertil Steril* 1984;42:216–222.

Bedolla-Tovar N, Rahman SA, Cekan SZ, Diczfalusy E: Assessment of the specificity of norethindrone radioimmunoassays. *J Steroid Biochem* 1978;9:561–567.

Bellman O, Duhme HJ, Gerhards E: In vitro studies on enzymatic cleavage of steroid esters. *Acta Endocrinol* 1976;81:839–853.

Bergink W, Bos ES, Klosterboer H et al.: Comparison of the metabolic effects of desogestrel and levonorgestrel in low-dose oral contraceptives. In: *Oral Contraceptives and Lipoproteins.* Geneva: International Health Found, 1983

Bergink W, Assendorp R, Kloosterboer L et al. :Pharmacokinetics of orally administered desogestrel. *Am J Obstet Gynecol* 1990;163:2132–2137.

Braselton WE, Lin TJ, Mills TM et al.: Identification by GC-MS of norethindrone and metabolites in humans. *J Steroid Biochem* 1977;8:9–18.

Braselton WE, Lin TJ, Ellegood JO et al.: Accumulation of norethindrone in plasma during short- and long-term administration. *Am J Obstet Gynecol* 1979;133:154–160.

Brenner PF, Mishell DR, Stanczyk F, Goebelsmann U: Serum levels of levonorgestrel, FSH, LH, estradiol and progesterone after taking oral contraceptives containing norgestrel. *Am J Obstet Gynecol* 1977;129:133–140.

Breuer H: Metabolic pathways of contraceptive drugs. In: *Pharmacology of Steroid Contraceptive Drugs*. Garattini S, Berendes HW (eds). New York: Raven Press, 1977.

Brody SA, Turkes A, Goldzieher JW: Pharmacokinetics of three bioequivalent norethindrone/mestranol and three norethindrone/ethinyl estradiol formulations. *Contraception* 1989;40:269–284.

Cerbon MA, Pasapera AM, Segal RG et al.: Variable expression of the uteroglobin gene after administration of norethindrone and its metabolites. *J Steroid Biochem* 1990;36:1–6.

Camaggi CM, Strocchi E, Canova N et al.: Medroxyprogesterone acetate plasma levels after multiple high-dose administration. *Cancer Chemother Pharmacol* 1985;14:229–231.

Colton FB: Steroids and "the Pill": Early research at Searle. *Steroids* 1992;57:624–630.

Cook CE, Twine ME, Tallent CR et al: Norethynodrel metabolites in human plasma and urine. *J Pharm Exp Therap* 1972;183:197–205.

Cook CE, Karim A, Forth J et al: Ethynodiol diacetate metabolites in plasma. *J Pharmacol Exp Ther* 1973;185:696–702.

Cook CE, Truman J, Dickey MC et al.: Norethindrone plasma levels in human subjects. *Life Sci* 1975;15:1621–1629.

Cooke ID, Back DJ, Shroff NE: Norethisterone concentrations in breast milk during ethynodiol diacetate administration. *Contraception* 1985;31:611–619.

Cornette JC, Kirton KT, Duncan GW: Measurement of medroxyprogesterone acetate by radioimmunoassay. *J Clin Endocrinol Metab* 1971;33:459–466.

DeJongh DC, Hribar JD, Littleton P et al.: Identification of some human metabolites of norgestrel. *Steroids* 1968;11:649–666.

Dennerstein L, Fotherby K, Burrows G et al.: Plasma levels of ethynyloestradiol and norgestrel during hormone replacement therapy. *Maturitas* 1980;2:147–154.

Dibbelt L, Knuppen R, Jutting G et al.: Group comparison of serum ethinylestradiol, SHBG and CBG levels in women using low-dose oral contraceptives. *Contraception* 1991;43:1–21.

Dikkeschie LD, Van Veelen H, Nagel GT et al.: Determination of medroxyprogesterone acetate in serum by GC/MS. *J Chromatog* 1985;345:1–10.

Düsterberg B, Tack JW, Krause W, Hümpel M: Pharmacokinetics and biotransformation of gestodene in man. In: *Gestodene*. Elstein M, (ed). Carnforth, England: Parthenon Publishing Group Ltd, 1987, pp. 35–44.

El-Raghy I, Back DJ, Makeram M et al.: Pharmacokinetics of oral contraceptives in Egyptian women. *Contraception* 1986;33:379–384.

Fotherby K: Metabolism of synthetic steroids in animals and man. *Acta Endocr* 1974a;(Suppl)185:119–142.

Fotherby K: Metabolism of 19-norsteroids to oestrogenic steroids. In: Proc 2nd Intern Norgestrel Symp. Excerpta Med Int Congr Series 344, 1974b, pp. 30–34.

Fotherby K: Pharmacokinetics of norethisterone oenanthate and its effects on ovarian function. In: Workshop on Fert Contr, Royal Soc Med Int Symp Series no.31 1980, pp. 73–80.

Fotherby K: Factors affecting the duration of action of norethisterone oenanthate. *Contracept Deliv Syst* 1981;2:249–257.

Fotherby K: Variability of pharmacokinetic parameters for contraceptive steroids. *J Steroid Biochem* 1983;19:817–820.

Fotherby K: A new look at progestogens. *Clin Obstet Gynaecol* 1984;11:701–722.

Fotherby K: Pharmacokinetics of progestational compounds. *Maturitas* 1986;8:123–132.

Fotherby K; Interactions of contraceptive steroids with steroid-binding proteins and the clinical implications. *NY Acad Sci* 1988a;538:313–324.

Fotherby K: Clinical pharmacology of gestagens. In: *Female Contraception*. Rünnebaum B, Rabe T, Kiesel L (eds). Berlin: Springer-Verlag, 1988b, pp. 122–128.

Fotherby K: Potency and pharmacokinetics of gestagens. *Contraception* 1990a;41:533–550.

Fotherby K: Pharmacokinetics gestagens: some problems. *Am J Obstet Gynecol* 1990b;163:323–328.

Fotherby K: Intrasubject variability in the pharmacokinetics of ethynyloestradiol. *J Steroid Biochem* 1991b;38:733–736.

Fotherby K: Pharmacokinetics and pharmacodynamics in drug development. In: Proc workshop on oral contracept and cardiovasc dis. Zatuchni GI, Elstein M (eds). Dordrecht: Kluwer Acad Publ, 1991a; vol 7, Suppl 3, pp. 107–115.

Fotherby K, Benagiano G, Toppozada HK et al.: A preliminary pharmacological trial of CycloProvera. *Contraception* 1982;25:261–273.

Fotherby K, Howard G, Shrimanker K et al.: Plasma levels of norethisterone after single and multiple injections of norethisterone oenanthate. *Contraception* 1978;18:1–6.

Fotherby K, James F: Metabolism of synthetic steroids. In: *Adv Steroid Biochem Pharmacol*. Briggs MH, Christie GA (eds). London: Academic Press, 1972, pp. 67–165.

Fotherby K, Koetsawang S: Metabolism of injectable contraceptive steroids in obese and thin women. *Contraception* 1982;26:51–58.

Fotherby K, Koetsawang S, Mathrubutham M: Pharmacokinetic study of different doses of depomedroxyprogesterone acetate. *Contraception* 1980;22:527–536.

Fotherby K, Shrimanker K, Abdel-Rahman HA et al.: Rate of metabolism of norethisterone in women from different populations. *Contraception* 1979;19:39–45.

Fotherby K, Warren RJ: Bioavailability of contraceptive steroids from capsules. *Contraception* 1976; 14:261–267.

Fotherby K, Warren RJ, Shrimanker K et al.: Plasma levels of norethisterone by radioimmunoassay and GC-MS. *J Steroid Biochem* 1979;10:121–122.

Garza-Flores J, Diaz-Sanchez V, Bedolla-Tovar N, Lozano-Ruy A: A rapid and sensitive radioimmunoassay for norethisterone. *Steroids* 1983;41:693–701.

Garza-Flores J, Menjivar M, Cardenas M et al.: Further studies on the antigonadotrophic mechanism of action of norethisterone. *J Steroid Biochem Molc Biol* 1991;38:89–93.

Gerhards E, Hecker W, Bellman O: Kinetics and metabolism of norethisterone oenanthate after intramuscular injection. *Arzneim-Forsch* 1976;26:1611–1614.

Gerhards E, Hecker W, Hitze H et al.: Metabolism of norethisterone and norgestrel in man. *Acta Endocrinol* 1971;68:219–248.

Goebelsmann U: Pharmacokinetics of contraceptive steroids in humans. In: *Contraceptive Steroids*: Pharmacology and Safety. Gregoire AT, Blye RT (eds). New York: Plenum Press, 1986, pp. 67–112.

Goebelsmann U, Hoffman D, Chiang S, Woutersz T: Bioavailability of levonorgestrel and ethinylestradiol administered as a low-dose oral contraceptive. *Contraception* 1986;34:341–351.

Goebelsmann U, Stanczyk FZ, Brenner PF et al.: Serum norethindrone concentrations after norethindrone enanthate injection. *Contraception* 1979;19:283–313.

Gupta G, Ostermann J, Santen R, Bardin CW: The effect of protocol design and the metabolic clearance rate and volume of distribution of medroxyprogesterone acetate. *J Clin Endocrinol Metab* 1979; 48:816–820.

Hammerstein J, Fotherby K, Goldzieher JW et al.: Clinical pharmacology of contraceptive steroids. *Contraception* 1979;20:187–199.

Hammond GL, Langley MS, Robinson PA et al.: Serum steroid binding protein concentrations during treatment with oral contraceptives containing desogestrel or levonorgestrel. *Fertil Steril* 1984;42:44–51.

Hasenack HG, Bosch AMG, Kaar K: Serum levels of 3-keto desogestrel after oral administration of desogestrel. *Contraception* 1986;33:591–596.

He CH, Shi YE, Liao DI et al.: Comparative crossover pharmacokinetic study on two types of postcoital contraceptive tablets containing levonorgestrel. *Contraception* 1990;41:557–567.

Hiroi M, Stanczyk F, Goebelsmann U et al.: Radioimmunoassay of medroxyprogesterone acetate after oral and intravaginal administration. *Steroids* 1975;26:373–386.

Howard G, Khan FS, Warren RJ, Fotherby K: Metabolism of norethisterone oenanthate in vivo and in vitro. *J Endocrinol* 1975a;65:20P–21P.

Howard G, Warren RJ, Fotherby K: Plasma levels of norethindrone in women receiving norethindrone enanthate. *Contraception* 1975b;12:46–52.

Hümpel M, Wendt H, Dogs G et al.: Comparison of pharmacokinetic parameters of levonorgestrel, lynestrenol and cyproterone acetate in women. *Contraception* 1977;16:199–215.

Hümpel M, Wendt H, Pommerenke G et al.: Pharmacokinetics of levonorgestrel and a possible first-pass effect in women. *Contraception* 1978;17:207–219.

Jeppsson S, Johansson EDB: Medroxyprogesterone acetate, estradiol, FSH and LH in blood after intramuscular injection of DepoProvera. *Contraception* 1976;14:461–469.

Jeppsson S, Johansson EDB, Ljungberg O, Sjoberg NO: Medroxyprogesterone acetate, estradiol, FSH and LH in women with MPA-induced amenorrhea. *Acta Obstet Gynecol Scand* 1977;56:43–48.

Jeppsson S, Gershagen S, Johansson EDB, Rannevik G: Plasma levels of medroxyprogesterone acetate, SHBG and gonadal steroids during long-term use of DepoProvera. *Acta Endocrinol* 1982;99:339–343.

Jenkins N, Fotherby K: Binding of norethisterone and norgestrel in human plasma. *J Steroid Biochem* 1980;13:521–527.

Juchem M, Pollow K: Binding of contraceptive progestogens to serum proteins and cytoplasmic receptor. *Am J Obstet Gynecol* 1990;163:2171–2183.

Jung-Hoffman C, Kuhl H: Interaction with the pharmacokinetics of ethinyl estradiol and progestogens. *Contraception* 1989;40:299–311.

Kaiser DG, Carlson RG, Kirton KT: GLC determination of MPA in plasma. *J Pharm Sci* 1974;63:420–424.

Kanluan T, Masironi B, Cekan SZ: On the validity of a levonorgestrel radioimmunoassay. *Clin Chim Acta* 1981;109:169–174.

Kamyab S, Fotherby K, Klopper AI: Metabolism of [4-^{14}C] norethisterone in women. *J Endocrinol* 1968;41:263–272.

Khan FS, Fotherby K: In vivo metabolism of norethisterone-3-oxime in rabbits. *J Steroid Biochem* 1978;9:229–232.

Khan FS, Fotherby K: In vitro hydrolysis of 19-norsteroid esters. *J Steroid Biochem* 1980;13:461–462.

Khan FS, Fotherby K: In vitro hydroxylation of norgestrel. *J Steroid Biochem* 1983a;19:1169–1172.

Khan FS, Fotherby K: Sulphation of contraceptive steroids. *J Steroid Biochem* 1983b;19:1657–1660.

Kiriwat O, Fotherby K: Pharmacokinetics of oral contraceptive steroids after morning or evening administration. *Contraception* 1983;27:153–160.

Kirton KT, Cornette JC: Return of ovulatory cyclicity after injection of Provera. *Contraception* 1974;10:39–45.

Kishimoto Y, Kraychy S, Ranney RE, Gantt CL: Metabolism of ethynodiol diacetate in women. *Xenobiotica* 1972;2:237–252.

Koetsawang S, Nukulkarn P, Fotherby K et al.: Transfer of contraceptive steroids in milk of women using long-acting gestagens. *Contraception* 1982;25:321–331.

Koetsawang S, Shrimanker K, Fotherby K: Blood levels of medroxyprogesterone acetate after multiple injections of DepoProvera or CycloProvera. *Contraception* 1979;20:1–4.

Kozyreff V: In: Proc Internat Symp on MPA. Cavalli F, McGuire WI, Panutti F et al. (eds). Excerpta Med, Amsterdam 1982, pp. 30–33.

Kuhl H: Pharmacokinetics of oral contraceptive steroids and drug interaction. *Am J Obstet Gynecol* 1990;163:2113–2218.

Kuhl H, Bremser HJ, Taubert HD: Serum levels and pharmacokinetics of norethindrone after ingestion of lynestrenol. *Contraception* 1982;26:303–315.

Kuhl H, Jung-Hoffman C, Heidt F: Serum levels of 3-ketodesogestrel and SHBG during treatment with ethynyl estradiol and desogestrel. *Contraception* 1988a;38:381–390.

Kuhl H, Jung-Hoffman C, Heidt F: Alterations in the serum levels of gestodene and SHBG during treatment with ethynyl estradiol and gestodene. *Contraception* 1988b;38:477–486.

Kuhnz W: Pharmacokinetics of levonorgestrel and gestodene in women. *Am J Obstet Gynecol* 1990; 163:2120–2127.

Kuhnz W, Al-Yacoub G, Fuhrmeister A: Pharmacokinetics of levonorgestrel in 12 women who received a single oral dose of 0.15mg levonorgestrel and, after a washout phase, the same dose during one treatment cycle. *Contraception* 1992;46:443–454.

Kuhnz W, Al-Yacoub G, Fuhrmeister A: Pharmacokinetics of levonorgestrel and ethinylestradiol in 9 women who received a low dose oral contraceptive over a treatment period of 3 months and, after a washout phase, a single oral administration of the same contraceptive formulation. *Contraception* 1992;46:455–469.

Lan PI, Aedo AR, Landgren BM et al.: Return of ovulation after a single injection of depot medroxyprogesterone acetate. *Contraception* 1984;29:1–16.

Landgren BM, Johannisson E, Aedo AR et al.: Effect of levonorgestrel in large doses on ovarian function. *Contraception* 1989;39:275–289.

Layne DS, Golab T, Arai K, Pincus G: Metabolic fate of ^{3}H-norethynodrel and ^{3}H-norethindrone in humans. *Biochem Pharmacol* 1963;12:905–911.

Lee GJ, Oyang MH, Bautista J, Kushinsky S: Determination of ethinyl estradiol and norethindrone by HPLC and radioimmunoassay. *J Liquid Chromatog* 1987;10:2305–2318.

Li QC, Hümpel M: Serum protein binding characteristics of cyproterone acetate, gestodene, levonorgestrel and norethisterone in rat, rabbit, dog, monkey and man. *J Steroid Biochem* 1990;35:319–326.

Madden S, Back DJ: Metabolism of norgestimate by human gastrointestinal mucosa and liver microsomes in vitro. *J Steroid Biochem* 1991;38:497–503.

Madden S, Back DJ, Orme ML: Metabolism of the contraceptive steroid desogestrel by human liver in vitro. *J Steroid Biochem* 1990;35:281–288.

Madden S, Back DJ, Martin CA, Orme ML: Metabolism of desogestrel by the intestinal mucosa. *Br J Clin Pharm* 1989;27:295–299.

Martin F, Jarvenpaa P, Kosunen K et al.: Ring A reduction of medroxyprogesterone acetate in biological systems. *J Steroid Biochem* 1980;12:491–497.

Mathrubutham M, Fotherby K: Medroxyprogesterone acetate in human serum. *J Steroid Biochem* 1981;14:783–786.

McGuire JL, Phillips A, Hahn D et al.: Pharmacologic and pharmacokinetic characteristics of norgestimate. *Am J Obstet Gynecol* 1990;163:2127–2131.

Milano G, Carlo G, Renee N et al.: Determination of medroxyprogesterone acetate in plasma by HPLC. *J Chromatog* 1982;232:413–417.

Mills TM, Lin TJ, Hernandez S et al.: Metabolic clearance rate of norethindrone. *Am J Obstet Gynecol* 1974;120:764–772.

Mills TM, Lin TJ, Braselton WE et al.: Metabolism of oral contraceptive drugs. *Am J Obstet Gynecol* 1976;126:987–992.

Morris SE, Cameron EHD: Radioimmunoassay system for norethindrone using ^{3}H and ^{125}I-labelled ligands. *J Steroid Biochem* 1975;6:1145–1150.

Mould GP, Read J, Edwards D, Bye A: A comparison of HPLC and radioimmunoassay measurement of medroxyprogesterone acetate. *J Pharm Biomed Anal* 1989;7:119–122.

Nair KM, Sivakumar B, Prema K, Rao BSN: Pharmacokinetics of levonorgestrel in Indian women. *Contraception* 1979;20:303–317.

Nieuweboer B, Tack J, Tauber U et al.: Development of a radioimmunoassay of a new progestagen, gestodene. *Contraception* 1989;40:313–323.

Nygren KG, Lindber P, Martinsson K et al.: Radioimmunoassay of norethindrone; plasma levels after administration to humans and monkeys. *Contraception* 1974;9:265–278.

Odlind V, Weiner E, Victor A, Johansson EDB: Plasma levels of norethindrone after oral administration of norethindrone and lynestrenol. *Clin Endocrinol* 1979;10:29–38.

Okerholm RA, Peterson FE, Keeley FJ et al.: Bioavailability of norethindrone in humans. *J Clin Pharmacol* 1978;13:35–39.

Orme ML, Back DJ, Breckenridge AM: Clinical pharmacokinetics of oral contraceptive steroids. *Clin Pharmacokin* 1983;8:95–136.

Ortiz A, Hiroi M, Stanczyk F et al.: Serum medroxyprogesterone acetate concentrations and ovarian function following injection of depomedroxyprogesterone acetate. *J Clin Endocrinol Metab* 1977;44:32–38.

Pala A, Benagiano G: A direct radio-iodination technique for radioimmunoassay of norethindrone. *J Steroid Biochem* 1976;7:491–496.

Palatsi R, Hirvensalo E, Liukko P et al.: Serum total and unbound testosterone and SHBG in female acne patients treated with oral contraceptives. *Acta Derem Venereol (Stockholm)* 1984;64:517–523.

Palmer KH, Ross FT, Rhodes LS, et al: Metabolism of antifertility steroids. I. Norethynodrel. *J Pharm Exp Therap* 1969;167:207–216.

Pannuti F, Camaggi CM, Strocchi E et al.: In: *Role of Medroxyprogesterone Acetate in Endocrine Related Tumors.* Pellegrini A, Rolustelli G, Pannuti F et al. (eds). New York: Raven Press, 1984, pp. 43–46.

Pannuti F, Martoni A, Lenaz GR: A possible approach to the treatment of metastatic breast cancer. *Cancer Treat Rep* 1978;62:499–504.

Pasqualini JR, Castellet R, Portois MC et al.: Radioimmunoassay of norethindrone. *Reproduccion* 1975;2:197–205.

Phillipou G, Frith RG: Specific quantitation of plasma medroxyprogesterone acetate by GC-MS. *Clin Chim Acta* 1980;103:129–133.

Phillips A, Hahn DW, McGuire JL: Relative binding affinity of norgestimate for human SHBG. *Steroids* 1990;55:373–375.

Prasad RNV, Fotherby K, Jenkins N, Ratnam SS: Single dose kinetics of norethisterone in lactovegetarians. *Singapore J Obstet Gynaec* 1981;12:59–67.

Prasad EVS, Nair KM, Sivakumar B et al.: Plasma levels of norethindrone in Indian women receiving norethindrone enanthate. *Contraception* 1982;23:497–506.

Prasad KVS, Narasimha Rao BS, Sivakumar B, Prema K: Pharmacokinetics of norethindrone in Indian women. *Contraception* 1979;20:77–90.

Ranney RE: Comparative metabolism of 17α-ethynyl steroids used in oral contraceptives. *J Toxicol Environ Health* 1977;3:139–166.

Read J, Mould GP, Stevenson D: High performance liquid chromatography of medroxyprogesterone acetate in human plasma. *J Chromatog Biomed Appl* 1985;341:437–444.

Reed MJ, Fotherby K, Peck JE, Gordon Y: Localisation of norethisterone in the reproductive tract of women. *J Endocrinol* 1973;59:569–577.

Reed MJ, Ross MS, Lai LC et al.: In vivo conversion of norethisterone to ethynyl oestradiol in perimenopausal women. *J Steroid Biochem* 1990;37:301–303.

Rossi E, Pascali E, Negrini P et al.: Estimation of medroxyprogesterone acetate by gas chromatography. *J Chromatog* 1979;169:416–421.

Royer ME, Ko H, Campbell JA et al.: Radioimmunoassay of medroxyprogesterone acetate using the 11α-hydroxy succinyl conjugate. *Steroids* 1974;23:713–730.

Sang GW, Fotherby K, Howard G et al.: Pharmacokinetics of norethindrone enanthate in humans. *Contraception* 1981;24:15–27.

Sankolli GM, Nair VK, Prasad KVS et al,: Influence of antisera on estimation of norethindrone and levonorgestrel. *J Steroid Biochem* 1979;11:1159–1165.

Sarkar NN, Laumas V, Agarwal N et al.: Norethindrone in serum after administration of norethindrone acetate. *Acta Obstet Gynecol Scand* 1983;62:71–76.

Saperstein S, Edgren RA, Ellis DJ et al.: Bioequivalence of norethindrone and ethynyl estradiol for two different weight tablets. *Contraception* 1986;33:547–557.

Saperstein S, Edgren RA, Lee GJ et al.: Bioequivalence of two oral contraceptives containing norethindrone and ethinyl estradiol. *Contraception* 1989;40:581–590.

Saxena BN, Shrimanker K, Grudzinkas JG: Levels of contraceptive steroids in breast milk and plasma of lactating women. *Contraception* 1977;16:605–613.

Shaw MA, Back DJ, Cowie AM, Orme ML: A non-chromatographic radioimmunoassay for 3-oxo-desogestrel. *J Steroid Biochem* 1985;22:111–113.

Shenfield GM, Griffin JM: Clinical pharmacokinetics of contraceptive steroids. *Clin Pharmacokin* 1991; 20:15–37.

Shi YE, He CH, Gu J, Fotherby K: Pharmacokinetics of norethisterone in humans. *Contraception* 1987; 35:465–475.

Shi Y, Zheng SM, Zhu Y et al.: Pharmacokinetic study of levonorgestrel used as a postcoital agent. *Contraception* 1988;37:359–369.

Shrimanker K, Akpoviroro J, Fotherby K, Watson J: Bioavailability of lynestrenol. *Arzneim Forsch* 1980;30:500–502.

Shrimanker K, Saxena B, Fotherby K: Radioimmunoassay of serum medroxyprogesterone acetate. *J Steroid Biochem* 1978;9:359–363.

Siekmann L, Siekmann A, Breuer H: Measurement by isotope dilution-mass spectrometry of ethynylestradiol and norethindrone. *Biomed Mass Spectr* 1980;7:511–514.

Singh H, Uniyal JP, Jha P et al.: Pharmacokinetics of norethindrone acetate in women. *Am J Obstet Gynecol* 1979;135:409–414.

Sisenwine SF, Kimmel H, Liu AL, Ruelius HW: Presence of DL, D and L-norgestrel and their metabolites in plasma of women. *Contraception* 1975;12:339–353.

Sisenwine SF, Kimmel H, Liu AL, Ruelius HW: Excretion and stereoselective biotransformation of norgestrel in women. *Drug Metab Dispos* 1975;3:180–188.

Sisenwine SF, Liu AL, Kimmel HB, Ruelius HW: Phenolic metabolites of norgestrel. *Acta Endocrinol* 1974;76:789–800.

Skouby SO, Jespersen J: Oral contraceptives in the nineties. *Am J Obstet Gynecol* 1990;163:273.

Song S, Chen JK, Yang PJ et al.: A pharmacokinetic and pharmacodynamic study of a "visiting pill" containing norethisterone. *Contraception* 1986;34:269–282.

Stanczyk F, Goebelsmann U: Use of iodohistamine-labelled steroid derivatives as ligands for radioimmunoassay. *J Steroid Biochem* 1981;14:53–62.

Stanczyk F, Hiroi M, Goebelsmann U et al.: Radioimmunoassay of levonorgestrel after oral and intravaginal administration. *Contraception* 1975;12:279–298.

Stanczyk F, Lobo RA, Chiang ST, Woutersz TB: Pharmacokinetic comparison of two oral contraceptives containing levonorgestrel and ethinyl estradiol. *Contraception* 1990;41:39–53.

Stanczyk F, Mroszczak EJ, Ling T et al.: Pharmacokinetics of norethindrone and ethinylestradiol administered in solution or as tablets. *Contraception* 1983;28:241–251.

Stanczyk F, Roy S: Metabolism of levonorgestrel, norethindrone and structurally related contraceptive steroids. *Contraception* 1990;42:67–96.

Stanczyk F, Brenner PF, Mishell DR et al.: A radioimmunoassay for norethindrone. *Contraception* 1978;18:615–628.

Stillwell WG, Stillwell RN, Horning EC: Analysis of norethindrone in plasma using GC-MS. *Steroids Lip Res* 1974;5:79–90.

Tauber U, Kuhnz W, Hümpel M: Pharmacokinetics of gestodene and ethinyl estradiol after oral administration. *Am J Obstet Gynecol* 1990;163:1414–1420.

Tauber U, Tack JW, Matthes H: Single dose pharmacokinetics of gestodene after intravenous and oral administration. *Contraception* 1989;40:461–479.

Tetsuo M, Axelson M, Sjovall J: Selective isolation procedures for GC-MS analysis of ethinyl steroids. *J Steroid Biochem* 1980;13:847–860.

Timmer CJ, Apter D, Voortman G: Pharmacokinetics of 3-ketodesogestrel and ethinyl estradiol released from vaginal rings. *Contraception* 1990;42:629–642.

Turkes A, Dyas J, Read GF, Riad-Fahmy D: A solid-phase enzyme immunoassay for norethindrone in saliva and plasma. *Steroids* 1980;35:445–457.

Turkes A, Read GF, Riad-Fahmy D: An enzyme immunoassay for norethisterone. *Contraception* 1982;25:505–514.

Urabe M, Yamamoto T, Toshiji S et al.: Aromatisation of norethisterone to ethynyl estradiol in human adult liver. *Steroids* 1987;50:607–608.

Utaaker E, Lundgren S, Kvinnsland S, Aakvaag A: Pharmacokinetics and metabolism of medroxyprogesterone acetate. *J Steroid Biochem* 1988;31:437–441.

Victor A, Johansson EDB: Pharmacokinetics of medroxyprogesterone acetate administered orally and intravaginally. *Contraception* 1976;14:319–326.

Victor A, Edqvist L, Lindberg P et al.: Plasma levels of levonorgestrel after oral or vaginal administration. *Contraception* 1975;12:261–278.

Viinikka L: Radioimmunoassay of a new progestagen ORG2969. *J Steroid Biochem* 1978;9:979–982.

Viinikka L, Ylikorkala O, Vikko R et al.: Metabolism of a new synthetic progestagen in female volunteers. *Acta Endocrinol* 1980;93:375–379.

Viinikka L, Ylikorkala O, Vihko R et al.: Metabolism of a new synthetic progestogen in female volunteers. *Europ J Clin Pharma* 1979;15:349–355.

Vose CW, Butler JK, Williams BM et al.: Bioavailability and pharmacokinetics of norethindrone after oral doses of ethynodiol diacetate. *Contraception* 1979;19:119–127.

Walls C, Vose CW, Horth CE, Palmer RF: Radioimmunoassay of norethindrone after ethynodiol diacetate administration. *J Steroid Biochem* 1976;7:511–516.

Warren RJ, Fotherby K: Radioimmunoassay of norethisterone and norgestrel. *J Endocrinol* 1974;62:605–618.

Warren RJ, Fotherby K: Unpublished PhD. Thesis, Univ. London, 1975a.

Warren RJ, Fotherby K: Iodine labelled ligands in the radioimmunoassay of synthetic progestins. *J Steroid Biochem* 1975b;6:1151–1155.

Warren RJ, Fotherby K: Metabolism of D- and L-norgestrel in humans. *Arzneim Forsch* 1975;25:964–965.

Watanabe H, Menzies JA, Jordan N, Loo JCK: HPLC-radioimmunoassay of norethindrone metabolite in plasma. *Contraception* 1983;28:337–342.

Watson TG, Stewart BJ: Radioimmunoassay of levonorgestrel in saliva. *Ann Clin Biochem* 1988;25:280–287.

Weiner E, Johansson EDB: Plasma levels of norethindrone after intramuscular injection of the enanthate. *Contraception* 1975;11:419–425.

Weiner E, Victor A, Johansson EDB: Plasma levels of norgestrel after oral administration. *Contraception* 1976;14:563–570.

Weintraub HS, Abrams LS, Patrick JE, McGuire JL: Disposition of norgestimate in the presence and absence of ethinyl estradiol in humans. *J Pharm Sci* 1978;67:1406–1408.

Werawatgoompa S, Vaivanijkul B, Leepipatpaiboon S et al.: Effect of norethisterone oenanthate on ovarian hormones in Thai women. *Contraception* 1980;21:299–309.

Yamamoto T, Kitawaki J, Shoroshita K et al.: The confirmation of norethisterone aromatisation in primary human hepatocytes. *Acta Obstet Gynec Jap* 1988;40:87–89.

Yoshiji S, Yamamoto T, Okada H: The aromatisation of norethisterone by human ovarian specimens. *Acta Obstet Gynec Jap* 1987;39:1422–1423.

Pharmacology of the Contraceptive Steroids,
edited by Joseph W. Goldzieher.
Raven Press, Ltd., New York © 1994.

8

Pharmacokinetics and Metabolism of Ethynyl Estrogens

Joseph W. Goldzieher

Department of Obstetrics and Gynecology, Baylor College of Medicine, Houston, Texas 77030

PHARMACOKINETICS

Methodology

Even at the present time, methodologic problems limit the reliability of pharmacokinetic analyses. Contraceptive doses of ethynyl estrogens have decreased over the years from around 80 to 100 μg in a single dose per day to around 30 to 35 μg. Although there is no evidence that multiples of this dose are metabolized differently, investigators persist in using conventional daily doses for their pharmacokinetic studies, thus straining the limits of detectability of the available analytical methods. The best antisera for radioimmunoassay cannot measure plasma levels 12 to 24 hours after single-dose administration with the sensitivity and specificity that is required. The concurrent administration of 19-norprogestins has raised considerable problems of specificity in the past. Ordinary criteria of cross-reactivity (i.e., specificity) are simply not good enough when 30 to 50 μg of ethynyl estradiol (EE) are accompanied by about 1,000 μg of a progestin that also has a 17α-ethynyl side chain. Various purification and separation procedures are required to eliminate these problems (Dyas et al., 1981; Bhavnani, 1991; Gallicano et al., 1991; Zacur et al., 1991). Additionally, nonspecific plasma blanks create a problem that is often not adequately addressed. These blank values may approach the levels of EE itself in the later stages of the elimination phase. Subtraction of an "average" blank derived from a plasma pool is unreliable, and variation of the blank from cycle day to cycle day (Dibbelt et al., 1991) in the same individual militates the use of extensive preassay purification procedures (Dyas et al., 1981). It is hoped that methods based on GC-MS will reach the required level of sensitivity in the near future; the problem of interference by metabolites, cross-reactive materials, and other substances contributing to the RIA blank will be eliminated. Such levels of sensitivity and specificity are necessary not only for fundamental kinetic studies but also for practical applications, as in the proof of bioequivalence of generic formulations and the reference product (Gallicano et al., 1991).

Pharmacokinetic Models

Although there are a score of pharmacokinetic studies of ethynyl estradiol, few of them have carried out a complete analysis. There appears to be a wide variation in the values for some parameters, as well as inconsistency in the notation used to describe them; often there is no explanation of how the parameters were calculated. Frequently, an insufficient number of samples was obtained; a theoretical analysis (Newburger et al., 1985) indicates that seven properly timed data points are a minimum: 0.5-, 1.0-, and 2.0-hr points for the absorption phase; 4- and 8-hr points for the α phase; and 12- and 24-hr points for the β phase, although with the importance of this latter time period for calculating AUC_{0-24} and the low values encountered with the doses usually administered, additional points appear necessary.

In most cases the pharmacokinetics have been said to fit a two-compartment open model after both oral and IV administration. One report in the literature (Hümpel et al., 1979) considers EE to behave as a three-compartment open model after IV administration and as a two-compartment model after oral dosage. The authors point out that the dichotomy arises from the fact that the second distribution phase (SDP) has a very short half-life, and may only be distinguishable after IV but not after oral administration. The average $t_{1/2}$ reported after IV administration is about 9 min. In 1 hr this phase will have gone through approximately seven half-lives. If only one data point has been obtained during this time period, the SDP cannot be identified and will merge with the other distribution phase. With oral administration, it may be impossible to identify the SDP. This will be particularly true if the absorption and distribution rate constants are very similar.

Identification of the elimination-phase rate constant β presents problems. Published data in many instances appear to be at or below the limit of sensitivity of the assay after about 12 hr. The assumption that the blood levels are zero simply because they are not detectable (or are zero by subtraction of an inappropriate blank value) is the cause of much of the variation in reported β values.

The reported elimination half-lives vary from 5.8 to 27 hr. The reason for this large variation is probably the assumption that the last two points measured are linear in a semilog plot; as discussed, it is essential to have more than two points to identify the terminal phase.

It is difficult to assign average values for the volume of distribution and clearance, since they have been reported in various ways. Further, Cp_{max}, A, B, and Co (Newburger and Goldzieher, 1985) will vary with the dose. The total area under the plasma concentration curve ($AUC_{0-\infty}$) is a most important parameter but is seldom calculated, AUC_{0-24} usually being considered adequate. Sometimes even AUC_{0-4} or AUC_{0-12} are used; their value is questionable. Usually these parameters are calculated by the trapezoidal rule; a matrix method has been published (Newburger et al., 1980).

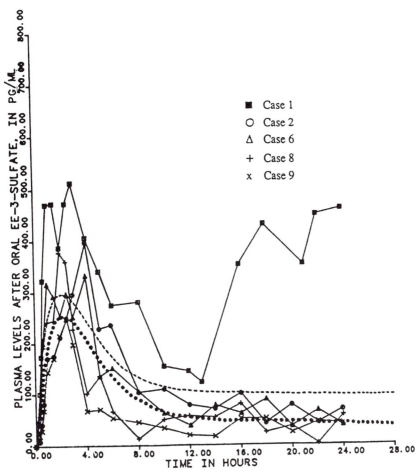

FIG. 1. Plasma EE levels after oral administration of the 3-sulfate. Note the "dumping" in Case 1. From Goldzieher et al., 1988.

None of the kinetic studies have taken into account the substantial first-pass effect that estrogens, including EE, undergo. The kinetics of compounds of this type should be analyzed by more appropriate but necessarily more complex procedures, such as that of Shepard and Reuning (1987) or Schumann et al. (1986). Additionally gallbladder dumping (see Fig. 1) will complicate attempts at kinetic analysis.

In examining the blood levels produced by a radiolabeled dose given IV, it is apparent that >95% of the EE or mestranol (MEE) radioactivity disappears from the circulation almost instantly, so that the kinetic compartments derived from blood level studies deal with an essentially trivial proportion of the administered dose. Moreover, the focus on blood levels promotes the tacit belief that they correlate with clinical effects, which (except for features such as dose-related nausea) is not necessarily the case. Receptor-mediated actions involve a variety of time constants, and effects on such mechanisms as inhibition of the hypothalamic-pituitary axis or

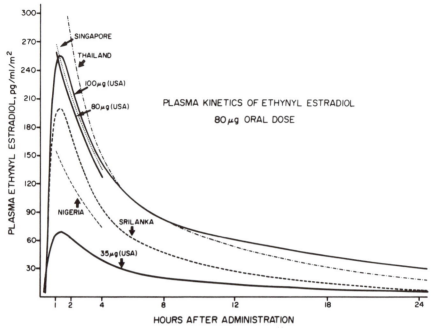

FIG. 2. Plasma EE profiles in various populations. From Goldzieher et al., 1980b.

on tissue changes (e.g., endometrium) depend on dose/duration inputs that are certainly not related to momentary blood levels in any simple fashion.

Pharmacokinetics

The micronized ethynyl estrogens in commercial oral contraceptive formulations or dissolved in weakly alcoholic (6%) solutions used in some studies are absorbed with great rapidity from the stomach; Speck et al. (1976) found that the $t_{1/2}$ even of coated tablets was 12 ± 10 min. This rapid gastric absorption, also observed in rats, suggests that vomiting is not likely to affect blood levels and efficacy unless the emesis occurs within a couple of hours after drug and food intake. Further absorption takes place in the upper intestine; Reed and Fotherby (1979) found, in gut loop preparations, that 90% of the drug was absorbed within 1 hr. Mangold et al. (1984) observed, furthermore, that formation of ethynyl estradiol sulfate takes place with great rapidity and efficiency in the upper small intestine; attempts to develop slow-release oral contraceptive formulations ran afoul of this phenomenon, which produced increased levels of EE sulfate and therefore substantially decreased the bioavailability of ethynyl estradiol (i.e., plasma levels). This was seen in a variety of experimental slow-release formulations. (Norethindrone, by contrast, not being sulfated to any extent, behaved in the expected slow-release fashion.)

After an IV bolus injection of radioactive EE or MEE, total plasma radioactivity peaks in about 30 min (Goldzieher and Kraemer, 1972), at which time about 7% of administered EE radioactivity and 1% of MEE radioactivity is present in the blood volume. Much of this is in the form of conjugated (glucuronide or sulfate) material.

Peak plasma levels of EE are attained in 60 to 120 min from an empty stomach (Orme et al., 1983). The peak plasma level of MEE itself, after oral administration, has been investigated in a study of 18-patients by Mangold et al. (1984). The MEE from an 80 μg tablet yielded average values of 1.9 hr for t_{max} and 121 pg/ml for C_{max}. In another study (Brody et al., 1989), the plasma EE levels seen with the administration of 50 μg MEE/norethindrone were equivalent to those produced by formulations containing 35 μg EE/norethindrone, both tablets prepared by the same manufacturers. This has important implications for epidemiological studies, which have invariably failed to categorize 50 μg mestranol oral contraceptives with low-dose (i.e., 35 μg) EE products, thus confounding attempts to evaluate allegedly dose-dependent adverse effects and other phenomena.

In some studies, the decline in plasma EE levels after a single oral dose is best described by a two-compartment model (Back et al., 1979; Humpel et al., 1979) while in others a three-compartment model provided a better fit (Goldzieher et al., 1980b). The situation is complicated by sudden changes in plasma levels due to enterohepatic recirculation and gallbladder dumping.

Plasma levels appear to be affected by body weight, diet, smoking, and possibly ethnic factors. Goldzieher et al. (1980a) studied plasma EE levels after single-dose administration of EE or MEE in Nigeria, Singapore, Thailand, Sri Lanka, and the U.S., (Fig. 2), while Fotherby et al. (1981) carried out similar studies in 14 centers throughout the world; a tenfold difference between extremes in AUC_{0-24} has been observed between various locations. Unfortunately, these studies were carried out before the large degree of interindividual variation was appreciated; consequently, the number of subjects studied per group is not as large as required, and interpretation of the variability between centers is to a certain extent confounded by this feature. However, studies of urinary metabolites (see section on EE metabolism) indicate that genuine metabolic differences existed between different localities.

The range of pharmacokinetic values for single-dose EE administration is shown in Table 1 (Newburger and Goldzieher, 1985); the data can be summarized as shown in Table 2.

Plasma EE concentrations during daily administration (so-called steady-state kinetics) have been examined by Dibbelt et al. (1991); changes between cycle days 1, 10, and 21 are shown in Table 3. There is no significant difference between the levels on cycle days 10 and 21. Interindividual differences are well illustrated by the data of Jung-Hoffmann and Kuhl (1990). While studies such as these have reported a progressive increase in plasma EE levels during the cycle of administration, other studies show that steady-state concentrations are reached after 3 to 4 days (Elstein et al., 1976; Cortes-Gallegos et al., 1979). EE is not bound to sex-hormone-binding globulin (SHBG), so the increase of SHBG concentration as a result of chronic estrogen administration does not affect plasma EE levels.

TABLE 1A. *Pharmacokinetic parameters*

Reference Species	1 Women	1 Women	14 Women	14 Women	2 Women
Dose (mcg)	30*	30	30	50	3000
Rte. of Admin.	Oral	IV	Oral	Oral	Oral
α (Hrs^{-1})					
$t_{1/2}\,\alpha$ (Hr)	1.1	0.5			2.4
A (pg/ml)					
β (Hrs^{-1})					
$t_{1/2}\,\beta$ (Hr)	7.3	9.0			13.1
B (pg/ml)					
$t_{1/2}\,(\gamma)$ (Hr)					
Ka (Hr^{-1})					
$t_{1/2}$ Ka (Hr)					
C (pg/ml)					
K_{12} (Hrs^{-1})					
K_{21} (Hr^{-1})					
K_{10} (Hr^{-1})					
t max (Hr)			1–2	1–2	
Cp max (Hr)	103		95–135	50–70	
AUC (pg·hr/ml)	794	1776			66100[g] 59200[h]
V_d (L)					6.0[i]
Clear. (L/Hr)					318[j]
Bioavailability (f)	0.44				
Metabolic clearance rate (L/24 hr)					
V_d (β)					
V_1/F (L)					

TABLE 1B. *Pharmacokinetic parameters*

Reference Species	9a Women	9b Women	9b Women	6 Women	15 Women	19 Women
Dose (mcg)	35[a]	80[b]	50[b]	89–136	50*	120*
Rte. of Admin.	Oral	Oral	Oral	Inf	Oral	Oral[m]
α (Hr^{-1})	0.48	0.66	0.57			
$t_{1/2}\,\alpha$ (Hr)	1.46	1.03	1.22			
A (pg/ml)	306	335	268			
β (Hr^{-1})	0.069	0.109	0.055			
$t_{1/2}\,\beta$ (Hr)	10.0	6.35	12.6		7.0	9.1
B (pg/ml)	52	110	26			
$t_{1/2}\,(\gamma)$ (Hr)						
Ka (Hr^{-1})	1.97	2.41	1.84			
$t_{1/2}$ (Ka) (Hr)	0.35	0.28	0.37			
C (pg/ml)	155	869	377			
K_{12} (Hr^{-1})	0.18	0.23	0.21			
K_{21} (Hr^{-1})	0.17	0.25	0.10			
K_{10} (Hr^{-1})	0.19	0.29	0.31			
t max (Hr)					1	1.5
Cp Max (Hr)					422	566
AUC (pg·hrs/ml)	915	1158	749			4879
V_d (L)	198[k]	235[k]	216[k]			
Clear. (L/Hr)	38[k]	69[k]	66[k]			
Bioavailability (f)				1345		
Metabolic clearance rate (L/24 Hr)						
V_d (β)						
V_1/F (L)						

[a]Subjects from Palo Alto, USA   [e]Administered as tablet Minovlar
[b]Subjects from Sri Lanka   [f]Administered as tablet Gynovlar
[c]Administered with antibiotic   [g]AUC 0–48 hours
[d]Administered with Rifampicin   [h]AUC 0–24 hours

reported in the literature

3 Women	3 Women	3 Women	3 Women	10 Women	10 Women	10 Women
50 IV	50 Oral	50^{e*} Oral	50^{f*} Oral	100 IV	100 Oral	3000 Oral
0.83				0.15		
6.75	5.8	8.2	6.8	1.3		1.5
				25.5	23.4	
						0.4
						2
636	136	105	142			7600
2510	1048	946	1200	5500		
3.79^{i}				1092		
375^{j}						
			0.48		0.43	

reported in the literature

19 Women	4 Rat	4 Rabbit	4 Rabbit	11 Women	11 Women	18 Women	5 Women	5 Women
120* Oral^{n}	100 IV	100 IV	100^{c} IV	50* Oral	50* Oral	50* Oral	50 Oral	50^{d} Oral
0.58		0.24	0.21			5.1	6.3	2.9
	0.26							
0.064				0.043	0.047			
9.4	1.5	1.7	1.5	8.0	7.3	2.7		
2.3						0.2		
				223	216			
						0.92		
1.5								
574		61330	37440	2772	2191	2100	1747	1014
4850		14.4	19.5			24		
		2.83^{l}	4.45^{l}					

^{i}Units of Lit/Kg
^{j}Units of ml/hr/Kg
^{k}Corrected for body surface
^{l}Units of ml/min—100 g/BW

^{m}Solution
^{n}Tablet
*Concomitant progestin administration
Reprinted from Newburger and Goldzieher, 1985.

TABLE 2. *Average values for pharmacokinetic parameters of ethynyl estradiol*

$t_{1/2}\,\alpha$	0.5–2.4 hr[a]
$t_{1/2}\,\beta$	13.1–27.0 hr
$t_{1/2}\,Ka$	0.2–0.4 hr
Bioavailability	0.38–0.48
K_{12}	0.182–0.249/hr
K_{21}	0.101–0.245/hr
K_{10}	0.193–0.309/hr
t_{max}	1–2 hr
Metabolic clearance rate	1345 L/hr
Plasma clearance	300–400 ml/hr/kg
Appar. volumn of distribution	2–5 L/kg

[a]Estimates have a wide range and need further documentation.

There is very large interindividual variation in the kinetic parameters, as might be expected from a drug with a first-pass effect and enterohepatic recirculation Fig. 3, Table 4. In the study of Brody et al. (1989), the interindividual variation of AUC for a single dose of 70 μg EE yielded a CV of 46.6%; for EE derived from 100 μg of mestranol it was 56.5%. The C_{max} value for the two formulations averaged 174 ± 59 and $17S \pm 72$ pg/ml, with CVs of 39% and 41%, respectively. The CVs of t_{max} were 37% and 44%. The values for k_{el} were 0.09 ± 0.09 and 0.15 ± 0.12, with CVs of 100% and 80%, respectively.

As pointed out previously by Fotherby (1982), the kinetics of norethindrone given concurrently with the estrogen do not behave in a parallel fashion. Some examples of this, from the study of Brody et al., are shown in Table 3.

Intraindividual variation in kinetics has been explored far less extensively, yet its importance is self-evident. In the study of Brody et al., a comparison was made between three monthly replications. For AUC_{0-24}, the standard deviation of the intraindividual variation was ± 425 for the 35 μg EE formulation and ± 404 for the 50 μg MEE formulation, with CVs of 41% and 42%, respectively.

There has been some discussion as to whether one steroid in the contraceptive formulation has any effect on the pharmacokinetics of the other. Jung-Hoffman and Kuhl (1989) claimed that the C_{max} and AUC of EE were decreased when EE was used with desogestrel as compared to being used with gestodene, but numerous studies by other investigators (Table 5) failed to find any difference. Brody et al. observed a difference in the pharmacokinetics of 1 mg norethindrone when given

TABLE 3. *Representative plasma AUC_{0-24} for repeated trials in the same individuals*

Subject	Ethynyl estradiol AUC			Norethindrone AUC		
	Trial 1	2	3	Trial 1	2	3
1	1002	431	855	29.2	23.1	49.3
2	1892	637	1390	79.7	77.2	91.7
3	657	1594	2122	90.3	86.3	88.0

Brody et al., 1989.

TABLE 4. *Recent measurements of AUC_{0-24} of ethynyl estradiol*

Reference	Dose	Route	AUC Cycle I	Cycle III
Dibbelt et al. 1991	30	p.o.CD1	829 ± 250	935 ± 397
		CD10	1078 ± 336	1113 ± 461
		CD21	1186 ± 354	1176 ± 505
Orme et al. 1991	30	i.v.	1280 ± 306	
		p.o.	867 ± 338	
Mangold et al. 1984	70	i.v.	1095 ± 169	
		p.o.	715 ± 169	
Brody et al. 1989	70	p.o.	1036 ± 483	

with 35 μg EE as compared to administration of EE with 50 μg MEE; this difference in EE/MEE formulations persisted throughout comparisons with the products of three different manufacturers, and did not appear to be due to interassay variation. However, the sets of clinical trials were carried out in spring and fall; although seasonal variation in norethindrone metabolism has not been reported, this might be a confounding factor. Confirmation is needed.

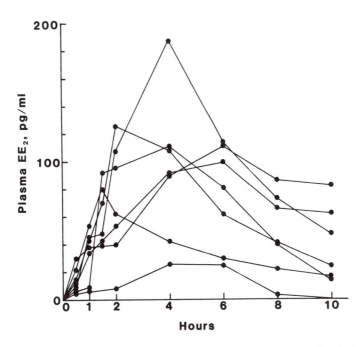

FIG. 3. Interindividual variation in plasma EE levels after administration of a single oral dose to women of a group matched for ethnicity, age, recent diet, and surroundings (temperature, activity, etc.) during the study.

TABLE 5. *Pharmacokinetic parameters of ethynyl estradiol (30–35μg) in the presence of various progestins*

Author	Progestin	C_{max}	AUC_{0-4}	AUC_{0-24}
Kuhnz	(G) gestodene	101 ± 28	308 ± 83	1002 ± 332
	(D) desogestrel	104 ± 28	315 ± 77	1001 ± 311
Kuhnz	G	111 ± 42	267 ± 97	726 ± 294
	D	175 ± 61	389 ± 166	943 ± 349
Back	G	146 ± 33	356 ± 18	925 ± 357
	D	165 ± 102	365 ± 96	914 ± 220
Hümpel	G	106 ± 38	305 ± 115	1264 ± 468
	D	129 ± 51	354 ± 139	1360 ± 541
Dibbelt	G	82 ± 22	224 ± 56	838 ± 235
	D	86 ± 26	228 ± 66	820 ± 264
Back	G		795 ± 206	
	D		614 ± 132	
	EE		867 ± 338	
Brody	(N) norethindrone + 70μg EE; formulations from three different manufacturers			
		171 ± 57		1809 ± 570
		178 ± 45		993 ± 220
		174 ± 59		1024 ± 454

Mestranol

Mestranol itself is biologically inactive until demethylated (Bolt and Bolt, 1974). Plasma kinetics are very similar to EE except for the t_{max} of EE derived from MEE, which averaged 1.9 ± 0.8 hr compared to 1.3 ± 0.5 for EE itself (Brody et al., 1989). With oral doses of 50 to 100 μg, mestranol was still detectable in plasma after 24 hr; the resultant EE levels were higher than those of the mestranol itself (Goldzieher et al., 1980a,b).

Brody et al. studied the plasma EE levels derived from formulations containing 50 μg mestranol and 1 mg norethindrone. The C_{max} of EE averaged 175 ± 72 pg/ml and the AUC_{0-24} averaged 963 ± 544, which was statistically indistinguishable from the AUC of 35 μg EE given under identical experimental conditions. Thus, 50 μg MEE produced the same EE exposure as 35 μg EE itself, a conversion efficiency of 70%. From a therapeutic point of view, therefore, 50 μg MEE oral contraceptives are equivalent to 35 μg EE pills, a finding that epidemiologists in particular have failed to appreciate.

In one study (Mills et al., 1974), the metabolic clearance rate of mestranol was found to be 1247 L/day, while another (Bird and Clark, 1973) found the MCR of mestranol at 1741 L/day to be higher than that of EE at 1345 L/day.

Bolt and Bolt (1974) observed that radiolabeled mestranol administered IV disappeared in an exponential manner from the plasma, with a half-life of about 0.7 hr. With ^{3}H-methoxy labeled MEE, the tritium was incorporated into body water in a manner described by two exponential functiors, with $t_{1/2}$ values of 0.83 and 20.4 hrs. Computer modeling of the data indicated that MEE was delayed in its entry into the circulation, and through indirect calculations it was inferred that $53.7 \pm 5.0\%$ of the MEE was demethylated to EE. This is lower than the value obtained by Brody et al. just mentioned.

Protein Binding

About 95% of plasma EE is bound, virtually all of it to albumin (Akpoviroro and Fotherby, 1980), with an equilibrium-association constant similar to that of estrone. EE is not bound to sex-hormone-binding globulin.

Tissue Distribution

Breast Milk

Nilsson et al. (1978) found no detectable EE levels in breast milk, and concluded on the basis of their assay parameters that a dose of 50 μg would yield about 10 ng EE per 600 ml milk per day. Similar calculations have been made by Wijmenga and Vander Molen (1969) on the basis of radioactively-labeled mestranol given to lactating women.

Total Tissue Radioactivity

Fotherby (1982) reported on the distribution of total tissue radioactivity (i.e., parent compound, metabolites, and conjugates) after administration of labelled EE. Assuming uniform distribution through all adipose tissue depots and that 18.8% of normal weight is adipose tissue, the following values were calculated for percent dose at 1 hr: uterus—0.9%, adipose tissue—28.2%, blood—8.8%; at 24 hr the values calculated were: uterus—0.2%, adipose tissue—6.8%, blood—1.6%.

First-pass Effect and Enterohepatic Recycling

Estrogens, including EE, are sequestered by the liver in the process of enterohepatic passage, resulting in decreased bioavailability. This problem has been studied by Back et al. (1979) and Hümpel et al. (1979). Comparison of oral and IV administration of 50 or 100 μg of EE yielded bioavailability values ranging from 20% to 65%, with an average of about 40%. This clearly accounts for a substantial part of the interindividual variation in plasma EE levels after oral administration. EE is rapidly conjugated to sulfuric or glucuronic acids (both in the 3- and 17-positions), and these compounds are returned to the GI tract by way of the bile. There, in turn, intestinal bacteria possessing sulfatase activity hydrolyse some of the EE sulfates and allow this biologically active material to be reabsorbed into the enterohepatic circulation. The use of antibiotics that affect intestinal flora and thereby might change this recirculation has not been observed to alter EE kinetics in a number of clinical studies. However, despite the lack of an obvious systematic interaction, anecdotal case reports of contraceptive failure exist. The antibiotic rifampicin affects EE metabolism by enzyme induction, not by antibacterial effects. (See section on EE metabolism.)

Ethynyl Estradiol Sulfates

Mono- and disulfates are the major circulating conjugates of both natural and synthetic estrogens. Their concentration in blood after oral administration is often an order of magnitude greater than that of the free (unconjugated) compound. Hydrolysis of the sulfates and enterohepatic recirculation of the free estrogens as well as their sulfates is an important feature of their pharmacokinetics. An example of gallbladder dumping of the sulfate is shown in Fig.1, Case 1.

It has been thought that the sulfates have a prolonged biological half-life and therefore may act as a reservoir from which significant quantities of free ethynyl estradiol might be regenerated. This question has been examined both in primates (Newburger et al., 1983) and humans (Goldzieher et al., 1988). Both the 3- and 17-sulfates were synthesized and administered orally and IV to ovariectomized women, and plasma levels of free and sulfoconjugated EE determined. The two sulfates have significantly different pharmacokinetic profiles (Fig. 4). EE-3-sulfate is cleared more rapidly from the central compartment; this may indicate that differences in protein-binding, tissue binding, metabolism, or distribution exist between the 3- and 17-sulfate. Only 3.4% of IV and 11.4% of orally administered 17-sulfate appeared in the blood as free EE. With the 3-sulfate, the proportions were 13.7% and 20.7%, respectively.

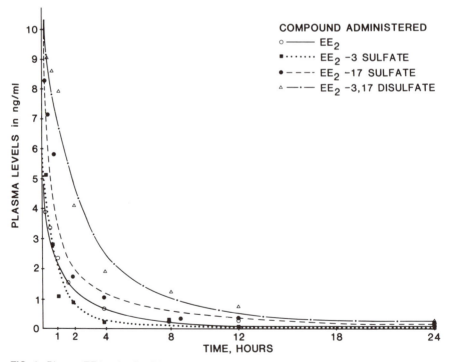

FIG. 4. Plasma EE levels after IV administration of EE or its various sulfates. (Goldzieher et al., 1988)

TABLE 6. *Pharmacokinetic parameters of ethynyl estradiol after intravenous or oral administration of the 3- or 17-sulfates*

Pharmacokinetic parameter	Units	Intravenous				Oral			
		EE-3-Sulfate		EE-17-Sulfate		EE-3-Sulfate		EE-17-Sulfate	
		Mean Data	SD	Mean Data	SD	Mean Data	SD	Mean Data	SD
Dose	µg	80	—	80	—	101.6	—	101.6	—
A	pg/mL	1623	372	8539	2182	7515	31734	872	3611
α	h^{-1}	1.90	0.75	1.18	0.317	0.549	0.133	0.239	0.191
$t_{1/2\alpha}$	h	0.36	0.19	0.59	0.12	1.3	0.41	2.9	2.3
B	pg/mL	454	175	747	244	106.8	110.6	75.6	28.4
β	h^{-1}	0.124	0.064	0.058	0.019	0.005	0.001	0.005	0.013
$t_{1/2\beta}$	h	5.59	4.13	11.93	2.70	139	16	139	45.7
C_0	pg/mL	2077	370	928	1943	7621	2004	948	3624
k_{21}	h^{-1}	0.513	0.312	0.148	0.061	0.596	0.149	0.840	0.239
k_{12}	h^{-1}	1.05	0.493	0.628	0.092	1.16	0.37	0.825	0.609
k_{10}	h^{-1}	0.460	0.108	0.462	0.180	2.50	1.13	1.50	1.19
$t_{1/2}\ k10$	h	1.51	0.436	1.5	2.7	325	86	446	134
AUC_{0-24}	pg·h/mL	4557	516	16959	3405	3.29	2.26	4.22	1.24
$AUC_{0-\infty}$	pg·h/mL	5191	1856	21187	3677	29.8	35.2	19.3	90.0
$AUMC_{0-24}$	pg·h/mL	30664	7649	97549	43299	33.5	31.7	34.0	15.2
$AUMC_{0-\infty}$	pg·h/mL	51099	67198	274472	92739	5.97	7.48	3.35	1.67
t	h	9.8	6.6	13	2.8	200	33.5	174	61.8
V_c	L	48.9	10.7	10.9	3.52	0.81	0.54	0.41	0.67
V_d	L	157.8	62.9	82.5	19.1	0.72	0.62	0.25	0.05
Cl	L/h	19.6	5.6	4.8	0.925	5.74	9.24	0.91	0.35

Goldzieher JW, Mileikowsky G, Newburgh J, Dorantes A, Stavchansky SA, 1988.

The pharmacokinetic parameters obtained after oral and IV administration of the two sulfates are shown in Table 6.

The differences after IV administration of the clearances and residence times presumably reflect tissue sequestration and/or the existence of other metabolic pathways for the disposition of the 3-sulfate, which appears to be more widely distributed than the 17-sulfate.

The absolute bioavailability was obtained by estimating the areas under the plasma concentration curves. It averaged $50.0 \pm 12.5\%$ for the 3-sulfate and $23 \pm 5.2\%$ for the 17-sulfate. Careful attention must be given to the terminal phase when enterohepatic recycling may confound the data. Based on AUC_{0-24}, approximately 11.7% of the orally-administered 17-sulfate appeared as free EE, while for the 3-sulfate the figure was 20.7%. With both sulfates, oral doses yielded a higher percentage of free EE than the IV doses, suggesting that the liver plays an important role. However, the conversion of either sulfate to free EE is not enough to represent a clinically significant reservoir.

REFERENCES FOR PHARMACOKINETICS

Akpoviroro J, and Fotherby, K. Assay of ethinyloestradiol in human serum and its binding to plasma protein. *J Steroid Biochem* 1980;13:773–9.

Back DJ, Breckenridge AM, Crawford FE, et al. An investigation of the pharmacokinetics of ethynylestradiol in women using radioimmunoassay. *Contraception* 1979;20:263–73.

Bhavnani BR. Analytical methodology for estimation of ethinyl estradiol following ingestion of oral contraceptives. *Adv Contraception* 1991;7(Suppl 3):116–39.

Bird CE, Clark AF. Metabolic clearance rates and metabolism of mestranol and ethynylestradiol in normal young women. *J Clin Endocrinol Metab* 1973;36:296–302.

Bolt HM, Bolt WH. Pharmacokinetics of mestranol in man in relation to its oestrogenic activity. *Europ J Clin Pharmacol* 1974;7:295–305.

Brody SA, Turkes A, Goldzieher JW. Pharmacokinetics of three bioequivalent norethindrone/mestranol 50 μg and three norethindrone/ethinyl estradiol-35 μg OC formulations: are "low-dose" pills really lower? *Contraception* 1989;40:269–84.

Cortes-Gallegos V, Carranco A, Sojo I, Navarrete M, Cervantes C, Parra A. Accumulation of ethinyloestradiol in blood and endometrium of women taking oral contraceptives—sequential therapy. *Fertil Steril* 1979;32:524–7.

Dibbelt L, Knuppen R, Jutting G, Heimann S, Klipping CO, Parikka-Olexih H. Group comparison of serum ethinylestradiol, SHBG and CBG levels in 83 women using two low-dose combination oral contraceptives for three months. *Contraception* 1991;43:1–21.

Dyas J, Turkes A, Read GF, Riad-Fahmy D. A radioimmunoassay for ethinyl estradiol in plasma incorporating an immunosorbent, pre-assay purification procedure. *Ann Clin Biochem* 1981;18:37–41.

Elstein M, Morris SE, Groom GV, Jenner DA, Scarisbrick JJ, Cameron EHD. Studies on low-dose oral contraceptives: cervical mucus and plasma hormone changes in relation to circulating d-norgestrel and 17α-ethynyl-estradiol concentrations. *Fertil Steril* 1976;27:892–9.

Fotherby K. Pharmacokinetics of ethynyloestradiol in humans. *Meth Find Exptl Clin Pharmacol* 1982;4:133–41.

Fotherby K, Akpoviroro J, Abdel-Rahman HA, et al. Pharmacokinetics of ethynylestradiol in women from different populations. *Contraception* 1981;23:489–96.

Gallicano KD, McGilveray IJ, Qureshi S, Nitchuk W, Chakraborty B, Boyed C. Situation paper: comparative bioavailability of oral contraceptive products. *Clin Biochem* 1991;24:107–11.

Goldzieher JW, Dozier TS, de la Pena A. Plasma levels and pharmacokinetics of ethynyl estrogens in various populations. II. Mestranol. *Contraception* 1980a;21:17–37.

Goldzieher JW, Dozier TS, de la Pena A. Plasma levels and pharmacokinetics of ethynyl estrogens in various populations. *Contraception* 1980b;21:1–16.

Goldzieher JW, Kraemer DC. The metabolism and effects of contraceptive steroids in primates. *Acta Endocrinol* 1972;166 (Suppl):389–421.

Goldzieher JW, Mileikowsky G, Newburger J, Dorantes A, Stavchansky SA. Human pharmacokinetics of ethynyl estradiol 3-sulfate and 17-sulfate. *Steroids* 1988;51: 64–79.

Hümpel M, Nieuweboer B, Wendt H, Speck U. Investigations of pharmacokinetics of ethinylestradiol to specific consideration of a possible first-pass effect in women. *Contraception* 1979;19:421–32.

Jung-Hoffmann C, Kuhl H. Interaction with the pharmacokinetics of ethinylestradiol and progestogens contained in oral contraceptives. *Contraception* 1989;40:299–312.

Jung-Hoffmann C, Kuhl H. Pharmacokinetics and pharmacodynamics of oral contraceptive steroids: factors influencing steroid metabolism. *Am J Obstet Gynecol* 1990;163:2183–97.

Kuhnz W, Back DJ, Power J, Schult B, Louton T. Concentrations of ethinyl estradiol in the serum of 31 young women following a treatment period of three months with two low-dose oral contraceptives in an intraindividual crossover design. *Hormone Res. [In press]*

Mangold DJ, Schlameus HW, Goldzieher JW, Doluisio JT, Newburger J. Development of orally active dosage forms for steroids. Contract N01-HD-7-28311 for the Contraceptive Development Branch, Center for Population Research, NICHD, Bethesda, Maryland. 1984.

Mills TM, Lin TJ, Hernandez-Ayup S, Greenblatt RB, Ellegood JO, Mahesh VB. The metabolic clearance rate and urinary excretion of oral contraceptive drugs. II.Mestranol. *Am J Obstet Gynecol* 1974;120:773–8.

Newburger J, Akwete A, Martin A. A simplified method to estimate area under the blood-plasma concentration vs. time curve. *J Clin Pharmacol* 1980;20:659–63.

Newburger J, Castracane VD, Moore PH Jr, Williams MC, Goldzieher JW. The pharmacokinetics and metabolism of ethynyl estradiol and its three sulfates in the baboon. *Am J Obstet Gynecol* 1983;146:80–7.

Newburger J, Goldzieher JW. Pharmacokinetics of ethynyl estradiol: a current view. *Contraception* 1985;32:33–44.

Nilsson S, Nygren K-G, Johansson EDB. Ethinyl estradiol in human milk and plasma after oral administration. *Contraception* 1978;17:131–9.

Orme ML'E, Back DJ, Breckenridge AM. Clinical pharmacokinetics of oral contraceptive steroids. *Clin Pharmacokin* 1983;8:95–136.

Orme M, Back DJ, Ward S, Green S. The pharmacokinetics of ethynylestradiol in the presence and absence of gestodene and desogestrel. *Contraception* 1991;43:305–16.

Reed MJ, Fotherby K. Intestinal absorption of synthetic steroids. *J Steroid Biochem* 1979;11:1107–12.

Schumann W, Hillesheim HG, Gira G. Model systems for pharmacokinetics of steroid drugs subject to enterohepatic circulation. *Exp Clin Endocrinol* 1986;87:118–124.

Shepard TT, Reuning RH. An equation for the systemic availability of drugs undergoing simultaneous enterohepatic cycling, first-pass metabolism, and intestinal elimination. *Pharm Res* 1987;4:195–200.

Speck V, Wendt H, Schultze PE, Jentsch D. Bioavailability and pharmacokinetics of cyproterone acetate-^{14}C and ethinylestradiol-^{3}H after oral administration as a coated tablet. *Contraception* 1976;14: 151–7.

Wijmenga HC, vander Molen HJ. Studies with 4-^{14}C mestranol in lactating women. *Acta Endocrinol* 1969;61:665–7.

Zacur HA, Linkins S, Chang V, Smith B, Kimball AW, Burkman R. Ethinyl estradiol and norethindrone radioimmunoassay following Sephadex LH-20 column chromatography. *Clin Chim Acta* 1991;204: 209–16.

METABOLISM

As soon as estrogens reach the gut wall, metabolic alteration begins (Diczfalusy et al., 1961). The effect on *natural* estrogens has been summarized by Adlercreutz et al. (1979). Portal vein sampling after EE administration has been carried out by Back et al. (1990); it showed that 44% ± 5% of the dose is altered by the gut within 60 min, compared to about 25% by the liver in the same interval. EE undergoes relatively more sulfation than estradiol, for which glucuronidation predominates (Back et al., 1981, 1982). *In vitro* studies of intestinal wall metabolism using an Ussing chamber showed that, after 2 hr, 56.6% ± 11.4% of EE remained unaltered, 33.3% ± 12.4% was conjugated with sulfuric acid, and 2.1% was glucuronidated. There was little steroid on the serosal side (Rogers et al., 1987).

Gut flora, which are mostly confined to the large intestine, are capable of hydrolyzing estrogen conjugates. Hydrolysis of EE conjugates is performed primarily by *clostridia* A bacteria according to one unpublished study (Chapman, 1981). However, while antibiotics have a profound effect on intestinal bacteria, they seem to have very little clinical effect, in part due to rapid development of antibiotic resistance (Orme and Back, 1990). These findings are in keeping with the low level of recycling of EE sulfates (see section on pharmacokinetics). Changes in diet affect the spectrum of microorganisms; whether this has any bearing on the geographical differences in EE metabolism (especially the nature of conjugates) that have been observed (Williams and Goldzieher, 1979) is speculative. Moreover, since the recycling of EE conjugates does not appear to be a major factor, the effect of diarrhea on contraceptive efficacy should not be a concern; there is only anecdotal speculation to support this idea.

First-pass Effect and Enterohepatic Recycling

This subject has been reviewed regarding the steroids by Adlercreutz et al. (1979) and Hümpel et al. (1979), and for recycled drugs generally by Chen and Gross (1979).

Cargill et al. (1969) found 26% to 28% of an administered EE dose in the bile during 100 hr of collection. Maggs et al. (1983) observed 28% to 43% of orally administered EE-radioactivity in the bile in the first 24 hr after administration; 70% to 90% was present in conjugate form. Sahlberg et al. (1981) found that glucuronides were mostly conjugated to the A-ring, and sulfates to the D-ring. Reed et al. (1972a,b) found up to 30% of the administered dose excreted in the feces, while Speck et al. (1976) found 53% in feces collected over 7 to 10 days.

The route and quantity of excretion of EE and MEE in nonhuman species has been reviewed (Goldzieher and Kraemer, 1972; Helton and Goldzieher, 1977; Ranney, 1977; Newburger et al., 1983).

The effect of the liver on the EE and metabolites delivered to it consists primarily of further glucuronidation and sulfation, and of various enzymatic attacks on the

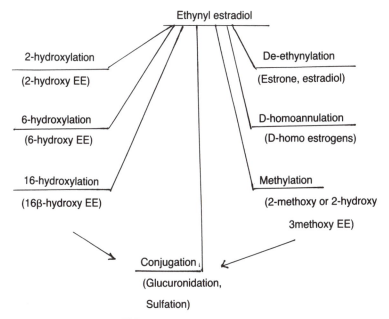

FIG. 5. Metabolic alterations of EE.

steroid moiety itself. As might be expected, there is a great deal of individual variability in the conjugation of EE by the liver (Helton et al., 1977). Conjugation has been investigated in a large number of human liver samples *in vitro* by Temellini et al. (1991). Age and sex of the donor made no difference, except that the proportion of sulfotransferase activity seemed to decrease with age. Glucuronyltransferase activity ranged between 12.6 and 242 pmol $min^{-1}mg^{-1}$ protein, with a mean of 96.8 ± 47.9 and a very large coefficient of variation of 49.5%. Sulfotransferase activity ranged from 14.4 to 98.2 pmol $min^{-1}mg^{-1}$ with a mean of 43.7 ± 18.6 and a coefficient of variation of 41.1%. A unimodal distribution was observed for both enzyme activities. The ratio of these two activities per liver ranged from 0.05 to 2.92, with a coefficient of variation of 70.9%. In general, there was a prevalence of hepatic glucuronidation over sulfation in the majority of individuals. Clearly, there is an enormous range of hepatic EE conjugation activity from individual to individual. The reasons for this are speculative.

The major forms of alteration of the steroid itself involve oxidative attacks at the 2,6, and 16-positions, de-ethynylation, and d-homoannulation of ring A (Fig. 5). Insight into these activities may be gained by examination of urinary metabolites. Many investigators have studied the route and pattern of excretion of metabolites following oral or IV administration of EE and MEE (Wijmenga and Vander Molen, 1969; Kappus et al., 1972; Helton and Goldzieher, 1977). Total urinary excretion of labeled metabolites of ^{3}H- or ^{14}C- EE or MEE varied from 22.6% to 58.7% during 5 days after administration, with no significant difference between the oral or IV routes. K.I.H. Williams (1969), and Longcope and Williams (1975) found 29% to

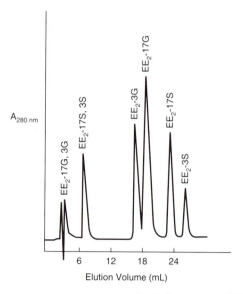

FIG. 6. Sephadex chromatography elution pattern of EE conjugates.

43% of an oral dose of labeled mestranol in the urine over 8 days of collection, which agreed with the report of 10% to 27% excretion over 5 days after an IV dose (Kulkarni and Goldzieher, 1970). A semilog plot of urinary excretion versus time yielded a straight line (i.e., exponentially decreasing output). With proper precautions against bacterial hydrolysis, essentially all of the urinary radioactivity is in the form of conjugated metabolites.

The EE conjugates expected in urine can be separated (Fig. 6) by Sephadex chromatography (Williams, Helton and Goldzieher, 1975; Helton, Williams and Goldzieher, 1976; Williams and Goldzieher, 1980). These correspond to the 3-glucuronides, the 17-glucuronides, the 3,17-diglucuronides, and mixed conjugates (sulfo-glucuronide diconjugates, sulfates). Resolution of urinary extracts is imperfect, but the patterns (which may change over the first 3 days) are of interest (Fig. 7). Enzymatic hydrolysis with liver glucuronidase and *helix pomatia* phenolsulfatase liberates 95% of urinary radioactivity. Analysis of the proportions of the various types of conjugates excreted by women from various countries (Williams and Goldzieher, 1980) showed consistent geographic differences in the proportion of 3- or 17-mono and 3,17-diglucuronides (Fig. 8). Sulfates comprised a relatively small proportion of the urinary conjugates, and analytical studies of the sulfate types have not been performed.

These observations, together with the results of studies of the metabolites (deconjugated) of EE and MEE (see next paragraph) support the conclusion that the phar-

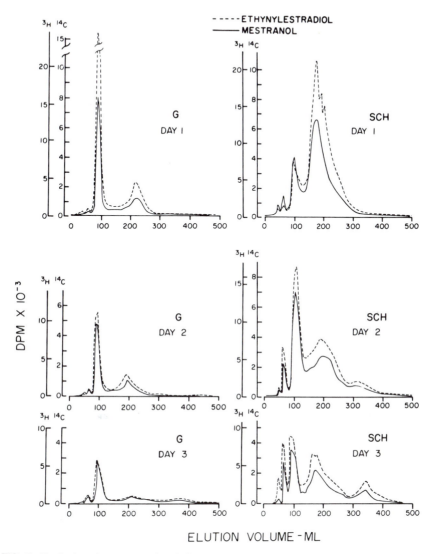

FIG. 7. Sephadex chromatography elution patterns on 3 consecutive days in two American subjects.

macokinetic differences between the various populations studied by Goldzieher et al. (1980) and Fotherby et al. (1981) were not merely statistical aberrations due to interindividual variability in small subsets of women.

After enzyme hydrolysis of the urinary conjugates, the freed EE and MEE metabolites have been separated by high-pressure liquid chromatography (Fig. 9), followed by definitive identification of the radiolabeled metabolites of both com-

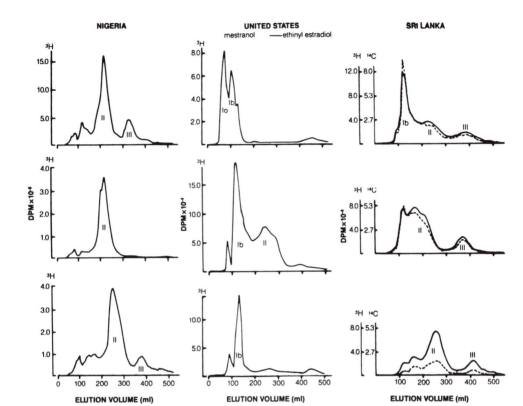

FIG. 8. Elution patterns in women from three countries. In Nigeria, conjugates grouped in Peak II predominate, while in U.S. subjects most of the radioactivity was in the Peak I area. Women from Sri Lanka showed a more general distribution of radioactivity.

pounds (Williams, Helton, and Goldzieher, 1975; Williams and Goldzieher, 1979). As expected, both intact and demethylated metabolites of MEE were observed; oxidation of the EE molecule that formed the 2-, 6-, and 16-hydroxy compounds was also seen (Fig. 10). Compared to the metabolism of estradiol itself, the presence of the 17α-ethynyl group in EE hinders oxidation at this site, causing proportionately greater oxidative activity at the 2- and 6- positions. The 2-hydroxylation of EE is catalyzed by cytochrome P450 3A4 (which is not induced by smoking), whereas 2-hydroxylation of estradiol involves cytochrome P450 IA2 (which is induced by smoking); this helps to explain why smoking influences estradiol but not EE metabolism (Orme et al., 1989; Forrester et al., 1992). The 2-hydroxy metabolites (Ball and Knuppen, 1990) have an extremely short half-life: their clearance is an order of magnitude greater than that of noncatechol estrogens (Kono et al., 1980), which accounts for the low and probably clinically insignificant plasma levels. Some removal of the ethynyl group also occurs, with the formation of estrone, estradiol, and d-homoestradiol (Fig. 5). In our studies of metabolites in the

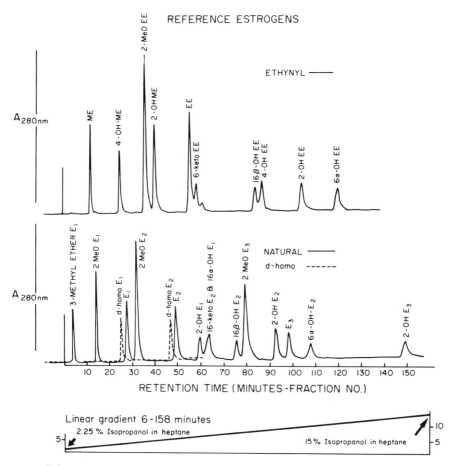

FIG. 9. Resolution of EE metabolites by high-pressure liquid chromatography.

urines of four women, the percent de-ethynylation of EE ranged from 14% to 35%. When EE and MEE were administered simultaneously, proportionately less de-ethynylation of MEE was observed.

The metabolism of EE differs qualitatively and quantitatively from individual to individual (Fig. 10; Williams and Goldzieher, 1980). In nearly all instances, unaltered EE is the major steroid metabolite; in some individuals, the sum of the oxidatively altered metabolites exceeds that of EE itself. There was no difference in the pattern of metabolites in never-users versus long-term users of oral contraceptives; further, no qualitative differences in the metabolite excretion pattern between the first and subsequent days of EE administration were observed. When tracer doses of both EE and MEE were given simultaneously, women tended to differ in the proportions of various metabolites derived from the two sources.

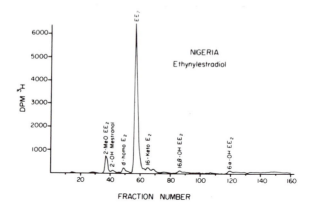

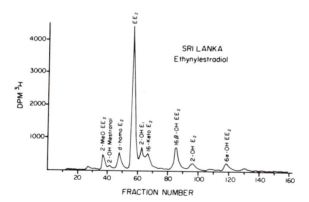

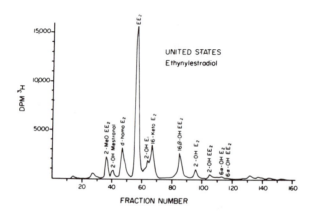

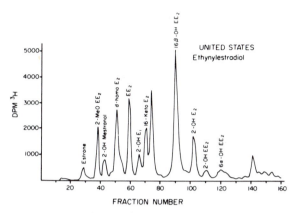

FIG. 10. Patterns of EE metabolites in women of several countries. The typical Nigerian pattern is excretion chiefly of EE itself; more oxidative metabolites are seen in the Sri Lankan pattern, and by far the most extensive oxidative metabolism are seen in a maximal (left) and average (right) U.S. pattern. These findings, together with differences in the conjugate patterns, underscore the ethnic differences.

Quite consistent differences were observed from country to country in the character of the metabolites (geographic differences in the types of conjugation were discussed previously). The variety and quantity of oxidative metabolites were least in Nigeria, intermediate in Sri Lanka, and highest in U.S. women, for whom high-metabolite and average-metabolite patterns are shown (Figure 10). In this regard, EE and MEE behaved similarly. Since oxidative attack occurs almost entirely in the liver, this suggests geographic differences in hepatic enzyme activity. Whether these differences originate in ethnic, dietary, or other factors is entirely speculative.

REFERENCES FOR INTERMEDIATE METABOLISM

Adlercreutz H, Martin F, Jarpenpaa P, Fotsis T. Steroid absorption and enterohepatic recycling. *Contraception* 1979;20:201–23.

Back DJ, Breckenridge AM, Crawford FE, MacIver M, Orme ML'E, Rowe PH, Watts MJ. An investigation of the pharmacokinetics of ethynylestradiol in women using radioimmunoassay. *Contraception* 1979;20:263–73.

Back DJ, Breckenridge AM, Ellis A, MacIver M, Orme ML'E, Rowe PH. The in vitro metabolism of ethinylestradiol, mestranol and levonorgestrel by human jejunal mucosa. *Brit J Clin Pharmacol* 1981;11:275–78.

Back DJ, Breckenridge AM, MacIver M, et al. The gut wall metabolism of ethinyloestradiol and its contribution to the pre-systemic metabolism of ethinyloestradiol in humans. *Brit J Clin Pharmacol* 1982;13:325–30.

Back DJ, Madden S, Orme ML. Gastrointestinal metabolism of contraceptive steroids. *Am J Obst Gynec* 1990;163:138–145.

Ball P, Knuppen R. Formation, metabolism, and physiologic importance of catecholestrogens. *Am J Obstet Gynec* 1990;163:2163–70.

Cargill DI, Steinetz BG, Gosnell E, et al. Fate of ingested radiolabelled ethynyloestradiol and its 3-cyclopentyl ether in patients with bile fistulas. *J Clin Endocrinol Metab* 1969;29:1051–61.

Chapman CR. Absorption and metabolism of steroid prodrugs, 1981. [*in press*]

Chen GH-S, Gross JF. Pharmacokinetics of drugs subjects to enterohepatic circulation. *J Pharmacol Sci* 1979;68:792–4.

Diczfalusy E, Franksson C, Martinsen B. Oestrogen conjugation by the human intestinal tract. *Acta Endocrinol* 1961;38:59–72.

Forrester LM, Henderson CJ, Glancey MJ, et al. Relative expression of cytochrome P450 isoenzymes in human liver and association with the metabolism of drugs and xenobiotics. *Biochem J* 1992;281:359–68.

Fotherby K, Akpoviroro J, Abdel-Rahman HA, et al. Pharmacokinetics of ethynylestradiol in women from different populations. *Contraception* 1981;23:489–96.

Goldzieher JW, Dozier TS, de la Pena A. Plasma levels and pharmacokinetics of ethynyl estrogens in various populations. *Contraception* 1980;21:1–16.

Goldzieher JW, Dozier TS, de la Pena A. Plasma levels and pharmacokinetics of ethynyl estrogens in various populations.II. Mestranol. *Contraception* 1980;21:17–37.

Goldzieher JW, Kraemer DC. The metabolism and effects of contraceptive steroids in primates. *Acta Endocrinol* 1972;166[Suppl]:389–421.

Helton ED, Goldzieher JW. The pharmacokinetics of ethynyl estrogens. A review. *Contraception* 1977; 15:255–84.

Helton ED, Simmons R, Meltz ML, Goldzieher JW. Variability in conjugates of ethynylestradiol produced by in vitro incubation of human liver tissues. *Contraception* 1977;16:257–60.

Helton D, Williams MC, Goldzieher JW. Human urinary and liver conjugates of 17α-ethynylestradiol. *Steroids* 1976;27:851–67.

Hümpel M, Nieuweboer B, Wendt H, Speck U. Investigations of pharmacokinetics of ethynyl estradiol to specific consideration of a possible first-pass effect in women. *Contraception* 1979;19:421–32.

Kappus H, Bolt HM, Remmer H. Demethylation of mestranol to ethynylestradiol in vitro and in vivo. *Acta Endocrinol* 1972;71:374–84.

Kono S, Brandon D, Merriam GR, Loriaux DL, Lipsett MB. Low plasma levels of 2-hydroxyestrone are consistent with its rapid metabolic clearance. *Steroids* 1980;36:463–71.

Kulkarni BD, Goldzieher JW. A preliminary report on urinary excretion pattern and method of isolation of ^{14}C-ethynylestradiol metabolites in women. *Contraception* 1970;1:47–55.

Longcope C, Williams KC. The metabolism of synthetic estrogens in non-users and users of oral contraceptives. *Steroids* 1975;25:121–33.

Maggs JL, Grimmer SFM, Orme ML'E et al. The biliary and urinary metabolites of [^{3}H]17α-ethynylestradiol in women. *Xenobiotica* 1983;13:421–31.

Newburger J, Castracane VD, Moore PH Jr, Williams MC, Goldzieher JW. The pharmacokinetics and metabolism of ethynyl estradiol and its three sulfates in the baboon. *Amer J Obstet Gynecol* 1983;146: 80–7.

Orme ML, Back DJ. Factors affecting the enterohepatic circulation of oral contraceptive steroids. *Amer J Obstet Gynecol* 1990;163:2146–52.

Orme ML, Back DJ, Ball S. Interindividual variation in the metabolism of ethynyl estradiol. *Pharmacol Ther* 1989;43:251–60.

Ranney RE. Comparative metabolism of 17α-ethinyl steroids used in oral contraceptives. *J Toxicol Environ Health* 1977;3:139–66.

Reed MJ, Fotherby K, Steele SJ. Metabolism of ethynylestradiol in man. *J Endocrinol* 1972a;55:351–61.

Reed MJ, Fotherby K, Steele SJ, Addison J. In vivo and in vitro metabolism of ethynyloestradiol. *Proc Soc Endocrinol* 1972b;53:28–9.

Rogers SM, Back DJ, Orme ML. Intestinal metabolism of ethynyloestradiol and paracetamol *in vitro*: studies using Ussing chambers. *Brit J Clin Pharmacol* 1987;23:727–34.

Sahlberg BL, Axelson M, Collins DJ, Sjövall J: Analysis of isomeric ethynylestradiol glucuronides in urine. *J Chromatog* 1981;217:453–61.

Temellini A, Giuliani L, Pacifici GM. Interindividual variability in the glucuronidation and sulfation of ethinyloestradiol in human liver. *Brit J Clin Pharmacol* 1991;31:661–64.

Wijmenga HC, vander Molen HJ. Studies with 4-^{14}C mestranol in lactating women. *Acta Endocrinol* 1969; 61:665–67.

Williams KIH. The metabolism of radioactive 17α-ethynylestradiol 3-methyl ether (mestranol) by women. *Steroids* 1969;13:539–44.

Williams MC, Goldzieher JW. Chromatographic patterns of urinary ethynyl estrogen metabolites in various populations. *Steroids* 1980;36:255–82.

Williams MC, Goldzieher JW. The metabolism of the ethynyl estrogens. Preparative HPLC profiling of radiolabelled urinary estrogens. In: Hawk GL, ed. *Biological/biomedical applications of liquid chromatography II*. New York: Marcel Dekker; 1979:395–409.

Williams MC, Helton ED, Goldzieher JW. The urinary metabolites of 17α-ethynylestradiol-9,11-^{3}H in women. Chromatographic profiling and identification of ethynyl and non-ethynyl compounds. *Steroids* 1975;25:229–46.

Pharmacology of the Contraceptive Steroids,
edited by Joseph W. Goldzieher.
Raven Press, Ltd., New York © 1994.

9

Long-Acting Contraceptives

Francesco M. Primiero and Giuseppe Benagiano

*First Institute of Obstetrics and Gynecology, University la Sapienza,
Policlinico Umberto I, Rome, 00161, Italy*

When hormonal methods of fertility were first introduced in the developing world it was not appreciated how strongly cultural, socioeconomic, and psychological factors could interfere with the overall acceptability and use-effectiveness of a contraceptive regimen. This lack of appreciation caused the practical failure of many international efforts to organize family planning in Asia or Africa. The need for hormonal methods based on long-acting substances—agents administered at long intervals that provided protection against pregnancy without forcing users to adhere strictly to a daily administration schedule—stems from these considerations.

In order to obtain a prolonged duration of action of a steroid hormone, three major approaches have been used. First, a novel molecule can be synthesized, as for example the preparation of esters in which the steroid is conjugated with a fatty acid (Dorfman and Shipley, 1956; Junkmann and Witzel, 1958), or the synthesis of enol-ether derivatives (Meli et al., 1963).

A second approach involves changes in the physical form of the steroid that allows slow dissolution at the site of injection, such as the formulation of medroxyprogesterone acetate as microcrystals (Babcock et al., 1958).

The third option is the use of polymeric devices, nonbiodegradable (Dzuik and Cook, 1966) or biodegradable (Benagiano and Gabelnick, 1979), implanted subcutaneously or administered as an injection and capable of releasing the active compound during matrix erosion or by diffusion across the polymeric membrane.

Following 25 years of worldwide research efforts, more than seven million women are currently using long-acting injectable or implantable contraceptives, and this number is increasing (WHO, 1990).

INJECTABLE CONTRACEPTIVES

Two major types of long-acting injectable contraceptive preparations have been tested clinically since 1963. The first contains a long-acting progestin alone and is intended to protect women against pregnancy for several months. The second type is an estrogen-progestin combination, and is designed to inhibit fertility for about 30 days.

TABLE 1. *Injectable hormonal preparations that have been studied in clinical trials for control of human fertility*

Preparation	Dose (mg)	First utilized by
Progestin alone (monthly)		
17 α-hydroxyprogesterone caproate	500	Siegel (1963)
17 α-hydroxy-19-norprogesterone caproate	200	Jurgensen and Taubert (1969)
Dihydroxyprogesterone acetophenide	200	Taymor et al. (1964)
Medroxyprogesterone acetate	50	Coutinho et al. (1966)
Norethindrone enanthate	25	Chavez and Garcia (1969)
20β-hydroxy-19-norprogesterone phenyl-propionate	50	Farkas and Szontagh (1972)
Lynestrenol phenylpropionate	50	Ruiz-Velasco and Alisedo-Aparicio (1972)
Progestin alone (two- or three-monthly)		
Depot-medroxyprogesterone acetate	150	Coutinho et al.; Zañartu et al. (1966)
Norethindrone enanthate	200	Zañartu and Navarro (1966)
Estrogen alone (monthly)		
Estradiol unducelate	30	El-Mahgoub and Karim (1972)
Estrogen-progestin combinations (monthly)		
17 α-hydroxyprogesterone caproate	500	Siegel (1963)
+ estradiol valerate	10	
Medroxyprogesterone acetate	150	
+ estradiol polyphosphate	40	Zañartu et al 1966
Medroxyprogesterone acetate	25	Coutinho and de Souza (1968)
+ estradiol cypionate	5	
Medroxyprogesterone acetate	50	Scommegna et al. (1970)
+ estradiol cypionate	10	
Medroxyprogesterone acetate	100	Goisis and Oppo (1975)
+ estradiol valerate	20	
Dihydroxyprogesterone acetophenide	150	Reifenstein et al. (1965)
+ estradiol enanthate	10	
Dihydroxyprogesterone acetophenide	150	Cappello (1975)
+ estradiol 3-benzoate,17β-butyrate	10	
dl-Norgesterel	25	de Souza and Coutinho (1972)
+ estradiol hexahydrobenzoate	5	
Norethindrone enanthate	30	Karim and El-Mahgoub (1971)
+ estradiol unducelate	50	
Norethindrone enanthate	50	WHO (1988)
+ estradiol valerate	5	

A list of the principal compounds or combinations that have been utilized clinically as injectable contraceptives is given in Table 1. Of all of these preparations, only two progestins and three estrogen-progestin combinations have reached the premarketing or marketing stage.

Long-acting Progestins

The pilot study of Siegel (1963) first utilized a steroid (17α-hydroxyprogesterone caproate) as a long-acting injectable contraceptive. In 1966 Zañartu et al. first re-

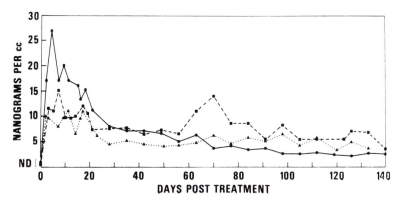

FIG. 1. Plasma levels of MPA in humans following intramuscular injection of 150 mg DMPA (after Cornette et al., 1971).

ported on the use of depot medroxyprogesterone acetate. Intensive testing of a variety of progestational agents followed these studies; however, only two compounds, depot-medroxyprogesterone acetate and norethindrone enanthate, are marketed worldwide today.

Depot-medroxyprogesterone Acetate

Depot-medroxyprogesterone acetate (DMPA) is an aqueous micronized suspension of medroxyprogesterone acetate (MPA), a synthetic progestin derived from natural progesterone. Following I.M. injection, there is a slow release of the drug from the microcrystals of steroid, thus providing contraceptive protection that lasts several months.

Early radioimmunoassay investigations of the pharmacokinetics of DMPA at the standard dose of 150 mg showed high initial plasma concentrations of the steroid and its metabolites, with peak levels ranging between 10 and 27 ng/ml; concentrations above 1 ng/ml can be maintained for periods up to 150 days (Cornette et al., 1971; Schwallie, 1974), as shown in Fig. 1. More recently, investigators utilizing gas chromatography/mass spectrometry found absolute plasma concentrations 5 to 10 times lower than previously obtained (Jeppsson and Johansson, 1976) (see Fig. 2), probably because specificity now excluded crossreacting conjugated steroids. The new levels ranged between 0.9 and 2.7 ng/ml (Kaiser et al., 1974). These data have been confirmed by several authors (Frick et al., 1977; Hiroi et al., 1975; Royer et al., 1974; Shrimanker et al., 1978; Werawatgoompa et al., 1979). Rosenfield (1974) suggested that the high initial release of MPA from the site of injection may produce a shock to the hypothalamus, with the resultant effect lasting 3 to 4 months. More recent pharmacodynamic studies do not confirm this hypothesis, showing that only the preovulatory LH surge is suppressed, while basal levels of LH and FSH are not lowered to the same degree by DMPA as they are by medium-dosage oral contraceptives (Goldzieher et al., 1970). In addition, the pituitary gland responds

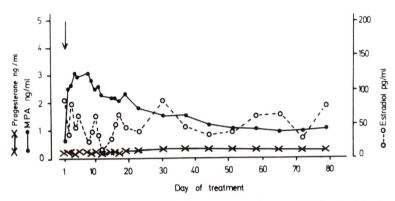

FIG. 2. Plasma levels of MPA, estradiol, and progesterone in a subject following injection of 150 mg DMPA (after Jeppsson and Johansson, 1976).

normally to GnRH stimulation, indicating a normal priming of the hypophysis by endogenous GnRH (Toppozada et al., 1978). This responsiveness to GnRH injection is not affected even after long-term use. Finally, Ortiz et al. (1977) and Fotherby et al. (1980) have demonstrated that ovarian function is fully resumed when MPA plasma concentrations fall <100 pg/ml, as shown in Fig. 3.

The standard contraceptive dose of DMPA in clinical trials is 150 mg, suspended in 1.5 ml and given every 90 days. In a study of the pharmacokinetics of different doses of DMPA in Thai women, however, Fotherby et al. (1980) found that no significant difference in serum levels of MPA was evident if a dose of 100 mg was injected instead of the usual 150 mg. These data were confirmed by Bassol et al. (1984), who administered DMPA in various doses to 20 Mexican women. These observations have raised the hope that, at least in some ethnic groups, a lower dosage could be used, with a possible decrease in dose-related effects on the bleeding pattern. In a recent WHO-sponsored multicenter trial comparing the 100 and 150 mg regimens, no statistically significant difference was observed in terms of contraceptive effectiveness (WHO, 1986). The rates for all medical and nonmedical reasons for discontinuation were comparable, with a lower incidence of amenorrhea in the 100 mg group. In spite of that, the introduction of the 100 mg dose in clinical use was not recommended before additional pharmacokinetic data from different populations became available (Hall and d'Arcangues, 1988).

The dose-reduction studies carried out in Mexico City and Bangkok clearly demonstrated what had already been observed with oral agents: certain injectable steroids such as DMPA show different pharmacokinetic profiles in different populations. A comparative analysis of these studies is shown in Fig. 4.

In 1980 McDaniel et al. reported from Chiang Mai that an increase in the pregnancy rate occurred with DMPA when a locally manufactured formulation of the drug was utilized. It was found that the microcrystal particles were smaller and dissolved more rapidly. Preliminary data from a study conducted in Thailand and

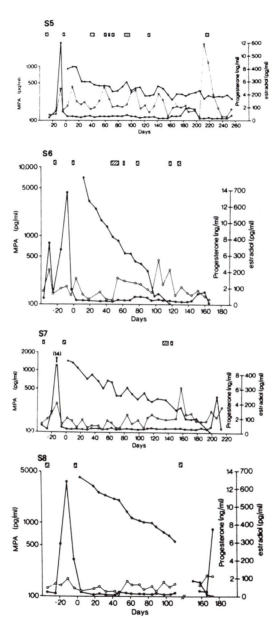

FIG. 3. Plasma levels of MPA, estradiol, and progesterone in Swedish subjects who received an injection of DMPA on day 0. Hatched bars denote days of menstruation (after Fotherby et al., 1980).

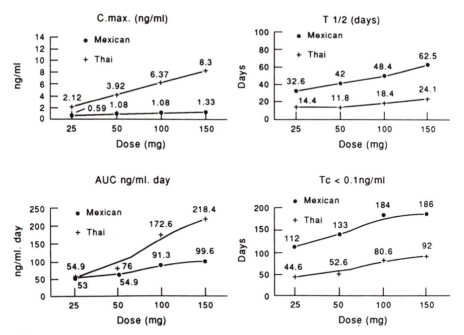

FIG. 4. Comparison of maximum concentration in serum (C_{max}), elimination half-life ($T_{1/2}$), area under the serum concentration curve (AUC), and time to reach MPA serum levels below 0.1 ng/ml (Tc<0.1 ng/ml) of different doses of DMPA in Mexican and Thai women (after Garza-Flores et al., 1991).

Mexico confirmed the differences previously observed in different populations, and also suggested that the particle size of DMPA is a major factor influencing the duration of action and hence the contraceptive protection (Garza-Flores et al., 1991).

Clinical experience with DMPA (150 mg) given every 3 months is reported in Table 2. Using the standard dosage, DMPA proved to be a very effective contraceptive, with most of the studies reporting pregnancy rates at 12 months not exceeding 0.5 per 100 woman-years.

Menstrual bleeding patterns are, without doubt, one of the most important determinants of the acceptability of hormonal contraceptive methods. The large experience of WHO obtained through a variety of multicenter studies has clearly demonstrated that sociocultural factors greatly influence women's perceptions of what represents an acceptable bleeding pattern (Snowden and Christian, 1983). However, irrespective of the different emphasis that changes in bleeding patterns may have in different sociocultural milieus, the majority of women wish to have an unchanged, regular pattern of bleeding episodes while using the contraceptive method. For this reason, alterations in bleeding patterns constitute one of the most common causes of method discontinuation (Odlind and Fraser, 1990).

If one tries to figure out the factors that determine which bleeding pattern results

TABLE 2. Clinical experience with depot-medroxyprogesterone acetate (150 mg) given every 3 months

Authors	Number of subjects	Total woman-months	Pregnancy rate (per 100 woman-years)
Bloch (1971)	7,335	38,714	0.35
Brat (1971)	584	4,677	0.77
Brun et al. (1972)	173	1,341	0
Chinnatamby (1971)	1,000	18,261	0.4
Dodds (1972)	1,883	38,599	0.1
El-Mahgoub et al. (1972)	231	4,671	0
Jeppsson (1972)	139	1,251	0
Jones and Lonky (1971)	86	1,200	0
Koetsawang et al. (1974)	886	24,399	1.2
Mishell et al. (1971)	312	5,377	0
Powell and Seymour (1971)	1,123	14,000	0.34
Rice-Wray et al. (1972)	256	5,662	0
Rosenfield (1974)[a]	23,851	485,112	—
Rubio-Lotvin (1973)	594	30,132	0
Rubio and Gonzales (1970)	100	1,892	0
Schwallie (1974)	11,500	208,894	0.31
Scutchfield et al. (1971)	723	5,067	0.23
Soichet (1969)	298	4,130	0.29
Tyler (1970)	238	2,621	0
Vikar et al. (1972)	277	1,111	0
WHO (1977)	846	4,782	0.7
WHO (1982)	1,589	19,730	0.2
WHO (1983)	1,587	20,550	0.4
WHO (1986)	607	5,429	0
WHO (1986 (100mg)	609	5,507	0.44
Zañartu and Onetto (1972)	561	22,000	0.22
Zartman (1970)	480	4,528	0

[a]Reporting data from McDaniel and colleagues in Chiang Mai.

from the use of a given hormonal contraceptive, it can be seen that these factors depend on the influence of both exogenous and endogenous steroids on ovarian function and endometrium. In theory, any changes in the normal hormonal profile should cause bleeding irregularities. Experience shows that this is not the case, since contraceptive formulations containing an estrogen produce fewer bleeding disturbances than progestin-only methods. The overall picture is further complicated by the existence of racial and individual differences. Significant variations in ovarian and endometrial sensitivity to equal or equipotent doses of contraceptive steroids can cause differences within a given hormonal contraceptive.

There is no doubt that injectable long-acting progestin-only contraceptives have the most disturbing effect on menstrual patterns; in a recent evaluation Belsey (1988b) found that DMPA caused the greatest deviation from normal. In the first 3-month reference period, only 10% of users showed regular menstrual patterns; in the fourth reference period amenorrhea was present in 40%. With this agent, great interindividual as well as intraindividual differences exist, resulting in a totally unpredictable bleeding pattern that has been called "menstrual chaos." There is no tendency to normalize with prolonged use (Belsey, 1988b). Most clinical trials report an incidence of amenorrhea at 1 year of 30% to 50%, with reports of incidences approaching 90% in very long-term users.

Norethindrone Enanthate

Following the discovery that esterification with fatty acids prolongs the action of a steroid alcohol (Junkmann, 1954), Junkmann and Witzel (1957) first synthesized norethindrone enanthate (NET-EN) by esterifying with heptanoic acid the hydroxyl group at carbon-17 of norethindrone (NET). Animal studies clearly indicate that the progestational activity of NET is substantially prolonged when injected in this form (Boschann and Kur, 1957; Davis and Wied, 1957).

Formulation as an oil solution and the need for the ester to be hydrolyzed in order to obtain the active progestin molecule complicate the bioavailability of this long-acting contraceptive. In addition, the presence of plasma and tissue esterases greatly influences the duration of action of NET-EN among different animal species; in rabbits extensive hydrolysis occurs in plasma, liver, kidney, gut wall, and muscle, whereas only negligible degradation takes place after incubation with human plasma, muscle, or fat (Back et al., 1981). In humans, the release of NET-EN from fat storage occurs both in free and conjugated form; following a single injection of the standard 200 mg dose, the ester is still detectable in the blood after 40 days (Sang et al., 1981).

The pharmacokinetic profile of NET-EN was first investigated by Gerhards et al., (1976), who administered the steroid ester labeled with tritium; maximum plasma concentration of the label was found between 1 and 2 weeks after injection. It has been calculated that 50% to 60% of the injected radioactivity is eliminated within 6 weeks.

Radioimmunoassay of free NET shows that, following the I.M. injection of 200 mg, peak plasma concentrations are obtained within 1 week (see Fig. 5) (Fotherby et al., 1980; Goebelsman et al., 1979, Howard et al., 1975; Weiner and Johansson, 1975; Zalanyi et al., 1984), with a rapid decline to almost undetectable levels within 50 to 70 days (Goebelsman et al., 1979; Weiner and Johansson, 1975).

Ethnic differences may affect the pharmacokinetics of NET-EN: a pilot study carried out under the auspices of WHO showed definite differences between Swedish and Indian women (Fotherby et al., 1980). In three of the four subjects recruited in Stockholm, plasma levels of NET-EN became undetectable within 25 to 46 days after the injection, whereas in the women from New Delhi, NET-EN disappeared from circulation between 33 and 71 days after injection. Within 100 days, free NET became undetactable in all 4 Swedish subjects, but it took more than 120 days for its disappearance in all Indian women. In spite of the small number of subjects, the difference was statistically significant. Interestingly, no difference was found be-

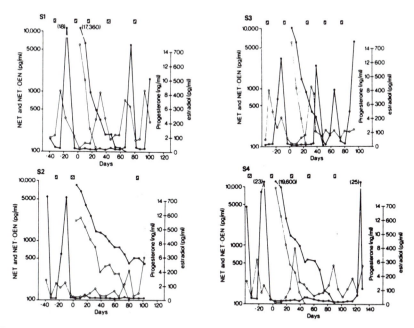

FIG. 5. Plasma levels of NET, NET-EN, estradiol, and progesterone in Swedish subjects who received an injection of NET-EN on day 0. Hatched bars denote days of menstruation (after Fotherby et al., 1980).

tween Swedish and Indian women in the pharmacokinetics of DMPA, used for comparison in the same study.

When a dose higher than the standard 200 mg is injected, there is an augmentation of the initial peak serum level; NET plasma concentrations, however, rapidly return to levels comparable to those obtained with the standard dosage (Hammerstein et al., 1979). For this reason no substantial prolongation of action can be achieved by simply increasing the dose. In spite of its short circulating half-life, some accumulation of NET-EN may occur if repeated injections of 200 mg are given at 70-day intervals, possibly because of a reduction in the metabolism of the steroid ester in the plasma and at the sites of storage (Fotherby et al., 1978) (see Fig. 6).

Like other 19-norprogestins, NET exhibits a high affinity for sex-hormone-binding globulin, the synthesis of which is directly inhibited by this ester at the hepatic level. This is why total NET or NET-EN serum concentrations are not a reliable parameter when comparing the pharmacokinetic profile and the pharmacodynamic effects, and separate measurements of both bound and unbound fractions should always be made (Hammerstein et al., 1979).

In a recent study, Joshi et al. (1989) found no statistical difference in NET plasma levels whether the injection was given in the gluteal or in the deltoid region. It

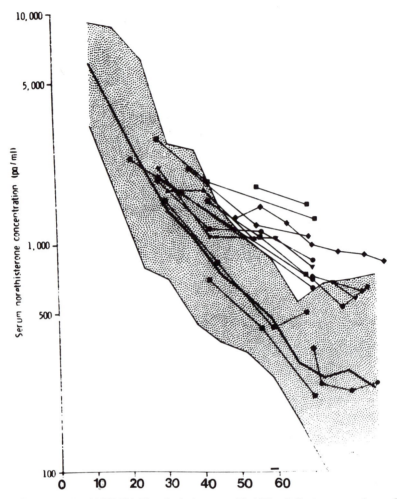

FIG. 6. Serum levels of NET-EN. The shaded area and bold line indicate mean values ± SD in 15 women after the first injection. (▼ --- ▼) values for women who received five injections; (● --- ●) six injections; (▲ --- ▲) seven injections; (■ --- ■) eight injections; (♦ --- ♦) 11 injections (after Fotherby et al., 1978).

seems, therefore, that differences in the amount of subcutaneous fat at the two sites do not affect circulating levels of NET.

When NET-EN was introduced in clinical practice, it was hoped that the standard dose of 200 mg would ensure protection for a period of 90 days (Zañartu and Navarro, 1966). Unfortunately, a marked increase in pregnancy rate was soon observed during the third month postinjection (Larrañaga and Kesserü, 1968; Zañartu and Onetto, 1972). For this reason, several investigators suggested other administration regimens: every 84 days (Larrañaga and Kesserü, 1968; Rice-Wray et al.,

TABLE 3. *Clinical experience with norethindrone enanthate (NET-EN) administered in various regimens*

Regimen and investigators	No. of subjects	Total woman-months	Pregnancy rate (per 100 woman-years)
90 days			
Chinnatamby (1971)	520	4,391	2.3
Larrañaga and Kesserü (1968)[a]	1,036	10,630	1.58
Rice-Wray et al. (1973)[b]	112	1,337	c
Zañartu and Onetto (1972)	130	2,300	5.2
84 days			
Ali and Jalil (1978)	109	951	d
El Mahgoub (1980)[e]	115	2,424	
El Mahgoub and Karim (1972)	171	4,329	0
Kesserü et al. (1973)	1,844	21,730	1.49
Swenson et al. (1980)	106	—	6 of 106
Toppozada et al. (1973)	86	739	—
WHO (1977)	832	5,048	3.6
70 days			
Howard et al. (1980)	324	3,503	1.3
60 and then 84 days			
Giwa-Osagie et al. (1978)	295	1,606	0
Virutamasen et al. (1980)	126	1,351	5.9
WHO (1983)	796	10,035	1.4
60 days			
WHO (1983)	789	10,361	0.4

[a]In an unspecified number of cases, the injection schedule was shortened to 84 days during treatment.
[b]Women were treated at 90-day intervals for 1,069 cycles and at 84-day intervals for 308 cycles.
[c]There were five pregnancies, in all women who received a subsequent injection 1 to 6 days late.
[d]The authors reported that the drug "was found to be almost 100% effective."
[e]Treatment was started at 7 to 42 days postpartum.

1973); every 60 days for the first 6 months and then every 84 days (Benagiano et al., 1977); every 70 days (Howard, 1976). Clinical experience with 200 mg NET-EN administered in various regimens is reported in Table 3.

According to available informaion, the 60-day regimen seems to be preferable, as it yields a lower pregnancy rate without worsening the bleeding pattern, at least as judged by the dropout rate for bleeding problems (WHO, 1983).

Published data indicate that bleeding patterns in users of NET-EN are more acceptable than those who use DMPA; comparative studies have shown that significantly fewer women on NET-EN report amenorrhea, or discontinue for that reason as compared to those using DMPA (WHO, 1978, 1983). In particular, in a large study at 12 months, DMPA produced significantly more amenorrhea than NET-EN (given at 200 mg every 60 days throughout, or every 60 days for the first 6 months and then every 84 days); approximately 50% versus 30%, respectively. At 24 months the incidence of amenorrhea was 30% in the NET-EN 84 group, 40% in the NET-EN 60 group, and 60% in the DMPA group (WHO, 1983).

Estrogen-progestin Monthly Combinations

When administered alone, long-acting progestins are known to cause an almost complete disruption of menstrual cyclicity. For this reason, since the early 1960s, estradiol valerate was added to 17α-hydroxyprogesterone caproate; the resulting estrogen-progestin long-acting contraceptive virtually eliminated breakthrough bleeding (Siegel, 1963).

During the last 30 years more than six monthly injectable preparations have been subjected to clinical trials; only one of them is currently marketed in a few countries. The fear of possible adverse long-term effects of long-acting estrogens has hindered the diffusion of this type of injectable contraceptive; this untested notion prompted the WHO to promote a new research effort to develop monthly combinations utilizing short-acting estrogens (WHO, 1981). Studies on the pharmacokinetic profiles and pharmacodynamic effects of estrogens alone (Oriowo et al. 1980) and various dosage combinations of the progestins and the estrogens have shown that the optimal dosages are: 25 mg DMPA plus 5 mg estradiol cypionate (ECY), and 50 mg NET-EN plus 5 mg estradiol valerate.

Depot-medroxyprogesterone Acetate Plus Estradiol Cypionate (Cyclofem)

Cyclofem, initially developed by a U.S. pharmaceutical company that later discontinued research on new contraceptives, contains a combination of DMPA (25 mg) and ECY (5 mg), and is administered on a monthly basis by deep I.M. injection. The problem created by the fact that ECY is formulated as an oily solution, whereas MPA is available as a microcrystalline aqueous suspension, was resolved by the manufacturer by suspending both the MPA microcrystals and micronized estradiol cypionate particles in an aqueous medium. Following the injection, even taking into account marked individual variations due to different clearance rates, peak plasma concentrations of estradiol are reached after 4 days; levels then decrease to pretreatment values within 11 days (Oriowo et al., 1980), as indicated in Fig. 7.

Since the duration of action of ECY is less than 1 month, these data clearly show that accumulation of the estrogenic component over the long term is unlikely. Oriowo et al. (1980) found that, after the injection of ECY 5 mg, peak plasma levels are higher than the physiological preovulatory surge, suggesting the possibility of a further decrease in the monthly dosage. These data, however, were not confirmed by a more recent study (Aedo et al., 1985) that found that the maximum level of E_2 concentration was of the same order as the normal preovulatory rise (see Fig. 8).

The first investigation of the pharmacokinetic profile of DMPA given at the dose of 25 mg was carried out in five Thai women and showed that, in four of the subjects, MPA was still detectable in plasma for more than 5 weeks (Fotherby et al., 1980). Another study sponsored by WHO and conducted in 11 subjects from different countries found that plasma concentrations of MPA were highest within the first

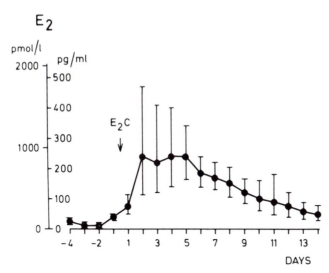

FIG. 7. Plasma levels of estradiol (E_2) in nine subjects before and after the intramuscular administration of 5.0 mg of estradiol cypionate in arachis oil. Geometric mean values and 95% confidence limits (after Oriowo et al., 1980).

10 days, then decreased slowly with time (Fotherby et al., 1982). In some subjects, however, low values were observed at the end of 1 month, whereas concentrations up to 1 ng/ml were still present in some at the end of the 30-day period, as illustrated in Fig. 9. MPA became undetectable between 28 and 62 days after the third and the sixth injections. A third investigation carried out in Stockholm and published in 1985 showed that, in four of eight normally menstruating women, MPA levels were detectable for 30 to 50 days; in the others, MPA was still measurable after 70 to 90 days (Aedo et al., 1985).

Norethindrone Enanthate Plus Estradiol Valerate (HRP 102)

HRP 102 contains a combination of 50 mg NET-EN and 5 mg estradiol valerate (EV); it is manufactured as a 1 ml oily solution by Schering AG, Berlin. In order to assess the pharmacokinetic properties of EV, Oriowo et al. (1980) administered 5 mg of the ester in 1 ml arachis oil. Peak plasma levels of estradiol were reached within about 2 days; increased levels of estradiol lasted 7 to 8 days (see Fig. 10).

When comparing the pharmacokinetic profile of estradiol cypionate, estradiol valerate and estradiol benzoate, the authors concluded that the valerate yielded the most predictable pharmacokinetic behavior, in contrast to the marked intersubject variation with both cypionate and the benzoate. Aedo et al. (1985) have compared the pharmacokinetic and pharmacodynamic properties of Cyclofem and HRP 102; they found that the exogenous estradiol peak with HRP 102 was not only higher

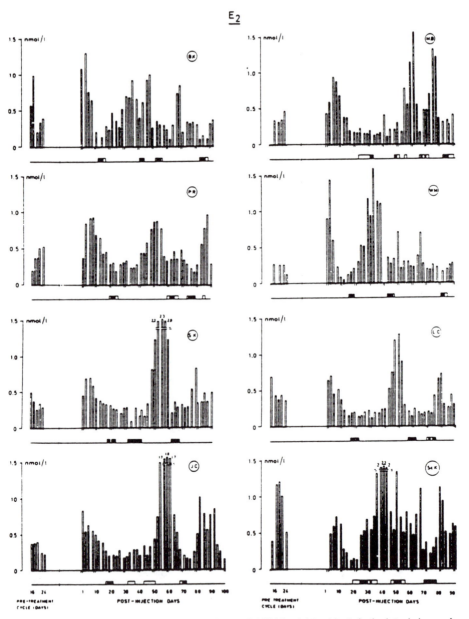

FIG. 8. Peripheral plasma levels (nmol/L) of estradiol (E_2) in eight subjects in the luteal phase of a pretreatment cycle and during 90 days following the third consecutive injection of Cyclofem. Open bars: spotting; filled bars: bleeding (after Aedo et al., 1985).

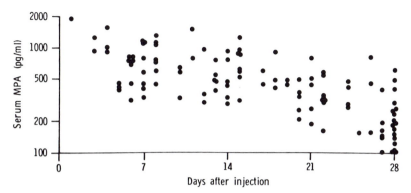

FIG. 9. Serum MPA concentrations at various times after injection of Cyclofem on day 0 (after Fotherby et al., 1982).

than that obtained after Cyclofem (geometric mean levels 428 versus 242 pg/ml), but also higher than the normal preovulatory E_2 surge. This suggests that the cypionate could have the advantage over the valerate of producing lower plasma E_2 concentrations while retaining contraceptive efficacy.

In a large randomized multicenter clinical trial sponsored by WHO and published in 1988, the contraceptive effectiveness of Cyclofem and HRP 102 was compared. A total of 2,320 women were admitted to the study; the accumulated experience was 10,969 woman-months with Cyclofem and 10,608 woman-months with HRP 102.

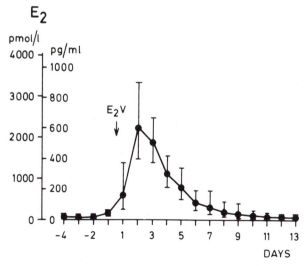

FIG. 10. Plasma levels of estradiol (E_2) in nine subjects before and after the intramuscular administration of 5.0 mg of estradiol valerate in arachis oil. Geometric mean values and 95% confidence limits (after Oriowo et al., 1980).

No pregnancy was reported in the Cyclofem group, while there were two pregnancies in the HRP group, giving, for the latter combination, a cumulative life-table rate of 0.2% at 12 months. No difference was found between the two regimens in terms of overall discontinuation rates—35.5% for Cyclofem and 36.8% for HRP 102 (WHO, 1988).

Dihydroxyprogesterone Acetophenide Plus Estradiol Enanthate

Among the progestin derivatives of $16\alpha,17\alpha$-dihydroxyprogesterone synthesized in 1961 by Fried et al., dihydroxyprogesterone acetophenide (DHPA), also called algestone, was found capable of preventing pregnancy when administered to adult female rats (Lerner et al., 1964). In order to combine high and prolonged progestational activity (i.e., contraceptive efficacy) with good cycle control, a combination of DHPA and estradiol enanthate (EEN) was tested in various doses. The best results were obtained by combining 150 mg DHPA with 10 mg EEN (Reifenstein et al., 1965).

The combination of 10 mg EEN with 150 mg DHPA was given extensive clinical testing in the late 1960s and then withdrawn by the manufacturer, presumably because of some negative animal toxicological data (Benson, 1970). This combination, however, or closely related products, are still being manufactured by small pharmaceutical companies and marketed in Spain and Latin America. In Mexico, up to 300,000 women per year have been using preparations containing this ester (Hall and Fraser, 1983).

Gual et al. (1973), studying the metabolic fate of the two steroids in this preparation, found that traces of the injected labels remained in the circulation throughout the treatment period. In particular, traces of labeled EEN were found in blood 60 days after injection, although the authors did not report for how long they could detect labeled DHPA. This created some concern about a possible accumulation of the estrogen over time.

In order to assess whether diminution of the DHPA/EEN combination to half dose still retains its contraceptive efficacy without compromising bleeding patterns, Recio et al. (1987) carried out a pharmacodynamic comparison of the two doses 150 mg DHPA/10 mg EEN versus 75 mg DHPA/5 mg EEN. Both dosages were able to inhibit ovulation, although the half-dose combination induced a disruption of the bleeding pattern. Serum estradiol levels peaked at day 8.1 for the full dose and 6.5 for the half-dose, with maximum E_2 concentrations in the full-dose group doubling those observed in subjects from the half-dose group.

In a further study conducted in long-term exposed women compared with non-users, Schiavon et al. (1988) demonstrated that baseline serum E_2 concentrations, as determined prior to DHPA/EEN injection, did not exhibit significant differences, while higher baseline estrone levels were found in long-term users. The exogenous E_2 peak occurred significantly earlier in chronic users (4.2 versus 6.3 days), but no significant difference was found in the maximum E_2 postinjection levels between the two groups; there was a complete return to pretreatment values in both groups by day 30 after administration.

All published studies concur that the preparation is an effective contraceptive. In more than 32,000 woman-months of experience reported, not a single pregnancy has been reported (Benagiano, 1977). This extraordinarily high efficacy is consistent with pharmacokinetic evidence that the dosage of estrogen is excessive (Gual et al., 1973) and that the combination causes complete suppression of ovarian activity (Hall and Fraser, 1983).

A different bleeding pattern is observed with monthly injectables containing both estrogen and progestin than with the progestin-only formulations. In a recent comparative clinical evaluation of the two monthly preparations available today (Cyclofem and HRP 102), no statistically significant difference was found in bleeding irregularity incidence (WHO, 1989). Bleeding and spotting days and episodes were significantly more frequent during the first reference period, with the first bleed occurring approximately 15 days after the first injection; this was to be expected in view of the pharmacokinetics of the estrogenic component. Normal patterns were present about 70% of the time in subsequent observations. Among the 30% who were classified as having unacceptable menstrual patterns, infrequent bleeding and irregular bleeding were the most common abnormalities. No particular trend could be detected except for the improvement from the first to the second observation period. A good correlation between discontinuations and bleeding patterns was observed.

POLYMERIC DEVICES

The discovery that polydimethylsiloxane (PDS) rubber films (commercially known as silastic) are permeable to various gases such as oxygen, carbon dioxide, and nitrous oxide opened a new era in the administration of substances for pharmacological purposes; drugs embedded in silatic tubings and inserted subcutaneously would have a prolonged release.

In 1966, Dzuik and Cook first applied this new delivery system to steroid hormones. They discovered that a variety of steroids, including estradiol, progesterone, testosterone, and cortisol, would pass through silastic capsules into a saline solution at constant rates over a period of several days. They used PDS capsules to reduce the incidence of estrus in ewes by more than 50%. The same year, addressing the World Congress of Fertility and Sterility, Segal (1967) proposed the application of this new technology to human contraception and predicted that the new method, based on the absorption of microdoses of synthetic progestins from an implanted capsule, would be effective for months or years as a protection against pregnancy, without interfering with ovulation or the regularity of menses. The subsequent year Segal and Croxatto (1967) presented conclusive animal data on the antifertility activity of estrogens and progesterone encapsulated in polysilicone.

Development of this method is mostly due to activities sponsored and supported

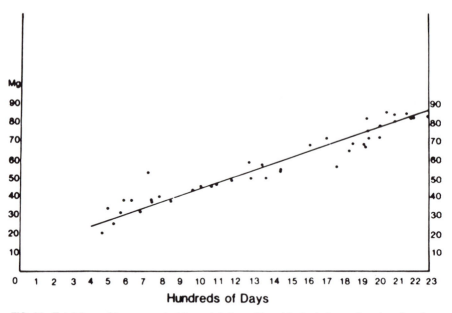

FIG. 11. Total dose of levonorgestrel (in mg) delivered to subjects during various lengths of use of Norplant subdermal implants (after Diaz et al., 1984).

by the Population Council. It is a *non biodegradable* delivery system. In the search of the best polymer to use, it was discovered that only certain membranes are permeable to steroids; out of eight membranes studied using progesterone, only PDS was highly permeable (Kincl et al., 1968).

NORPLANT

The Norplant, developed by the Population Council, has been used by more than 60,000 women in more than 50 countries throughout the world and is currently registered in 23 countries including the United States (Bardin and Sivin, 1992).

Norplant-1

The Norplant-1 contraceptive system consists of six silastic capsules (2.4 mm × 34 mm), each containing 36 mg levonorgestrel, to be inserted under the skin (usually of the ventral portion of the forearm) under local anesthesia, utilizing a trocar.

In order to determine the daily dose of levonorgestrel (LNG) delivered and the life span of the implants, Croxatto and his coworkers (Diaz et al., 1984) measured the steroid remaining in capsules removed after different lengths of use. The average dose per day was calculated by dividing the total amount of drug delivered by

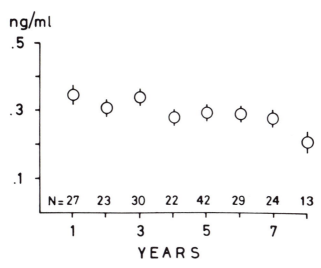

FIG. 12. Levonorgestrel plasma levels during long-term use of Norplant subdermal implants. Each symbol represents the mean ± SE of the averages calculated for the sampling runs of each year (after Diaz et al., 1984).

the number of days *in situ*. The total amount of LNG delivered by implants removed between days 500 and 2,000 of use is shown in Fig. 11.

The amount delivered in the first 500 days was approximately 30 mg, an estimated average daily dose of 60 µg. Between days 500 and 2,000 the rate of the delivery was constant, with an estimated average dose of about 30 µg/day. Nash et al. (1978) showed that there is a higher daily delivery rate of 100 µg during the first months after insertion. This may be due to multiple factors: a local inflammatory process may induce a higher rate in the first days; later, the organization of a thin layer of fibrous tissue may, in fact, stabilize the release rate (Ermini et al., 1973). Then, for the first year, the release rate averages from 50 to 80 µg/day; finally, from the second through the sixth year of use, the release rate is approximately 30 to 35 µg/day (Robertson et al., 1983).

When monitoring plasma LNG levels during Norplant-1 use, Croxatto et al. (1981) found that the concentrations were between 3 and 4 ng/ml during the first 3 years and then declined, with lowest levels observed during the eighth year (range: 0.02 to 0.35 ng/ml). The overall picture suggests a slight time-related decrease (see Fig. 12).

The plasma concentration of LNG shows considerable variation depending on individual factors such as clearance rate and body weight; the levels in a given individual, however, remain relatively constant. The variability has also made it difficult to detect any difference in the plasma levels obtained with the original Norplant and the marketed (Norplant System™) form with less filler in the silicone rubber.

Because of this variability in both serum LNG levels and the individual's response to progestins, serum levels by themselves may only suggest the level of risk of pregnancy in a given woman. Mean concentrations associated with the occurrence of an unwanted pregnancy have been 210 ± 60 (SD) pg/ml (Bardin, 1992). This observation must be contrasted against the fact that, in clinical studies, 20% of all women had one or more values below 200 pg/ml, in spite of an annual gross pregnancy rate of less than 1%.

In order to investigate the mechanism of action of Norplant, blood samples were collected from a randomly selected group of users several times a week for 6 weeks (Bardin, 1992). The results showed that ovulation appeared to be suppressed in some women but not in others. The percentage of women with elevated serum progesterone levels suggested that ovulation increased with longer duration of Norplant use. After 3 to 5 years of use, approximately 50% of the samples were either compatible with ovulation or of uncertain classification. However, a more intense study conducted in a subset of Norplant users who had regular menstrual periods showed that most women with presumptive evidence of ovulation had progesterone levels 50% lower than the normally ovulating controls; in addition, the midcycle surge of LH was blunted, even though cyclic estradiol secretion by the ovary continued (Alvarez-Sanchez et al., 1986). Faundes et al. (1991) examined 31 women who had insertions 13 to 77 months before study; almost half the cycles were anovulatory and all the rest had some form of endocrine dysfunction—diminished gonadotropin surge, luteal phase insufficiency, and estradiol profiles different from the controls. Segal et al. (1991) used a highly sensitive immunoenzymatic assay to test for β-hCG in 32 women after 2 to 7 years of Norplant use. All the results were negative, whether the cycles were anovulatory or ovulatory. These results suggest that some women using Norplant either do not ovulate but secrete progesterone from a luteinized unruptured follicle or have an ovulation followed by an inadequate luteal phase.

During the first and second years, only 0.2% and 0.5%, respectively, of all continuing users became pregnant. During years 3 to 5 the pregnancy rate rose to over 1%, with differences among women of differing weights. In particular, women who weighed 70 kg or more had the highest pregnancy rate (Table 4). When the implant was left *in situ* for more than 5 years, the yearly pregnancy rate rose to 2.5% to 3.0% for all users. Fifty percent of all pregnancies occurred in the 3 to 5 year interval. The decrease in efficacy in women of higher body weight after 3 years prompted a reformulation of the silicone rubber to one containing less filler. This improved contraceptive efficacy materially; whereas with the original silastic the pregnancy rate was 3.9 per 100 users over 5 years (based on studies in 2,970 women), the new tubing yielded a 5-year pregnancy rate of only 1.1, based on studies in 400 women using the Norplant System™ device.

The bleeding pattern in the majority of women using Norplant is characterized by frequent, irregular, and/or prolonged bleeding during the first 12 months of use (Faundes et al., 1978). Several studies confirmed that, unlike other progestin-only methods, bleeding patterns with Norplant improve with time; indeed, the most altered patterns and most terminations for menstrual reasons occur during the first

TABLE 4. Annual and 5-year cumulative pregnancy rates per 100 Norplant users by weight class*

Weight class	Year					Cumulative
	1	2	3	4	5	
<50 kg	0.2	0	0	0	0	0.2
50–59	0.2	0.5	0.4	2.0	0.4	3.4
60–69	0.4	0.5	1.6	1.7	0.8	5.0
≥70	0	1.1	5.1	2.5	0	8.5
All	0.2	0.5	1.2	1.6	0.4	3.9

*Norplant, not Norplant System™.

year (Sivin et al., 1983; Olsson et al., 1988). In one study (Olsson et al., 1988), while 26% of the women abandoned the method for menstrual problems during the first year, only 6% discontinued during the second year and no terminations for menstrual problems occurred in the third year. Bardin et al. (1987), analyzing bleeding patterns in a group of women using Norplant for up to 5 years, found that in the first year 34% of them had 97 or more bleeding days and 15% had at least one episode longer than 15 days. At 5 years, the figures were 19% and 7%, respectively. Amenorrhea, defined as no bleeding for at least 90 days, occurred in 26% at 1 year and in 15% at 3 years. The progressive improvement in bleeding patterns is probably determined by the return of ovulatory or ovulatory-like cycles which, in turn, reflects the decrease in hormone release rate. In order to correlate the bleeding patterns with the endocrine response, 15 women who had been using Norplant-2 for more than 3 years were monitored with hormonal assays and ultrasonography for assessment of ovarian function. Among these women, six had ovulatory-like patterns, six had signs of follicular activity, and three signs of inadequate luteal activity, with regular menstrual patterns in all cases (Olsson and Odlind, unpublished data quoted by Odlind and Fraser, 1990).

Norplant-2

In order to enhance primary acceptability and ease of placement and removal, a second generation system (Norplant-2) has now been designed. It consists of two 2.4 mm × 44 mm rods in which LNG is homogeneously dispersed and covered by a layer of silastic. When plasma levels of LNG were compared in women utilizing either Norplant or Norplant-2, no significant difference was found between the two groups (Olsson et al., 1987) (see Fig. 13). However, when considering the biologically active form of levonorgestrel, expressed as "free LNG index" and calculated as the ratio between LNG and sex-hormone-binding globulin (SHBG), this index was significantly lower in users of Norplant-2, probably because of a higher initial release of LNG from Norplant-1, causing a reduced SHB capacity (Olsson et al., 1987).

A comparative evaluation of the contraceptive effectiveness carried out in the U.S. in 250 subjects for 4,464 months of use did not show any significant differ-

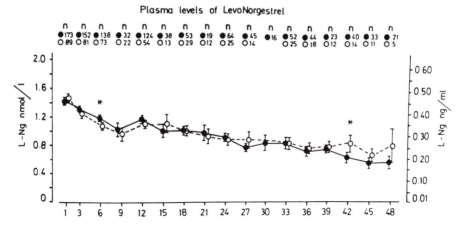

FIG. 13. Plasma levels of levonorgestrel during use of Norplant implants (open circles) and two covered rods (filled circles); mean ± SEM. * = p<0.05 (after Olsson et al., 1987).

ence, with only one pregnancy occurring in the Norplant-1 group (Pasquale et al., 1987). In another study of 240 women conducted in Sweden, no pregnancy was recorded among women using Norplant-1 during the first 3 years of use, with two pregnancies observed among users of Norplant-2. This difference was not statistically significant. During the fourth year, however, four pregnancies occurred in the Norplant-2 group and none among the Norplant-1 users (Olsson et al., 1988).

Bleeding irregularities, which are the major cause for rejection of Norplant, vary with the type of device. Shoupe et al. (1992) have compared the patterns with the original Norplant-1, with the reduced-filler Norplant (Norplant System), and Norplant-2. With the original model, bleeding irregularity was the typical pattern in 66.3% of users, regular cycles in 26.6%, and amenorrhea in 7.1%. With the Norplant System, irregular cycles were the characteristic pattern in 69.3%, regular cycles in 10.7%, and amenorrhea in 20.0%. With Norplant-2, the frequencies were 73.6% irregular, 9.2% regular, and 16.1% amenorrhea. Thus, the bleeding patterns with Norplant System and Norplant-2 are essentially identical. The lower incidence of regular cycles with both Norplant System and Norplant-2 suggests that LNG levels on the average are higher than with the original Norplant, and are associated with much less chance of follicular activity and endogenous progesterone secretion.

It has been a puzzle that Norplant System users, after 2 to 3 years, tend to have a higher percentage of regular cycles and more signs of ovarian follicular activity, whereas plasma levonorgestrel levels remain essentially constant. Brache et al. (1992) have shown that SHBG levels are below normal for the first 18 months of Norplant use (thereby increasing the amount of unbound levonorgestrel in the plasma) and return to normal during the last 3 years. This correlates with their observation of 12% of some degree of luteal activity during the first 2 years, in-

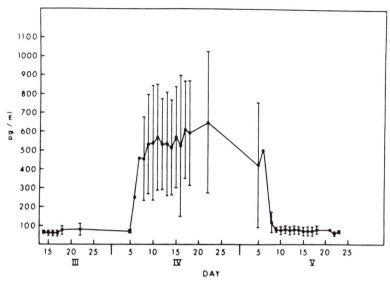

FIG. 14. Plasma concentrations (means and SD) of levonorgestrel for cycles 3,4, and 5 of the phase 1 clinical evaluation where the Capronor was implanted during the fourth cycle (after Ory et al., 1983).

creasing to 44% in the later years when free levonorgestrel levels are lower. These events are not reflected in the total plasma levonorgestrel level.

Capronor

During the early 1970s the WHO Special Programme of Research in Human Reproduction, soon joined by the U.S. National Institutes of Health, initiated work aimed at developing more sophisticated systems which, once inserted in the body, need not be retrieved because they would be self-degrading. These are known as biodegradable delivery systems (Benagiano et al., 1979).

The goal of the Capronor project—developed by the Research Triangle Institute, with support from the National Institute of Child Health and Human Development (NICHD)—was to design a single tubular implant capable of releasing a quantity of LNG sufficient to block ovulation for 1 year. The device was then expected to biodegrade during the following year. After an initial review of potential polymers, poly-(-caprolactone) (PCL) was ultimately selected as the material of choice because of its availability, permeability, biodegradability, and biocompatibility.

PCL maintains its physical integrity in spite of continuous random scission of the polymer chain until the drug supply is exhausted. Eventually, the molecular weight decreases because of the formation of monomers and oligomers; further metabolization leads to carbon dioxide and water. Compared with silastic, PCL releases LNG at a rate 10 times faster, thus requiring less surface area and only one capsule. In a phase 1 clinical evaluation lasting no more than 30 days, eight ovulatory women were implanted with Capronor. The blood profiles for LNG are shown in Fig. 14.

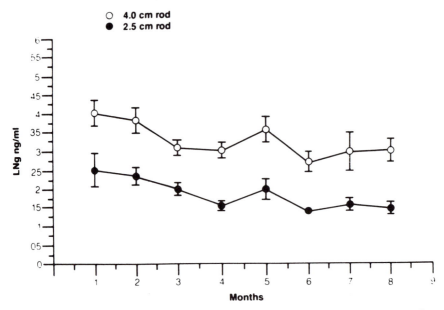

FIG. 15. Levonorgestrel levels in two groups of women receiving either 25 mm or 40 mm Capronor capsules (after Darney et al., 1989).

Although fairly large intersubject variations were observed, blood levels generally remained constant during one single cycle, with mean plasma concentrations between 450 and 650 pg/ml. Seven out of eight treated cycles were anovulatory (Ory et al., 1983). The serum levels of LNG, however, were somewhat lower than expected from *in vitro* release studies. An additional pharmacokinetic/pharmacodynamic study was undertaken by WHO, aimed at assessing the dose-response of the system by inserting either one or two 25 mm devices and by using a new 40 mm device releasing approximately 100 mg/day World Health Organization, unpublished data. All women receiving either two 25 mm devices or one 40 mm device showed suppression of ovulation during the treatment period; two out of 17 women with a single 25 mm implant appeared to have ovulated. Increasing the length of the device to 40 mm resulted in higher LNG levels, with mean plasma concentrations between 600 and 900 pg/ml.

In a recent clinical study conducted in California (Darney et al., 1989) 32 women received a 40 mm capsule containing 21.6 mg LNG and 16 subjects received a 25 mm capsule containing 12 mg LNG. Serum LNG levels were significantly lower in the 25 mm group (see Fig. 15).

Ovulation occurred in all cycles in the 25 mm group and in 26% of cycles in the 40 mm group. It was concluded that LNG levels with the shorter capsule were too low for reliable contraception.

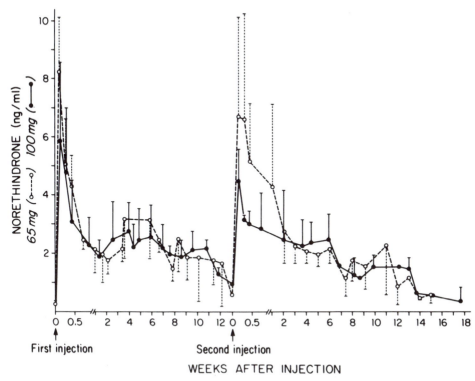

FIG. 16. Mean serum NET levels (±SD) in women injected with either 65 mg (filled circles) or 100 mg (open circles) NET contained in biodegradable microspheres (after Singh et al., 1989).

Poly(d,l-lactide-co-glycolide) Norethindrone Microcapsules

The homopolymers poly(lactic acid) (PLA) and poly(glycolic acid) (PGA) and copolymers thereof, poly(lactide-co-glycolide) (PLGA) have been utilized to prepare, by a solvent-evaporation microencapsulation process, injectable mircospheres of NET crystals homogeneously dispersed throughout the polymer excipient.

Following preliminary animal studies with PLA microcapsules (Beck et al., 1980), a second generation system made of PLGA was developed. This system exhibited a more convenient two-phase release profile of norethindrone; there was an initial phase characteristic of diffusional release, followed by a secondary increase in the serum NET levels due to microcapsule biodegradation (Beck et al., 1983). This biphasic release profile represents a significant improvement over the single-phase profile, with higher serum NET levels during the second half of the treatment interval to reduce the chance of contraceptive failure. In a recent phase II clinical study, 17 women were injected with PLGA microspheres containing either 65 or 100 mg NET. No significant difference was observed in the maximum serum

NET levels, which occurred, for both dose groups, within 24 hours after injection. During the 90-day period after the I.M. administration, average serum NET levels were 1 to 3 ng/ml, with no statistical difference between the two groups. The mean serum NET concentrations returned to nonspecific Radio Immuno Assay basal levels 100 days after the second injection (see Fig. 16) (Singh et al., 1989). Ovulation was inhibited in all women and the contraceptive efficacy was 100% during this study.

REFERENCES

Aedo A-R, Landgren B-M, Diczfalusy E. Pharmacokinetic and pharmacodynamic investigations with monthly injectable contraceptive preparations. *Contraception* 1985;31:453.

Ali MN, Jalil MA. Further study on the effect of norethisterone enanthate, an injectable contraceptive, on body functions. *Bangladesh Med Res Counc Bull* 1978;4:63.

Alvarez-Sanchez F, Brache V, Tejada AS, Faundes A. Abnormal endocrine profile among women with confirmed or presumed ovulation during long-term Norplant use. *Contraception* 1986;33:111.

Babcock JC, Gutsell ES, Herr ME, et al. 6α-methyl-17α-hydroxyprogesterone 17-acetates: a new class of potent progestins. *J Am Chem Soc* 1958;80:2902.

Back AM, Breckenridge C, Chapman CR, et al. Studies on the enzymatic cleavage of norethisterone oenanthate. *Contraception* 1981;23:125.

Bardin CW, Sivin I. Norplant: the first implantable contraceptive. In: Sitruk-Ware R, Bardin CW, eds. *Contraception: newer pharmacologic agents, devices, and delivery systems.* New York: Marcel Dekker Inc.; 1992;23.

Bardin CW, Sivin I, Nash H, et al. Norplant contraceptive implants. In: Diczfalusy E, Bygdeman M, eds. *Fertility regulation today and tomorrow,* New York: Raven Press; 1987;143.

Bassol S, Garza-Flores J, Cravioto M, et al. Ovarian function following a single administration of depot medroxyprogesterone acetate (DMPA) at different doses. *Fertil Steril* 1984;42:216.

Beck LR, Pope VZ, Cowsar DR, Lewis DH, Tice TR. Evaluation of a new three-month injectable contraceptive microsphere system in primates (baboon). *J Contracept Deliv Syst* 1980;1:79.

Beck LR, Pope VZ, Flowers CE Jr, et al. Poly(DL-lactide-co-glycolide)/norethisterone microcapsules: an injectable biodegradable contraceptive. *Biol Reprod* 1983;28:186.

Belsey EM. Task force on long-acting systemic agents for fertility regulation. The association between vaginal bleeding patterns and reason for discontinuation of contraceptive use. *Contraception* 1988a; 38:207.

Belsey EM. Task force on long-acting systemic agents for fertility regulation. Vaginal bleeding patterns among women using one natural and eight hormonal methods of contraception. *Contraception* 1988b; 38:81.

Benagiano G. Long-acting systemic contraceptives. In: Diczfalusy, ed. *Regulation of human fertility. WHO Symposium,* Moscow: Scriptor: Copenhagen; 1977;323.

Benagiano G, Gabelnick HL. Biodegradable systems for sustained release of fertility-regulating agents. *J Steroid Biochem* 1979;11:449.

Benagiano G, Gray R, Parker R, et al. Multinational comparative clinical evaluation of contraceptive effectiveness of norethisterone oenanthate injected every 60 to 84 days. In: *Progress of Seventh Asian Congress of Obstetrics and Gynaecology.* Bangkok: 1977;203.

Benagiano G, Schmitt E, Wise D, Goodman M. Sustained release hormonal preparations for the delivery of fertility-regulating agents. *J Polymer Sci* 1979;66:129.

Benson RC. Discussion in: Keifer WS, Lee AF, Scott JC. A clinical evaluation of a monthly injection for fertility control. *Am J Obstet Gynecol* 1970;107:410.

Bloch B. Depot medroxyprogesterone acetate (depo-provera) as a contraceptive preparation. *S Afr Med J* 1971;45:777.

Boschann HW, Kur S. Uber die wirkung des 17-aethinyl-nortestosteron-oenanthats, eines neuen gestagens mit depotcharakter auf das menschliche endometrium und das atrophishe vaginal epithel. *Geburtshilfe Frauenheilkd* 1957;17:928.

Brache V, Alvarez-Sanchez F, Faundes A et al: Free levonorgestrel index and its relationship with luteal activity during long-term use of Norplant implants. *Adv Contraception* 1992;8:319.

Brat TM. Acceptability of depo-provera as a reliable contraceptive method. *Exc Med Internat Congr Series* 1971;243:291(abst).

Brun G, Delotte H, Laffont G. Utilisation de la médroxyprogestérone à titre contraceptif. *Rev Fr Gynecol.* 1972;67:67.

Cappello F. Uso di un estroprogestinico parenterale come inibitore dell'ovulazione in singola somministrazione mensile. *Minerva Ginecol* 1975;27:964.

Chavez A, Garcia L. Estudio de gestagenos inyectables de deposito, dosis unica mensual, como tratamiento anticoncepcional. *Congr Bolivariano Endocrinol*, Lima, Peru. 1969;44.

Chinnatamby S. A comparison of the long-acting contraceptive agents norethisterone oenanthate and medroxyprogesterone acetate. *Austr N Z J Obstet Gynaecol* 1971;11:233.

Cornette JC, Kirton KT, Duncan JK. Measurement of medroxyprogesterone acetate (provera) by radioimmunoassay. *J Clin Endocrinol Metab* 1971;33:459.

Coutinho EM, de Souza JC. Conception control by monthly injections of medroxyprogesterone suspension and a long-acting oestrogen. *J Reprod Fertil* 1968;15:209.

Coutinho EM, de Souza JC, Csapo AI. Reversible sterility induced by medroxyprogesterone injections. *Fertil Steril* 1966;17:261.

Croxatto HB, Diaz S, Miranda P, Elamsson K, Johansson EDB. Plasma levels of levonorgestrel in women during long-term use of norplant. *Contraception* 1981;23:197.

Darney PD, Monroe SE, Klaisle CM, Alvarado A. Clinical evaluation of the capronor contraceptive implant: Preliminary report. *Am J Obstet Gynecol* 1989;160:1292.

Davis ME, Wied GL. Long-acting progestational agents: 17-ethinyl-19-nortestosterone enanthate, 17α-hydroxyprogesterone caproate, and 17α-hydroxyprogesterone acetate. *Geburtshilfe Frauenheilkd* 1957;17:916.

de Souza JC, Coutinho EM. Control of fertility by monthly injections of a mixture of norgestrel and a long-acting estrogen. *Contraception* 1972;5:395.

Diaz S, Pavez M, Miranda P, et al. Performance of Norplant® subdermal implants in clinical studies in Chile. In: Zatuchni GL, Goldsmith A, Shelton JD, Sciarra JJ, eds. *Long-acting contraceptive delivery systems.* Philadelphia: Harper & Row; 1984;482.

Dodds GH. A report of the clinical findings and two year follow-up on 1,883 women treated by 3-monthly injections of depo-provera. In *Proceedings of Vth Asian Obstetrics and Gynecology Congress.* Jakarta, Indonesia: 1971;761.

Dorfman RI, Shipley RA. *Androgens, biochemistry, physiology and clinical significance.* New York: John Wiley and Sons; 1956.

Dzuik PJ, Cook B. Passage of steroids through silicone rubber. *Endocrinol* 1966;78:208.

El-Mahgoub S. Body weight and cycle control of injectable contraceptives. *J Reprod Med* 1980;24:119.

El-Mahgoub DS, Karim MC. The long-term use of injectable norethisterone enanthate as a contraceptive. *Contraception* 1972;6:21.

Ermini M, Carpino F, Russo M, Benagiano G. Studies on sustained contraceptive effects with subcutaneous polydimethylsiloxane implants. 3. Factors affecting steroid diffusion *in vitro* and *in vivo.* *Acta Endocrinol (Kobenh)* 1973;73:360.

Farkas M, Szontagh FE. Clinical experiences concerning the intramuscular contraceptive oxogestone. *Acta Eur Fertil* 1972;3:37.

Faundes A, Brache V, Tejada AS, et al. Ovulatory dysfunction during continuous administration of low-dose levonorgestrel by subdermal implants. *Fertil Steril* 1991;56:27.

Faundes A, Sivin I, Stern J. Long acting implants. An analysis of menstrual bleeding patterns. *Contraception* 1978;18:355.

Fotherby K, Benagiano G, Toppozada HK, et al. A preliminary pharmacological trial of the monthly injectable contraceptive, cycloprovera. *Contraception* 1982;25:261.

Fotherby K, Howard G, Shrimanker K, Elder M, Bye PGT. Plasma levels of norethisterone after single and multiple injections of norethisterone oenantate. *Contraception* 1982;18:1.

Fotherby K, Saxena BN, Shrimanker K, et al. A preliminary pharmacokinetics and pharmacodynamic evaluation of depot-medroxyprogesterone acetate and norethisterone oenantate. *Fertil Steril* 1980; 34:131.

Frick J, Bartsch G, Jakes G. Radioimmunoassay of ethinyl norgestrienone (R2323) and medroxyprogesterone acetate (MPA) and their clinical applicability. *Urol Res* 1977;5:55.

Fried J, Sabo F, Grabowich P, et al. Progestationally active acetals and ketals of 16-alpha, 17-alpha-dihydroxyprogesterone. *Chem Industr* 1961;April 15:465.

Garza-Flores J, Hall PE, Perez-Palacios G. Long-acting hormonal contraceptives for women. *J Steroid Biochem Mol Biol* 1991;40:697.

Gerhards E, Hecker W, Bellman O. Studies on the kinetics and metabolism of 17-heptanoyl-17-ethinyl-4-oestren-3-one-^{3}H (norethisterone enanthate) in humans following intramuscular injection. *Arzneimittelforschung* 1976;26:1611.

Giwa-Osagie OF, Savage J, Newton JR. Norethisterone enanthate as an injectable contraceptive: use of a modified dose schedule. *Br Med J* 1978;1:1660.

Goebelsmann U, Stanczyk FZ, Brenner FP, et al. Serum norethindrone (NET) concentrations following intramuscular NET enanthate injection: effect upon serum LH, FSH, estradiol and progesterone. *Contraception* 1979;19:283.

Goisis M, Oppo GT. Block of gonadotrophin activity with a long-acting estro-progestogen. *Atti Accad Med Lombarda* 1975;30:126.

Goldzieher JK, Kleber J, Moses L, Rathmacher RP. A cross sectional study of plasma FSH and LH in women using sequential combination and injectable steroid contraceptives over long periods of time. *Contraception* 1970;2:225.

Gual C, Perez-Palacios G, Perez AE, et al. Metabolic fate of long acting injectable estrogen-progestogen contraceptive. *Contraception* 1973;7:21.

Hall PE, d'Arcangues C. Long-acting methods of fertility regulation, World Health Organization: Special Programme of Research, Development and Research Training in Human Reproduction (1988). *Res Hum Reprod, Biennial Rep* 1986–1987;129.

Hall PE, Fraser IS. Monthly injectable contraceptives. In: Mishell DR, ed. *Long-acting steroid contraception.* New York: Raven Press: 1983;65.

Hammerstein J, Fotherby K, Goldzieher JW, Johansson EDB, Schwartz U. Clinical pharmacology of contraceptive steroids: report on a workshop conference held in Igls, Austria, May 4–7, 1978. *Contraception* 1979;20:187.

Hiroi M, Stanczyk FZ, Goebelsmann U, Brenner PF, Lumkin ME, Mishell DR, Jr. Radioimmunoassay of serum medroxyprogesterone acetate in women following oral and intravaginal administration. *Steroids* 1975;26:373.

Howard G. Injectable contraception. *J Matern Child Hlth* 1976;8:10.

Howard G, Blair M, Fotherby K, Howell R, Elder MG, Bye P. Clinical experience with intramuscular norethisteron oetanoate as a contraceptive. *J Obstet Gynecol* 1980;1:53.

Howard G, Warren RJ, Fotherby K. Plasma levels of norethisterone in women receiving norethisterone oetanoate intramuscularly. *Contraception* 1975;12:45.

Jeppsson S. Experience with depo-medroxyprogesterone acetate (depo-provera) as a contraceptive agent. *Acta Obstet Gynecol Scand* 1972;51:257.

Jeppsson S, Johansson EDB. Medroxyprogesterone acetate, estradiol, FSH, LH in peripheral blood after intramuscular administration of depo-provera to women. *Contraception* 1976;14:461.

Jones JR, Lonky S. Use of injectable contraceptives immediately post-partum. *NY State J Med* 1971; 71:2279.

Joshi JV, Hazari KT, Shah RS, et al. Serum progesterone and norethisterone levels following injection of norethisterone enanthate in different sites and doses. *Steroids* 1989;53:751.

Junkmann K. Uber protrahiert wirksame gestagene. Naunyn Schmiedbergs. *Arch Exp Pathol Pharmakol* 1954;223:244.

Junkmann K, Witzel H. Chemie und pharmakologie von steroidhormonestern. *Zeitschr Vit Hormon Fermentforschunde* 1958;9:97.

Jurgensen O, Taubert HD. Klinische beobachtungen über die wirkung des depot-gestagens 17-hydroxy-19-norprogesteronecapronat bei frauen mit eumenorrhoe. *Klin Wochenschr* 1969;47:162.

Kaiser DG, Carlson RC, Kirton KT. GLC determination of medroxyprogesterone acetate in plasma. *J Pharm Sci* 1974;63:420.

Karim M, El-Mahgoub. Conception control by cyclic injections of norethisterone enanthate and estradiol unducelate. *Am J Obstet Gynecol* 1971;110:740.

Kesserü-Koss E, Hurtado-Koo H, Larrañaga-Leguia A, Scharff HJ. Fertility control with norethindrone enanthate, a long-acting parenteral progestogen. *Acta Eur Fertil* 1973;4:203.

Kincl FA, Benagiano G, Angee I. Sustained release hormonal preparations. 1. Diffusion of various steroids through polymer membranes. *Steroids* 1968;11:673.

Koetsawang S, Srisupandit S, Srivanaboon S, et al. Intramuscular depot-medroxyprogesterone acetate for contraception. *J Med Ass Thailand* 1974;57:396.

Larrañaga A, Kesserü E. Dos anos de experiencia clinica con el enantato de noretisterona como anticonceptivo inyectable de deposito. *Ginecol Obstet (Peru)* 1968;14:209.

Lerner LJ, Yiacas E, Bianchi A, et al. Effect of the acetophenide derivative of 16 alpha, 17 alpha-dihydroxyprogesterone acetophenide on the estrous cycle, mating and fertility in the rat. *Fertil Steril* 1964;15:63.

McDaniel EB, Gray RH, Pardthaisong T. Method failure pregnancy rates with depo-provera and local substitute. *Lancet* 1980;1:1293.

Meli A, Wolff A, Howarth WL. The mechanism by which 3-esterification with cyclopentyl alcohol enhances the oral activity of ethinyl oestradiol. *Steroids* 1963;2:417.

Mishell DR, Kharam D, Seward P. Experience with three-monthly injection of depo-medroxyprogesterone acetate as a contraceptive agent. *Exc Med Internat Congr Series* 1971;234:295 (abst).

Nash HA, Robertson DN, Moo Young AJ, Atkinson LE. Steroid release from silastic capsules and rods. *Contraception* 1978;18:367.

Odlind V, Fraser IS. Contraception and menstrual bleeding disturbances: a clinical overview. In: D'Arcangues C, Fraser, IS, Newton JR, Odlind V, eds. *Contraception and mechanisms of endometrial bleeding*. Cambridge: Cambridge University Press: 1990;5.

Olsson SE, Odlind V, Johansson EDB, Nordström M-L. Plasma levels of levonorgestrel and free levonorgestrel index in women using norplant® implants or two covered rods. *Contraception* 1987;35:215.

Olsson SE, Odlind V, Johansson EDB, Sivin I. Contraception with Norplant implants and Norplant-2 (two covered rods). *Contraception* 1988;37:61.

Oriowo MA, Landgren BM, Stenstrom B, Diczfalusy E. A comparison of the pharmacokinetic properties of three estradiol esters. *Contraception* 1980;21:415.

Ortiz A, Hiroi M, Stanczyk FZ, Goebelsmann U, Mishell DR, Jr. Serum concentrations and ovarian function following intramuscular injection of depo-provera. *J Clin Endocrinol Metab* 1977;44:32.

Ory SJ, Hammond CB, Yancy SG, Hendren RW, Pitt CG. The effect of a biodegradable contraceptive capsule (capronor) containing levonorgestrel on gonadotropin, estrogen, and progesterone levels. *Am J Obstet Gynecol* 1983;145:600.

Pasquale SA, Brandeis V, Cruz RI, Kelly S, Sweeney M. Norplant contraceptive implants: rods versus capsules. *Contraception* 1987;36:305.

Powell LC, Seymour RG. Effect of depo-medroxyprogesterone acetate as a contraceptive agent. *Am J Obstet Gynecol* 1971;110:36.

Recio R, Garza-Flores J, Schiavon R, et al. Pharmacodynamic assessment of dihydroxyprogesterone acetophenide plus estradiol enanthate as a monthly injectable contraceptive. *Contraception* 1987;33:579.

Reifenstein EC, Jr, Pratt TE, Hartzell KA, Shafer WB. Artificial menstrual cycles induced in ovulating women by monthly injection of progestogen-estrogen. *Fertil Steril* 1965;16:652.

Rice-Wray E, Gutierrez J, Godorovsky J, Maqueo M, Goldzieher JW. Injectable contraceptives in family planning: clinical experience in 14,958 cycles. *Adv Plann Parenth* 1973;8:103.

Rice-Wray E, Gutierrez J, Godorovsky J, Maqueo M, Goldzieher JW. Injectable contraceptives in family planning: clinical experience in 14,948 cycles. *Exc Med Internat Congr Series* 1972;271:103.

Robertson DN, Sivin I, Nash HA, Braun J, Dinh J. Release rates of levonorgestrel from silastic capsules, homogeneous rods and covered rods in humans. *Contraception* 1983;27:483.

Rosenfield AG. Injectable long-acting progestogen contraception: a neglected modality. *Am J Obstet Gynecol* 1974;120:537.

Royer ME, Ko H, Campbell JA, Murray HC, Evans JS, Kaiser DG. Radioimmunoassay of serum medroxyprogesterone acetate (provera) using the hydroxy succinyl conjugate. *Steroids* 1974;23:713.

Rubio E, Gonzales RA. Contraception with medroxyprogesterone acetate: a follow-up of 1981 cycles. *Proc Sixth World Congr Fertil Steril, Tel Aviv* 1968. 1970:27.

Rubio-Lotvin B. Anticonceptivos de deposito: evaluaccion de diversos esquemas terapeuticos. Experiencia de 8 anos de uso. *Prensa Med Mexicana* 1973;38:435.

Ruiz-Velasco V, Alisedo-Aparicio LE. Efectos colaterales de los anticonceptivo de deposito. *Prensa Med Mexicana* 1972;37:25.

Sang GW, Fotherby K, Howard H, Elder M, Bye PG. Pharmacokinetics of norethisterone oenanthate in humans. *Contraception* 1981;24:15.

Schiavon R, Benavides S, Oropeza G, et al. Serum estrogens and ovulation return in chronic users of a once-a-month injectable contraceptive. *Contraception* 1988;37:591.

Schwallie PC. Experience with depo-provera as an injectable contraceptive. *J Reprod Med* 1974;13:113.

Scommegna A, Lee AW, Borushek S. Evaluation of an injectable progestin-estrogen as a contraceptive. *Am J Obstet Gynecol* 1970;107:1147.

Scutchfield FD, Long WN, Corey B, Tyler CW. Medroxyprogesterone acetate as an injectable female contraceptive. *Contraception* 1971;3:21.

Segal SJ. Future prospects in contraception. *Exc Med Internat Congr Series* 1967;132:1028.

Segal SJ, Alvarez-Sanchez F, Brache V, et al. Norplant implants: the mechanism of contraceptive action. Fertil Steril 1991;56:273.

Segal SJ, Croxatto H. Single administration of hormones for long-term control of reproductive functions. *23rd Annual Meet Am Fertil Soc* 1967.

Shrimanker K, Saxena BN, Fotherby K. A radioimmunoassay for serum medroxyprogesterone acetate. *J Steroid Biochem* 1978;9:359.

Siegel I. Conception control by long-acting progestogens: preliminary report. *Obstet Gynecol* 1963;21: 666.

Singh M, Saxen BB, Graver R, Ledger WJ. Contraceptive efficacy of norethindrone encapsulated in injectable biodegradable poly-dl-lactide-co-glycolide microspheres: phase II clinical study. *Fertil Steril* 1989;52:973.

Sivin I, Diaz S, Holma P, Alvarez-Sanchez F, Robertson DN. A four-year clinical study of Norplant implants. *Stud Fam* Plann 1983;14:184.

Snowden R, Christian B. *Patterns and perception of menstruation*. London: Croom Helm; 1983:

Soichet S. Depo-provera (medroxyprogesterone acetate) as a female contraceptive. *Int J Fertil* 1969; 14:33.

Swenson I, Khan AR, Jahan FA. A randomized single blind comparative trial of norethindrone enanthate and depo-medroxyprogesterone acetate in Bangladesh. *Contraception* 1980;21:207.

Taymor ML, Plank ST, Yahia C. Ovulation inhibition with a long-acting parenteral progestogen-estrogen combination. *Fertil Steril* 1964;15:653.

Toppozada HK, Khowessah M, Youssef HA, Salch FM. A study on injectable contraceptives. *Bull Alexandr Fac Med* 1973;9:35.

Toppozada M, Parmar C, Fotherby K. Effect of injectable contraceptive depo-provera and norethisterone oenanthate on pituitary gonadotropin response to luteinizing hormone-releasing hormone. *Fertil Steril* 1978;30:545.

Tyler ET. A contraceptive injection study employing medroxyprogesterone acetate suspension. *Proc Sixth World Congr Fertil Steril, Tel Aviv, 1968.* 1970;197.

Vikar KD, Kora SJ, Dikshit SS, Bodkya MJ. Long-acting injectable therapy for fertility control. *J Reprod Fertil* 1971;27:305.

Virutamasen P, Nitichai Y, Tangkeow P, Kankeerati W, Rienpraiura D, Boonsiri B. A clinical and metabolic study of norethisterone enanthate in Thai women. *Contraception* 1980;22:397.

Weiner E, Johansson ED. Plasma levels of norethindrone after i.m. injection of 200 mg of norethindrone enanthate. *Contraception* 1975;11:414.

Werawatgoompa S, Pongpradit T, Leepipatpaiboon S, Sukanthanak A. Radioimmunoassay for serum medroxyprogesterone acetate in Thai women receiving injectable DMPA contraceptive. *Contraception* 1979;20:319.

World Health Organization, Expanded Programme of Research, Development and Research Training in Human Reproduction, Task Force on Long-acting Systemic Agents for Fertility Regulation. Multinational comparative clinical evaluation of two long-acting injectable contraceptive steroids: norethisterone oenanthate and medroxyprogesterone acetate. 1. Use-effectiveness. *Contraception* 1977;15:513.

World Health Organization, Special Programme of Research, Development and Research Training in Human Reproduction. Research in Human Reproduction, Biennial Report. 1988–1989:17.

World Health Organization, Special Programme of Research, Development and Research Training in Human Reproduction, Task Force on Long-acting Systemic Agents for Fertility Regulation. Multinational comparative clinical evaluation of two long-acting injectable contraceptives: norethisterone enanthate given in two dosage regimens and depot-medroxyprogesterone acetate. A preliminary report. *Contraception* 1982;25:1.

World Health Organization Special Programme of Research, Development and Research Training in Human Reproduction. Task Force on Long-acting Systemic Agents for Fertility Regulation (1978). Multinational comparative clinical evaluation of two long-acting injectable contraceptive steroids: norethisterone oenanthate and medroxyprogesterone acetate. 2. Bleeding patterns and side-effects. Contraception 17:395.

World Health Organization, Special Programme of Research Development and Research Training in Human Reproduction. *Tenth Ann Rep* 1981.

World Health Organization, Task Force on Long-acting Systemic Agents for Fertility Regulation, Special Programme of Research, Development and Research Training in Human Reproduction. A multi-centered pharmacokinetic, pharmacodynamic study of once-a-month injectable contraceptives. I. Different doses of HRP102 and of depoprovera. *Contraception* 1987;36:441.

World Health Organization, Task Force on Long-acting Systemic Agents for Fertility Regulation, Special Programme of Research, Development and Research Training in Human Reproduction. A multi-centered phase III comparative study of two hormonal contraceptive preparations given once-a-month by intramuscular injection. I. Contraceptive efficacy and side effects. *Contraception* 1988;37:1.

World Health Organization Task Force on Long-acting Systemic Agents for Fertility Regulation Special Programme of Research, Development and Research Training in Human Reproduction. A multicentered phase III comparative clinical trial of depot-medroxyprogesterone acetate given three-monthly at doses of 100 mg or 150 mg: 1. contraceptive efficacy and side effects. *Contraception* 1986;34:223.

World Health Organization, Task Force on Long-acting Systemic Agents for Fertility Regulation, Special Programme of Research, Development and Research Training in Human Reproduction. A multi-centered phase II comparative study of two hormonal contraceptive preparations given once-a-month by intramuscular injection. II. the comparison of bleeding patterns. *Contraception* 1987;40:531.

World Health Organization Task Force on Long-acting Systemic Agents for Fertility Regulation Special Programme of Research, Development and Research Training in Human Reproduction. Norethisterone enanthate given in two regimens and depot-medroxyprogesterone acetate, final report. *Contraception* 1983;28:1.

World Health Organization, Task Force on Long-acting Systemic Agents for Fertility Regulation, Special Programme of Research, Development and Research Training in Human Reproduction (1989) A multicentred phase II comparative study of two hormonal contraceptive preparations given once-a-month by intramuscular injection: II. The comparison of bleeding patterns. Contraception 40:531.

Zalanyi S, Landgren BM, Johannisson E. Pharmacokinetics, pharmacodynamic and endometrial effects of a single dose of 200 mg norethisterone enanthate. *Contraception* 1984;30:225.

Zañartu J, Navarro C. Long-acting progestogens in fertility control. *Exc Med Internat Congr Series* 1966; 122:150.

Zañartu J, Onetto E. Long-acting injectable progestogens in human fertility control. *Clin Proc I Internat Meet Planned Parenth Fed, South-East Asia and Oceania Regional Med Scientif Congr, Sydney, Australia,* 1972:65.

Zartman ER. Long-acting injectable contraception with medroxyprogesterone acetate. *Proc Sixth World Congr Fertil Steril, Tel Aviv* 1968:229.

Pharmacology of the Contraceptive Steroids,
edited by Joseph W. Goldzieher.
Raven Press, Ltd., New York © 1994.

10

The Hypothalamo-Pituitary-Ovarian System

Joseph W. Goldzieher

*Department of Obstetrics and Gynecology, Baylor College of Medicine,
Houston, Texas 77030*

GONADOTROPINS

The regulation of pulsatile gonadotropin secretion by the hypothalamo-pituitary system and the controlling influences of steroid hormones are in the domain of classical neurophysiology and will not be addressed here. There are many excellent chapters and reviews dealing with this subject, including the problems of interpretation due to variable similarities and differences between species (El Etreby et al., 1979; Brann and Mahesh, 1991). Both estrogenic and progestational substances have biphasic effects (i.e., stimulating or inhibiting secretion, and release of FSH and LH); moreover, the interactions, which are time- and dose-dependent, are extremely complex. Additionally, metabolites such as catechol estrogens and the 5α-dihydro metabolites of progesterone (Putnam-Roberts et al., 1992) are biologically active and must be taken into consideration. This active-metabolite problem raises important, as yet unsolved, questions regarding the role of metabolites of synthetic estrogens and progestins administered for fertility control.

With regard to estrogens used in fertility control, ethynylated compounds appeared fortuitously, originating as contaminants from the process used in synthesizing norethynodrel, for example. A trivial amount (to a chemist) of 1.5% of a 10 mg dose of norethynodrel represented 150 μg of mestranol—to a biologist, a far from trivial amount of a potent estrogen. In any event, the amount of estrogen included was standardized for the purpose of menstrual cycle control. However, the Mexico City group (see Historical section, Goldzieher) was unwilling to take it for granted that ethynyl estrogens were qualitatively similar (i.e., as weak as) other estrogens insofar as pituitary inhibition of gonadotropin secretion was concerned, and clinical studies (Gual et al., 1967, Goldzieher et al., 1975) quickly showed that the ethynyl group greatly potentiated the antigonadotropic activity of estradiol. Workers in this field, not appreciating this point, later attempted to formulate oral contraceptives with "natural" estrogens, and the results were disastrous. In fact, the ethynyl estrogen dosage studies showed that, had the original progestin dosage (10 mg nor-

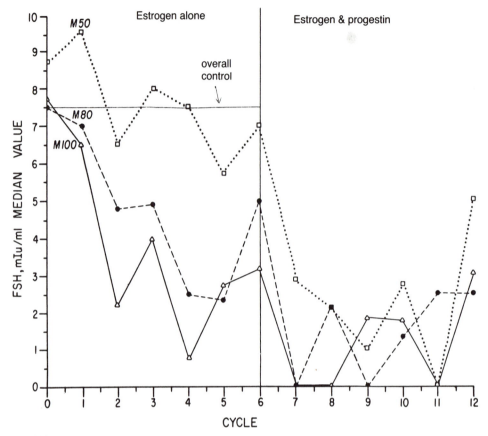

FIG. 1. Median values for plasma FSH in groups of subjects receiving cyclic estrogen therapy for six cycles, followed by six cycles during which a synthetic progestin was added. Mestranol at 50, 80, and 100 μg/day. Goldzieher et al., 1976 by permission.

ethynodrel or norethindrone administered daily for contraceptive purposes) been *totally inert*, the estrogen "contaminant" would have been a fully effective contraceptive anyway! An additional unexpected feature emerged in subsequent studies of lower-dose estrogen-progestin combinations—namely that the ethynyl estrogens and the 19-norprogestins acted synergistically in the inhibition of pituitary gonadotropin secretion, thereby making possible the highly effective, very-low-dose contraceptive formulations in use at the present time. Neither of these pharmacologically important properties was foreseen, and they were only belatedly appreciated by the manufacturers of contraceptive formulations.

The effect on plasma FSH and LH levels of cyclic ethynyl estrogens given alone showed in general a progressive dose-dependent decline and eventually a stabilization during six successive 21-day cycles. As shown in Figs. 1 to 4, the addition of

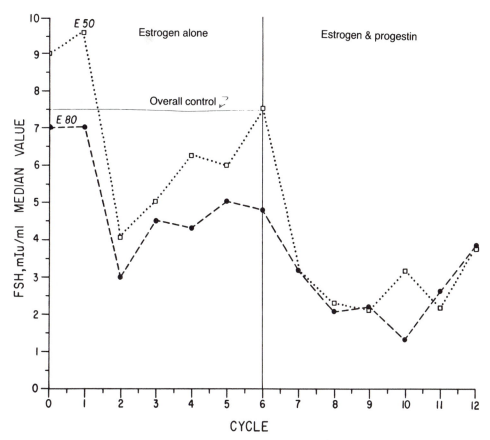

FIG. 2. Median plasma FSH values in groups of subjects receiving cyclic estrogen therapy for six cycles, followed by six cycles during which a synthetic progestin was added to the regimen. Ethynyl estradiol at 50 and 80 µg/day. Goldzieher et al., 1976 by permission.

a progestational agent for six additional cycles dramatically increased gonadotropin inhibition (Goldzieher et al., 1975). However, even with the high doses used in this study, occasional high or very high plasma FSH or LH levels were seen even in very-long-term users. (Figs. 5 and 6). These did not represent preovulatory surges (Swerdloff and Odell, 1969). One can only speculate that they resulted from subjects' failure to take medication reliably, resulting in "rebound" phenomena that had also been observed by others at the end of various treatment regimens.

On the basis of this purely estrogenic inhibition of ovulation, "sequential" contraceptive regimens were developed that typically used 80 µg of mestranol daily for 21 days, with a progestin such as chlormadinone acetate or dimethisterone added during the last 5 to 8 days of medication. Studies that formed part of an experience of 11,730 cycles examined the level of urinary pregnandiol in 185 single samples,

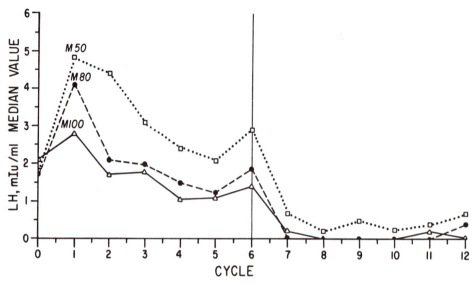

FIG. 3. Median LH values for plasma FSH in groups of subjects receiving cyclic estrogen therapy for six cycles, followed by six cycles during which a synthetic progestin was added. Mestranol at 50, 80, and 100 µg/day. Goldzieher et al., 1976 by permission.

yielding an incidence of 2.2% elevations (Goldzieher et al., 1964); however, these did not necessarily indicate actual ovulation or potentially fertile cycles, and the contraceptive use-effectiveness was remarkably high for these populations. The side effects of such estrogen doses warranted attempts at dosage reduction, and it became clear that levels below 50 µg mestranol were not sufficiently protective (the high degree of inter- and intraindividual variation in pharmacokinetics was not appreciated at that time). Historically, some abnormal endometria reported (incorrectly) as endometrial carcinoma in mestranol/dimethisterone sequential users, plus toxicology studies of huge doses of chlormadinone and related C_{21} steroids in beagle dogs, impelled the FDA to request withdrawal of the sequential formulations from the market. Experts of the World Health Organization (WHO) were unanimous in declaring the beagle dog an inappropriate animal model for the study of progestational compounds, but formulations with these and other C_{21}-steroids never reappeared in America although they are still used elsewhere in the world. Of course, the continuing pressure to lower steroid dosages in contraceptive formulations eventually made estrogen-only sequential regimens obsolete.

Estrogen/progestin Combinations

Figures 1 and 2 clearly demonstrate the more powerful gonadotropin-suppressive effect of the estrogen-progestin combination. This action is thought by some to occur mainly in the hypothalamus or higher in the CNS (Kastin et al., 1972; Vandenberg et al., 1974), while others conclude that the action is mainly a direct sup-

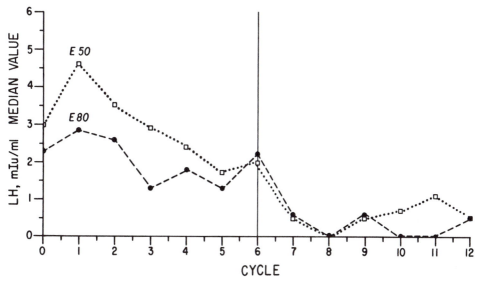

FIG. 4. Median plasma LH values in groups of subjects receiving cyclic estrogen therapy for six cycles, followed by six cycles during which a synthetic progestin was added to the regimen. Ethynyl estradiol at 50 and 80 μg/day. Goldzieher et al., 1976 by permission.

pressive effect on the pituitary gonadotrophs (Baker et al., 1973; Robyn et al., 1974; Perez-Lopez et al., 1975; Krog et al., 1976). Dericks-Tan et al. (1983) carried out a double GnRH stimulation test in users of a 30 μg oral contraceptive (OC) on days 8 to 11 of use. Both the immediate response of LH and the second response (indicating subsequent synthesis and release) were decreased, and this persisted during the treatment-free period. Acute FSH release was unaffected but replenishment of depleted stores was reduced. FSH inhibition did not extend into the treatment-free period, when the response actually exceeded the control response. This pattern remained unchanged in the third and sixth cycle of OC use. The authors had previously emphasized the dose-dependency of these phenomena (Dericks-Tan et al., 1976). With 50 μg estrogen formulations (Spellacy et al., 1980; Wan et al., 1981), decreased basal FSH and LH levels were observed, as was blunting of the response to GnRH. Wan et al. found little impact of a 20 μg OC, whereas de Leo et al. (1991), using a similar estrogen dosage for six cycles, found an elevation in LH response but an inhibition of FSH response to GnRH. With the lower ethynyl estradiol (EE) dosages (Van der Vange et al., 1985), gonadotropins tended to normalize promptly in the off-pill interval, but Rubinstein et al. (1978) still detected suppression on off-days 2 to 3 with a 50 μg OC. However, Craft et al. (1975) found it had normalized by post-pill day 14.

Mishell et al. (1977) and Scott et al. (1978) found considerable variability among long-term users: initial values of FSH and LH were suppressed only in about 75% of subjects, with the LH response to GnRH diminished in 80%, and FSH in 90%. They remarked upon the degree of individual variation. This may be attributable to interindividual variation in the pharmacokinetics of the contraceptive steroids themselves, or to intrinsic variability in hypothalamopituitary responses. All investigators agree that basal FSH and LH levels do not predict the response to GnRH, and that the length of OC use has no effect on the gonadotropin response, but that different formulations have different effects. With equal estrogens, Wan et al. (1981) found 1 mg norethindrone to be equivalent to 0.5 mg levonorgestrel; Dericks-Tan and others feel that the estrogen component is the major influence on the gonadotropic response.

Virtually nothing has been done to explore the gonadotropin dynamics of multiphasic preparations; however, the nature of ovarian activity with these preparations (see following section) suggests much less suppression of gonadotropin levels, although it can be assumed from the low conception rate that effective ovulatory surges are interdicted.

Ovarian activity obviously reflects the gonadotropic and steroid milieu to which it is exposed. Logically, the higher the dosage of the OC, the greater the inhibition of gonadotropins and the less the follicular activity. As the dosage has been decreased, there is more ovarian activity as evidenced by higher prevailing estradiol levels and sonographic evidence of follicular maturation. Van der Vange et al. (1985) carried out an intensive study of ovarian ultrasound and peripheral endocrine parameters with seven different monophasic and multiphasic formulations including levonorgestrel, norethindrone, desogestrel, gestodene, and cyproterone acetate. The estrogen content ranged from 30 to 40 µg EE. According to ultrasound, over 50% of cycles showed follicles >10 mm, and in about 30% of cycles follicles >18 mm in diameter were observed. In over 55% of the tested cycles, serum estradiol levels reached those of the early follicular phase. Fifteen cycles showed evidence of insufficient luteinization and 15 were suspected of being ovulatory. A comparison of the seven products on this small scale (10 women per group) showed that monophasic desogestrel and triphasic gestodene suppressed ovarian function to a greater extent than the other formulations, while monophasic levonorgestrel possessed an intermediate position. Other sonographic studies of triphasic OCs that have been carried out also show a certain degree of follicular activity (Elstein and Killick, 1985). More such studies are in progress, chiefly because of a gratuitous claim (eventually shown to be incorrect) that ovarian cysts requiring surgical intervention were more common in users of multiphasic formulations.

The responsiveness of gonadotropes to GnRH after discontinuation of combined OCs has been mentioned above. Van der Spuy et al. (1990) observed gonadotropin and estradiol dynamics for 8 hours at the start and the end of the placebo week after combination OC use (50 µg, 30 µg monophasics and a triphasic were examined). By day 7 of placebo, gonadotropin concentrations and pulse patterns had normalized, but estradiol levels were still lower than at corresponding times in a control cycle. Gillmer et al. (1978) reported persistent suppression during the pill-free week, though not to the degree seen during OC use. They found that women who failed to bleed at the end of the pill cycle had higher gonadotropin and estradiol levels than those who menstruated, and hypothesized that less pituitary inhibition and more follicular activity resulted in better endometrial stimulation and less likelihood of withdrawal bleeding. Klein and Mishell (1977) followed endocrine parameters for 2 months following OC discontinuation. They found that the follicular phase was prolonged, with the ovulatory LH surge occurring generally 21 to 28 days after the last pill. Otherwise, the patterns and levels of all hormones were indistinguishable from those of normal ovulatory subjects, clearly indicating the absence of any "hangover" effects.

Progestin-only "Minipills"

The use of continuous microdose (0.5 mg) chlormadinone acetate as an oral contraceptive was reported by Martinez-Manautou in 1966. Subsequent studies with other progestins confirmed the contraceptive effect, despite the fact that ovulatory levels of progesterone were observed in 60% of chlormadinone cycles. Examination of plasma gonadotropins showed erratic patterns; however, ovulatory spikes of LH

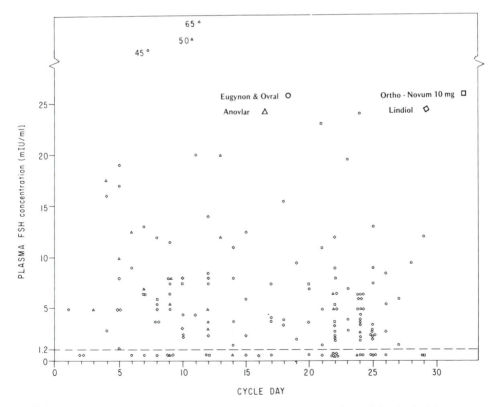

FIG. 5. Levels of plasma FSH in fertile women using .05 mg ethynylestradiol or 0.06–0.075 mg mestranol and 0.5 mg norgestrel or 2.5 mg lynestrenol or 4 mg norethindrone acetate or 10 mg norethindrone for 5 to 12 yrs. by menstrual cycle day. (From Goldzieher et al., 1976 by permission.)

and FSH were absent. Ovarian function reflected this milieu: in a study with daily 300 µg norethindrone, Landgren et al. (1979) found suppression of LH and FSH peaks in all users, as follows: 1) 16% showed no follicular or luteal activity, although the FSH level was not depressed; 2) 23% showed some follicular but no luteal activity, and depressed LH levels were characteristic; 3) 21% showed normal follicular development but inadequate luteinization; and 4) 40% showed normal follicular growth, with normal estradiol and progesterone levels. Moghissi et al. (1973) had made identical observations on gonadotropin dynamics. Similar observations have been made with lynestrenol, a norethindrone pro-drug (Friedrich et al., 1975). The erratic behavior of LH levels with a range of doses of ethynodiol diacetate has been illustrated by Mishell and Odell (1971).

The nongonadotropic effects of microdose contraception are described in Chapter 12.

Few studies of the effect of progestins on the Fallopian tubes have been carried out. Coutinho et al. (1973) found that tubal motility was depressed during progestin use, and the cyclic changes that occur during normal ovulatory cycles were abolished. El-Mahgoub et al. (1972) described changes seen after the use of injectable progestins.

Long-acting Oral Agents

A weekly dose of a progestin (R2323-ethylnorgestrienone) was briefly evaluated by Niaraki et al. (1981). Results were mixed: some ovulatory gonadotropin patterns were seen, but in other instances the ovulatory peaks and luteal progesterone production were suppressed. Little has been heard about this compound recently.

A combination of quinestrol (the 3-cyclopentyl enol ether of EE) and quingestanol (the 3-cyclopentyl enol ether of norethindrone acetate) was studied briefly as a possible contraceptive pill to be given once monthly. Efficacy and side effects were unsatisfactory. This combination suppressed cyclic fluctuations of FSH, while estrogen and LH levels were often at preovulatory levels; nevertheless, breakthrough ovulations and pregnancies occurred in some instances (Nudemberg et al., 1973).

Long-acting Injectable Agents

The gonadotropin dynamics with the use of depo-Provera and other injectables are described in Chapter 9. Detailed studies of GnRH response have not been carried out. Early work (Goldzieher et al. 1970) reported cross-sectional studies indicating that there was little alteration in dynamics except for elimination of the ovulatory surge. Plasma FSH values, assayed immediately before the next injection, remained in the normal range, and were occasionally at the preovulatory surge level (Fig. 8). LH values, while depressed to 65% of control at the end of the first injection period, gradually rose into the normal range during the 27-month observation period (Fig. 7). Various studies have shown that estradiol levels remain around the early follicular range; thus, no hypoestrogenic state occurs.

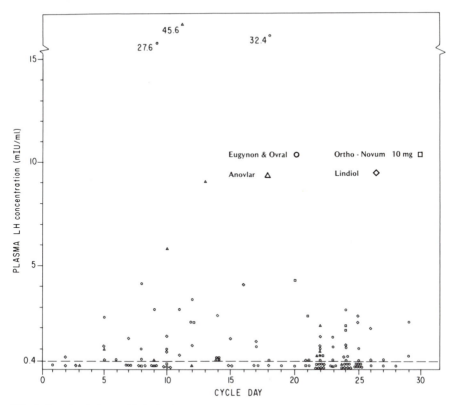

FIG. 6. Levels of plasma LH in fertile women using 0.05 mg ethynylestradiol or 0.06–0.075 mg mestranol and 0.5 mg norgestrol or 2.5 mg lynestrenol or 4 mg norethindrone acetate or 10 mg norethindrone for 5 to 12 yrs. by menstrual cycle day.

GROWTH HORMONE

Hansen and Weeke (1974), Hausman et al. (1976), and others observed no effect of combined OC use on fasting GH levels or GH response following insulin or glucose infusion. Others (Spellacy et al., 1967; Davidson and Holzman, 1973) have observed increased response. Since it is known that estrogen increases fasting GH levels as well as response to stimuli, Mishell et al. (1977) believe that the estrogen/ progestin balance in various formulations determines the ultimate GH blood level and response to stimuli.

PROLACTIN

Estrogens are known to increase prolactin secretion in rodents, and there is considerable evidence that the same occurs in humans (Franks, 1983). Results have been equivocal in OC users; for example, Abu-Fadil et al. (1976) observed an increase in plasma levels, while Spellacy et al. (1978) did not. Both of these studies were cross-sectional, with the problems attendant to such a design; a longitudinal study of 126 normal women by Hwang et al. (1986) found a trivial elevation (from 8.9 ng/ml to 10.9 ng/ml at 12 months). The relation of opioids to such changes is controversial (Snowden et al., 1986). Buckmann and Peake (1973) and Mishell et al. (1977) reported augmented prolactin secretion following a stimulus with thyrotropin-releasing hormone (TRH) or phenothiazine in combined OC users. However, another study found no effect in users of OCs with levonorgestrel or cyproterone acetate (Bellmann et al., 1978). Medroxyprogesterone acetate was said to increase prolactin (PRL) response to the suckling stimulus in lactating women (Mishell et al., 1977). Direct implantation of norethindrone or norethynodrel into the hypophyseal pars distalis of rats caused a local hypertrophy of prolactin cells and reduction in size of LH-cells. Medroxyprogestrone was ineffective. In such studies, however, one must be wary of extrapolation from one species to another.

The known effect of estrogen on prolactin, and anecdotal clinical observations of women who remained amenorrheic after OC use and showed elevated prolactin levels, brought about the invention of the syndrome of "post-pill amenorrhea." This *post hoc* fallacy was put to rest by a number of investigations (Shy et al., 1983; Pituitary Adenoma Study Group, 1983).

The Ovary

Maqueo et al. (1972) examined ovarian biopsies from 125 women who had used high-dose combination or sequential OCs for 2 to 91 months. The follicular system

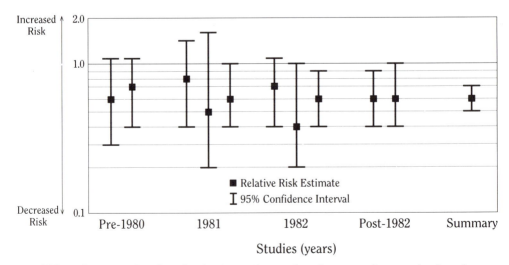

FIG. 7. Case control studies of oral contraceptives and ovarian cancer, by year, showing relative risk estimate and 95% confidence intervals.

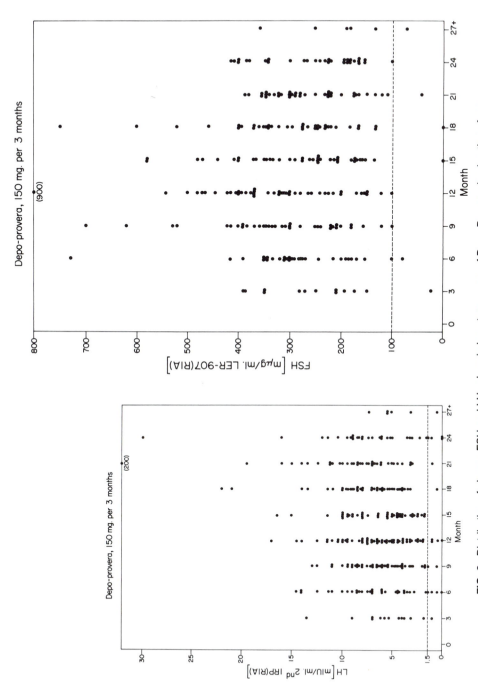

FIG. 8. Distribution of plasma FSH and LH values in long-term users of Depo-Provera, by duration of use.

showed inactivity, as expected, and except for some cortical fibrosis, no unexpected pathology was seen. Unexpectedly, long-term case-control studies have revealed a decrease in incidence of epithelial ovarian cancer in users of high-dose OCs (WHO, 1989; the Cancer and Steroid Hormone Study (CASH) Study, 1987). This finding has been consistent in all epidemiologic studies (Fig. 7). The reduction in relative risk approaches 0.5 in a relatively short time, although less than 1 year of use may have no effect (Gross et al., 1992). With increased duration of use, relative risks approaching 0.3 have been reported after 10 or more years. Moreover, the protective effect persists for at least 15 years after OC discontinuation (Prentice and Thomas, 1987).

REFERENCES

Abu-Fadil S, DeVane G, Siler TM, Yen SS. Effects of oral contraceptive steroids on pituitary prolactin secretion. *Contraception* 1976;13:79–85.

Baker BL, Eskin TA, Lawrence LN. Direct action of synthetic progestins on the hypophysis. *Endocrinol* 1973;92:965–72.

Bellmann O, Broschen-Zywietz C, Fichte K. Stimulation of prolactin and TSH secretion by TRH in long-term oral contraceptive users. *Arch Gynäk* 1978;225:31–42.

Brann DW, Mahesh VB. Regulation of gonadotropin secretion by steroid hormones. *Frontiers Neuroendocr* 1991;12:165–207.

Buckmann MT, Peake GT. Estrogen potentiation of phenothiazine-induced prolactin secretion in man. *J Clin Endocrinol Metab* 1973;37:977.

The Cancer and Steroid Hormone Study of the Centers for Disease Control and the National Institute of Child Health and Human Development. The reduction in risk of ovarian cancer associated with oral contraceptive use. *N Engl J Med* 1987;316:650–5.

Coutinho EM, et al. The effect of a continuous low dose progestin on tubal and uterine motility. *Int J Fertil* 1973;18:161.

Craft I, Foss GL, Warren RJ, Fotherby K. Effect of norgestrel administered intermittently on pituitary-ovarian function. *Contraception* 1975;12:589–98.

Davidson MB, Holzman GB. Role of growth hormone on the alteration of carbohydrate metabolism induced by oral contraceptive agents. *J Clin Endocrinol Metab* 1973;36:246–55.

DeLeo V, Lanzetta D, Vanni AL, et al. Low estrogen oral contraceptives and the hypothalamopituitary axis. *Contraception* 1991;44:155–61.

Dericks-Tan JSE, Koch P, Taubert HD. Synthesis and release of gonadotropins: effect of an oral contraceptive. *Obstet Gynecol* 1983;62:687–90.

Dericks-Tan JSE, Krog W, Aktories K, Taubert HD. Dose-dependent inhibition by oral contraceptives of the pituitary to release LH and FSH in response to stimulation with LH-RH. *Contraception* 1976; 14:171–81.

El Etreby MF, Gräf KJ, Neumann F. Evaluation of effects of sexual steroids on the hypothalamic-pituitary system of animals and man. *Arch Toxicol* 1979;[Suppl 2]:11–39.

El-Mahgoub S, Karim M, Ammar R. Long term effects of injected progestogens on the morphology of human oviducts. *J Reprod Med* 1972;8:288–92.

Elstein M, Killick S. Ovarian follicular development in patients taking the combined oral contraceptive pill. *Arch Gynecol* 1985;237[Suppl]:331.

Friedrich E, Keller E, Jaeger-Whitegiver ER, et al. Effects of 0.5mg of lynestrenol daily on hypothalamic-pituitary-ovarian function. *Am J Obstet Gynecol* 1975;122:642–9.

Franks S. Regulation of prolactin secretion by oestrogens: physiological and pathological significance. *Clin Sci* 1983;65:457–62.

Gillmer MDG, Fox EJ, Jacobs HS. Failure of withdrawal bleeding during combined oral contraceptive therapy: amenorrhea on the pill. *Contraception* 1978;18:507–13.

Goldzieher JW, Becerra C, Gual C, et al. New oral contraceptive. *Am J Obstet Gynecol* 1964;90:404–11.

Goldzieher JW, de la Pena, Chenault CB, Woutersz T. Comparative studies of the ethynyl estrogens used in oral contraceptives II. antiovulatory potency. *Am J Obstet Gynecol* 1975;122:619–24.

Goldzieher JW, de la Pena A, Chenault CB, Woutersz TM. Comparative studies of the ethynyl estrogens used in oral contraceptives III. Effect on plasma gonadotropins. *Am J Obstet Gynecol* 1976;122:625–36.

Goldzieher JW, Kleber JW, Moses LE, Rathmacher RP. A cross-sectional study of plasma FSH and LH levels in women using sequential, combination, or injectable steroid contraceptives over long periods of time. *Contraception* 1970;2:225–48.

Gross TP, Schlesselman JJ, Stadel BV, et al. The risk of epithelial ovarian cancer in short-term users of oral contraceptives. *Am J Epidemiol* 1992;136:46–53.

Gual C, Becerra C, Rice-Wray E, Goldzieher JW. Inhibition of ovulation by estrogens. *Am J Obstet Gynecol* 1967;97:443–447.

Hansen AP, Weeke J. Fasting serum growth hormone levels and growth hormone responses to exercise during normal menstrual cycles and cycles of oral contraceptives. *Scand J Clin Lab Invest* 1974;34:199–205.

Hausmann L, Goebel KM, Zehner J. Influence of an oral contraceptive (ethinyl estradiol/d-norgestrel) on growth hormone and insulin secretion. *Schweiz Med Wochschr* 1976;106:1470–4.

Hwang PLH, Ng CSA, Cheong ST. Effect of oral contraceptives on serum prolactin: a longitudinal study in 126 normal premenopausal women. *Clin Endocrinol* 1986;24:127–33.

Kastin AJ, Schally AV, Gual C, Arimura A. Release of LH and FSH after administration of synthetic LH-releasing hormone. *J Clin Endocrinol Metab* 1972;34:753.

Klein TA, Mishell DR Jr. Gonadotropin, prolactin and steroid hormone levels after discontinuation of oral contraceptives. *Am J Obstet Gynecol* 1977;127:585–9.

Krog, W, Aktories K, Dericks-Tan JSE, Taubert HD. Dose-dependent inhibition by oral contraceptives of the pituitary to release LH and FSH in response to stimulation with LHRH. *Contraception* 1976;15:171.

Landgren B-M, Balogh A, Shin MW, Diczfalusy E. Hormonal effects of the 300 μg norethisterone (NET) minipill. 2. daily gonadotropin levels in 43 subjects during pretreatment cycle and during the second month of NET administration. *Contraception* 1979;20:585–605.

Martinez-Manautou, J, Cortez V, Giner J et al. Low dose progestogen as an approach to fertility control. *Fertil. Steril* 1966;17:49.

Maqueo M, Rice-Wray E, Calderon JJ, Goldzieher JW. Ovarian morphology after prolonged use of steroid contraceptive agents. *Contraception* 1972;5:177–85.

Mishell DR Jr, Kletzky OA, Brenner PF, et al. The effect of contraceptive steroids on hypothalamo-pituitary function. *Am J Obstet Gynecol* 1977;128:60–74.

Mishell DR Jr, Odell WD. Effect of varying dosages of ethynodiol diacetate upon serum luteinizing hormone. *Am J Obstet Gynecol* 1971;109:140–9.

Moghissi KS, Syner FN, McBride LC. Contraceptive mechanism of microdose norethindrone. *Obstet Gynecol* 1973;41:585–94.

Niaraki MA, Moghissi K, Borin K. The effect of a synthetic progestogen, ethylnorgestrienone, on hypothalamic-pituitary-ovarian function, cervical mucus, vaginal cytology and endometrial morphology. *Fertil Steril* 1981;35:284–8.

Nudemberg F, Kothari M, Karam K, Taymor ML. Effects of the "pill-a-month" on the hypothalamic-pituitary-ovarian axis. *Fertil Steril* 1973;24:185–90.

Perez-Lopez FR, L'Hermite M, Robyn C. Gonadotropin hormone releasing tests in women receiving hormonal contraception. *Clin Endocrinol* 1975;4:477.

Pituitary Adenoma Study Group. Pituitary adenomas and oral contraceptives: a multicenter case control study. *Fertil Steril* 1983;39:753–60.

Prentice RL, Thomas DB. On the epidemiology of oral contraceptives and disease. *Adv Cancer Res* 1987;49:285ff.

Putnam-Roberts C, Brann DW, Mahesh VB. Role of 5α-reduction in progesterone's ability to release FSH in estrogen-primed ovariectomized rats. *J Steroid Chem Mol Biol* 1992;42:875–82.

Robyn C, Schondorf H, Jurgenson O, et al. Oral contraception can decrease the pituitary capacity to release gonadotropins in response to synthetic LH-releasing hormone. *Arch Gynaekol* 1974;216:73.

Rubinstein L, Moguilevsky J, Leiderman S. The effect of oral contraceptives on the gonadotropin response to LHRH. *Obstet Gynecol* 1978;52:571–4.

Scott JA, Brenner PF, Kletzky OA, Mishell DR. Factors affecting gonadotropin function in users of oral contraceptive steroids. *Am J Obstet Gynecol* 1978;130:817–21.

Shy KS, McTiernan AM, Daling JR, Weiss NS. Oral contraceptive use and the occurrence of pituitary prolactinoma. *JAMA* 1983;249:2,204–7.

Snowden EU, Khan-Dawood FS, Dawood MY. Opioid regulation of pituitary gonadotropins and prolactin in women using oral contraceptives. *Am J Obstet Gynecol* 1986;154:440–4.

Spellacy WN, Carlson KL, Schade SL. Human growth hormone levels in normal subjects receiving an oral contraceptive. *JAMA* 1967;202:451–4.

Spellacy WN, Kalra PS, Buhi WC, Birk SA. Pituitary and ovarian responsiveness to a graded gonadotropin releasing factor stimulation test in women using a low-estrogen or a regular type of oral contraceptive. *Am J Obstet Gynecol* 1980;137:109–15.

Spellacy WM, Mahan CS, Buhi WC, Dumbaugh VS. Plasma prolactin levels and contraception: oral contraceptives and intrauterine devices. *Contraception* 1978;17:71–7.

Swerdloff RL, Odell WD. Serum luteinizing and follicle stimulating hormone levels during sequential and nonsequential contraceptive treatment of eugonadal women. *J Clin Endocrinol Metab* 1969;29:157–63.

Van der Spuy ZM, Sohnius U, Pienaar CA, Schall R. Gonadotropin and estradiol secretion during the week of placebo therapy in oral contraceptive pill users. *Contraception* 1990;42:597–609.

Van der Vange N, Bruinse HW, Bennink HJT, et al. Is ovarian activity inhibited during low dose oral contraceptive use? *Arch Gynecol* 1985;237:331.

Vandenberg G, DeVane G, Yen SSC. Effects of exogenous estrogen and progestin on pituitary responsiveness to synthetic luteinizing-hormone releasing factor. *J Clin Invest* 1974;53:1750.

Wan LS, Ganguly M, Weiss G. Pituitary response to LHRH stimulation in women on oral contraceptives: a followup dose-response study. *Contraception* 1981;24:229–34.

World Health Organization Collaborative Study of Neoplasia and Steroid Contraceptives. Epithelial ovarian cancer and combined oral contraceptives. *Int J Epidemiol* 1989;18:538–45.

Pharmacology of the Contraceptive Steroids,
edited by Joseph W. Goldzieher.
Raven Press, Ltd., New York © 1994.

11

The Female Breast

Fritz K. Beller

*Department of Obstetrics and Gynecology, University of Iowa College of Medicine,
Iowa City, Iowa 52242*

Since there are almost no data available, the endocrinology of the human female breast remains an enigma. Nearly all conclusions have been derived from animal experimentation or epidemiological studies. This may explain the difficulty in interpreting data regarding the influence of estrogen and progesterone on breast cancer.

The biology is poorly understood and speculations run high. Although there is interest in fibrocystic change, the underlying mechanisms responsible for the size, form, and magnitude of the breast have received little attention. Extensive data on animal experimentation were summarized recently by Bässler (1978 and 1986), and Neville and Daniel (1987). A variety of hormones are influential, predominantly estrogens, progesterone, and prolactin. T_3 and T_4 are involved, as is aldosterone. The interaction during human embryological development is unknown.

Estrogens are considered in general as proliferative hormones that stimulate growth. The current knowledge of systemic hormonal effect on mammogenesis comes primarily from classical endocrine ablation/replacement studies in rats and mice. Daniel and Silberstein (1987) concluded that estrogen may act directly as a ductal mammogen. It is assumed that estrogens stimulate ductal growth and increase progesterone receptors (Haslam et al., 1987). Progestins are said to stimulate ductal branching and lobuloaveolar development (Assairi et al. 1974). Vorherr (1986) has summarized this into a scheme (Fig. 1).

Although it is believed that estrogens act directly as ductal mammogens, they may also act solely as local agents promoting local synthesis of unidentified mitogen (Daniel and Silberstein, 1987). Estrogens also induce progesterone receptor concentration and play a key role in mammary growth *in vivo* (for a review, see Leung et al., 1976).

Progesterone does not appear to be required for ductal elongation, but the development of alveoli is dependent on this hormone in rats and mice (Freeman and Topper, 1978; Lyons and Li, 1988). On the other hand, Topper and Freeman (1980) believe that progesterone is required for the estrogen activity on lobuloalveolar development.

Estrogen → Development of ductal epithelium → Decreasing concentration of receptors

----

Progesterone → proliferation of alveolar lobular system.

FIG. 1. Influence of estrogen and progesterone on elements of breast tissue. (From Vorherr 1986 with permission).

In conclusion, Haslam (1987) stated that estrogens and progesterone are clearly required for the promotion of mammary growth *in vivo*. In the case of estrogen, specific cellular hormone receptors are present in both the epithelial and stromal components of the gland. The ability of estrogens to regulate progesterone receptors appears to be due to a direct effect of the hormone on the epithelial cells. The mitogenic effects of estrogen, on the other hand, are expressed in both the epithelium and the stroma.

THE BREAST AT BIRTH

The very high estrogen and progesterone activity in pregnancy crosses the placental barrier and must be effective on the fetal tissue. Indeed, almost 70% of newborn females (a male/female distribution is not known) demonstrate a slight growth of the breast (without reaching the budding stage). In approximately 30%, a few drops of colostrum can be expressed. This was observed by German midwives in the middle 19th century and described as an enigma, "Hexenmilch," (witch's milk). This phenomenon is believed to be a reflection of estrogen reaching the fetus, but there are no data available. Two weeks after birth, the enlargement of breast tissue subsides to the normal flat appearance, supporting the idea that it was related to estrogen.

THE BREAST FROM BIRTH TO PUBERTY

After the hormonal activity of pregnancy on the female breast has subsided, the breast remains "silent" until puberty (Bässler, 1978). Exceptions occur in two pathological conditions: premature menarche and precocious puberty. Premature menarche is a condition in which breast growth is stimulated at age 4 to 6 for unknown reasons, but with little change in endocrinology. However, it may reflect a low estrogen effect in a magnitude of 20 to 30 pg/ml (Stolecke, 1989). Precocious puberty is the onset of secondary sex characteristics before age 9. Thelarche is present (Fig. 2).

PUBERTY

Twenty-five years ago, Tanner was the first to study the development of sexual characteristics in a longitudinal fashion. His observations on the female breast and on hair growth of the pubes, based on 145 girls, have been accepted universally as

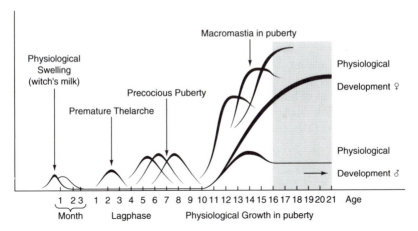

FIG. 2. The development of the female breast. (From Bassler 1978 with permission.)

Tanner Stages I to V. Tanner observed that thelarche begins a few months (11.1 years) before pubarche (11.6 years), which begins before menarche (12.5 years). Beller et al. (1991) repeated the longitudinal study on more than 800 girls in central Europe 25 years after Tanner. They confirmed the original data, and included axillary hair growth in their observations and noted that axillarche develops before menarche. In their group, breast growth had ceased 2 years after menarche.

There are no endocrine data available to understand these endocrine developments. In fact, breast measurements are lacking in the literature, and one has to refer to textbooks by artists to find discussions on breast size and proportions. Therefore, at present there is no evidence to indicate that hormone use at puberty could make a breast smaller or larger.

Primary ovarian failure is associated with failure of breast growth stimulation, as in Turner's syndrome, gonadal agenesis, or 46 XX or 46 XY. There are exceptions if islands of ovarian tissue have emerged. The McCune-Albright syndrome is an example with endocrine ovarian activity in which breast growth has been observed.

INFLUENCES DURING THE MENSTRUAL CYCLE

A few studies indicate that there is a cyclical change in proliferative activity of the breast during the menstrual cycle (Anderson et al., 1983; Mauvais-Jarvis et al., 1982; Potten et al., 1988; Going et al., 1988). However, the cycle acts in a way opposite to the endometrium. Proliferation is higher in the second phase of the cycle, after ovulation, and therefore is under the influence of progesterone. The change is also considerably less pronounced than in the endometrium. The breast changes size during the cycle, presumably because of endogenous estrogen activity causing edema. Milligan et al. (1975) have shown that the breast increases in size from 15 to 30 cm^3 in the premenstrual phase and returns to its original volume during menses. This change is believed to be the result of water retention in the stroma and infiltration of connective tissue with lymphoid and plasma cells. The breast is smallest during days 4 to 7 of the cycle, when endogenous estrogen is lowest (Dabelow, 1957).

Biopsy specimens of human breast tissue obtained in the luteal phase of the menstrual cycle exhibited higher DNA synthesis in ductal epithelium than specimens in the follicular phase (Masters et al., 1977; Meyer, 1977).

PREGNANCY

Breast growth has not been completed after puberty, and the full development of the mammary gland is believed to be completed at the end of the first pregnancy (Mauvais-Jarvis et al., 1982; Moolgarkar et al., 1979). Estrogen and progesterone increase to very high levels during normal pregnancy. It is assumed that estradiol (E_2) is one of the hormones necessary for growth and epithelial proliferation of the human breast (Topper and Freeman, 1980). The breast increases in size, turgor, and water content. Estrogens may mediate the mammary gland response to lactogenic hormones. It is believed that progesterone prevents premature lactation (for review see Kuhn, 1977). Following delivery the breast regresses to prepregnancy size.

LACTATION

Transfer of Contraceptive Steroids to Breast Milk

The literature has been reviewed by Nilsson and Nygren (1979), and Fraser (1991). Using radiolabeled steroids, Wijmenga and van der Molen (1969) found 0.02% to 0.04% of administered mestranol-radioactivity dose per 100 ml milk, totaled over 4 days. Pincus et al. (1966) gave 5 mg labeled doses of norethynodrel or ethynodiol diacetate and recovered only 0.004% to 0.13% of the radioactivity in milk over a 4-day collection. In users of norethindrone oral contraceptives (OCs), studies by radioimmunoassay yielded undetectable levels in half the subjects at 4 hours, levels to 790 pg/ml at 4 hours, and 287 pg/ml at 24 hours (Saxena et al., 1977; Toddywalla et al., 1980; Adey et al., 1982). With 30 μg levonorgestrel doses, milk levels ranged from undetectable (Nilsson et al., 1977) to 135 pg/ml (Thomas 1984). With 50 μg doses, Toddywalla et al. (1980) found levels of 50 to 200 pg/ml at 2 to 3 hours and no detectable levels at 4 hours. Overall, it is estimated that 0.1% to 1.0% of the steroid dose appears in the milk. How much of this material is still biologically active is speculative. With Depo-Provera, Benagiano and Primiero (1983) have estimated that 0.2 μg per kg body weight is ingested by the infant immediately after the mother's Depo-Provera injection, falling to less than 0.08 μg by the end of the injection period. Norplant users have concentrations of 23 to 311 pg/ml of levonorgestrel in the milk (Diaz et al., 1985).

The American Academy of Pediatrics (1981) assumes that a newborn would ingest 10 pg of ethinyl estradiol daily if the OC content was 50 μg. This is in a range similar to the amount of natural estrogens taken up by mothers who have not taken OCs. Regarding norgestrel in milk, a plasma ratio of 0.15 was calculated (Nilsson et al., 1977). For lynestrenol a ratio of 0.16 has been calculated (Van der Molen, 1969).

Effect on Milk Composition

The WHO multicenter study (1988) compared a monophasic OC with two progestin-only contraceptives up to 6 months postpartum. With a 30 μg ethynyl estradiol/levonorgestrel (EE/LNG) formulation, they confirmed previous observations of a reduction in milk volume, a deficit in calories, and widespread changes in minerals. However, these changes were not reflected in any criterion of infant growth at 24 weeks, in spite of the study's 80% likelihood of detecting a minimum difference of 400 to 500 g in infant weight at 24 weeks. Various speculations were offered to account for the chemical changes in milk quantity and composition, and the entire absence of any effect on infant nutrition and welfare. Nevertheless, the WHO Task Force reiterates the recommendation to avoid combined OCs during the first weeks or months of lactation. Toddywalla et al. (1977) found a slight decrease in fat and calcium content but, interestingly, this was nullified by the addition of 10 μg EE to the formulation. Progestin-only minipills apparently have no effect on milk quantity or quality (Gupta et al., 1974; Lonnerdal et al., 1980; Delgado-Betancourt et al., 1984; WHO, 1988). The effect of injectable progestins on milk composition is uncertain; various studies report increases, no change, or decreases in lactose, protein, or lipid quantities (Abel-Kader et al., 1976; Koetsawang, 1977; Toddywalla et al., 1977; Ali and Jalil, 1978). No differences were found between the progestin-only minipill and DMPA by the WHO Task Force (1988). The observed changes are most probably insignificant from the practical point of view. The American Academy of Pediatricians (1981) has reviewed a possible decrease of milk production and decreased composition of nitrogen and protein, and considered the magnitude to be very low. It may be of consequence only in malnourished mothers, an issue that requires further research in third-world countries.

Effect on the Neonate

Extensive studies show no deleterious effects (Delgado-Betancourt et al., 1984; WHO, 1984,1988), and occasionally even beneficial effects (Jimenez et al., 1984; McCann et al., 1989), of oral or injected contraceptive steroid formulations. Neonatal weight gain, and growth and development in childhood have been unaffected (Koetsawang et al., 1984; WHO, 1984,1988). Only one study with a low-dose combined OC showed a transient reduction in weight and weight gain (Diaz et al., 1983; Croxatto et al., 1983). Wilson and Brent (1981) considered the risk to the fetus for nongenital malformations very small, if it exists at all (see chapter 27).

BENIGN BREAST DISEASE

Breast Growth

There is only one paper that indicates an attempt to stimulate breast growth by estrogens and progesterone. Lauritzen (1989) gave a bimonthly I.M. injection of 40 mg estradiol valerate + 250 mg 17-hydroxyprogesterone acetate once a week for as long as 15 to 20 weeks. The estrogen dose corresponds to four times the proliferation dose on the endometrium. Among 224 patients, 65 responded with an increase in size, whereas 30% failed. In 40%, the response declined after termination of treatment. Receptor sides for E and P in the breast were found by Savitt and Durant (1981).

Fibrocystic Change

Various data accumulated in epidemiological studies address the influence of steroid hormones on breast tissue. The problem is that benign breast disease as summarized under the term fibrocystic disease in the U.S. (a term which should not be used anymore, Consensus Conference 1986), Aberrations of Normal Development and Involution (ANDI) in England (Hughes et al., 1989), and Mastopathia in Germany is not a single well-defined disease (Kodlin et al., 1977) but consists of a variety of changes that are not interrelated (e.g., fibrosis, fibroadenoma, cystic mastitis, adenosis, intraductal papillomas, mastalgia or mastodynia, and nipple discharge, to name only a few). It is said that fibrocystic change is a condition of estrogen dominance (Vorherr, 1985; Schindler, 1989; Mauvais-Jarvis et al., 1982). However, this conclusion is based on unsubstantiated epidemiological data. Fibrocystic change is associated more frequently with monophasic cycles. Moreover, an imbalance between estrogen and progesterone is said to be pathogenetic (Sitruk-Ware et al., 1979); however, there are no data to substantiate this statement.

Interestingly, monophasic cycles have not been related to the size of the breast. However, it is known that breasts increase in size in the premenopause; this is believed to be a reflection of estrogen effect with less-than-normal progesterone influence.

Epidemiological studies have consistently shown a strongly negative association (i.e., a protective effect) between OC use and benign breast disease (Vessey et al., 1972; Fasal and Pfaffenbarger, 1975; Ory et al., 1976; Pastides et al., 1983; Franceschi et al., 1984; Hislop and Threlfall, 1984; Odenheimer et al., 1984). In the study of Ory et al. (1976), 1 to 12 months of use did not decrease the risk of hospital admission for breast disease (i.e., biopsy); thereafter, risk was reduced by 30% with 13 to 24 months of use, and 65% by more than 25 months of use. Other studies found the negative association to begin 2 to 5.5 months after use. Rohan et al. (1992) examined the relationship of OC use and type of cytology found at biopsy. In this Australian case-control study, there was a 60% reduction of risk in current users; further reduction occurred with increasing duration of use. There was little variation in risk with total duration of use, use before first pregnancy, and years since first and last use. Nor was there any change in risk of various types of atypia, which does not support the hypothesis of Cole (1977) that OCs might increase the risk of "premalignant" forms of atypia and decrease the risk of "non-premalignant" forms. Some authors have indicated a negative association between OCs and benign breast disease with increasing length of use, starting after 2 to 5.5 years (Fasal and Pfaffenberger, 1975; Franceschi et al., 1984; Haagensen, 1986; Hislop and Threifall, 1984; Odenheimer et al., 1984; Pastides et al., 1983; Vessey et al., 1972).

The protective effect lasts after terminating treatment from a few months to a year (Fasal and Pfaffenberger, 1975; Franceschi et al., 1984; Vessey et al., 1972). According to Boynton et al. (1981), the response of fibroadenomas requires less time than that of fibrocystic disease. Long-term benefits were reported also by Canny et al. (1988), Franceschi et al. (1984), Hislop et al. (1984), and Vessey et al. (1972).

Boynton et al. (1981) and the Royal College of General Practitioners' study (1974) found no association with estrogen dose and type of progestational agents. However, the lowest risk with confirmed cystic disease was obviously in users of OCs containing the highest progestin dose. In a recent analysis by Berkowitz et al. (1984), the risk was not decreased in women taking OCs containing 20 to 50 μg of ethinyl estradiol. It may therefore be that the protective effect is exerted with the higher dose OCs only. This view has to be substantiated by further studies. No differences were found in fibroadenomas (Fechner, 1970; Prechtel, 1974).

The conclusion drawn from these data is that OCs in higher doses protect against benign breast disease, an effect that may be lost using lower doses. There is, however, no detrimental effect and no data to infer that benign breast disease is a precursor of breast cancer. Relation to breast cancer is present when there is epithelial hyperplasia affecting the small ducts and the terminal ductal lobular unit (Black and Chabron, 1969; Dupont and Page, 1985; Hutchinson et al., 1984; Page et al., 1978; WHO, 1991).

When the histopathological grading of Black and Chabron (1969) was used, LiVolsi et al. (1983) and Pastides et al. (1983) found a decreased proliferation in women taking OCs; it was assumed that protection from fibrocystic disease due to use of OCs is greater in women with higher atypia. Brown (1970) and Goldenberg et al. (1968) indicate that there is a relationship between OCs and epithelial hyperplasia in fibroadenomas, but these studies were uncontrolled. No difference between the proliferative rates of terminal ductal cells and benign breast tissue was found (Meyer, 1977; Potten et al., 1988; Going et al., 1988) or in fibroadenomas after OC use (Meyer, 1977; Anderson et al., 1983). LiVolsi et al., (1978) found a procedure by OCs only if atypia was held as absent.

Preliminary data do not suggest an adverse effect of progesterone on the risk of developing breast cancer (Korenman, 1980; Clavel et al., 1985; Vorherr, 1986). This is not the place to discuss the data on estrogen and breast cancer, because a number of problems cloud the facts. A long time period exists between exposure to a carcinogen and development of a malignant disease. Theoretically, OCs could act as an initiator, transforming a normal cell into a malignant cell. The other possibility is that they promote the growth of a transformed but latent cancer cell. Initiation may require more than 30 years between exposure and clinical expression, whereas the effects of promotion are evident in a shorter period of time. Many authors agree that, in breast cancer, the steroid hormones promote rather than initiate tumor growth (Vorherr, 1981; Thomas, 1984; Lipsett, 1986). A few cancers pertain to young women, but this issue is difficult to address because of small numbers. At age 25 the incidence of breast cancer is estimated to be three per 100,000 women. At age 35 the incidence is 75 per 100,000 in the U.S (Boring, 1991). In general, the following conclusions can be drawn:

1. Long-term use of oral contraceptives during the reproductive years is not associated with a significant increase in the risk of breast cancer after age 45. There is a possibility that exposure to early hormonal contraception confers some degree of protection against postmenopausal breast cancer.

2. There has been consistent failure to demonstrate an increased risk of breast cancer with OC use in women with positive family histories of breast cancer, or in women with proven benign breast disease (Stadel et al., 1986; Murray et al., 1989).

3. There is a possibility that a young subgroup of women who use oral contraception early and for a long time (4 years or more) have a slightly increased risk of breast cancer before the age of 45, a relative risk of less than 1.5. This possibility is derived from studies with older, higher-dose oral contraceptives.

4. A detailed analysis of the epidemiological studies and factors related to the breast cancer problem has been undertaken by the Committee on the Relationship Between Oral Contraceptives and Breast Cancer, and published by the National Institute of Medicine (1991). The appendix addressing the issue of evidence regarding occurrence in younger women states, "The one conclusive statement that can be made concerning the sum of the epidemiological evidence regarding a relationship between OCs and breast cancer . . . is the remarkable lack of consistency in the findings." With respect to the overall issue, "OCs as they have been used to date have caused little or no overall increase in the risk of breast cancer in women in developed countries. Risks in women of all ages combined have not been appreciably enhanced by more than a decade of exposure or after a potential latent period of up to two decades. . . . Limited information suggests that OCs (whether used before or after a benign lesion) may enhance the risk of breast cancer in young women with a prior history of benign breast disease but not in older women with such a history . . . Limited evidence suggests that the use of OCs near the time of menopause may increase a woman's risk of breast cancer . . . further investigation of this issue is warranted."

5. The WHO Collaborative Study of Neoplasia and Steroid Contraceptives conducted a hospital-based case-control study of Depo-Provera use in three developing countries. The relative risk of breast cancer in women who had ever used Depo-Provera was 1.21 (95% C.L. = 0.96–1.52). Risk was increased only within the first 4 years of exposure, mainly in women under 35 years of age. A causal inference from this finding, in conjunction with the further observations, is biologically quite implausible. Risk did not increase with duration of use and was not increased in women who had started to use the agent more than 5 years previously. The negative findings are in agreement with a study from New Zealand (Paul et al., 1989).

CONCLUSION

Estrogens are most likely ductal growth stimulators, whereas progesterone may be involved in alveolar development. The interaction of the various hormones in puberty and pregnancy in the human is not known.

Estrogens promote the growth of breast size. When given with progestins, OCs are not related to benign breast disease in any form. In fact, they appear protective to a certain degree.

There is no overall significant association between OCs and breast cancer, but various subsets of women need to be examined further.

REFERENCES

Abdel-Kader MM, Abdel-Aziz MT, Bahgat R. Effect of some progestational steroids in lactation in Egyptian women II. Chemical composition of milk during the first year of lactation. *J Biosoc Sci* 1976;8:49–56.

Adey T, Brown JB, Fotherby K. Norethisterone concentrations in milk of lactating women using a progestogen-only pill. *J Obstet Gynaecol* 1982;3:112–3.

Ali MN, Jalil MA. Further study on the effect of norethisterone enanthate, an injectable contraceptive, on body functions. *Bangladeshi Med Res Council Bull* 1978;14:63–70.

American Academy of Pediatricians, Committee on Drugs. Breast feeding and contraception. *Pediatrics* 1981;68:138–40.

Anderson TJ, Ferguson DJP, Raab GM. Cell turnover in the "resting" human breast: influence of parity, contraceptive pill age and laterality. *Brit J Cancer* 1983;46:376.

Assairi L, Delouis C, Houdebine LM, et al. Inhibition by progesterone of the lactogenic effect of prolactin in the pseudopregnant rabbit. *Biochem J* 1974;144:245–52.

Bässler R. Pathology and endocrine disorders. *Verhdlg Dtsch Ges Pathol.*

Bässler R. *Pathologie der brustdrüse.* Berlin: Springer Verlag; 1978:736–40.

Beller FK, Borsos A, Kieback D, et al. Geschlechtsentwicklung: die Entwicklung der secundären Geschlechtsmerkmale-die tannerstadien. 25 Jahre später. *Zentrbl Gynaec* 1991;113:499.

Benagiano B, Primiero FM. Long-acting progestogens in human fertility regulation. In, Benagiano G, Zulli P, Diczfalusy E, eds. *Progestogens in therapy.* New York: Raven Press; 1983:191–210.

Berkowitz GS, Kelsey JL, LiVolsi VA, et al. Oral contraceptive use and fibrocystic breast disease among pre- and postmenopausal women. *Am J Epidemiol* 1984;120:87.

Black MM, Chabon AB: In-situ carcinoma of the breast. *Pathol Ann* 1969;4:185.

Boring CC, Squires TS, and Tong T: Cancer statistics 1991. *CA* 1991;41:19.

Boynton LA, Vessey MP, Flavel R, et al. Risk factors for benign breast disease. *Am J Epidemiol* 1981;113:203.

Brown JM. Histological modification of fibroadenoma of the breast associated with oral hormonal contraceptives. *Med J Austral* 1970;1:276.

Canny PF, Berkowitz GS, Kelsey JL, et al. Fibroadenoma and the use of exogenous hormones: a case-control study. *Am J Epidemiol* 1988;127:454.

Clavel F, Benhamon E, Sitruk-Ware R, et al. Breast cancer and oral contraceptives: a review. *Contraception* 1985;32:533.

Cole PT. Oral contraceptives and breast neoplasia. *Cancer* 1977;39:1,906–1,908.

Committee on the Relationship Between Oral Contraceptives and Breast Cancer. Oral contraceptives and breast cancer. National Institute of Medicine; Washington, D.C.: National Academy Press; 1991: pp. 9–17

Consensus Conference. Is fibrocystic disease of the breast precancerous? *Arch Pathol Lab Med* 1986;110:171.

Croxatto HB, Diaz S, Perlata O, et al. Fertility regulation in nursing women IV. *Contraception* 1983;27: 13–25.

Dabelow A. Die Milchdrüse. In: Bargmann W, ed. *Handbuch der mikroskopischen anatomie der menschen.* Berlin: Springer; 1957:277.

Daniel W, Silberstein GB. Postnatal development of the rodent mammary gland. In: Neville MC, Daniel CW, eds. *The mammary gland*. New York: Plenum Press; 1987:17.

Delgado-Betancourt J, Sandoval JC, Sanchez F. Influence of exluton and the multiload Cu-250 IUD on lactation. *Contracept Deliv Syst* 1984;5:91–5.

Diaz S, Herreros C, Juez G, et al. Fertility regulation in nursing women VII. Influence of norplant levonorgestrel implants on lactation and infant growth. *Contraception* 1985;32:53–73.

Diaz S, Peralta O, Juez G, et al. Fertility regulation in women III. Short-term influence of a low dose combined oral contraceptive upon lactation and infant growth. *Contraception* 1983;27:1–11.

Dupont W, Page DL. Risk factors in breast cancer in women with proliferative breast disease. *N Engl J Med* 1985;312:146.

Fasal E, Pfaffenberger RS. Oral contraceptives as related to cancer and benign lesions of the breast. *JNCI* 1975;55:767.

Fechner RE. Fibrocystic disease in women receiving oral contraceptive hormones. *Cancer* 1970;25:1,332.

Fentiman IS, Caleffi M, Braun K, et al. Double blind controlled trial of tamoxifen therapy for mastalgia. *Lancet* 1986;1:287.

Franceschi S, LaVecchia C, Parazzini F, et al. Oral contraceptives and benign breast disease: a case control study. *Am J Obstet Gynecol* 1984;149:602.

Freeman CS, Topper YJ. Progesterone is not essential to the differentiative potential of mammary gland epithelium in the mouse. *Endocrinol* 1978;103:186.

Going JJ, Anderson TV, Battersby S, et al. Proliferative and secretory activity in human breast during natural and artificial menstrual cycles. *Am J Pathol* 1988;130:193.

Goldenberg VE, Wiegenstein L, Mottet NK. Florid breast fibroadenomas in patients taking hormonal oral contraceptives. *Am J Clin Pathol* 1968;49:52.

Gupta AN, Mathus VS, Garg SK. Effect of oral contraceptives on quality and quantity of milk secretion in human beings. *Indian J Med Res* 1974;62:964–70.

Haagensen CD. The relationship of gross cystic disease of the breast and carcinoma. *Am Surg* 1958:375,2,977.

Haslam SZ. Role of sex steroid hormones in normal mammary gland function. In: Neville MC, Daniel AW, eds. *The mammary gland*. New York: Plenum; 1987:499.

Hislop TG, Threlfall WJ. Oral contraceptives and benign breast disease. *Am J Epidemiol* 1984;120:273.

Hughes LE, Mansell RE, Webster DJT. *Benign disorders and diseases of the breast*. London: Bailliere Tindall; 1989:25–36.

Hutchinson WB, Thomas DB, Hamlin WJ, et al. Risk of breast cancer in women with benign breast disease. *JNCI* 1984;65:13.

Jimenez J, Ochoa M, Paz Soler M, et al. Long-term followup of children breast fed by mothers receiving depo-medroxyprogesterone acetate. *Contraception* 1984;30:523–33.

Kodlin D, Winger EE, Morgenstern NL, et al. Chronic mastopathy and breast cancer. *Cancer* 1977;39:2,603.

Koetsawang S. Injected long-acting medroxyprogesterone acetate: effect on human lactation and concentrations in milk. *J Med Assoc Thail* 1977;60:57–66.

Koetsawang S, Boonyaprakob V, Suvanichati S, et al. Long-term study of growth and development of children breast fed by mothers receiving depo-provera during lactation. In: Zatuchni G, Goldsmith A, et al. eds. *Long-acting contraceptive delivery systems*. Philadelphia: Harper and Row; 1984:378–87.

Korenman S. The endocrinology of breast cancer. *Cancer* 1980;46:874.

Kuhn NJ. Lactogenesis: The search for trigger mechanisms in different species. In: Parker M, ed. *Comparative aspects of lactation*. New York: Academic Press; 1977:165.

Lauritzen CH. Hormonelle substitutions therapie Brustvergrösserung. In: Beller FK and Seitzer D, eds. 7th Ann Meet German Soc Serol. Mühlheim, Germany: HUF; 1989:39.

Leung BS, Wench JM, Reiney CG. Estrogen receptors in mammary glands and uterus of mice during pregnancy. *J Steroid Biochem* 1976;7:88–95.

Lipsett MB. Steroids and carcinogenesis. In: Gregoire RT, Blye RT., eds. *Contraceptive steroids: pharmacology and safety*. New York: Plenum Press; 1986:215.

LiVolsi VA, Stadel BV, Kelsey JL, et al. Fibrocystic breast disease in oral contraceptive users: a histopathological evaluation of epithelial atypia. *N Engl J Med* 1978;299:381–85.

Lonnerdal B, Forsum E, Hambraeus L. Effect of oral contraceptives on composition and volume of breast milk. *Am J Clin Nutr* 1980;33:816–24.

Lyons WR, Li CH, Johnson RE. The hormonal control of mammary growth and lactation. *Recent Progr Horm Res* 1958;14:219–23.

Masters JRW, Drijle JO, Scavisbeck JJ. Cyclic variation of DNA synthesis in human breast epithelium. *JNCI* 1977;58:1,263.

Mauvais-Jarvis P, Sitruk-Ware LR, Williams GT, et al. The effect of age and menstrual cycle upon proliferative activity of the normal human breast. *Breast Cancer Res Treat* 1982;2:139.

McCann MF, Moggia AV, Higgins JE, et al. The effects of a progestin-only oral contraceptive (levonorgestrel 0.03 mg) on breast feeding. *Contraception* 1989;40:635–48.

McGonigle KF, Huggins GR. Oral contraceptives and breast disease. *Fertil Steril* 1991;56:799.

Meyer JS. Cell proliferation in normal human breast ducts, fibroadenomas, and the ductal hyperplasias as measured by nuclear labelling with tritiated thymidine. *Hum Pathol* 1977;8:67.

Milligan D, Drife J, Short RV. Changes in breast volume during the menstrual cycle and after oral contraceptives. *Br Med J* 1975;4:494.

Moolgarkar SH, Day NE, Stevens RG. Two stage model for carcinogenesis: epidemiology of breast cancer in females. *JNCI* 1979;65:1,347.

Murray B, Schlesselman JJ, Stadel BV, et al. Oral contraceptives and breast cancer risk in women with a family history of breast cancer. *Am J Obstet Gynecol* 1989;73:977.

Neville MC, Daniel CHW. *Mammary gland*. New York: Plenum Press; 1987:

Nilsson S, Nygren KG. Transfer of contraceptive steroids to human milk. *Res Reprod* 1979;11:1–2.

Nilsson S, Nygren KG, Johansson EDB. Norgestrel concentrations in maternal plasma, milk and child plasma during administration of oral contraceptives to nursing women. *Am J Obstet Gynecol* 1977;129:178–84.

Odenheimer DJ, Zunzunegu MV, King MC, et al. Risk factors for benign breast disease: a case-control study of discordant twins. *Am J Epidemiol* 1984;120:565.

Ory H, Cole P, MacMahon B, Hoover R. Oral contraceptives and reduced risk of benign breast diseases. *N Engl J Med* 1976;294:419.

Page DL, Zwaag RV, Rogers LW, et al. Relation between component parts of fibrocystic disease complex and breast cancer. *JNCI* 1978;61:1055.

Paul C, Skegg DCG, Spears GFS. Depo-medroxyprogesterone acetate (depo-provera) and risk of breast cancer. *Br Med J* 1989;299:759–62.

Pastides H, Kelsey JL, LiVolsi VA, et al. Oral contraceptive use and fibrocystic breast disease with special reference to its histopathology. *JNCI* 1983;71:5.

Pincus G, Bialy G, Layne DS, et al. Radioactivity in the milk of subjects receiving radioactive 19-norsteroids. *Nature* 1966;2:924–25.

Potten CS, Watson RV, Williams GT, et al. The effect of age and menstrual cycle upon proliferative activity of the normal human breast. *Br J Cancer* 1988;56:163.

Prechtel K. Allgemeine erläuterungen zur Histomorphologie von Brustdrüsenerkrankungen. *Fortschr Med* 1974;92:374–80.

Prechtel K. Ovulation and mammary changes in sexually mature women. 8th International Congress, International Academy Path, Mexico City, Mexico, May 18, 1970. *Program Supplement*. 1970;1 (abst).

Roberts MM, Jones V, Elton RA, et al. Risk of breast cancer in women with history of benign disease of the breast. *Br Med J* 1984;288:275.

Rohan TE, L'Abbe KA, Cook MG. Oral contraceptives and risk of benign proliferative epithelial disorders of the breast. *Int J Cancer* 1992;50:891–4.

Royal College of General Practitioners. *Oral contraceptives and health*. New York: Pitman; 1974:

Russo J, Russo IH. Development of the human mammary gland. In: Neville MC, Daniel AW, eds. *The mammary gland*. New York: Plenum; 1987:67.

Sarrif AM, Durant JR. Evidence that estrogen-receptor negative, progesterone-receptor positive breast and ovarian carcinomas contain estrogen receptor. *Cancer* 1981;48:1,215.

Saxena BF, Shrimanker K, Grudzinskas JG. Levels of contraceptive steroids in breast milk and plasma of lactating women. *Contraception* 1977;16:605–13.

Schindler, AE. Etiologie und epidemiologie und gutartiger veränderungen der brust. *Gynäk* 1989;22: 212.

Sitruk-Ware R, Sterkers N, Mauvais-Jarvis P. Benign breast disease: hormonal investigation. *Obstet Gynecol* 1979;53:457–60.

Stadel BV, Schlesselman JJ. Oral contraceptive use and the role of breast cancer with a prior history of benign disease. *Am J Epidemiol* 1986;123:373.

Stoleke H. Hormone und brustdrüsenentwicklung. In: Beller FK, Seizer D, eds. 7th Scient Meet, German Soc Serol, Muhlheim, Germany: HUF; 1989:26.

Thomas DB. Do hormones cause breast cancer? *Cancer* 1984;53:595.

Toddywalla VS, Mehta S, Katayn DV, et al. Release of 19-nortestosterone-type of contraceptive steroids through different drug delivery systems into the serum and breast milk of lactating women. *Contraception* 1980;21:217–23.

Topper YJ, Freeman CS. Multiple hormone interactions in the developmental biology of the mammary gland. *Physiol Rev* 1980;60:1,049.

Van der Molen HJ, Hart PG, Wijmenga HG. Studies with 4-^{14}C-mestranol in normal and lactating women. *Acta Endocrinol* 1969;61:255–74.

Vessey MP, Doll R, Sutton PM. Oral contraceptives and breast neoplasia: a retrospective study. *Br Med J* 1972;3:719.

Vorherr H. *The breast: morphology, physiology and lactation.* New York: Academic Press; 1974:

Vorherr H. *Breast cancer.* Baltimore: Urban-Schwarzenberg; 1980:

Vorherr H. Development of the female breast. In: Vorherr H, ed. *The breast.* New York: Academic Press; 1974:1–18.

Vorherr H. Endocrinology of breast cancer. *Maturitas* 1987;5:113.

Vorherr H. Fibrocystic non disease [Letter] *N Engl J Med* 1985;312:1,258.

Vorherr H. Fibrocystic breast disease: pathology, pathomorphology, clinical picture, and management. *Am J Obstet Gynec* 1986;154:161.

Vorherr H. Hormones and prostaglandins in relation to breast cancer. In: Ngasawa KA, ed. *Hormone-related tumors.* Berlin: Springer; 1981:165.

Wijmenga HG, Van der Molen HJ. Studies with 4-^{14}C-mestranol in lactating women. *Acta Endocrinol* 1969;61:655–77.

Wilson JG, Brent RL. Are female sex hormones teratogenic? *Am J Obstet Gynecol* 1981;141:567–80.

World Health Organization. Collaborative study of neoplasia and steroid contraceptives. *Lancet* 1991;338:833–8.

World Health Organization. WHO Task Force on Oral Contraceptives. Effects of hormonal contraceptives on breast milk composition and infant growth. *Stud Fam Plann* 1988;19:361–9.

World Health Organization. WHO Task Force on Oral Contraceptives. Effects of hormonal contraceptives on milk volume and infant growth. *Contraception* 1984;30:505–22.

Pharmacology of the Contraceptive Steroids,
edited by Joseph W. Goldzieher.
Raven Press, Ltd., New York © 1994.

12

The Lower Reproductive Tract

*Elisabeth Johannisson and †Ivo Brosens

*Laboratory of Analytical and Quantitative Cytology, International Committee for
Research in Reproduction, CH-1208 Geneva, Switzerland and †Department of Obstetrics
and Gynecology, University Hospital Gasthuisberg, B-300 Leuven, Belgium

The endometrium, cervix, and vagina are all target organs for the sex steroids. In principle, estrogens stimulate the proliferative activity in these target organs. The progestins are considered to counteract the estrogen-induced proliferation and to transform the estrogen-primed cells into histologically mature types that are prepared to meet the needs of their final function. When progestins are administered alone or as a sequential regimen, the effect on the target organs is likely to be different from that observed in the usual combined oral contraceptive (OC) treatment. It may then be more closely related to the dosage and time of exposure. In the present review, the effect of exogenously administered estrogens and progestins on the endometrium, cervix, and vaginal epithelium will be described when given alone or in combination.

EFFECT OF EXOGENOUS ESTROGENS WITHOUT ADDITIONAL PROGESTINS

Endometrium

Estrogen-only therapy has been used primarily for gonadal dysgenesis, pituitary deficiency, and menopausal complaints. When exogenous estrogens are administered alone from the first day of the menstrual cycle in women of fertile age, the preovulatory phase is prolonged, the secretion of FSH significantly suppressed, and the development of the corpus luteum inhibited until the estrogen administration is discontinued (Dallenbach-Hellweg, 1980a). Treatment with high doses of estrogens in the early postovulatory phase has been reported to be followed by severe stromal edema (Egger and Kindermann, 1980). Long-term estrogen treatment may give rise to cystic glandular hyperplasia (Greenblatt and Zarate, 1967; Ober and Bronstein, 1967). In the mid-1970s, several studies reported a significant relationship between unopposed estrogen administration and endometrial hyperplasia (Ziel and Finkle,

1976; Antunes et al., 1979; Gray et al., 1977). Both the duration of treatment and the size of dose seemed to be important. In postmenopausal women exposed to unopposed long-term use of estrogens, the risk of developing endometrial adenocarcinoma from endometrial abnormalities was increased by a factor of 2.9 (Peterson et al., 1988) However, more recent studies have revealed that the proliferative activity of the endometrium in postmenopausal women is correlated not only with the dosage and duration of estrogen administration but also with the route of administration. Moyer (1990) reported that women exposed to percutaneous estradiol for 6 months had less endometrial hyperplasia than women using injectable estradiol or daily administration of 1.25 mg conjugated equine estrogens.

In a randomized, crossover study, endometrial and vaginal response to transdermal estradiol was compared with the effect of oral administration of 1.25 mg conjugated estrogens daily and 2 mg estradiol valerate daily (Johannisson et al., 1988). By objective assessment of DNA synthesis in the endometrial cells—differentiating between the cell nuclei in "resting" phase and those synthesizing deoxyribonucleic acid—a significant increase of DNA synthesis was found during treatment with conjugated equine estrogens compared to transdermal estradiol and estradiol valerate. Slight proliferative activity was found in the endometrium of women using the transdermal estrogen, as well as in the mucosa of women using estradiol valerate when compared with the pretreatment control samples. The daily administration of 1.25 mg conjugated equine estrogens therefore seems to induce a significantly higher estrogen-stimulated proliferative activity than the oral administration of 2 mg estradiol valerate per day or the transdermal release of 50 μg of 17β-estradiol per 24 hours. The increase in the number of cells synthesizing DNA as well as the increase in DNA content per cell nucleus following the use of equine estrogens was paralleled by a significantly higher karyopyknotic (or maturation) index in the vaginal epithelium. This finding seems to reflect the difference between the chemical activity (i.e., potency and bioavailability) of various estrogens as to the response of the target organs. It also reflects the specific effect on target organs other than the endometrium (e.g., the cervical and the vaginal epithelium).

Endocervix

During the reproductive years, the morphologic appearance of the endocervix varies with the physiologic status. The endocervix is lined by an epithelium that is histologically different from that of the endometrium. Already in 1959, Fluhmann described the nature and development of the human endocervix and emphasized that the endocervix was composed of an "intricate system of tunnels and clefts that give an illusory impression of glands." The glands and the stroma of the endocervix respond to endogenous sex steroids (Sjöwall, 1938), and cyclic changes in the production of cervical mucus support this theory. Estrogen enhances mucus production and increases the proportion of mucus-containing cells in both the upper and lower cervical segments (Gaton et al., 1982). The endocervical secretion induced by estrogens is watery and consists of carbohydrate-rich glycoproteins of the mucoid type (Schumacher, 1970). The specific reaction induced by estrogens in the endocervix reflects the presence of estrogen receptors similar to those of the endometrium. The relationship between estrogen dosage and the reaction of the endocervical epithelial cells is still incompletely understood. However, from animal experiments (Galand et al., 1971) it is clear that the DNA-synthesizing phase of the mitotic cycle is measurably shortened following administration of estrogen, thereby indicating increased proliferative activity.

Exocervix and Vaginal Epithelium

The exocervix as well as the vagina are covered by squamous epithelium, which normally never reaches the stage of full cornification observed in the skin. This epithelium is a sensitive target organ for sex steroids. It is well established that increasing circulating levels of estrogens are reflected in the vaginal epithelium by an increased number of superficial squamous epithelial cells having a pyknotic nucleus. A significant correlation has been found between the number of superficial cells having a pyknotic nucleus and the level of urinary estrogens, provided that 17-ketosteroid and pregnanediol excretion remains low and unchanged (Johannisson et al., 1961). The definition of the karyopyknotic index is the number of mature squamous cells with pyknotic nuclei per 100 squamous epithelial cells. It can therefore be concluded that the vaginal epithelium reacts to estrogen stimulation by increased maturation of the squamous epithelial cells. It is likely that the squamous epithelium of the exocervix reacts like the vaginal epithelium, but the dose relationship between the maturation of the cells of exocervix and the circulating level of estrogens has not been fully investigated.

THE EFFECT OF CONTRACEPTIVE STEROIDS: PROGESTIN-ONLY PREPARATIONS

Endometrium

As with the estrogens, the effect of progestins on the endometrium depends upon the dose, duration of treatment, potency of the particular progestin, and route of administration. The effect of progestins is further complicated by the prerequisite of appropriate estrogen priming of the target organ cells.

When progesterone is released from a vaginal delivery system at a rate of 1.4 mg/24 hr in the very early preovulatory phase (cycle days 2 to 6), there is little if any effect on the appearance of the endometrium at cycle day 6 (Xing et al., 1983). When the same amount of progesterone is released in the late preovulatory phase (cycle days 7 to 11), the endometrial structure becomes significantly different from the control cycle day 11 (Xing et al., 1983). It is likely that the lack of progesterone effect on the endometrium in the early preovulatory phase reflects the receptor concentration, which has been reported to be lower than the concentration of estradiol receptors in the early proliferative phase (Baulieu et al., 1980). Therefore, there is reason to believe that progesterone receptors are synthesized in a gradual way in the endometrium following an initial priming by endogeneous estrogen, and that the endometrium can only respond to progesterone when a certain level of specific receptors is available. It is noteworthy that the premature release of progesterone from cycle days 7 to 11, with approximately a sixfold increase in plasma progesterone, gave rise to a significant increase in the ratio of the length of follicular to luteal phases (Xing et al., 1983).

The dose-response effect on the lower genital tract following oral administration of medroxyprogesterone acetate (MPA) has been demonstrated by Zalànyi and co-workers (1986). The progestin was administered during the preovulatory phase at three different dose levels (2.5 mg, 5 mg, and 10 mg per day) for 4 days starting on cycle days 7 to 10. The lowest dose did not influence the hormonal profile or the length of the cycle. The higher doses of MPA affected the hormonal profile but the length of the cycle was not shortened or prolonged. On the other hand, the endometrial tissue obtained at cycle day 10 in all three experimental groups revealed significant changes when compared to control samples obtained at the same cycle. The histological pattern was morphometrically assessed and statistically analyzed. As shown in Table 1, the endometrium displayed significant changes that could be related to the MPA dose. The lowest dose of MPA (2.5 mg $\times$ 4) produced an increase of the basal vacuolation of the glandular cells ($p < 0.01$). With 5 mg MPA for 4 days, the basal vacuolation of the glandular epithelium was also increased. In addition, there was now diminished pseudostratification of the glands ($p < 0.01$). When 10 mg was given from cycle days 7 to 10, the influence on the histology of the endometrium included not only the increase in basal vacuolation ($p < 0.01$) but also a significant decrease in the number of stromal mitoses (< 0.05) when compared to control biopsies. The pseudostratification of the glandular epithelium had completely disappeared. Therefore, the use of morphometric methods to assess the dose-response effect of the progestins on this target organ can be of great utility.

Injection of the depot preparation (DMPA) in a single dose of 150 mg has been reported to suppress ovulation for 5 months or more (Fotherby et al., 1980; Pardthaisong et al., 1980; Lan et al., 1984). The suppression of ovarian activity was also reflected in the endometrium, which revealed atrophy or completely suppressed proliferative activity as long as 16 weeks after the injection (Lan et al., 1984). This study also revealed that two of eight women started to show active proliferation of the endometrium 25 weeks after the single injection. In some subjects, an endometrial biopsy obtained 33 weeks after injection still revealed an abnormal endometrial appearance in spite of low or undetectable plasma levels of MPA.

The use of progestin-only preparations is usually reflected in irregular menstrual bleedings. In the study by Lan et al. (1984), irregular bleeding episodes were found throughout the period of observation. Usually the bleeding episodes occurred in women with suppressed proliferative activity of the endometrium, but they also occurred in women with an atrophic uterine mucosa. No signs of cellular atypia or malignancy were found (Lan et al., 1984).

Whether the 19-norprogestins differ from the 17-acetoxyprogestins in their endometrial effects qualitatively or merely quantitatively is unknown. However, the pharmacodynamic effects of the norprogestins have been reported to vary between

TABLE 1. *Effect of graded doses of medroxyprogesterone acetate (MPA) on some morphometric indices in endometrial biopsies taken on cycle day 11; MPA was administered on cycle days 7 to 10 (Geometric mean values and ranges)*

Index	2.5 mg (n = 4)		5.0 mg (n = 5)		10 mg (n = 6)	
	Control	Treatment	Control	Treatment	Control	Treatment
No. of glands/ mm²	12.9 (10.5–17.0)	13.2 (10.5–16.8)	15.3 (9.10–10.5)	12.3 (8.40–15.0)	15.2 (10.8–28.0)	13.2 (8.40–31.0)
Diameter of glands (μ)	27.9 (23.8–37.6)	30.0 (19.6–41.0)	28.8 (26.1–33.8)	43.2 (30.3–61.5)	24.9 (21.4–33.5)	31.3* (23.3–42.5)
Glandular epithelial height (μ)	20.2 (16.8–24.4)	21.1 (17.7–23.5)	20.7 (17.9–23.8)	22.3 (20.7–25.0)	19.9 (17.9–22.5)	19.8 (17.6–23.7)
Glandular mitoses (per 1000 cells)	15.5 (11.5–27.8)	4.61 (0.5–12.5)	15.9 (12.2–18.6)	4.58*** (2.8–8.2)	15.9 (7.9–22.9)	3.61 (0–16.0)
Vacuolated glandular cells (per 1000 cells)	17.0 (10.5–41.0)	410** (230–574)	11.5 (1.4–40.0)	584** (348–836)	5.0 (0–45.5)	378** (97–682)
Stromal mitoses (per 1000 cells)	3.1 (1.30–9.0)	1.0 (0–4.6)	1.8 (1.3–3.4)	0.98 (0.1–2.8)	4.25 (0.8–21.0)	0.72* (0.1–5.0)
Pseudostratification (score)	0.32 (0–1.0)	0.32 (0–1.0)	1.15 (1.0–2.0)	0.1** (0–1.0)	1.26 (1.0–2.0)	0*** (0–0)
Edema (score)	1.99 (1.7–2.2)	1.98 (1.7–2.5)	1.92 (1.5–2.2)	1.90 (1.6–2.2)	1.49 (0.5–2.2)	1.50 (0.5–2.3)

*P<0.05 **P<0.01 ***P<0.001

the compounds—probably a matter of potency (Greenblatt and Zarate, 1967). The pharmacodynamics of the 19-norprogestins have been more extensively studied than those of the acetoxyprogestins with regard to effects on the lower genital tract. In one investigation, the daily administration of 300 μg norethindrone for 2 months resulted in great variability in the ovarian response among the 68 women participating in the study (Landgren and Diczfalusy, 1980). Based on the hormonal levels characterizing a normal ovulatory cycle, four types of ovarian reactions were recognized; 1) no follicular and no luteal function (18%) (type A); 2) marked follicular activity but no luteal function (18%) (type B); 3) normal follicular activity but inadequate luteal function (25%) (type C); and 4) hormonally normal follicular and luteal function (40%) (type D). However, irrespective of ovarian function, significant morphologic changes were found in the endometrium. As displayed in Table 2, norethindrone reduced the number of endometrial glands (P<0.001), diminished the glandular diameter (P<0.001) and reduced DNA-synthesis in the endometrial cells (P<0.001). (Johannisson et al. 1982). The effect on the glands and the stroma of the endometrium was accompanied by significant changes of the subepithelial cells. As illustrated in Fig. 1, most capillaries revealed contraction of the cytoplasm with increased electron density in the electron microscope. Furthermore, a significant increase in the number of plasmolemmal vesicles occurred after 2 months' oral administration of 300 μg NET per day (Fig. 2). Simultaneously with the morphologic changes in the endometrium, the number of irregular bleeding episodes

TABLE 2. *Indices of endometrial activity before (control) and during the second month of administration of the 300μg norethisterone (NET) minipill in women with and without intermenstrual bleeding during treatment. Geometric mean values with 95% confidence limits.*

Endometrial index	Bleeders		Nonbleeders		All subjects	
	Control	NET	Control	NET	Control	NET
No. of glands (1)	3.2	1.5 (c)	3.3	1.3 (c)	3.2	1.4 (d)
	(2.6–3.9)	(0.7–3.0)	(2.9–3.7)	(0.6–2.8)	(2.7–3.8)	(0.7–2.9)
	(n = 12)	(n = 12)	(n = 8)	(n = 8)	(n = 20)	(n = 20)
Glandular diame-	84.9	26.1 (d,e)	79.7	50.6 (b,e)	82.7	34.5 (d)
ter (μm)	(72.3–99.7)	(14.5–45.7)	(66.1–96.0)	(30.8–82.9)	(69.7–98.0)	(18.4–64.6)
	(n = 11)	(n = 11)	(n = 8)	(n = 8)	(n = 19)	(n = 19)
Double-stranded	24.9	21.9 (d)	23.4	20.6 (d)	24.2	21.3 (d)
polynucleotides	(22.7–27.3)	(19.1–25.1)	(21.1–25.9)	(18.1–23.5)	(21.8–26.7)	(18.6–24.3)
per nucleus (2)	(n = 12)	(n = 12)	(n = 11)	(n = 11)	(n = 23)	(n = 23)
Deoxyribonucleic	19.4	17.8 (d)	19.7	17.6(d)	19.5	17.7 (d)
acid per	(17.2–21.8)	(15.7–20.1)	(17.7–22.1)	(15.5–19.9)	(17.5–21.8)	(15.7–19.9)
nucleus (2)	(n = 12)	(n = 12)	(n = 12)	(n = 12)	(n = 24)	(n = 24)
No. of plasmolem-	8.9	13.5 (b)	7.7	14.3 (c)	8.4	13.9 (d)
mal vesicles (3)	(5.5–14.4)	(8.1–22.4)	(4.7–12.5)	(10.8–19.1)	(5.2–13.6)	(9.1–21.1)
	(n = 12)	(n = 12)	(n = 9)	(n = 9)	(n = 21)	(n = 21)
Endothelial con-	34.9	51.9 (a)	24.6	52.2 (a)	30.4	51.9 (b)
traction (4)	(19.0–64.2)	(26.1–103.3)	(10.2–59.3)	(24.1–113.1)	(14.5–62.9)	(25.7–104.8)
	(n = 12)	(n = 12)	(n = 9)	(n = 9)	(n = 21)	(n = 21)

(1) = No. of transversally sectioned glands per microscopic field (× 400).
(2) = Expressed in ethidium bromide fluorescence units.
(3) = In arterial and venular capillary endothelial cells.
(4) = Percentage of endothelial cells of the venules showing contraction.
(a) = Not significant
(b) = p<0.05
(c) = p<0.01
(d) = p<0.001 when compared with the control samples
(e) = Difference between bleeders and non-bleeders, p<0.01

was increased. It was concluded that the endometrial changes might represent a potential predisposing factor for intermenstrual bleeding and spotting. However, no direct correlation was found between ovarian response and endometrial reaction. Nor was any correlation found between irregular menstrual bleedings and the ovarian response to norethindrone.

The effects of low-dose progestins (mainly 19-norprogestin compounds) have been repeatedly reviewed (Maqueo et al., 1964, 1970; Moghissi and Marks 1971; Flowers et al., 1974; Maqueo, 1980). Most of these studies have shown that continuous oral administration of small doses of progesterone or synthetic progestins suppresses proliferative activity of the endometrium, sometimes to the point of complete atrophy (Richart and Ferenczy, 1974; Dallenbach-Hellweg, 1980b). A major problem with a number of these studies is that the investigators did not measure ovarian reaction *pari passu* with the endometrial changes. In women using low-dose progestin-only OCs, anovulatory and quasi-ovulatory cycles often occur in haphazard sequence; therefore, conclusions assuming that there are only synthetic-progestin effects on the endometrium may be in error.

The endometrial effect of oral administration of various progestins cannot be extrapolated to other types of delivery systems. Many systems provide a decreased dose level at a constant, sustained release. The various 19-norprogestins may very well exert qualitatively different effects on the endometrium. Whitehead and co-

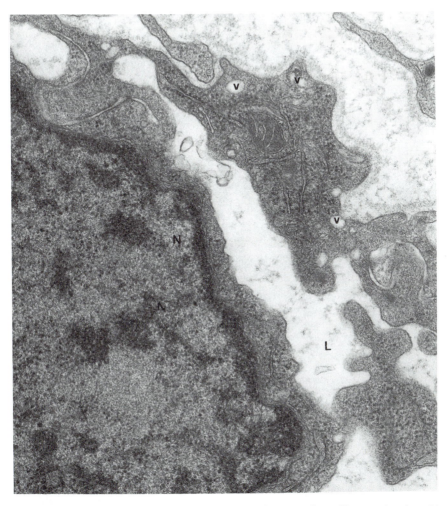

FIG. 1. Part of an endothelial cell showing contraction of the cytoplasm. The cytoplasmic matrix has a high optical density with plasmolemmal vesicles (V) scattered in the periphery. N = nucleus, L = capillary lumen (70'000 ×).

Prentice R L, Thomas D B. On the epidemiology of oral contraceptives and disease. *Advances Cancer Research* 1987;49:285–401.

workers (1981, 1982), and King and Whitehead (1984) studied the effect of four different progestins on the morphology, DNA synthesis, estradiol dehydrogenase activity, and epithelial labeling index in the endometrium of postmenopausal women primed with estrogen. As displayed in Table 3, each progestin elicited a specific chemical and morphological profile. Therefore, the chemical properties of individual progestins also have to be taken into consideration when used as contraceptives. It was considered that other 19-norprogestins might be equally efficient in contraceptive terms but provoke less intermenstrual bleeding. Several new deriva-

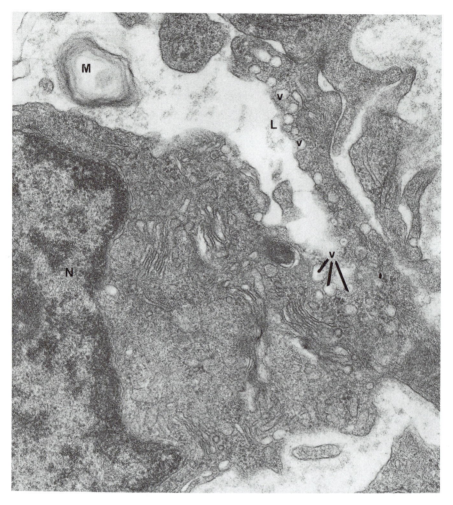

FIG. 2. Part of an endothelial cell showing a large number of plasmolemmal vesicles (V) in the periphery of the cytoplasm. N = nucleus, L = capillary lumen, M = myelin figure (70'000 ×)

Prentice R L, Thomas D B. On the epidemiology of oral contraceptives and disease. *Advances Cancer Research* 1987;49:285–401.

Beral V, Hannaford P, Kay C. Oral contraceptive use and malignancies of the genital tract. Results from The Royal College of General Practioners' Oral Contraception study. *Lancet* 1988;2:1,331–5.

Ebeling K, Nischan P, Schindler C H. Use of oral contraceptives and risk of invasive cervical cancer in previously screened women. *Int J Cancer* 1987;39:427–30.

tives of levonorgestrel have been marketed in various formulations, but definitive comparative studies of bleeding performance are not available.

The fluctuating plasma levels of progestins following oral administration were at one time considered to be responsible for irregular menstrual bleedings. In order to avoid this side effect, it was felt that the development of a new delivery system assuring a constant (i.e., zero order) release of progestins might prevent the irregu-

TABLE 3. *Mean (± SD) morphological changes in the endometrium before and during the use of a vaginal device releasing norethisterone at a rate of 50 and 200 μg/24 hours and levonorgestrel at 10, 20 and 25 μg/24 hours. Biopsies obtained in a control cycle (C) and after 6 and 10 weeks' use*

Type of device	Number of glands/mm²			Diameter of glands (μm)			Glandular epithelial height (μm)		
	C	6	10	C	6	10	C	6	10
Norethisterone 50 μg/24 hours (n = 7)	21.1 ± 10.5	22.1 ± 11.3	28.4 ± 15.9	42.7 ± 16.0	30.7 ± 13.9	49.1 ± 22.2	21.8 ± 5.1	19.9 ± 1.8	18.6 ± 5.1
Norethisterone 200 μg/24 hours (n = 7)	19.4 ± 6.6	16.5 ± 10.0	9.5[a] ± 5.9	54.4 ± 18.7	25.6[b] ± 17.3	23.7[b] ± 10.8	20.0 ± 3.4	18.3 ± 2.9	18.5 ± 3.5
Levonorgestrel 10 μg/24 hours (n = 5)	25.2 ± 9.9	16.0 ± 10.3	15.5 ± 4.5	61.1 ± 6.5	41.9 ± 12.1	29.9 ± 16.6	16.9 ± 3.0	18.4 ± 3.4	18.7 ± 2.0
Levonorgestrel 20 μg/24 hours (n = 5)	15.5 ± 2.5	11.6 ± 5.6	13.7 ± 8.0	58.6 ± 25.2	28.4[a] ± 11.4	25.9[a] ± 5.3	19.1 ± 5.2	23.4 ± 5.8	19.2 ± 3.6
Levonorgestrel 25 μg/24 hours (n = 15)	22.8 ± 9.6	16.9 ± 9.8	16.0 ± 13.2	54.4 ± 17.2	21.4[c] ± 11.6	24.4[c] ± 12.7	18.0 ± 4.9	19.2 ± 3.4	18.2 3.6

Notes:
[a] $P < 0.05$ when compared with the control sample
[b] $P < 0.01$ when compared with the control sample
[c] $P < 0.001$ when compared with the control sample

lar bleeding episodes and improve the acceptability of an otherwise efficient contraceptive method. Several delivery systems were proposed; vaginal rings, subdermal implants, and intrauterine devices providing a constant local release of progestin. They, as well as various types of injectables, underwent extensive testing.

The Effect of Various Delivery Systems

Taking into account that oral administration is metabolically different from local administration, and that steroid released from vaginal rings, intrauterine devices, subdermal implants, or long-acting injectables is also kinetically different, the route of administration as well as specific dose-response differences between individual steroids must be carefully considered. When administrated locally, norethindrone released from vaginal rings shows a clear dose-related effect on the endometrium (Landgren et al., 1979). Vaginal rings releasing 50 μg norethindrone per 24 hours induced a suppression of luteal function in four cycles out of 20. Thirteen of 14 biopsies revealed normal cyclic endometrial changes. However, in women using a vaginal ring releasing 200 mg norethindrone per 24 hours for 10 weeks, luteal function was suppressed in 13 out of 22 cycles. In 11 out of 14 biopsies, endometrium showed predecidual or atrophic changes associated with a significant decrease in the number of endometrial glands (Landgren et al., 1979).

Studies of vaginal rings releasing levonorgestrel at a rate of 20 μg/day for periods up to 10 weeks revealed an effect on the endometrium less constant than that of norethindrone. Usually the histologic pattern varied between normal secretory, irregular secretory, and suppressed (Landgren et al., 1982). During observations in subjects given either norethindrone or levonorgestrel rings, no signs of adenomatous hyperplasia were found in any biopsies.

A multiple-compartment vaginal ring system for independently adjusting release of contraceptive steroids has also been developed; preliminary studies were carried out with 3-ketodesogestrel and ethynyl estradiol (De Leede et al., 1986). Other rings with various progestins with or without EE are also under study (Alvarez-Sanchez et al., 1992).

Another way to administer progesterone or synthetic progestins as a long-acting contraceptive is the use of IUDs releasing the steroid at a reasonably constant rate. Scommegna et al. (1970) first reported endometrial suppression in 34 human volunteers after 12 weeks' use of intrauterine progesterone. In 1974, Martinez-Manautou and coworkers published a study on clinical findings in women using a device releasing progesterone at 20, 30, and 60 μg per day. The study included 617 fertile women who were followed for 1 to 12 months. Biopsies showed a clear dose-response effect: approximately 70% of the women using the device releasing 60 μg/day showed suppressed activity of the endometrium, whereas only 30% of women exposed to 20 μg/day release had suppressed endometria. In 1975, Martinez-Manautou and coworkers extended these studies in women exposed to systems releasing progesterone at six dose levels. Endometrial biopsies were taken following 2 to 10 months of exposure. They reported that 332 out of 402 biopsies showed suppressed proliferation with predecidual reaction in the stroma. Further investigations by Johannisson et al. (1977) revealed that the insertion of a progesterone IUD releasing 65 μg/day decreased the DNA content per endometrial cell nucleus significantly after 6 to 7 months of use. These data clearly confirm a suppression of proliferative activity in spite of circulating levels of endogenous steroids commensurate with normal ovarian function. More detailed studies of human endometrial epithelial cells have shown that progesterone, chlormadinone, and medroxyprogesterone induced nuclear differentiation, giant mitochondria, and glycogen accumulation. Norethindrone, norethynodrel, ethynodiol diacetate, dimethisterone, and norgestrel failed to induce nucleolar differentiation, although enlarged mitochondria and glycogen accumulation were seen (Uniyal et al., 1977).

Other studies have examined the nature of the intrauterine environment under the influence of progesterone. Uterine washings had an inhibitory effect on the oxygen uptake, glucose utilization, and peptidase activity of human spermatozoa, more prominently at a release rate of 50 μg compared to a rate of 30 μg/day. Such washings also inhibited the in vitro capacitation of rabbit spermatozoa (Hagenfeldt, 1976).

There may be other direct effects on spermatozoa. Progesterone (as well as lynestrenol and norethynodrel) reduced the motility of washed sperm (Hyne et al.,

1978). Norethynodrel affects the oxidative metabolism of sperm at a concentration of 32 μg/ml and the glycolytic metabolism at 320 ug/ml. At these high concentrations there may be a change in membrane permeability, with consequent loss of cofactors essential for sperm metabolism associated with motility. Progesterone released from an IUD has an effect on sperm oxygen uptake and glucose utilization, as well as on tetracycline binding and release processes (Rosado et al., 1974).

In spite of these multitudinous actions, the need to improve the hormone-releasing IUD was evident. A more potent and long-acting progestin, levonorgestrel, was introduced and a T-shaped device was designed (Nilsson et al., 1975). One device released levonorgestrel at 20 μg/day and the other at 40 μg/day (Nilsson et al., 1978). After exposure for 74 to 118 days (mean = 96 days), the histologic picture of the endometrium was uniform, revealing predecidual changes in the stroma and atrophic glands with a low epithelial lining and no signs of mitotic activity.

Levonorgestrel is also used in the Norplant system (see chapter 9). One of us (Johannisson) has studied a large number of these endometria. Compared to normal endometria that have an average of 19.3 ± 4.4 glands/mm^2, Norplant endometria vary between 8.5 and 11.2, the number remaining fairly constant over 30 months. Glandular diameter was in the same range as seen during the normal proliferative phase. Glandular epithelium height was in the same range as in normal midsecretory phase of the cycle. About 50% of the endometria were suppressed and 10% to 20% were atrophic; these changes appeared to diminish after 19 to 24 months of use. Decidual reaction was scanty. As in other instances of irregular bleeding, the relation to endometrial morphology was uncertain.

Endocervix

In fertile women, the morphologic appearance of the endocervix varies during the menstrual cycle. It is lined by an epithelium histologically different from that of the endometrium. However, at the borderline with the endometrium, cellular elements of "glands" can be recognized. The number of ciliated cells also is significantly increased when compared to the endometrium.

During the 10 years that low-dose progestin preparations have been in use either as oral contraceptives, or locally applied progestin-releasing intrauterine, intracervical or vaginal devices, no increase in the rate of endocervical adenomatous hyperplasia has been reported. Preliminary results from a study on the distribution of the DNA content per nucleus in isolated endocervical cells following the use of a vaginal ring releasing 200 μg norethindrone for 6 and 10 weeks showed that most cell nuclei were nonproliferating and that distribution of DNA content per nucleus was similar to that of the endometrium in the same subject. There is evidence that the endocervix reacts to estrogens and progestins in a way similar to the endometrium (Maqueo et al., 1966; Moghissi and Marks, 1971). Estrogen administration enhances mucus production and increases the proportion of mucus-containing cells, both in the upper and lower cervical segments. A significant decrease in the percentage of mucus-containing epithelial cells occurs in women treated with MPA (Gaton et al., 1982) or other progestins. Scanty, thick cervical mucus is a typical effect of oral or parenteral progestin administration. With Norplant, for example, mucus could be obtained in only about 30% of attempts, and sperm penetration is extremely poor.

It was therefore felt that the cervix could be exposed to a steroid-releasing device in a way similar to that of the endometrium. Such a device could alter the properties of the cervical mucus and prevent sperm penetration. Cohen et al. (1970) applied progesterone-containing silastic capsules in the endocervix for one to two cycles and demonstrated a marked decrease in the amount of cervical mucus. An intracervical device releasing levonorgestrel at a rate of 10 µg/day was investigated by El Mahgoub (1982). Endometrial and cervical biopsies were obtained from 30 out of 64 subjects during 3 years of use. After six cycles, the cervical material showed mild to moderate leukocytic and plasma cell infiltration, and endocervical epithelial height was significantly lower than that of the controls. Furthermore, the cervical clefts appeared empty, with minimal amounts of mucus. These changes were more pronounced after 3 years of use, when a marked reduction in the number and size of the endocervical crypts was observed. The epithelium lining was stunted and the stroma was atrophic. The intracervical levonorgestrel-releasing IUD also affected the endometrium and after 3 years of use, the uterine mucosa showed a uniform suppressed proliferation and atrophic changes in the stroma. No systemic effects of the intracervical levonorgestrel device releasing 20 µg/day were observed by Ratsula (1987,1989) and Ratsula and coworkers (1988). A high expulsion rate was reported during the first 6 months of use, and irregular bleeding appeared to be a major problem and the main reason for removals. In a follow-up study after two years' use, no major problem with respect to infection or malignant changes was reported (Ratsula, 1989).

Exocervix

Progesterone itself will cause cervical mucus to become scanty, viscous, and cellular, with low Spinnbarkeit and no ferning. The proteins, enzymes, and electrolytes, but not the pH or the trace elements, are altered, and sperm penetration is inhibited. A single dose of 0.5 mg megestrol acetate affects mucus penetrability within 4 hours; the effect wears off after a day (Cox, 1968). Comparable changes are induced by 19-norprogestins whether administered orally, intravaginally, or by various devices. The evanescence of this effect undoubtedly accounts for the low contraceptive effectiveness of "minipills".

Wright et al. (1978) claim that the effect of levonorgestrel also occurs within 4 hours and continues for about 20 hours, but confirmatory data on the effects on mucus of a single exposure to a minipill are surprisingly scanty. Moghissi et al. (1973), Wright et al. (1970), and others have shown that minipill contraception is not due to cervical or endometrial changes alone. Studies of ovarian function indicate some interference with ovulation, but also major effects on progesterone production by luteal tissue: urinary pregnanediol excretion is severely depressed. Studies of the FSH and LH peaks during such cycles indicate that ovarian malfunction appears to be attributable to effects of these progestin exposures on gonadotropin secretion.

There are few data regarding the administration of progestins alone and the incidence of cervical dysplasia or carcinoma. In 2,409 women using intrauterine devices and 1,684 women using long-acting injectable progestins, Dabancans et al. (1974) concluded that the risk of developing cervical carcinoma in subjects using long-acting injectables was not significantly different from women using IUDs after 6 years of observation. No data are available on the long-term effect of vaginal, endocervical, and intrauterine release of progestins on the exocervix.

COMBINED ESTROGEN-PROGESTIN PREPARATIONS

The effect of combined OCs on the lower genital tract is reasonably predictable from the pharmacological actions of the main components. Apart from the well-recognized variability between women and in the same woman between cycles and different parts of the genital tract, the absolute and relative dosage of the pill, schedule of dosage, and duration of use are determining factors. More difficult to determine is the contraceptive significance of these changes.

Endometrium

Early, high-dose OCs such as 150 μg mestranol/10 mg norethynodrel preparations produced such unusual effects that a Mayo Clinic pathologist, unaware of the biopsied patient's OC use, diagnosed endometrial sarcoma because of the extensive stromal hyperplasia. With other formulations, both combined and sequential, and using 80 to 50 μg estrogen and substantial doses of progestin, extensive endometrial biopsy studies were undertaken (Rice-Wray et al., 1963; Maqueo et al., 1963; Maqueo et al., 1964). After an initial stage of secretory changes, the endometrial glands underwent involution while the stroma showed edema, pseudodecidual changes, and dilatation of the vascular sinusoids, which seemed to be related to the progestin dose. An involuted endometrium eventually developed and remained essentially unchanged even during OC use for a decade or longer (Maqueo et al., 1970a). Here, as with the more recent low-dose formulations, there was no correlation between breakthrough bleeding and endometrial morphology. Regeneration of these suppressed endometria occurred promptly (Maqueo et al., 1970b). With sequential agents containing 80 μg mestranol and chlormadinone acetate, the morphology resembled a cycle day 19 endometrium with variable degrees of stromal edema; this picture persisted during several years of use (Maqueo et al., 1964).

With current combined OCs containing 50 μg of EE or the equivalent in mestranol, the effect is again apparent from the first treatment cycle. Endometrial proliferation is inhibited so that at midcycle the endometrium is thinner than normal, with poorly developed glands showing little or no mitotic activity and no pseudostratification. The weak secretory effect of the progestin in some of the glands provokes a premature and irregular subnuclear vacuolization. Later in the cycle, the inadequately estrogen-primed endometrium is unable to produce a full secretory response and, in the absence of enhancement of the progestational effect, the glands undergo involution and atrophy during the remainder of the cycle. The stroma appears edematous from cycle day 10 to 20, but the edema gradually regresses towards the end of the cycle. The stroma also is inadequately primed by estrogen, and the predecidual changes during the last week of the cycle are less developed and more focal in the superficial layer than during the normal cycle. Under these conditions the spiral arterioles are poorly developed but the venules may be ectatic. At the end of the cycle, the endometrium shows hypoplasia with small inactive glands, a variable and inadequate predecidual reponse, inconspicuous spiral arterioles, and ectatic venules. After a number of cycles the antiestrogenic action of the progestin tends to dominate, and the endometrium becomes atrophic with poor gland elements, an edematous fibroblastic stroma, and occasional foci of predecidua with granulocytes (K+ cells). The sinusoidal or ectatic venules are presumed to be the origin of the spotting experienced by some women. On the other hand, withdrawal bleeding at the end of an OC cycle is usually short in duration and small in amount. This bleeding depends on the relative dose of estrogen and progestin; high-dose formulations abbreviate and diminish bleeding, whereas triphasic formulations produce less of these effects. The very low-dose formulations containing 30 μg of EE or less also have relatively little hemostatic effect.

The latest generation of OCs have less inhibitory effect on the endometrium; for example, an OC containing 35 μg EE/250 μg norgestimate suppressed proliferative activity less than progestin-only formulations (Rabe et al., 1986). Similar findings have been reported with other new progestins. The use of triphasic formulations seems to produce a relatively normal cyclic pattern in the endometrium (Brosens et al., 1982). However, early progestational effects and rather hypoplastic growth could still be observed (Wynants and Ide, 1986). Almost normal cycle behavior has been reported in women using a "normophasic" regimen (Luikku and Kortesluoma, 1983; van de Walle and Demol, 1984). The endometrium is characterized by a better development and more balanced ratio between endometrial glands and stroma, thereby imitating the normal physiological changes occurring in the uterine mucosa during the normal cycle (Wynants and Ide, 1986).

There have been innumerable studies on the pattern of endometrial bleeding resulting from various formulations and regimens of oral contraceptives. As pointed out in Chapter 29 (Edelman & Goldzieher) and more recently by Rosenberg and Long (1992), comparisons are extremely difficult to evaluate because of: 1) differences in definitions of bleeding, spotting, amenorrhea, etc.; 2) experimental protocols and manner of evaluation; and 3) exclusion/inclusion/separation of first-time users versus switchover subjects, etc. Even with the earliest high-dose formulations, there were such differences between groups observed in large multicentered studies who used the same oral contraceptive (Hines and Goldzieher, 1969), that true differences between different formulations would have been very difficult to detect. Two general observations emerged from this wealth of data: 1) levonorgestrel generally gave better cycle control than norethindrone and 2) the longer the use was continued, the better the cycle control tended to be. How much of the latter was due to dropout of subjects with bleeding problems or switching of such subjects to other formulations by their managing physicians has not been properly evaluated.

Recently, Rosenberg and Long (1992) reviewed the literature on cycle control with the newer low-dose formulations and found highly variable rates of bleeding problems, just as was reported in the older literature with high-dose formulations. After 6 months of use, the prevalence of spotting varied from 0% to 8.5%, breakthrough bleeding from 0% to 12.2%, and amenorrhea from 0% to 5.8%. As a generalization, they found that formulations with gestodene did better than desogestrel and possibly levonorgestrel.

Presumably, the newer agents follow the same general principles that were observed with the earlier formulations: in individuals with heavy and/or prolonged bleeding one favored high-dose monophasic OCs, which are known to diminish and abbreviate menstrual flow; in women who had comfortable cycles, lower dose monophasics tended to be favored; and in women who tended to have short, light cycles or a tendency toward amenorrhea under monophasic OC use, the multiphasics were favored. These general rules were of course modified by individual tolerance (e.g., adolescents and women of low body weight tend to develop nausea more easily than others, which indicates use of the lowest-estrogen formulation available), and by regulatory-agency and other pressures to lower OC dose as much as possible. Whether this latter philosophy is not at times counterproductive, as in the case of possibly decreasing the important noncontraceptive benefits of OC use, is a matter for debate.

Uterine Receptivity

On the basis of morphology, the endometrium seen with low-dose combined OCs appears to be sufficiently aberrant to prevent nidation. However, the natural occurrence of ectopic implantation demonstrates the intrinsic invasiveness of human trophoblast. It has been suggested that the endometrium has a mechanism to control and limit trophoblastic invasion. The term "implantation window" has been introduced for that stage of the reproductive process when the egg has become a blastocyst and the endometrium has optimal receptivity for implantation. For obvious reasons, much of the understanding of the hormonal control of implantation is derived from animal studies. It is certain that all species require a progesterone-primed uterus to permit implantation. The postovulatory triad of glandular epithelium comprising subnuclear glycogen, giant mitochondria, and nuclear channel system (NCS) is likely to be implicated in implantation. The NCS is believed to participate in the regulatory mechanism of the glandular epithelium. It was recently found that the NCS is not formed in anovulatory cycles or under low-dose progestin therapy (Spornitz, 1992). However, the need for estrogen in all species is controversial since estrogen secretion from the ovary cannot always be demonstrated.

Recent experimental work in monkeys suggests that estrogen is necessary to establish implantation in the primate (Ravindranath and Moudgal, 1987, 1990). The factors that determine whether the environment is receptive, neutral (the embryo can survive for a limited time, but not implant) or hostile (the embryo cannot survive or implant) are still not well understood. In IVF programs, the determination of the optimal time for transfer is critical. Mandelbaum et al. (1990) inadvertently treated some women with a luteal phase supplement of progesterone from the time of HCG administration rather than from the day of transfer, and observed a highly significant decline in clinical pregnancy rate from 21% to 12%. These data suggest that: 1) embryos older than the uterus should survive better than those younger than the uterus, or 2) an underdeveloped endometrium is less resistant to implantation than an "overripe" one, which is the case for an endometrium under the influence of combined OCs.

POSTCOITAL CONTRACEPTIVES

Contraception with "morning-after" pills was introduced in the 1970s. Haspels reported on the effects of high doses of estrogens given within 72 hours of coital exposure in 3,016 women (1976), and Dixon et al. reviewed the results of such "interception" with various types and doses of estrogen in 1980. The mechanism of action of these compounds, whether on tubal transport or endometrium, is not well understood. The effectiveness of high estrogen dosage is rated at 84% (Trussell and Stewart, 1992). Speculations regarding the high-dose combined OCs include suppression of ovulation (Ling et al., 1979), altered luteal function (Ling et al., 1983), and interference with the endometrial environment (Van Santen and Haspels, 1980; Azadian-Boulanger et al., 1976). Kubba et al. (1986) found a reduction in receptor concentration and isocitrate dehydrogenase (a progestin-sensitive enzyme), supporting the idea of an endometrium-mediated effect. The effectiveness of such regimens is estimated at better than 75% (Trussell and Stewart, 1992). Due to the severe side effects of these high estrogen doses, alternatives were sought, and Yuzpe et al. (1982) reported on the effectiveness of 100 μg EE and 500 μg levonorgestrel, repeated after 12 hours. The side effects were still substantial, but less than those with the estrogen-only regimen. More recently, the antiprogestational steroid mifepristone (RU 486) has been tested for the same purpose. A single dose of 600 mg mifepristone lowered the incidence of nausea, vomiting and other side effects still further, but caused delay in the onset of the next menses more frequently—42% vs. 13% (Glasier et al., 1992). A randomized trial of the Yuzpe regimen versus mifepristone yielded a raw pregnancy rate of 2.62% (95% confidence limits, 0.86% to 6.0%) with the former and 0% (0% to 1.87%) with the latter, a significant difference.

Mifepristone is also under investigation as an antiovulatory agent when given during the follicular phase. The results are complex, and dose- and timing-dependent. Mifepristone can block imminent midcycle gonadotropin surges and delay subsequent folliculogenesis, thus lengthening the duration of the menstrual cycle (Collins and Hodgen, 1986). There is a great deal of current investigative activity into mifepristone and other antiprogestins with different pharmacokinetic properties.

MALIGNANCIES

Endometrial Carcinoma

The factors that influence the incidence of spontaneous endometrial cancer are: 1) international variation (lowest in China, Japan, India, and the Philippines at 2 to 4 per 1,000 women through age 74, to 20 to 30 per 1,000 in U.S. whites, Canadians, and certain Pacific islanders); 2) age; 3) anovulation and nulliparity; 4) early age at menarche and late age at menopause; 5) obesity; and 6) positive family history.

Over a dozen epidemiological studies (reviewed by Schlesselman, 1991) are remarkably consistent in finding a protective effect (Fig. 3). The risk before age 60 is reduced by about 38% with 2 years of use, while 4, 8, and 12 years of use confer an estimated risk reductions of 51%, 64%, and 70%, respectively. The histological type of endometrial malignancy does not appear to affect this protective effect. Since these estimates do not correct for the increasing incidence of hysterectomy in older women, the protective effect is undoubtedly underestimated. The data of most of these studies apply to women who used the older "high-dose" formulations, and the degree of protection afforded by current OCs remains to be established. Since parity itself is a protective factor, the effect of OCs is less pronounced in women of increasing parity. The duration of this protection, after termination of OC use, appears to persist for at least 15 years. From the epidemiological perspective of overall *lifetime* risks, this protective effect—a 7% reduction—appears inconsequential (Schlesselman, 1991); however, endometrial cancer is one of the major reproductive tract cancers, and the possibility of prophylaxis by means of a few years of OC use should not be taken lightly.

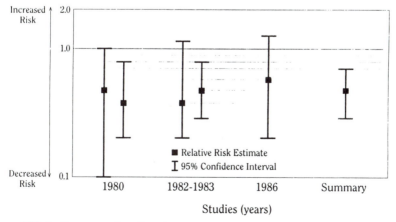

FIG. 3. Case-control studies of oral contraceptives and endometrial cancer.

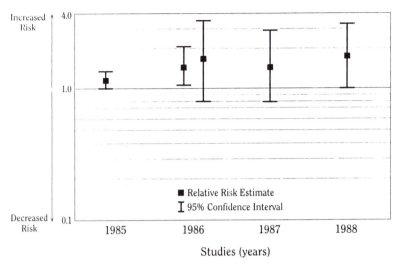

FIG. 4. Case-control studies of oral contraceptives and invasive cervical cancer.

Cervical Carcinoma

The issue of OC use and cervical neoplasia has been reviewed by Brinton (1991). This is an extremely thorny problem because of the confounding effects of socioeconomic status, sexual behavior (e.g., age at first coitus, number of partners, and prevalence of various sexually transmitted diseases (STDs), especially certain papillomaviruses in the population), and the biasing effect of Pap smear screening, which differs between OC users and nonusers (who may or may not use condoms). Issues of study design and analysis also arise (Brinton, 1991). The observed relative risks are shown in Fig. 4. Several relatively well-controlled studies suggest that a 2-fold risk persists in those who use OCs for 5 years or more. A possible promotional effect is suggested by higher risk with recent use.

REFERENCES

Alvarez-Sanchez F, Brache V, Jackanicz T, Faundes A. Evaluation of four different contraceptive vaginal rings: steroid serum levels, luteal activity, bleeding control and lipid profiles. *Contraception* 1992;46:387–98.

Antunes CM, Stolley PD, Rosenshein NB, et al. Endometrial cancer and estrogen use. *N Engl J Med* 1979;300:9.

Azadian-Boulanger G, Secchi J, Laraque F, et al. Action of midcycle contraceptive (R2323) on the human endometrium. *Am J Obstet Gynecol* 1976;125:1,049.

Baulieu E-E, Mortel R, Robel P. Receptors in human endometrium: regulatory and pathophysiological aspects. In: Diczfalusy E, Fraser IS, Webb FTG, eds. *WHO symposium on steroid contraception and mechanisms of endometrial bleeding*. Bath/Heidelberg/New York: Pitman Press Ltd; 1980:266–90.

Beral V, Hannaford P, Kay C. Oral contraceptive use and malignancies of the genital tract. Results from The Royal College of General Practitioners' Oral Contraception Study. *Lancet* 1988;ii:1331–35.

Brinton LA. Oral contraceptives and cervical neoplasia. *Contraception* 1991;43:581–96.

Brosens I, Klerckx P, de Groote A, et al. The hormonal effect of a triphasic oral contraceptive (trinor-diol, triphasil) on the endometrium and cervical mucus. In: Brosens I, ed. *New considerations in oral contraception.* New York: Biomed Inform Corp, 1982:181–9.

Cohen MR, Pandya GN, Scommegna A. The effects of an intracervical steroid-releasing device on the cervical mucus. *Fertil Steril* 1970;21:715–23.

Collins RL, Hodgen GD. Blockade of the spontaneous midcycle gonadotropin surge in monkeys by RU486: a progesterone antagonist or agonist? *J Clin Endocrinol Metab* 1986;63:1,270–1,276.

Cox HJE. The precoital use of minidosage progestogens. *J Reprod Fertil* 1968;5 (Suppl):167.

Dabancens A, Prado R, Larraguibel R, Zanartu J. Intraepithelial cervical neoplasia in women using intrauterine devices and long-acting injectable progestogens as contraceptives. *Am J Obstet Gynecol* 1974;119:1,052–6.

Dallenbach-Hellweg G. The influence of contraceptive steroids on the histological appearance of the endometrium. In: Diczfalusy E, Fraser IS, Webb FTG eds. *WHO Symposium on steroid contraception and mechanisms of endometrial bleeding.* Bath/Heidelberg/New York: Pitman Press Ltd; 1980a:153–173.

Dallenbach-Hellweg G. Morphological changes induced in the human uterus and Fallopian tube by exogenous estrogens. In: Dallenbach-Hellweg G, ed. *Functional morphologic changes in female sex organs induced by exogenous hormones.* Berlin/Heidelberg/New York: Springer-Verlag; 1980b:39–44.

De Leede LGJ, Govers CPM, De Nijs H. A multi-compartment vaginal ring system for independently adjustable release of contraceptive steroids. *Contraception* 1986;34:589–602.

Dixon GW, Schlesselman JJ, Ory HW, Blye RP. Ethinylestradiol and conjugated estrogens as postcoital contraceptives. *JAMA* 1980;244:1,336–9.

Ebeling K, Nischan P, Schindler CH. Use of oral contraceptives and risk of invasive cervical cancer in previously screened women. *International Journal of Cancer* 1987;39:427–30.

Egger H, Kindermann G. Effects of high estrogen doses on the endometrium. In: Dallenbach-Hellweg, G., ed. *Functional morphologic changes in female sex organs induced by exogenous hormones.* Berlin/Heidelberg/New York: Springer-Verlag; 1980:51–61.

El Mahgoub S. Long-term intracervical contraception with a levonorgestrel device. *Contraception* 25:357–374, 1982.

Flowers CE, Wilborn WH, Enger J. Effects of quingestanol acetate on the histology, histochemistry, and ultrastructure of the human endometrium. *Am J Obstet Gynecol* 1974;120:589–612.

Fluhmann CF. The glandular structures of the cervix uteri during pregnancy. *Am J Obstet Gynecol* 1959;78:990–7.

Fotherby K, Koetsawang S, Mathrubutham M. Pharmacokinetic study of different doses of depo-provera. *Contraception* 1980;22:527–36.

Galand P, Leroy F, Chretien J. Effect of oestradiol on cell proliferation and histological changes in the uterus and vagina of mice. *J Endocrinol* 1971;49:243.

Gaton E, Zejdel L, Bernstein D, et al. The effect of estrogen and gestagen on the mucus production of human endocervical cells: a histochemical study. *Fertil Steril* 1982;38:580–5.

Greenblatt RB, Zarate A. Endometrial studies following quinestrol administration. *Intl J Fertil* 1967;12:187.

Hagenfeldt K. The modes of action of medicated intrauterine devices. *J Reprod Fertil* 1976;25 (Suppl):117.

Haspels AA. Interception: postcoital estrogens in 3016 women. *Contraception* 1976;14:375–81.

Hyne RV, Murdoch RN, Boettcher B. The metabolism and motility of human spermatozoa in the presence of steroid hormones and synthetic progestogens. *J Reprod Fert* 1978;53:315.

Johanisson E, Gemzell A, Diczfalusy E. Effect of a single injection of human pituitary follicle-stimulating hormone on urinary estrogens and the vaginal smear in amenorrheic women. *J Clin Endocrinol Metab* 1961;21:1,068–78.

Johannisson E, Landgren B-M, Diczfalusy E. Endometrial morphology and peripheral steroid levels in women with and without intermenstrual bleeding during contraception with the 300 µg norethisterone (NET) minipill. *Contraception* 1982;25:13–29.

Johannisson E., Landgren B-M, Diczfalusy E. Endometrial and vaginal response to three different oestrogen preparations administered by the transdermal and oral routes. *Maturitas*, 1988;10:181–92.

Johannisson E, Landgren B-M, Hagenfeldt K. The effect of intrauterine progesterone on the DNA-content in isolated human endometrial cells. *Acta Cytol* 1977;21:441–6.

King RJB, Whitehead MI. Progestin action in relation to the prevention of endometrial abnormalities. In: Raynaud JP, Ojasoo T, Martini L, eds. *Medical management of endometriosis*. New York: Raven Press; 1984:67.

Kubba AA, White JO, Guillebaud J, Elder MG. The biochemistry of human endometrium after two regimens of postcoital contraception: a dl-norgestrel/ethinylestradiol combination or danazol. *Fertil Steril* 1986;45:512–6.

Kurunmäki H, Toivonen J, Lähteenmäki PLA, Luukkainen T. Pituitary and ovarian function and clinical performance during the use of a levonorgestrel-releasing intracervical contraceptive device. *Contraception* 1984;29:31–43.

Lan PT, Aedo A-R, Landgren B-M, et al. Return of ovulation following a single injection of depo-medroxy-progesterone acetate: a pharmacokinetic and pharmaco-dynamic study. *Contraception* 1984; 29:1.

Landgren B-M, Diczfalusy E. Hormonal effects of the 300 µg norethisterone (NET) minipill. 1. daily steroid levels in 43 subjects during a pretreatment cycle and during the second month of NET administration. *Contraception* 1980;21:87–113.

Landgren B-M, Johannisson E, Masironi B, Diczfalusy E. Pharmacokinetic and pharmacodynamic effects of small doses of norethisterone released from vaginal rings continuously during 90 days. *Contraception* 1979;19:253–71.

Landgren B-M, Johannisson E, Masironi B, Diczfalusy E. Pharmacokinetic and pharmacodynamic investigations with vaginal devices releasing levonorgestrel at a constant near zero order rate. *Contraception* 1982;26:567.

Landgren B-M, Oriowo MA, Diczfalusy E. Pharmacokinetic and pharmacodynamic studies with vaginal devices releasing norethisterone at a constant near zero order rate. *Contraception* 1981;24:29.

Ling WY, Robichaud A, Zayid I, et al. Mode of action of dl-norgestrel and ethinylestradiol combination in postcoital contraception. *Fertil Steril* 1979;32:297.

Ling WY, Wrixon W, Zayid I, et al. Mode of action of dl-norgestrel and ethinylestradiol combination in postcoital contraception. I. effect of postovulatory administration on ovarian function and endometrium. *Fertil Steril* 1983;39:292.

Luikku J, Kortesluoma M. Normophasic preparation containing progestagen desogestrel and ethinylestradiol. *Contracept Deliv Syst* 1983;4:61–66.

Mandelbaum J, Junca AM, Plachot M et al. The implantation window in humans after fresh or frozen-thawed embryo transfers. In: Mashiach S, Ben-Rafael Z, Laufer N, Schenker JG eds. *Advances in Assisted Reproductive Technologies*. New York: Plenum; 1990;729–35.

Maqueo M. Vascular and perivascular changes in the endometrium of women using steroidal contraceptives. In: Diczfalusy E, Fraser IS, Webb FTG, eds. *WHO symposium on steroid contraception and mechanisms of endometrial bleeding*. Bath/Heidelberg/New York: Pitman Press Ltd; 1980:138–152.

Maqueo M, Azuela JC, Calderon JJ, Goldzieher JW. Morphology of the cervix in women treated with synthetic progestins. *Am J Obstet Gynecol* 1966;96:994–8.

Maqueo M, Becerra C, Munguia H, Goldzieher JW. Endometrial histology and vaginal cytology during oral contraception with sequential estrogen and progestin. *Am J Obstet Gynecol* 1964;90:395–400.

Maqueo M, Gorodovsky J, Rice-Wray E, Goldzieher JW. Endometrial changes in women taking hormonal contraceptives for periods up to ten years. *Contraception* 1970a;1:115–29.

Maqueo M, Rice-Wray E, Gorodovsky J, and Goldzieher JW. The effect of contraceptive steroids on endometrial sinusoids and the failure of these changes to correlate with breakthrough bleeding or systemic vascular effects. *Contraception* 1970b;2:283–8.

Maqueo M, Perez-Vega E, Goldzieher JW, et al. Comparison of the endometrial activity of 3 synthetic progestins used in fertility control. *Am J Obstet Gynecol* 1963;85:427–32.

Maqueo M, Rice-Wray E, Gorodovsky J, Goldzieher JW. Endometrial regeneration in patients discontinuing oral contraceptives. *Fertil Steril* 1970;21:224–9.

Martinez-Manautou J, Aznar RJ, Maqueo M, et al. Uterine therapeutic system for long-term contraception II. clinical correlates. *Fertil Steril* 1974;25:922–6.

Martinez-Manautou J, Maqueo M, Aznar RM, et al. Endometrial morphology in women exposed to uterine systems releasing progesterone. *Am J Obstet Gynecol* 1975;121:175–9.

Moghissi KS, Marks C. Effects of microdose norgestrel on endogenous gonadotropic and steroid hormones, cervical mucus properties, vaginal cytology and endometrium. *Fertil Steril* 1971;22:424.

Moghissi KS, Syner FN, McBride LC. Contraceptive mechanism of microdose norethindrone. *Obstet Gynecol* 1973;41:585–93.

Moyer DL. Endometrial tolerance with cutaneous administration of estradiol. In: Dusitsin N, Notelovitz

M, eds. *Physiological hormone replacement therapy*. Carnforth, New Jersey: The Parthenon Publishing Group; 1990:65–71.

Nilsson CG, Johansson EDB, Jackanicz T, Luukkainen T. Biodegradable polylactate as a steroid-releasing polymer: intrauterine administration of d-norgestrel. *Am J Obstet Gynecol* 1975;122:90–5.

Nilsson CG, Luukkainen T, Arko H. Endometrial morphology of women using a levonorgestrel-releasing intrauterine device. *Fertil Steril* 1978;29:397–401.

Ober WB, Bronstein SB. Endometrial morphology following oral administration of quinestrol. *Intl J Fertil* 1967;12:210.

Pardthaisong T, Gray RH, McDaniel EB. Return of fertility after discontinuation of depot-medroxyprogesterone acetate and intrauterine devices in Northern Thailand. *Lancet* 1980;1:509–12.

Peterson H, Lee N, Rubin G. Genital neoplasia. In: Mishell D, ed. *Menopause. Physiology and pharmacology*. Chicago: Year Book Medical Publications; 1988:275.

Prentice RL, Thomas DB. On the epidemiology of oral contraceptives and disease. *Advances in Cancer Research* 1987;49:285–401.

Rabe T, Leppien G, Kiesel G, et al. Licht und elektronenmikroskopische veränderungen des endometriums unter einnahme eines norgestimathaltigen oralen kontraceptivums (cilest). *Geburtsh Frauenheilk* 1986;46:883.

Ratsula K. Clinical performance of a levonorgestrel-releasing intracervical contraceptive device during the first year of use. *Contraception* 1987;36:659–66.

Ratsula K. Clinical performance of a levonorgestrel-releasing intracervical contraceptive device during the first two years of use. *Contraception* 1989;39:187–93.

Ratsula K, Toivonen J, Lähteenmäki P, Luukkainen T. Plasma levonorgestrel levels and ovarian function during the use of a levonorgestrel-releasing intracervical contraceptive device. *Contraception* 1988;39:195–204.

Ravindranath N, Moudgal NR. Effect of a specific estrogen antibody on pregnancy establishment in the bonnet monkey (macaca radiata). *Fertil Steril* 1990;54:1,162–7.

Ravindranath N, Moudgal NR. Use of tamoxifen, an antiestrogen, in establishing a need for oestrogen in early pregnancy in the bonnet monkey (macaca radiata). *J Reprod Fertil* 1987;81:327–36.

Rice-Wray E, Aranda-Rosell A, Maqueo M, Goldzieher JW. Comparison of the long-term endometrial effects of synthetic progestins used in fertility control. *Am J Obstet Gynecol* 1963;87:429–33.

Richart RM, Ferenczy A. Endometrial morphologic response to hormonal environment. *Gynecol Oncol* 1974;2:180–97.

Rosado A, Hicks JJ, Aznar R, et al. Intrauterine contraception with the progesterone-T device. *Contraception* 1974;9:39.

Rosenberg MJ, Long SC. Oral contraceptives and cycle control: a critical review of the literature. *Avd Contracept* 1992;8 (pt 1):35–45.

Schlesselman JJ. Oral contraceptives and neoplasia of the uterine corpus. *Contraception* 1991;557–80.

Schumacher CFB. Biochemistry of cervical mucus. *Fertil Steril* 1970;21:697.

Scommegna A, Lee AW, Borushek S. Evaluation of an injectable progestin-estrogen as a contraceptive. *Am J Obstet Gynecol* 1970;107:1,147–54.

Sjöwall A. Studies of cervical mucosa during menstrual cycle, childhood, sterility and some hormonal disorders. *Acta Obstet Gynecol Scand* 1938;(Suppl 4):18.

Spornitz UM. The functional morphology of the human endometrium and decidua. *Adv Anat Embryol Cell Biol* 1992;124:1–99.

Trussell J, Stewart F. The effectiveness of postcoital hormonal contraception. *Fam Plann Perspect* 1992;24:262–4.

Uniyal JP, Bucksee K, Bhargava BL, et al. Binding of norgestrel to receptor proteins in the human endometrium and myometrium. *J Steroid Biochem* 1977;8:1,183.

Van de Walle J, Demol R. Contraceptive oral normophasique à base de désogestrel. *Ars Medici* 1984;36 (19/20):1765–73.

Van Santen MR, Haspels AA. Interfering with implantation by postcoital estrogen administration I. endometrium histology. *Prog Reprod Biol* 1980;7:310.

Vessey MP, McPherson K, Lawless M, Yeates D. Neoplasia of the cervix uteri and contraception: a possible adverse effect of the pill. *Lancet* 1983;2:930–4.

Webb, AMC, Russell J, Elstein M. Comparison of Yuzpe regimen, danazol, and mifepristone (RU486) in oral postcoital contraception. *Br Med J* 1992;305:927–30.

Whitehead MI, Townsend PT, Pryse-Davies J, et al. Effects of oestrogens and progestins on the biochemistry and morphology of the postmenopausal endometrium. *N Engl J Med* 1981;305:1,599.

Whitehead MI, Townsend PT, Pryse-Davies J, et al. Effects of various types and dosages of progestogens on the postmenopausal endometrium. *J Reprod Med* 1982;27;539.

Wright SW, Fotherby K, Davies JE. The effect of d- and l-norgestrel on penetration of cervical mucus by sperm. *Rev de Med* 1978;4:153–5.

Wright SW, Fotherby K, Fairweather F. Effects of daily small doses of norgestrel on ovarian function. *J Obstet Gynaecol Br Commonw* 1970;77:65–8.

Wynants P, Ide P. Endometrial morphology during a normophasic and a triphasic regimen: a comparison. *Contraception* 1986;33:149–57.

Xing S, Johannisson E, Landgren B-M, Diczfalusy E. Pituitary, ovarian and endometrial effects of progesterone released prematurely during the proliferative phase. *Contraception* 1983;27:177–93.

Yuzpe AA, Smith RP, Rademaker AW. A multicenter clinical investigation employing ethinylestradiol combined with dl-norgestrel as a postcoital contraceptive agent. *Fertil Steril* 1982;37:508.

Zalànyi S, Aedo A-R, Johannisson E, et al. Pituitary, ovarian and endometrial effects of graded doses of medroxyprogesterone acetate administered on cycle days 7 to 10. *Contraception* 1986;33:567–78.

Ziel HK, Finkle WD. Association of estrone with the development of endometrial carcinoma. *Am J Obstet Gynecol* 1976;124:735.

Pharmacology of the Contraceptive Steroids,
edited by Joseph W. Goldzieher.
Raven Press, Ltd., New York © 1994.

13

The Adrenal Gland

*†Steven M. Petak and †Emil Steinberger

*Department of Pharmacology, and †Texas Institute for Research in Reproductive Medicine and Endocrinology, and University of Texas School of Medicine at Houston, Houston, Texas 77054

The effects of oral contraceptives on adrenal function can be both direct and indirect. There is a large body of evidence suggesting that there are direct effects on the steroidogenic pathways in the adrenals and on the regulatory mechanisms of the pituitary-adrenal axis. The indirect effects relate to hepatic production of steroid binding proteins. These various effects are complicated by the fact that: 1) oral contraceptives (OCs) contain both estrogenic and progestational agents, each having distinct and sometimes opposite effects; 2) the various formulations contain different types of estrogenic and progestational agents that produce different effects and interactions; 3) there are different amounts of the hormones and different ratios of estrogenic-to-progestational activity; and 4) the various progestational agents can act as estrogen antagonists or agonists, and may exhibit varying degrees of androgenic or glucocorticoid activities.

EFFECTS ON THE HYPOTHALAMIC-PITUITARY AXIS

Hypothalamic-pituitary regulation of adrenal function is concerned with control of cortisol and androgen production. Mineralocorticoids are regulated primarily by the renin-angiotensin-aldosterone system. Adrenal medullary function is more appropriately classified as neuroendocrine.

The adrenocorticotropic hormone (ACTH) regulates cortisol and androgen secretion. There may exist a distinct hormone—cortical androgen-stimulating hormone (CASH)—that may also be involved in regulation of adrenal androgens (Parker and Odell, 1980). ACTH production is in turn regulated by corticotropin-releasing hormone (CRH) produced by the hypothalamus. A negative feedback mechanism operating at the hypothalamic-pituitary level, involving blood cortisol levels, regulates ACTH production. Thus the hypothalamic-pituitary axis interactions maintain appropriate blood cortisol levels via a negative feedback mechanism. There is a physiologic diurnal variation in blood cortisol levels, with the nadir near midnight and the maximum level at approximately 8 AM.

Both the estrogens and progestins produce distinct and specific effects on mechanisms involved with the physiologic control of blood cortisol levels.

Effect of Estrogens

Estrogens down-regulate type I corticoid receptors in the anterior pituitary of female rats (Ferrini et al., 1990). This mechanism could modify the negative feedback regulation of the hypothalamic-pituitary axis and influence cortisol production. Estradiol may also influence ACTH production via a distinct stimulatory effect on pituitary cells. Redei and Li (1991) have shown that estradiol increases basal ACTH secretion in cultured rat anterior pituitary cells. Whether this mechanism operates in humans remains to be determined.

Progestins

Synthetic progestins exhibit glucocorticoid-like activity that varies with the type of progestational agent and its concentration. Medroxyprogesterone acetate (MPA) has significant glucocorticoid activity (Hellman et al., 1975) that may be of sufficient magnitude to exert a negative feedback effect, and cause a decrease in plasma ACTH levels as well as lower cortisol levels. An OC containing norethindrone and mestranol has also been shown to exert a negative feedback effect on ACTH secretion, possibly due to intrinsic glucocorticoid activity (Carr et al., 1979). Early studies by Mestman et al. (1968) of a combination OC demonstrated no impairment of pituitary-adrenal axis function after ACTH stimulation lent an impaired metopirone response. Natural progesterone is apparently devoid of glucocorticoid and negative feedback activity.

Integrated Effects

Estrogens and progestins appear to exert opposite effects on the hypothalamic-pituitary-adrenal axis. Estrogens may augment ACTH release by down-regulating pituitary glucocorticoid receptors, while progestins tend to decrease ACTH release via their glucocorticoid activity. The effect of a combination of the two depends on the specific estrogens and progestins used, and the dose, as well as the ratio.

THE ADRENAL GLAND

Estrogens and progestins have markedly different direct effects on the function of the adrenal gland, and varying effects on the kinetics involved in maintenance of appropriate circulating steroid levels which are affected by production rates, peripheral metabolism, excretion patterns, and the binding characteristics of steroids while they are circulating in the blood.

Estrogens

Estrogen has a profound effect on the production of cortisol-binding globulin (CBG) by the liver, and also a direct effect on adrenal steroidogenesis.

Plasma Cortisol Levels

Ninety percent of plasma cortisol is bound to CBG, also known as transcortin. This protein has high affinity but limited binding capacity. Complete saturation occurs at a plasma level of about 20 μg/dl with about 10% free cortisol. At higher concentrations free cortisol increases nonlinearly to about 30%, with the remainder being bound to albumin, which has low affinity but high capacity (Anderson, 1974). During pregnancy, the serum levels of cortisol may increase by 300% in the last trimester. Estrogen therapy increases CBG synthesis by the liver. The higher levels of binding protein provide an increased number of binding sites that account for the typically elevated levels of cortisol found in patients on estrogen therapy.

Total blood cortisol levels are also increased in women using OCs, presumably due to stimulation of CBG production by the estrogenic component. Biologically, it is the level of unbound cortisol that is important. While most studies clearly demonstrate an increase in plasma CBG and total cortisol levels, whether or not free cortisol levels are also elevated remains a controversial issue. Early studies (Bulbrook et al., 1973) demonstrated increased total cortisol but no change in unbound cortisol. Using salivary cortisol levels as an index of free cortisol, Evans et al. (1984) demonstrated an increase in total cortisol values while salivary cortisol levels were not significantly different from normal. More recently, others reported increased free plasma and salivary cortisol levels (Meulenberg et al., 1987). None of the women in these studies demonstrated clinical evidence of hypercortisolism. The changes in plasma CBG, total cortisol, and salivary cortisol levels appear to be dose dependent. The use of OCs containing less than 35 μg estrogen appears to be associated with increased plasma CBG levels and unchanged levels of total and salivary cortisol (Scott et al., 1990).

In a study by van der Vange et al. (1989), seven low-dose OCs with different progestin types and quantity all caused similar increases in CBG levels. A preparation with cyproterone acetate caused a greater increase in CBG than the other combinations.

Adrenal Steroidogenesis

In hypophysectomized rats, estradiol alone does not affect adrenal production of corticosterone but potentiates the effect of ACTH (Colby and Kitay, 1974). In women, OCs also appear to augment adrenal cortisol responsiveness to ACTH stimulation. This effect is probably estrogen related (Fujimoto et al., 1986; Mestman et al., 1968). The mechanism of increased adrenal sensitivity to ACTH in the presence of estrogens is unclear. Studies in rats suggest that cytochrome P-450 may be increased in the setting of estrogen therapy (Purvis et al., 1973). Whether or not similar mechanisms operate in humans is unknown.

The effects of acute and chronic estrogen therapy on the activity of adrenal 3β-hydroxysteroid dehydrogenase have been studied in ovariectomized women (Anderson and Yen, 1976). The ratio of Δ^5 to Δ^4 steroids was no different in patients on or off estrogen therapy. Furthermore, an increased availability of Δ^5 substrate created by infusing ACTH also resulted in no differences in steroidogenesis. Thus, *in vitro* studies showing inhibition of 3β-hydroxysteroid dehydrogenase by estrogen (Sobrinho et al., 1971) appear not to be significant in humans *in vivo*.

Fonzo et al. (1967) demonstrated increased *in vitro* activity of 11β-hydroxylase of rat adrenals in the presence of estrogens. With estrogen administration *in vivo*, the corticosterone production decreased and ACTH levels rose. The increase in ACTH was attributed to the negative feedback mechanism associated with the decreased corticosterone levels; however, a direct effect of estrogen on the pituitary could not be excluded. Fujimoto et al. (1986) reported increased cortisol response to ACTH in women on ethynodiol diacetate/ethynyl estradiol (EE). Wallace et al. (1957) demonstrated increased levels of urinary 17-hydroxycorticosteroids in women using OCs after a 6-hour infusion of ACTH. It is possible that increased 11β-hydroxylase activity may explain these findings, but further studies are needed. One would assume that an increase in free cortisol levels would signal to the pituitary the need for further reductions in ACTH production. If estrogens act to down-regulate corticoid receptors in the anterior pituitary in women, as has been demonstrated in animals (Ferrini et al., 1990), this pituitary set point may be unresponsive to the increased levels of free cortisol.

Mineralocorticoids

One of the clinically apparent effects of estrogens and estrogen-containing OCs is fluid retention. In some cases, increases in blood pressure may also occur.

Estrogens are capable of increasing the activity of the renin-angiotensin-aldosterone system, which results in fluid retention. Estrogen may also have an effect on urine output. Atrial natriuretic peptide (ANP) acts to increase urine output and limit fluid retention. Women using OCs have higher ANP and plasma renin activity levels than nonusers. There was no significant difference in aldosterone levels between 35 μg EE estradiol OC users and nonusers (Davidson et al, 1988).

Goldhaber et al. (1984) studied plasma renin substrate, plasma renin activity, and plasma aldosterone levels in healthy women using OCs. He found a threefold increase in levels of plasma renin substrate, with no change in plasma renin activity, plasma aldosterone levels, or blood pressure. These findings indicate that, in normal women, compensatory mechanisms are capable of maintaining normal blood pressure.

Estrogen increases the production of aldosterone-binding globulin (ABG) by the liver. Nowaczynski et al. (1978) demonstrated greatly increased aldosterone binding but no difference in total aldosterone concentrations between OC users and nonusers. The significance of this finding with respect to hypertension and fluid retention is not known.

Adrenal Androgens

Estrogen has a permissive, dose-related effect on adrenal production of androgens. Oophorectomized women have significantly lower dehydroepiandrosterone sulfate (DHEAS) levels than premenopausal women. After 4 weeks of treatment with 0.625 mg conjugated equine estrogens (Premarin) in postmenopausal women, there were no significant changes in DHEAS levels. After 4 weeks of a daily 2.5 mg dose, however, the DHEAS levels rise significantly (Lobo et al., 1982). These data suggest that maintenance of the 3β-ol and 17,20 desmolase activity needed for androgen production may be estrogen dependent.

Only 1% to 3% of the blood testosterone and estradiol circulate in biologically active, unbound form. Two circulating macromolecules bind sex steroids: 1) albumin, a low-affinity, high-capacity binding protein, and 2) sex-hormone-binding globulin (SHBG), a high-affinity, low-capacity binding protein that binds testosterone preferentially over estradiol (Anderson, 1974). In women, SHBG levels are twofold greater than in men, and testosterone concentrations are much lower; thus, SHBG has many available binding sites. Estrogens stimulate and androgens inhibit SHBG production. With increased estrogen stimulation of SHBG, the unbound testosterone concentration decreases. Contrariwise, an increased androgen concentration will lower SHBG levels and increase the unbound testosterone concentration, possibly producing a clinical state of hyperandrogenism. Thus, by increasing SHBG synthesis, estrogen may have a major effect on biologically active androgen in circulation and may produce a prominent clinical effect.

EFFECT OF PROGESTINS

Cortisol Levels

As discussed in the previous section, some synthetic progestational agents have glucocorticoid activity. Therefore, they can decrease adrenal cortisol production via a negative feedback mechanism. Natural progesterone does not appear to have glucocorticoid activity.

Steroidogenesis

Norgestrel, ethynodiol diacetate, and norethindrone-containing OCs are capable of reducing circulating DHEAS, pregnenolone, and 17α-hydroxypregnenolone levels, either by a decrease in ACTH stimulation or by a direct effect (e.g., by inhibiting the cytochrome P450 mixed-function oxidase [Fern et al., 1978]).

Mineralocorticoids

Progesterone has antialdosterone effects. Some progestational agents are capable of binding to the aldosterone receptor; for example, gestodene is an aldosterone receptor antagonist (Pollow et al., 1989; Hoppe, 1988). The estrogen component of OCs stimulates plasma renin activity (PRA) and angiotensin II activity, but progestins do not stimulate the renin-angiotensin axis (Soveri et al., 1977).

Effect of Progestins or Estrogen-progestin Combinations on Adrenal Androgens

Different progestational agents have different effects on SHBG production. Medroxyprogesterone acetate lowers SHBG levels in both men and women (Forest et al., 1972). Norgestrel also lowers SHBG levels (Victor et al., 1977). The effects of norethindrone on SHBG are not clear. Key et al. (1989) demonstrated a decreased SHBG concentration in women on norethindrone only. Odlind et al. (1980) demonstrated that norethindrone alone has no effect on SHBG-binding capacity, but is capable of blocking the SHBG-binding capacity increase induced by EE (Granger et al., 1982). SHBG levels appear to remain relatively constant throughout the menstrual cycle; the rate of response to changes in sex hormone levels may be too slow to produce significant changes. SHBG levels rise five- to tenfold during pregnancy, and accompany a two- to fourfold rise in testosterone. The route of administration of estrogen-progestin combinations is important. Following oral administration, EE norethindrone will increase SHBG by 92%; EE norgestrel will increase it by only 12%. If estrogen norethindrone preparations are administered by vaginal ring, SHBG levels decrease about 16%. Whether these differences have clinical significance is uncertain. The effect of norgestrel on SHBG-binding capacity appears to be greater. A decrease in SHBG levels of up to 31% compared with baseline has been demonstrated by Granger et al. (1982). Many 19-nor progestational agents such as norethindrone exhibit intrinsic androgenicity, while 17α-hydroxyprogesterone acetate derivatives such as cyproterone acetate often act as antiandrogens. These agents also act to a variable extent as estrogen agonists. Norethindrone and norgestrel do not bind androgen receptors. In addition, norethindrone and norgestrel do not bind to SHBG and therefore would displace less testosterone from the binding protein (Granger et al., 1982). Therefore, the more androgenic progestational agents can affect free testosterone levels by decreasing levels of SHBG as well as by displacing testosterone from SHBG binding sites, making them unavailable for testosterone binding.

Hirsute women with elevated testosterone levels treated with an OC containing norethindrone and 0.05 mg mestranol showed a reduction in testosterone levels of about 73% (Wiebe et al., 1984). The level of DHEAS was also decreased about 41%. The fall in circulating testosterone is due mainly to a decrease in ovarian steroid secretion. The suppression of adrenal DHEAS has been postulated to be due to a decrease in ACTH secretion because of an increase in free cortisol or decreased clearance. This effect can be considered similar to, but not as pronounced as, the use of low-dose glucocorticoid suppression therapy for adrenal hyperandrogenism (Steinberger et al., 1990). Estrogen by itself has been shown to increase or have a neutral effect on DHEAS levels (Lee et al., 1975; Anderson et al., 1976). Nonhirsute women were studied before and after 4 to 5 months of various OCs. 35 μg EE and 1 mg norethindrone resulted in a 39% decrease in DHEAS levels. Thirty-five μg EE and 0.4 mg norethindrone resulted in a 30% decrease. These results did not differ statistically. Thirty μg EE and 150 μg levonorgestrel produced no change in DHEAS levels. Levonorgestrel implants also fail to change DHEAS levels (Klove et al., 1984; Murphy et al., 1990).

The changes in SHBG production and binding capacity reflect the combined properties of the estrogen and progestational agent. The net effect is dependent on the estrogen/androgen balance of the preparation. This may explain why estrogen-norgestrel combinations lower SHBG and occupy SHBG-binding sites, while estrogen/norethindrone-containing agents increase SHBG levels with little change in binding capacity, and therefore increase binding capacity of SHBG for circulating testosterone.

TESTING OF ADRENAL FUNCTION

The baseline cortisol levels in OC users are significantly elevated, complicating pituitary-adrenal axis diagnostic studies. Suppression of cortisol levels following an overnight dexamethasone suppression test is incomplete in patients on OCs and is related to the estrogen dose. The effect of estrogen on this test may persist for up to 1 month after discontinuation of OCs. Thus, caution should be exercised when interpreting dexamethasone suppression tests in women recently on OCs. Furthermore, urinary free cortisol levels are increased, while 17-hydroxycorticosteroids and 17-ketosteroids are often decreased in OC users (Lucis et al., 1972; Weindling et al., 1974; Miale et al., 1974). Since the half-life of CBG is about 5 days, cortisol levels gradually rise during the first half of OC therapy cycles and then fall when the cycle is terminated. However, the normal circadian rhythm of cortisol is preserved in OC users (Dommisse et al., 1985; Tiller, 1988).

SUMMARY

Oral contraceptives can alter adrenal function at multiple levels. The increased hepatic production of CBG, ABG, and SHBG is caused by estrogens and variably affected by the progestational agent, depending on its structure and concentration. The progestational agent may exhibit specific androgenic, estrogenic, mineralocorticoid, and glucocorticoid-agonist or antagonistic activity. Estrogen increases the total circulating bound cortisol levels and availability of free-testosterone-binding sites, while some progestational agents impair the estrogen-mediated increase in SHBG levels and bind to SHBG, directly displacing free testosterone. Pituitary regulation of adrenal function may be altered by the glucocorticoid activity of some progestational agents. This alteration results in a decreased ACTH level and decreased production of cortisol and adrenal androgens. Furthermore, estrogens may modify the feedback loop through down-regulating the pituitary glucocorticoid type I receptor, making the pituitary less responsive to negative feedback from the adrenal. The estrogen may stimulate adrenal responsiveness to ACTH stimulation, resulting in increased cortisol production in the setting of low ACTH levels. This effect does not appear to increase the sensitivity of the adrenal androgen pathway to the same extent, as DHEAS levels are only modestly decreased. The modestly increased free cortisol does not appear to have any pathological effect but can affect laboratory testing for Cushing's syndrome.

REFERENCES

Anderson DC. Sex-hormone binding globulin. *Clin Endocrinol* 1974;3:69.

Anderson DC, Yen SSC. Effects of estrogens on adrenal 3-beta-hydroxysteroid dehydrogenase in ovariectomized women. *J Clin Endocrinol Metab* 1976;43:561.

Bulbrook RD, Herian M, Tong D, Hayward JL, Swain MC, Wang DY. Effect of steroidal contraceptives on levels of plasma androgen sulphates and cortisol. *Lancet* 1973;628.

Carr BR, Parker CR Jr, Madden JD, MacDonald PC, Porter JC. Plasma levels of adrenocorticotropin and cortisol in women receiving oral contraceptive steroid treatment. *J Clin Endocrinol Metab* 1979; 49:346.

Colby HD, Kitay JI. Interaction of estradiol and ACTH in the regulation of adrenal corticosterone production in the rat. *Steroids* 1974;24:527.

Davidson BJ, Rea CD, Valenzuela GJ. Atrial natriuretic peptide, plasma renin activity, and aldosterone in women on estrogen therapy and with premenstrual syndrome. *Fertil Steril* 1988;50:743.

Dommisse CS, Hayes PE, Kwentus JA. Effect of estrogens on the dexamethasone suppression test in nondepressed women. *J Clin Psychopharmacol* 1985;5:315.

Edgren RA, Sturtevant FM. Potencies of oral contraceptives. *Am J Obstet Gynecol* 1976;125:1029.

Evans PJ, Peters JR, Dyas J, Walker RF, Riad-Fahmy D, Hall R. Salivary cortisol levels in true and apparent hypercortisolism. *Clin Endocrinol* 1984;20:709.

Fern M, Rose DP, Fern EB. Effect of oral contraceptives on plasma androgenic steroids and their precursors. *Obstet Gynecol* 1978;51:541.

Ferrini M, Magarinos A, De Nicola A. Oestrogens down-regulate type I but not type II adrenal corticoid receptors in rat anterior pituitary. *J Steroid Biochem* 1990;35:671.

Fonzo D, Mims RB, Nelson DH. Estrogen influence on pituitary and adrenal function in the rat. *Endocrinology* 1967;81:29.

Forest MG, Bertrand J. Studies of the protein binding of dihydrotestosterone in human plasma (in Different physiological conditions and effect of medroxyprogesterone). *Steroids* 1972;19:197.

Fujimoto VY, Villanueva AL, Hopper B, Moscinski M, Rebar RW. Increased adrenocortical responsiveness to exogenous ACTH in oral contraceptive users. *Adv Contracept* 1986;2:343.

Gaillard RC, Riondel A, Muller AF, Herrmann W, Baulieu EE. RU 486: a steroid with antiglucocorticosteroid that only disinhibits the human pituitary-adrenal system at a specific time of day. *Proc Natl Acad Sci USA* 1984;81:3879.

Givens JR, Andersen RN, Wiser WL, Fish SA. Dynamics of suppression and recovery of plasma FSH, LH, androstenedione and testosterone in polycystic ovarian disease using an oral contraceptive. *J Clin Endocrinol Metab* 1974;38:727.

Goldhaber SZ, Hennekens CH, Spark RF, et al. Plasma renin substrate, renin activity, and aldosterone levels in a sample of oral contraceptive users from a community survey. *Am Heart J* 1984;107:119.

Goldzieher JW, Chenault CB, De La Pena A, Tazewell SD, Kraemer DC. Comparative studies of the ethynyl estrogens used in oral contraceptives: effects with and without progestational agents on the plasma androstenedione, testosterone, and testosterone binding in humans, baboons, and beagles. *Fertil Steril* 1978;29:388.

Granger LR, Roy S, Mishell DR. Changes in unbound sex steroids and sex hormone binding globulin-binding capacity during oral and vaginal progestogen administration. *Am J Obstet Gynecol* 1982; 144:578.

Hellman L, Yoshida K, Zumoff B, Levin J, Kream J, Fukushima DK. The effect of medroxyprogesterone acetate on the pituitary-adrenal axis. *J Clin Endocrinol Metab* 1975;42:912.

Hoppe G. Gestodene, an innovative progestagen. *Contraception* 1988;37:493.

Jung-Hoffmann C, Kuhl H. Divergent effects of two low-dose oral contraceptives on sex hormone-binding globulin and free testosterone. *Am J Obstet Gynecol* 1986;156:199.

Jung-Hoffmann C, Kuhl H. Interaction with the pharmacokinetics of ethinylestradiol and progestogens contained in oral contraceptives. *Contraception* 1989;40:299.

Key TJA, Pike MC, Moore JW, et al. The relationships of SHBG with current and previous use of oral contraceptives and oestrogen replacement therapy. *Contraception* 1989;39:179.

Kirschner MA, Jacobs JB. Combined ovarian and adrenal vein catheterization to determine the site(s) of androgen overproduction in hirsute women. *J Clin Endocrinol* 1971;33:199.

Klove KL, Roy S, Lobo RA. The effect of different contraceptive treatments on the serum concentration of dehydroepiandrosterone sulfate. *Contraception* 1984;29:319.

Lachelin GCL, Barnett M, Hopper BR, Brink G, Yen SSC. Adrenal function in normal women and women with the polycystic ovary syndrome. *J Clin Endocrinol Metab* 1979;49:892.

Lee PA, Kowarski A, Migeon CJ, Blizzard RM. Lack of correlation between gonadotropin and adrenal androgen levels in agonadal children. *J Clin Endocrinol Metab* 1975;40:664.

Lobo RA, Goebelsmann U, Brenner PF, Mishell DR. The effects of estrogen on adrenal androgens in oophorectomized women. *Am J Obstet Gynecol* 1982;142:471.

Lobo RA, Wellington LP, Goebelsmann U. Serum levels of DHEAS in gynecologic endocrinopathy and infertility. *Obstet Gynecol* 1981;57:607.

Lucis OJ, Lucis R. Oral contraceptives and endocrine changes. *Bull WHO* 1972;46:443.

Madden JD, Milewich L, Parker CR, Carr BR, Boyar RM, MacDonald PC. The effect of oral contraceptive treatment on the serum concentration of dehydroisoandrosterone sulfate. *Am J Obstet Gynecol* 1978;132:380.

Mestman JH, Anderson GV, Nelson DH. Adrenal-pituitary responsiveness during therapy with an oral contraceptive. *Obstet Gynecol* 1968;31:378.

Meulenberg PMM, Ross HA, Swinkels LMJW, Benraad TJ. The effect of oral contraceptives on plasma-free and salivary cortisol and cortisone. *Clin Chim Acta* 1987;165:379.

Miale JB, Kent JW. The effects of oral contraceptives on the results of laboratory tests. *Am J Obstet Gynecol* 1974;120:264.

Murphy AA, Cropp CS, Smith BS, Burkman RT, Zacur HA. Effect of low-dose oral contraceptive on gonadotropins, androgens, and sex hormone binding globulin in nonhirsute women. *Fertil Steril* 1990; 53:35.

Nowaczynski W, Murakami T, Richardson K, Genest J. Increased aldosterone plasma protein binding in women on combined oral contraceptives throughout the menstrual cycle. *J Clin Endocrinol Metab* 1978;47:193.

Odlind V, Weiner E, Vicrot A, Johansson EDB. Effects on sex hormone binding globulin of different oral contraceptives containing norethisterone and lynesterol. *Br J Obstet Gynaecol* 1980;87:416.

Parker LN, Odell WD. Control of adrenal androgen secretion. *Endocrine Reviews* 1980;1:392.

Plager J, Schmidt DG, Staubitz WJ. Increased unbound cortisol in the plasma of estrogen-treated subjects. *J Clin Invest* 1964;43:1066.

Pollow K, Juchem M, Grill MJ, et al. Gestodene: a novel progestin—characterization of binding to receptor and serum proteins. *Contraception* 1989;40:325.

Purvis JL, Canick JA, Mason JI, Estabrook RW, McCarthy JL. Lifetime of adrenal cytochrone P-450 as influenced by ACTH. *Ann NY Acad Sci* 1973;212:

Redei E, Li LF. Differential effects of estrogen and progesterone on ACTH secretion in vitro. 73rd Annual Meeting of the Endocrine Society. 1991; (abst) 55:44.

Scott EM, McGarricle HG, Lachelin GCL. The increase in plasma and saliva cortisol levels in pregnancy is not due to the increase in corticosteroid-binding globulin levels. *J Clin Endocrinol Metab* 1990;71:639.

Sobrinhi IG, Kase NG, Grunt JA. Changes in adrenocortical function of patients with gonadal dysgenesis after treatment with estrogen. *J Clin Endocrinol Metab* 1971;33:110.

Soveri P, Fyhrquist F. Plasma renin activity and angiotensin II during oral contraception. *Ann Clin Res* 1977;9:346.

Steinberger E, Rodriguez-Rigau LJ, Petak SM, Weidman ER, Ayala C. Glucocorticoid therapy in hyperandrogenism. *Balliere's Clin Obstet Gynaecol* 1990;4:457.

Tiller JWG, Maguire KP, Schweitzer I, et al. The dexamethasone suppression test: a study in a normal population. *Psychoneuroendocrinology* 1988;13:377.

van der Vange N, Blankenstein MA, Kloosterboer HJ, Haspels AA, Thijssen JHH. Effects of seven low-dose combined oral contraceptives on sex hormone binding globulin, corticosteroid binding globulin, total and free testosterone. *Contraception* 1989;41:345.

Victor A, Weiner E, Johansson EDB. Relation between sex hormone binding globulin and d-norgestrel levels in plasma. *Acta Endocrinol (Copenh)* 1977;86:430.

Wallace EZ, Silverberg HI, Carter AC. Effect of ethinyl estradiol on plasma 17-hydroxysteroids, ACTH responsiveness, and hydrocortisone clearance in man. *Proc Soc Exp Biol Med* 1957;95:805.

Weindling H, Henry JB. Laboratory test results altered by the pill. *JAMA* 1974;229:1,762.

Wiebe RH, Morris CV. Effect of an oral contraceptive on adrenal and ovarian androgenic steroids. *Obstet Gynecol* 1984;63:12.

Wild RA, Umstot ES, Andersen RN, Givens JR. Adrenal function in hirsutism. II. effect of an oral contraceptive. *J Clin Endocrinol Metab* 1982;54:676.

Pharmacology of the Contraceptive Steroids,
edited by Joseph W. Goldzieher.
Raven Press, Ltd., New York © 1994.

14

The Thyroid Gland

Joseph W. Goldzieher

*Department of Obstetrics and Gynecology, Baylor College of Medicine,
Houston, Texas 77030*

The effects of pregnancy and estrogen therapy on laboratory parameters of thyroid function are well known. The phases of the normal menstrual cycle also exert detectable effects (Beck et al., 1972). Consequently, thyroid studies were included in the early clinical trials of oral contraceptives, and the expected changes due to the estrogen-induced increase in TBG were observed (Hollander et al., 1963). The progestins themselves appeared to have no effect on these laboratory parameters (Winikoff, 1968; Olsson et al., 1986).

Studies of plasma TSH levels showed no change (Penttilä et al., 1983; Kuhl et al., 1985) or slight elevation (Weeke and Hansen, 1975). The thyroid-stimulating hormone (TSH) response to a thyroid-releasing hormone (TRH) challenge has been reported as unchanged (Penttilä et al., 1983) or augmented (Ramey et al., 1975). Gross et al. (1971) studied the effect of high doses of ethynyl estradiol (EE). A single dose of 100 to 500 μg acutely suppressed plasma TSH, while still larger doses (3,000 μg) directly inhibited thyroid hormone release. An "escape" from this inhibition occurred in 2 to 3 days, but there remained a blunting or absence of the normal diurnal pattern of thyroid hormone release.

Thyroid radioiodine studies in women using oral contraceptives (OCs) with 75 to 100 μg of EE for 3 months or up to 3 years showed no change in the 24-hour uptake as compared to controls (Irizzary et al., 1966). Starup and Friis (1967) also found no change in 4- and 24-hour uptake, while others found that OCs with either higher (Vega-de Rodriguez et al., 1972) or lower (Barsivala et al., 1974) estrogen doses had a lowering effect on 24-hour uptake.

Within a week of instituting combined OC use, serum T4 and other tests affected by the level of thyroxine-binding globulin (TBG) show a rise; these changes are reversed about 2 months after OC discontinuation (Weindling and Henry, 1974). In general, T4 and related levels are increased about 30% with 50 to 100 μg estrogen OCs, compared to an increase of about 100% at 36 weeks gestation (Knopp et al., 1985). Triphasic OCs containing 30 μg EE raise TBG by about 20%, with a consequent 40% elevation of total T4; free-T3 and reverse-T3 levels are unchanged (Kuhl et al., 1985). Progestin-only OCs or implants do not alter conventional plasma thyroid tests (Goolden et al., 1970) except for the impact of a slight decrease in the TBG level (Olsson et al., 1986).

Several prospective studies have examined the incidence of thyroid disorders in OC users. McTiernan et al. (1984) and Preston-Martin et al. (1987) found some overall positive association for thyroid cancer, but the risk did not increase with duration of OC use, suggesting that the association was not causal. The Royal College study (1978) found fewer cases of benign thyroid swelling, and hyper- and hypothyroidism in current OC users. Vessey et al. (1987) found no difference between OC users and controls in frequency of hospital admission for thyroid disorders. Nontoxic nodular goiter showed a statistically significant negative relationship with total duration of OC use.

REFERENCES

Barsivala V, Virkar K, Kulkarni RD. Thyroid functions of women taking oral contraceptives. *Contraception* 1974;9:305–14.

Beck RP, Fawcett DM, Morcos F. Thyroid function studies in different phases of the menstrual cycle and in women receiving norethindrone with and without estrogen. *Am J Obstet Gynecol* 1972;112:369–73.

Goolden AWG, Bateman DM, Pleehachinda R, Sanderson C. Thyroid function tests in women taking norgestrel. *Lancet* 1970;1:624.

Gross HA, Appleman MD Jr, Nicoloff JT. Effect of biologically active steroids on thyroid function in man. *J Clin Endocrinol Metab* 1971;33:242–8.

Hollander CS, Garcia AM, Sturgis SH, Selenkow HA. Effect of an ovulatory suppressant on the serum protein-bound iodine and the red-cell uptake of radioactive triiodothyrnine. *New Engl J Med* 1963; 269:501–4.

Irizzary S, Paniagua M, Pincus G, Janer JL, Frias Z. Effect of cyclic administration of certain progestin-estrogen combinations on the 24-hour radioiodine thyroid uptake. *J Clin Endocrinol Metab* 1966;26: 6–10.

Knopp RH, Bergelin RO, Wahl PW, et al. Clinical chemistry alterations in pregnancy and oral contraceptive use. *Obstet Gynecol* 1985;66:682–90.

Kuhl H, Gahn G, Romberg G, Althoff PH, Taubert HD. A randomized crossover comparison of two low-dose oral contraceptives upon hormonal and metabolic serum parameters II. Effects upon thyroid function, gastrin, STH, and glucose tolerance. *Contraception* 1985;32:97–107.

McTiernan AM, Weiss NS, Daling JR. Incidence of thyroid cancer in women in relation to reproductive and hormonal factors. *Am J Epidemiol* 1984;120:423–35.

Olsson SE, Wide L, Odlind V. Aspects of thyroid function during use of Norplant implants. *Contraception* 1986;34:583–7.

Penttilä IM, Makkonen M, Castren O: Thyroid function during treatment with a new oral contraceptive combination containing desogestrel. *Europ J Obstet Gynecol Reprod Biol* 1983;16:269–74.

Preston-Martin S, Bernstein L, Pike MC, Maldonado AA, Henderson BE. Thyroid cancer among young women related to prior thyroid disease and pregnancy history. *Brit J Cancer* 1987;55:191–5.

Ramcharan S, Pellegrin FA, Ray R, Hsu JP. The Walnut Creek Contraceptive Drug Study: a prospective study of the side effects of oral contraceptives. Vol.III. Bethesda, Maryland: National Institutes of Health, Bethesda MD; 1981.

Ramey JN, Burrow GN, Polackwich RJ, Donabedian RK. Effect of oral contraceptive steroids on the response of thyroid-stimulating hormone to thyrotropin-releasing hormone. *J Clin Endocrinol Metab* 1975;40:712–4.

Royal College of General Practitioners. Incidence of thyroid disease associated with oral contraceptives. *Br Med J* 1978;2:1,513.

Starup J, Friis T. Thyroid function in oral contraception. *Acta Endocrinol* 1967;56:525–32.

Vega-de Rodriguez G, Fuertes-de la Haba A, Pelegrina I. Thyroid status in long-term, high-dose oral contraceptive users. *Obstet Gynecol* 1972;39:779–83.

Vessey M, Villard-Mackintosh L, McPherson K, Yeates D. Thyroid disorders and oral contraceptives. *Br J Fam Plann* 1987;13:124–7.

Weeke J, Hansen AP. Serum TSH and serum T3 levels during normal menstrual cycles and during cycles on oral contraceptives. *Acta Endocrinol* 1975;79:431–8.

Weindling H, Henry JB. Laboratory test results altered by "The Pill". *JAMA* 1974;229:1,762–68.

Winikoff D. Oral contraceptives and thyroid function tests: the role of progestogens. *Med J Austral* 1968;2:13–8.

Pharmacology of the Contraceptive Steroids,
edited by Joseph W. Goldzieher.
Raven Press, Ltd., New York © 1994.

15

The Liver

M. H. Sillem and A. T. Teichmann

*Klinikum Aschaffenburg, University of Würzburg,
8750 Aschaffenburg, Germany*

Although not a classical target organ, the liver is influenced by sex steroids in numerous ways. This is true for both its morphological and functional aspects. Of the various functions of hepatic metabolism affected by contraceptive steroids, this chapter focuses primarily on biotransformation and secretion. It also covers the relations between contraceptive steroids and liver disease.

The liver is inevitably most involved if the steroids are administered orally, due to the first pass effect after intestinal absorption. In nonenteral forms of steroid contraception (depot progestin, vaginal ring), the impact on hepatic metabolism is less pronounced, yet the typical effects caused by the chemical structure of ethynyl estradiol (EE) are still present (Goebelsmann et al., 1985).

NORMAL ALTERATIONS DURING OC USE

Wide discrepancy exists between the variety of changes induced by the administration of contraceptive steroids on the one hand and the very rare instances where these changes gain any pathological importance. These effects are predictable, reproducible, and reversible. They include alterations in appearance, laboratory findings, and function. Both estrogen and androgen receptors are present in mammalian liver, whereas progesterone receptors are lacking (Eisenfeld and Aten, 1987).

Morphology

Upon ingestion of sex steroids, the size of the liver may increase to a variable degree. Concomitantly, liver blood flow is enhanced. Microscopically, the cytoplasm of the enlarged hepatocytes appears more eosinophilic, whereas basophilic segments of the rough endoplasmic reticulum are concentrated towards the biliary side of the cell. This phenomenon is called peribiliary basophilia of cytoplasm (Andree and Roschlau, 1987). Martinez-Manautou and coworkers (1970) found a moderately increased vesiculation of the rough and smooth endoplasmic reticulum, both in women given microdoses of progestins and in those using a combination progestin/estrogen OC. In the latter group, the vesiculation appeared more marked. Additionally, an elongation of mitochondria with cristalloid inclusions and fatty vacuolation was found. The latter phenomenon was more marked in combined and sequential types of OCs. In rats on EE, liver sinusoids show a persistent dilatation in the acinar inlet together with a sustained constriction of the acinar outlet (Raufman et al., 1980). Corresponding observations in humans are reported by Balasz (1988), who described sinusoidal dilatation in connection with proliferation and enhanced activity of sinusoidal endothelial cells in patients on OCs. All reported phenomena can be seen as expression of an altered hepatic metabolism under the influence of steroid hormones.

Laboratory Findings

In modern contraceptives containing low EE doses ($<35\mu g$) the parameters of liver function are very rarely raised to a pathological level. Numerous studies have been conducted and the results are somewhat contradictory. Walden et al. (1986) studied the effects of various estrogen-progestin combinations in 1,355 women. They attributed their observation of lowered bilirubin, alkaline phosphatase, and aspartate aminotransferase (SGOT) to estrogenic effects. Accordingly, the smallest bilirubin reductions were seen with progestin-dominant OCs. A WHO Task Force on oral contraceptives (Sadik et al., 1985) reported corresponding results for bilirubin and alkaline phosphatase in 847 women on either 1 mg norethindrone/35 μg EE or 150 μg levonorgestrel/30 μg EE; SGOT levels did not change significantly. Not surprisingly, with high-estrogen combinations more pathological values will be found (Larsson-Cohn, 1965). Consistently, an increase in bromsulphthalein retention is reported. Whereas this test reflects the excretion capacity, Metzner et al. (1990) suggest the ^{15}N ammonium test as a marker of partial metabolic performance of the liver. They found pathological values in 50% of women after long-term use of OCs. Table 1 gives an overview of the effects of contraceptive steroids on liver

TABLE 1. *C.S. and liver function tests*

Transaminases	variable	Sadik et al., 1985
y-Glutamyl-Transferase	increased	Taubert and Kuhl, 1981
Alkaline Phosphatase	decreased	Percival Smith and Sizto, 1983
		Sadik et al., 1985
		Odlind et al., 1982
Bilirubin	decreased	Sadik et al., 1985
		Knopp et al., 1985
		Walden et al., 1986
LDH	increased	Percival Smith and Sizto, 1983
		Dickerson et al., 1980
Bromsulphthalein Retention	increased	Larsson-Cohn, 1965
		Weindling and Henry, 1974

function tests in common use. Cyproterone acetate alone did not cause any structural or functional hepatic disturbances, even when used for a long duration and in high doses (Kaiser and Gruner, 1987). Equally, no substantial changes were seen in women on subdermal levonorgestrel (Shaaban et al., 1984).

Hepatic Metabolism

Although sex steroid receptors are frequently found in liver tissue, they do not seem to play an important role in the activation and degradation of these substances. The biological activity of mestranol depends on its being demethylated at position 3, a process that leads to EE. Ethynyl estradiol itself is to some extent found as EE-sulfate. Very small quantities of EE may be deacetylated, yielding estradiol and estriol. The major hepatic degradation pathway, however, is 2-hydroxylation by microsomal cytochrome P 450NF (= P 450 III A 4). This enzyme is influenced in several ways by a variety of pharmacological substances, a phenomenon that explains the complexity of interactions between EE and synthetic progestins and other drugs (Teichmann, 1990). The most important enhancing factor is enzyme induction. This may be effected by barbiturates and rifampicin. On the other hand, acetylenes and, in particular, steroids with a 17α-ethynyl group may cause a mechanism-based irreversible inhibition of cytochrome P 450NF. This mechanism is also called "suicide inactivation" (Guengerich, 1990). The molecular mechanism of this inhibition seems to be a covalent binding of the acetylene group to the heme prosthetic group of the enzyme, requiring nicotinamide adenine dinucleotide phosphate (NADPH) (Ortiz de Montellano and Kunze, 1980). In rat hepatocyte suspensions, a group of N-alkylated porphyrins ("green pigments") can be detected after incubation with these steroids, possibly as a reaction product (Blakey and White, 1986).

In addition to these rather strong influential factors, weak competitive and noncompetitive inhibitors exist. The influencing factors are summarized in Table 2.

The hydroxylation products just mentioned are also called catechol estrogens due to their prime affinity to O-methyl-transferase that inhibits catecholamine degradation. In phase II, the hydroxylation products then undergo conjugation with acids, (i.e., glucuronidation and sulfation). These conjugates then are excreted via bile or

TABLE 2. *Substances influencing cytochrome P 450_{NF} activity**

Induction	Rifampicin
	Phenytoin
	Barbiturates
Competitive Inhibition (weak)	Natural Steroids
	Norgestrel
Noncompetitive Inhibition (weak)	Primaquin
	Tolbutamide
"Suicide" Inhibition	Ethynyl Estradiol
	17alpha-Ethynyl Progestins
	Troleandomycin

*After Guengerich, 1990

urine; sulfates mostly occur in the bile. Simultaneously, the enzymes catalyzing this process are induced (Teichmann, 1990).

Due to their 17α-ethynyl group, estranes and gonanes are potent mechanism-based inactivators of cytochrome P 450NF. Back et al. (See Chapter 20) found that gestodene, 3-ketodesogestrel, norethindrone, and levonorgestrel are such inhibitors, respectively in decreasing order.

OCS AND LIVER DISEASE

Conditions Without Causal Relationship to OC Use

Although numerous diseases could be discussed in this category, very few gain practical importance in relation to hormonal contraception. This is due to their low incidence, either in general or during the reproductive years.

With acute viral hepatitis, the need for steroid contraception may be reduced. A negative impact on the course or outcome of the disease has not been proven (Schweitzer et al., 1975).

The relations between contraceptive hormones and porphyrin metabolism are not fully understood. However, the mean excretion of Δ-amino-laevulinic acid (Kosvelo et al., 1966) and urinary total coproporphyrin concentration in 26% of healthy volunteers on OCs (Burton et al., 1967) were measured as increased. Uroporphyrin decarboxylase activity is reduced in porphyria cutanea tarda and may be further decreased by administration of estrogens (Doss, 1983). Some women with acute intermittent porphyria experience a higher frequency of attacks in the second half of their menstrual cycle. Although they could be treated by the administration of sex hormones (Wetterberg, Perlroth, et al., 1965), contraceptive steroids are well-known to trigger porphyria cutanea tarda, particularly after long-term administration (Sixel-Dietrich and Doss, 1985; Meyer, 1983). Sex hormones are therefore generally considered to be contraindicated in the various forms of porphyria.

Conditions Associated with Contraceptive Steroids

Occlusion of postsinusoidal venules and veins, a condition commonly referred to as Budd-Chiari syndrome, has been related to OC use.

Peliosis hepatis has been known for some time to occur in patients on 17-alkylated androgens. The lesion consists of blood-filled cysts. It has also been observed in patients on OCs (Griffin and Wilson, 1983; van Erpecum et al., 1988). Vascular proliferation to the degree of liver hamartomas was observed by O'Sullivan and Wilding (1974). Zafrani et al. (1980) described a case of focal hemorrhagic necrosis of the liver, associated with marked changes of liver arterioles and small hepatic veins, in a woman with a 10-year history of OC use.

Evidence about the link between exogenous sex steroids and tumorigenesis is largely derived from animal experiments. Wanless and Medline (1983) described a rat model that uses diethylnitrosamine to induce malignant change; subsequently stilbestrol and EE promoted the development of hepatic neoplasms. Yager and Shi (1991) used a similar model to show that both EE and tamoxifen are able to promote tumor growth, whereas after simultaneous application of both substances, this effect did not occur. While this might suggest a receptor-specific mechanism, Pirovino and coworkers (1986) found human estrogen and progesterone receptors increased in only one case of focal nodular hyperplasia; in contrast, malignant liver tumors showed a low or nonmeasurable receptor content. Two more cases are reported by Hunt et al. (1985). Of two other possibilities of tumor promotion—the induction of liver growth through parenchymal hyperplasia or the induction of hepatic monooxygenases—Ochs and coworkers (1987) prefer the former possibility. This opinion might be further supported by Mathieu et al. (1989), who found a frequent association between hemangioma and focal nodular hyperplasia in women on OCs, whereas hepatic adenomas were not associated with this phenomenon. Finally, Purdy et al. (1983) reported experiments with moxestrol, the 11β-methoxy derivative of EE. This compound, as opposed to EE and stilbestrol, does not undergo the metabolic pathway to catechols or epoxides. In contrast to other estrogens, it does not cause neoplastic changes in transformed cell clones in vitro.

Two benign tumors of hepatocellular origin have been related to contraceptive steroids: hepatocellular adenoma (HCA) and focal nodular hyperplasia (FNH). The latter tumor seems to be a congenital dysplasia of liver tissue, consisting of normal hepatocytes arranged in groups around a single abnormally large artery without concomitant vein or bile duct. The surrounding parenchymal nodes result in macroscopically visible tumors. Hepatocellular adenoma normally occurs singularly, histologically consisting of homogeneous hepatocellular trabeculae with interposed sinusoids. There are no bile ducts (Andree and Roschlau, 1987). Whereas the statistical association between HCA and steroid contraception is widely accepted, disagreement exists with respect to FNH. (Smith and Fitz, 1984). Schild and coworkers (1987) reviewed 930 cases of focal nodular hyperplasia from their own experience and the literature. Within this group, 37.8% of women had taken female steroid hormones. Keeping in mind that, as a rough measure, about one third of women of reproductive age in industrial countries use OCs, this seems to be a strong argument against the proposed relationship.

Taking both conditions together, the estimated incidence ranges between one in 30,000 and one in 80,000 OC users per year (Hammerstein, 1987). The risk of developing an HCA seems to increase with dosage, duration of intake, and age. Among long-term users of OCs, the annual incidence is estimated at three to four per 100,000 (Rooks et al., 1979). However, simultaneous occurrence of both conditions has been reported (Friedman et al., 1984).

Spontaneous regression after discontinuance of steroid contraceptives has been observed in FNH (Pain et al., 1991).

Some statistical association seems to exist between hepatocellular carcinoma and long-term use of OCs. If no cirrhosis and no hepatitis B virus infection is present, the relative risk in women using OCs for 8 years or more was found to be 7.1

(Neuberger et al., 1986). The incidence is estimated to be thirteen hepatocellular carcinomas in one million OC users per year (Hammerstein, 1987). However, this association could not be shown in populations where hepatitis B virus is endemic (Molina et al., 1989; Kew et al., 1990). Not a single case of liver tumor has been registered by any of the major U.S. or British prospective studies over more than 2 decades.

Other tumors like rhabdomyosarcoma and hemangioendothelioma are even rarer, yet they have also been related to OC use (Palmer et al., 1989; Cote and Urmacher, 1990; Kelleher et al., 1989).

IMPACT OF CONTRACEPTIVE STEROIDS ON BILE FORMATION, STORAGE, AND EXCRETION

Quite unlike the effects described in the last section, OCs lead to alterations at all levels of the biliary system, gaining clinical relevance in a considerable proportion of women. Balász (1988) investigated the liver biopsies of 27 patients on OCs who were operated on because of uncomplicated cholelithiasis. None of these women showed any sign of liver dysfunction; concomitant liver disease was excluded. Yet the electron microscopic examination showed damaged bile canaliculi with severe alterations of the canalicular membranes. On the intracellular side of the membrane, actin-like filaments were seen, whereas in the lumina of the canaliculi an accumulation of granular, filamentous, lipoid material, or collagen fibers could be observed. In contrast to these morphological findings, King and Blitzer (1990) conclude from a review of the available experimental findings that estrogens act principally at the hepatocyte basolateral membrane to produce cholestasis by means of decreasing membrane fluidity and function of membrane-bound enzymes. This process reduces taurocholate and bromsulphthalein, as well as bilirubin excretion. Na, K-ATPase activity was found decreased, whereas AP and $Mg2^+$-ATPase was increased (Rosario et al., 1988). According to Kern et al. (1978), the reduction in bile acid synthesis and secretion leads to a secondary reduction in lecithin secretion, whereas cholesterol secretion is less dependent upon bile acid secretion. This imbalance results in a supersaturated (i.e., potentially lithogenic) bile composition.

Down et al. (1983) investigated bile composition during administration of various OCs. Whereas administration of EE and norgestrel in two different dosages led to a significant increase in the cholesterol saturation index, neither 30 μg of ethynyl estradiol alone nor together with 2.5 mg of norethindrone showed this effect. The authors state that the mechanism does not appear to involve bile acid metabolism, and conclude that the progestin norgestrel rather than the EE is responsible for the observed changes. Etchegoyen and coworkers (1983) found that 200 mg I.M. norethindrone enanthate every 2 months resulted in a slight although significant increase of the lithogenic index, while an oral combination of 150μg levonorgestrel and 30 μg EE did not; thus, these steroid contraceptives do not appear to constitute a risk factor in terms of gallstone formation.

According to the Boston Collaborative Drug Surveillance Program, the incidence of gallstones is twice as high during OC use as compared to controls not using OCs. More recent results from the Royal College Study (Kay, 1984) indicate that this is true only for the first 3 years of OC use. Strom et al. (1986) found that young women are at some risk of developing gallbladder disease during OC use. Shaffer et al. (1984) found that the administration of a synthetic progestin (medroxyprogesterone acetate) significantly impaired both gallbladder filling and emptying, and concluded that this could predispose to the formation of cholesterol gallstones.

Hyperbilirubinemia to the degree of clinical jaundice has been observed after administration of OCs. The exact mechanism is still not clear, although the effects just mentioned should contribute to this phenomenon. Persons at particular risk are women who have had intrahepatic cholestasis of pregnancy, and those suffering from a Dubin-Johnson syndrome or Rotor syndrome (Isselbacher, 1983). Reyes and coworkers (1981) concluded from bromsulphthalein retention studies that there might be a genetically determined abnormality in excretory function predisposing to cholestasis under high levels of estrogens, independent of pregnancy itself. Although not generally diseases of reproductive age, cholestasis and pruritus in primary biliary cirrhosis may also be aggravated.

S-adenosyl-L-methionine seems able to counteract most of the effects listed above, and reverse the oversaturation of biliary cholesterol and restore normal hepatocyte membrane fluidity (Almasio et al., 1990). This occurs possibly due to inactivation of catechol estrogens and methylation of membrane phospholipids that increase the liver plasma membrane fluidity (Di Padova et al., 1984).

CONCLUSIONS

Although exogenous sex steroids alter the appearance and function of liver tissue as described in the last section, only under certain rare circumstances do these alterations gain clinical importance. The changes discussed under morphology were seen as variations rather than pathology by most authors. However, Roschlau (1977) attributes transaminase elevations together with specific, exclusively structural changes as just discussed to OC intake, and claims that these may reach the degree of reactive hepatitis.

In vitro studies have revealed a number of reproducible hepatic effects of exogenous steroids, especially those with 17α-ethynyl groups. Yet due to the enormous intra- and interindividual variations in sex steroid metabolism, it is very difficult to draw conclusions from these findings in order to predict *in vivo* effects in individuals or even populations.

Concerning neoplastic changes and OC use, it should be stressed that these, particularly hepatomas, are very rare events; in fact, not a single case has been recorded in all the major epidemiological prospective studies (Vessey, 1989; Ramcharan et al., 1981).

In summary, the proliferative, enzyme-inducing and cholestatic effects of OCs are mostly harmless to the vast majority of women. However, 17-alkylated steroids in particular may produce serious disease in predisposed individuals.

REFERENCES

Abernethy DR, Greenblatt DJ, Shader RI. Imipramine disposition in users of oral contraceptive steroids. *Clin Pharmacol Ther* 1984;35:792–7.

Abernethy DR, Greenblatt DJ. Impairment of antipyrin metabolism by low-dose oral contraceptive steroids. *Clin Pharmacol Ther* 1981;29:106–10.

Abernethy DR, Greenblatt DJ, Divoll M, et al. Impairment of diazepam metabolism by low-dose estrogen-containing oral contraceptive steroids. *New Engl J Med* 1982;306:791–2.

Abernethy DR, Greenblatt DJ, Ochs HR, et al. Lorazepam and oxazepam kinetics in woman on lowdose oral contraceptives. *Clin Pharmacol Ther* 1983;33:628–32.

Abernethy DR, Todd EL. Impairment of caffeine clearance by chronic use of low-dose estrogen-containing oral contraceptives. *Eur J Clin Pharmacol* 1985;28:425–8..

Almasio P, Bartolini M, Pagliaro L, Coltorti M. Role of S-adenosyl-L-methionine in the treatment of intrahepatic cholestasis. *Drugs* 1990;40[Suppl 3]:111–23.

Balász M. Sinusoidal dilatation of the liver in patients on oral contraceptives. Electron microscopic study of 15 cases. *Exp Pathol* 1988;35:231–7.

Balász M. Intrahepatic biliary tract - oral contraceptives. Electron microscopic examinations of 27 surgical liver biopsies. *Exp Pathol* 1988;33:103–8.

Blakey DC, White NH. Destruction of cytochrome P-450 and formation of green pigments by contraceptive steroids in rat hepatocyte suspensions. *Biochem Pharmacol* 1986;35:1,561–7.

Boekenoogen SJ, Szefler SJ, Jusko WJ. Prednisolone disposition and protein binding in oral contraceptive users. *J Clin Endocrinol Metab* 1983;56:702–9.

Burton JL, Loudon NB, Wilson AT. Urinary coproporphyrin excretion and hepatic function in women taking oral contraceptives. *Lancet* 1967;2:1,326–27.

Carter DE, Goldman JM, Bressler R, et al. Effects of oral contraceptives on drug metabolism. *Clin Pharmacol Ther* 1973;15:22–31.

Cote RJ, Urmacher C. Rhabdomyosarcoma of the liver associated with long-term oral contraceptive use. Possible role of estrogens in the genesis of embryologically distinct liver tumors. *Am J Surg Pathol* 1990;14:784–90.

Crawford JS, Rudolfsky S. Some alterations in the pattern of drug metabolism associated with pregnancy, oral contraceptives and the newly born. *Br J Anaesth* 1966;38:446–54.

Dickerson J, Bressler R, Christian CD. Liver function tests and low-dose estrogen oral contraceptives. *Contraception* 1980;22:597.

Di Padova C, Tritapepe R, Di Padova F, et al. S-adenosyl-L-methionine antagonizes oral contraceptive induced bile cholesterol supersaturation in healthy women: preliminary report of a controlled randomized trial. *Am J Gastroenterol* 1984;79:941–4.

Doss M. Hereditärer uroporphyrindecarboxylase-defekt bei porphyria cutanea tarda durch hormonale kontrazeptiva. *Deutsch Med Wschr* 1983;108:1,857–8.

Down RHL, Whiting MJ, Watts JMcK, Jones W. Effects of synthetic oestrogens and progestagens in oral contraceptives on bile lipid composition. *Gut* 1983;24:253–9.

Eisenfeld AJ, Aten RF. Estrogen receptors and androgen receptors in the mammalian liver. *J Steroid Biochem* 1987;27:1,109–18.

Etchegoyen G, Wolpert E, Galvan E, et al. Effects of synthetic steroid contraceptives on biliary lipid composition of normal Mexican women. *Contraception* 1983;27:591–603.

Frey BM, Schaad JH, Frey FJ. Pharmacokinetic interaction of contraceptive steroids with prednisone and prednisolone. *Eur J Clin Pharmacol* 1984;26:505–11.

Frey BM, Frey FJ. The effect of altered prednisolone kinetics in patients with the nephrotic syndrome and women taking oral contraceptive steroids on human mixed lymphocyte cultures. *J Clin Endocrinol Metab* 1985;60:361–9.

Friedman LS, Gang DL, Hedberg SE, Isselbacher KJ. Simultaneous occurence of hepatic adenoma and focal nodular hyperplasia: report of a case and review of the literature. *Hepatology* 1984;4:536–40.

Gardner MJ, Jusko WJ. Effects of oral contraceptives and tobacco use on the metabolic pathways of theophylline. *Int J Pharmacol* 1986;33:55–64.

Gardner MJ, Tornatore KM, Jusko WJ, Kanarkowski R. Effects of tobacco smoking and oral contraceptive use on theophylline disposition. *Br J Clin Pharmacol* 1983;16:271–80.

Giles HG, Sellers EM, Naranjo CA, et al. Disposition of intravenous diazepam in young men and women. *Eur J Clin Pharmacol* 1981;20:207–13.

Goebelsmann V, Mashchak C, Mishell DR Jr. Comparison of hepatic impact of oral and vaginal administration of ethinyl estradiol *Am J Obstet Gynecol* 1985;151:868–77.

Greenblatt DJ, Shader RI, Franke K, et al. Kinetics of intravenous chlordiazepoxide: sex differences in drug distribution. *Clin Pharmacol Ther* 1977;22:893–903.

Greenblatt DJ, Allen MD, Harmatz JS, Shader RI. Diazepam disposition determinants. *Clin Pharmacol Ther* 1980;27:301–12.

Griffin JE, Wilson JD. Disorders of the testis. In: Petersdorf RG, Adams RD, Braunwald E, et al., eds. *Harrison's principles of internal medicine*. 10th ed. Tokyo: McGraw-Hill; 1983.

Guengerich FP. Inhibition of oral contraceptive steroid-metabolizing enzymes by steroids and drugs. *Am J Obstet Gynecol* 1990;163:2,159–63.

Gustavson, LE, Legler UF, Benet LZ. Impairment of prednisolone disposition in women taking oral contraceptives or conjugated estrogens. *J Clin Endocrinol Metab* 1986;62:234–7.

Hammerstein J. Gegenwärtiger stand des tumorrisikos bei der hormonalen kontrazeption. *Deutsch Med Wschr* 1987;112:897–9.

Herz R, Koelz HR, Haemmerli MP, Benes J, Blum AL. Inhibition of hepatic demethylation of aminopyrine by oral contraceptive steroids in humans. *Eur J Clin Invest* 1978;8:27–30.

Hooper WD, Bochner F, Eadie MJ, Tyrer JH. Plasma protein binding of diphenylhydantoin. Effects of sex hormones, renal and hepatic disease. *Clin Pharmacol Ther* 1974;15:276–82.

Hunt RF, Sali A, Kune GA. Oestrogen receptors in focal nodular hyperplasia of the liver. *Med J Aut* 1985;143:519–20.

Isselbacher KJ. Disturbances of bilirubin metabolism. In: Petersdorf RG, Adams RD, Braunwald E, et al., eds. *Harrison's principles of internal medicine*, 10th ed. Tokyo: McGraw-Hill; 1983.

Jacobs MB. Hepatic infarction related to oral contraceptive use. *Arch Intern Med* 1984;144:642–3.

Jochemsen R, van der Graaff M, Boeijinga JK, Breimer DD. Influence of sex, menstrual cycle and oral contraception on the disposition of nitrazepam. *Br J Clin Pharmacol* 1982;13:319–24.

Kaiser E, Gruner HS. Liver structure and function during long-term treatment with cyproterone acetate. *Arch Gynecol* 1987;240:217–24.

Kay CR. The Royal College of General Practitioners oral contraception study: some recent observations. *Clin Obstet Gynaecol* 1984;11:759–86.

Kendall MJ, Quarterman CP, Jack DB, Beeley L. Metoprolol pharmacokinetics and the oral contraceptive pill. *Br J Clin Pharmacol* 1982;14:120–2.

Kendall MJ, Jack DB, Quarterman CP, et al. Beta-adrenoceptor blocker pharmacokinetics and the oral contraceptive pill. *Br J Clin Pharmacol* 1984;17:87S–9S.

Kelleher MB, Iwatsuki S, Sheahan DG. Epitheloid hemangioendothelioma of liver. Clinicopathological correlation of 10 cases treated by orthotopic liver transplantation. *Am J Surg Pathol* 1989;13:999–1,008.

Kew MC, Song E, Mohammed A, Hodkinson J. Contraceptive steroids as a risk factor for hepatocellular carcinoma: a case control study in South African black women. *Hepatol* 1990;11:298–302.

King PD, Blitzer BL. Drug induced cholestasis: pathogenesis and clinical features. *Sem Liver Dis* 1990; 10:316–21.

Knopp RH, Bergelin RO, Wahl PP, et al. Clinical chemistry alterations in pregnancy and oral contraceptive use. *Obstet Gynecol* 1985;66:682.

Koch-Wester J, Sellers EM. Drug interactions with coumarin anticoagulants. *N Engl J Med* 1971;285: 487–98, 547–58.

Kosvelo P, Eisalo A, Toivonen I. Urinary excretion of porphyria precusors and coproporphyria in healthy females on oral contraceptives. *Br Med J* 1966;1:652–4.

Kozower M, Veatch L, Kaplan MM. Decrease clearance of prednisolone, a factor in the development of corticosteroid side effects. *J Clin Endocrinol Metab* 1974;38:407–12.

Larsson-Cohn U. Oral contraception and liver function tests. *Br Med J* 1965;1:1,414–5.

de Leacy EA, McLeay CD, Eadie MJ, Tyrer JH. Effects of subjects' sex and intake of tobacco, alcohol and oral contraceptives on plasma phenytoin levels. *Br J Clin Pharmacol* 1979;8:33–6.

Legler UF, Benet L. Marked alterations in dose-dependent prednisolone kinetics in women taking oral contraceptives. *Clin Pharmacol Ther* 1976;39:425–9.

Liu HF, Magdalou J, Nicolas A, et al. Oral contraceptives stimulate the excretion of clofibric acid glucuronide in women and female rats. *Gen Pharmacol* 1991;22:393–7.

MacLeod SM, Sellers EM. Pharmacodynamic and pharmacokinetic drug interactions with coumarin anticoagulants. *Drugs* 1976;11:461–70.

Madden S, Back DJ, Orme ML'E. Metabolism of the contraceptive steroid desogestrel by human liver in vitro. *J Steroid Biochem* 1990;35:281–8.

Marks LJ, Benjamin G, Duncan FJ, O'Sullivan VI. Comparative effects of ethinyl estradiol, 17-alpha-ethinyl-19-nortestosterone and methyl-testosterone on the plasma clearance of infused cortisol. *J Clin Endocrinol* 1961;21:826–32.

Martinez-Manautou J, Aznar-Ramos R, Bautista-O'Fanill J, Gonzales-Angulo A. The ultrastructure of liver cells in women under steroid therapy, II. contraceptive therapy. *Acta Endocrinol* 1970;65:207–21.

Mathieu D, Zafrani ES, Anglade MC, Dhumeaux D. Association of focal nodular hyperplasia and hepatic haemangioma. *Gastroenterol* 1989;97:154–7.

Metzner C, Jung K, Laue R, et al. Einsatz des stabilen stickstoffisotops 15N zur beurteilung des leberstoffwechsels bei hormonaler kontrazeption. *Leber-Magen-Darm* 1990;1:34.

Meyer VA. Porphyrias. In: Petersdorf RG, Adams RD, Braunwald E, et al., eds. *Harrison's Principles of Internal Medicine, 10th ed.* Tokyo: McGraw-Hill; 1983.

Meyer FP, Canzler E, Giers H, Walther H. Langzeituntersuchung zum einfluß von non-ovlon auf die pharmakokinetik von coffein im intraindividuellen vergleich. *Zentrbl Gynäkol* 1988;110:1449–54.

Miners JO, Grgurinovich N, Whitehead AG, et al. Influence of gender and oral contraceptive steroids on the metabolism of salicylic acid and acetylsalicylic acid. *Br J Clin Pharmacol* 1986;22:135–42.

Miners JO. Gender and oral contraceptive steroids as determinants of drug glucuronidation: effects on clofibric acid elimination. *Br J Clin Pharmacol* 1984;18:240–3.

Mitchell MC, Hanew T, Meredith CG, Schenker S. Effects of oral contraceptive steroids on acetaminophen metabolism and elimination. *Clin Pharmacol Ther* 1983:34:48–53.

Molina R, Martinez L, Salas O, et al. Combined oral contraceptives and liver cancer. *Int J Cancer* 1989;43:254–9.

Neuberger J, Forman D, Doll R, Williams R. Oral contraceptives and hepatocellular carcinoma. *Br Med J* 1986;292:1,355.

Ochs H, Dusterberg B, Günzel P, Schulte-Hermann RR. Effects of tumor promoting contraceptive steroids on growth and drug metabolizing enzymes in rat liver. *Cancer Res* 1986;46:1,224–32.

Ochs HR, Greenblatt DJ, Friedman H, et al. Bromazepam pharmacokinetics: influence of age, gender, oral contraceptives, cimitidine and propranolol. *Clin Pharmacol Ther* 1987;41:562–70.

Odlind V, Borglin NE, Christensen OJE, et al. Routine liver function testing during long-term administration of the oral contraceptive preparation 0,150 mg desogestrel plus 0,030 mg ethinyl estradiol to healthy female volunteers in Scandinavia. *Acta Obstet Gynecol Scand* 1982;111[Suppl]:43–6.

Ortiz de Montellano PR, Kunze KL. Self-catalyzed inactivation of hepatic cytochrome P-450 by ethinyl substrates. *J Biol Chem* 1980;225:5,578–85.

O'Sullivan JP, Wilding RP. Liver hamartomas in patients on oral contraceptives. *Br Med J* 1974;3:–10.

Pain JA, Gimson AES, Williams R, Howard ER. Focal nodular hyperplasia of the liver: results of treatment and options in management. *Gut* 1991;32:524–7.

Palmer JR, Rosenberg L, Kaufmann DW, et al. Oral contraceptive use and liver cancer. *Am J Epidemiol* 1989;130:878–82.

Patwardhan RV, Mitshell MC, Johnson RF, Schenker S. Differential effects of oral contraceptive steroids on the metabolism of benzodiazepines. *Hepatol* 1983;3:248–53.

Patwardhan RV, Desmond PV, Johnson RF, Schenker S. Impaired elimination of caffeine by oral contraceptive steroids. *J Lab Clin Med* 1980;95:603–8.

Percival Smith R, Sizto R. Metabolic effects of two triphasic formulations containing ethinyl estradiol and dl-norgestrel. *Contraception* 1983;28:189.

Perlroth MG, Mavver HS, Tschudy DP. Oral contraceptive agent and the management of acute intermittent porphyria. *JAMA* 1965;194:1,037–42.

Pirovino M, Walti E, Akorbiantz A, et al. Estrogen and progesterone receptors in human liver: does their analysis improve the understanding of benign liver tumors associated with oral contraceptive use? *Schweiz Med Wochenschr* 1986;116:971–3.

Purdy RH, Goldzieher JW, LeQuesne PW, et al. Active intermediates and carcinogenesis. In: Merriam GR, Lipsett MB, eds. *Catechol estrogens.* New York: Raven Press; 1983;123–140.

Purdy RH, Goldzieher JW. Toward a safer estrogen in aging. In: Intervention in the aging process part A: quantitation, epidemiology and clinical research. New York: Alan R. Liss Inc; 1983:247–266.

Ramcharan S, Pellegrin FA, Ray R, HSU JP. The Walnut Creek contraceptive drug study: a prospective study of the side effects of oral contraceptives. Vol III Washington, D.C.: U.S. Government Printing Office; 1981.

Raufman, JP, Miller DL, Gumucio JJ. Estrogen-induced zonal changes in rat liver tissue. *Gastroenterology* 1980;79:1,174–7.

Reyes H, Ribalta J, Gonzalez HC, et al. Sulfobromophthalein clearance tests before and after ethinyl estradiol administration, in women and men with a familial history of intrahepatic cholestasis of pregnancy. *Gastroenterology* 1981;81:226–31.

Roberts RK, Grice J, McGuffie C, Heilbronn L. Oral contraceptive steroids impair the elimination of theophylline. *J Lab Clin Med* 1983;101:821–5.

Roberts RK, Desmond PV, Wilkinson GR, Schenker S. Disposition of chlordiazepoxide: sex differences and effects of oral contraceptives. *Clin Pharmacol Ther* 1979;25:826–31.

Rooks JB, Ory HW, Ishak KG, et al. Epidemiology of hepatocellular adenoma: the role of oral contraceptive use. *JAMA* 1979;242:644–8.

Rosario J, Sutherland E, Zaccaro L, Simon FR. Ethinylestradiol administration selectively alters liver sinusoidal membrane lipid fluidity and protein composition. *Biochem* 1988;27:3,939–46.

Roschlau G. Leberveränderungen durch kontrazeptiva. *Deutsch Gesundheits Ws* 1977;32:2,271–4.

Routledge PA, Stargel WW, Kitchell BB, et al. Sex-related differences in the plasma protein binding of lidocain and diazepam. *Br J Clin Pharmacol* 1981;11:245–50.

Sadik W, Kovaes L, Pretnar-Darovec A, et al. A randomized double-blind study of the effects of two low-dose combined oral contraceptives on biochemical aspects. Report from a seven-centered study. *Contraception* 1985;32:223.

Schild, H, Kreitner KF, Thelen M, et al. Focal nodular hyperplasia of the liver in 930 patients. *ROFO Fortschr Geb Röntgenstr Nuklearmed* 1987;147:612–8.

Schweitzer K, Weiner JM, McDeak CM, Thursby MW. Oral contraceptives in acute viral hepatitis. *JAMA* 1975;233:979–80.

Shaaban MM, Elwan SI, el-Sharkawy MM, Farghaly AS. Effect of subdermal levonorgestrol contraceptive implants, norplant, on liver functions. *Contraception* 1984;30:407–12.

Shaffer EA, Taylor PJ, Logan K, et al. The effect of a progestin on gallbladder function in young women. *Am J Obstet Gynecol* 1984;148:504.

Shaw MA, Back DJ, Aird SA, Grimmer SF, Orme MC. Urinary concentrations of steroid glucuronides in women taking oral contraceptives. *Contraception* 1983;28:69–75.

Sixel-Dietrich F, Doss M. Hereditary uroporphyrinogen-decarboxylase deficiency predisposing porphyria cutanea tarda (chronic hepatic porphyria) in females after oral contraceptive medication. *Arch Dermatol Res* 1985;278:13–6.

Smith LH Jr, Fitz JG. Oral contraceptives and benign tumors of the liver. *West J Med* 1984;140:260–7.

Stoehr GP, Kroboth PD, Juhl RP, et al. Effect of oral contraceptives on triazolam, temazepam, alprazolam and lorazepam kinetics. *Clin Pharmacol Ther* 1984;36:683–90.

Strom BL, Tamragouri RN, Morse ML, et al. Oral contraceptives and other risk factors for gallbladder disease. *Clin Pharmacol Ther* 1986;39:335–41.

Teichmann AT. Kontrazeption. Ein kompendium für klinik und praxis. Stuttgart; *Wissenschaftl Verlagsgesellsch*; 1991.

Tephyly TR, Mannering GJ. Inhibition of drug metabolism by steroids. *Med Pharmacol* 1969;4:10–4.

de Teresa E, Vera A, Ortigosa J, et al. Interaction between anticoagulants and contraceptives: an unsuspected finding. *Br Med J* 1979;2:1,260–1.

Teunissen MWS, Srivastava AK, Breimer DD. Influence of sex and oral contraceptive steroids on antipyrine metabolite formation. *Clin Pharmacol Ther* 1982;32:240–6.

van Erpecum KJ, Janssens AR, Kreuning J, et al. Generalized peliosis hepatis and cirrhosis after long-term use of oral contraceptives. *Am J Gastroenterol* 1988;83:572–5.

Vessey MP. Oral contraception and cancer. In: Filshie M, Guilleband J, eds. *Contraception*. London: Butterworths; 1989:52–68.

Walden CE, Knopp RH, Johnson JL, et al. Effect of estrogen/progestin potency on clinical chemistry measures. The Lipid Research Clinics Program Prevalence Study. *Am J Epidemiol* 1986;123:517.

Wanless IR, Medline A. Role of estrogens as promoters of hepatic neoplasia. *Lab Invest* 1983;46:313.

Weindling H, Henry JB. Laboratory test results altered by the pill. *JAMA* 1974;229:1762–68.

Wetterberg L. Oral contraceptives and acute intermittent porphyria. *Lancet* 1964;2:1,178–9.

Yager JD, Shi YE. Synthetic estrogens and tamoxifen as promoters of hepatocarcinogenesis. *Prev Med* 1991;20:27–37.

Zafrani ES, Pinaudeau Y, Le Cudonnec B, et al. Focal hemorrhagic necrosis of the liver. A clinicopathological entity possibly related to oral contraceptives. *Gastroenterol* 1980;79:1,295–99.

Pharmacology of the Contraceptive Steroids,
edited by Joseph W. Goldzieher.
Raven Press, Ltd., New York © 1994.

16

Bone

Morris Notelovitz

*Women's Medical and Diagnostic Center and The Climacteric Clinic, Inc.
Gainesville, Florida 32607*

Approximately 70 to 80% of the mechanical strength of bone is attributed to its bone mineral content (Hui et al., 1989). In this context, oral contraceptives (OCs) may play an important role in preventing fractures in later life. The greater the bone mass accrued before menopause, the lesser the chance of developing osteoporosis subsequently. Sex steroids improve and maintain bone mass and, hence, bone strength.

BONE REMODELING

Bone is living tissue. "Old" bone is constantly being lost and replaced with healthier and stronger "new" bone. The process involved is known as the bone remodeling cycle and is described in detail elsewhere (Parfitt, 1987). In brief, remodeling is controlled by two classes of cells: (1) osteoclasts derived from mononuclear cells known as pre-osteoclasts (they line the bone-forming surface in the quiescent phase of the bone remodeling sequence); and (2) osteoblasts—specialized cells whose main function is to form new bone by the synthesis of bone matrix, a collagen-rich ground substance essential for the adherence of hydroxyapatite and other crystals. As illustrated in Fig. 1, there are five phases to the bone remodeling cycle: activation is said to take place somewhere in the adult skeleton every 10 seconds. The newly formed osteoclasts secrete an acid-like substance from their ruffle borders, thus dissolving and digesting the organic matrix and mineral of the underlying "old" bone. When the cavity has reached a pre-set depth, resorption at that site ceases and new monocyte-derived cells appear, form a cement surface that prevents further resorption, and attract osteoblasts into the cavity. The osteoblasts form "new" bone in two stages: matrix synthesis and mineralization. Under normal circumstances, resorption cavities are completely filled with new bone. However, a negative bone balance results if overactive osteoclasts create a resorptive cavity of excessive depth that is incompletely filled with new bone, or if subnormally functioning osteoblasts incompletely fill a resorption cavity of normal depth. The net result is the same—bone loss. Since the mechanism of bone loss is different, the

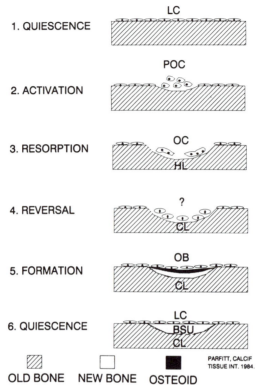

FIG. 1. The normal remodeling sequence in adult human cancellous bone. Schematic representation of successive events on the endosteal surface.

LC—lining cell. POC—preosteoclast (mononuclear). OC—osteoclast (multinucleated). HL—Howship's lacuna. CL—cement line (reversal line). OB—osteoblast. BSU—bone structural unit. Parfitt, 1987

treatment (prevention) should be directed either to inhibiting osteoclast activity or stimulating osteoblast and new bone formation. At present, there are no clinical tests that allow for this discrimination.

Estrogen therapy prevents bone loss and can, to a certain extent, replace lost bone mineral (Christiansen and Lindsay, 1990). The cellular mechanism is incompletely understood. Biochemical tests have suggested that estrogen inhibits osteoclast activity and, therefore, bone resorption. Yet, estrogen receptors are found in osteoblasts—the bone forming cells (Eriksen et al., 1988). Osteoblasts may indirectly control the resorptive activity of the osteoclast, possibly by Interleukin-1 activity. In addition, estradiol stimulates progesterone nuclear binding to osteoblasts. There are *in vitro* data showing that the positive action of progesterone on bone is enhanced by the presence of estradiol (Prior, 1990). In addition, progesterone displaces synthetic glucocorticoids from osteoblast cells (Chen et al., 1977) and glucocorticoids decrease bone formation by receptor-mediated inhibition of osteoblasts.

OSTEOPENIA AND OSTEOPOROSIS

One of the important events in the pathogenesis of osteoporosis is slow but progressive thinning of the trabecular plates in cancellous bone, prior to their eventual perforation, and loss of continuity and strength. Excessive thinning of the supporting horizontal and vertical structures of trabecular bone is known as osteopenia and may be considered a precondition to osteoporosis (Kanis, 1990).

Osteopenia is potentially reversible; therefore, its early recognition plays a key role in the ability of sex steroids to prevent osteoporosis. Osteopenia can be diagnosed clinically by any one of a number of bone density measures: 1) radiographic absorptiometry of the hand; 2) single photon absorptiometry of the far-distal and proximal radius, and the calcaneum; and 3) dual energy x-ray absorptiometry of the spine and hip. The merits and clinical applicability of these tests are discussed in greater detail elsewhere. (Cummings et al., 1990; Ross et al., 1988). Depending on the sensitivity and specificity of methods for identifying osteopenia, various levels of reduced bone mineral density have been specified. Based on the author's experience and a summary of the literature on the subject, a bone density value two standard deviations or more below peak bone mass, irrespective of the patient's age, is the most appropriate level to use as a predictor or risk factor for osteoporosis.

Women with athletic-induced amenorrhea tend to have low bone mass and a higher incidence of stress fractures (Marcus et al., 1985; Barrow and Saha, 1988). This association and the use of sex steroids to increase bone mass poses the question of whether OCs can be used to prevent stress fractures.

ESTROGEN, PROGESTINS AND BONE MASS IN POSTMENOPAUSAL WOMEN

Estrogen replacement therapy increases the bone mineral density of postmenopausal women and is associated with a significant reduction in osteoporosis-related fractures (Christiansen and Lindsay, 1990). Until recently, the effect of concomitant use of progestins was less clear, since most studies were based on indirect bone markers such as the urinary calcium/creatinine and hydroxyproline/creatinine ratios, and alkaline phosphatase. The overall conclusion was that an increase in bone formation occurred in women on progestins (Prior, 1990). A few studies have shown that progestins, used alone, do maintain and/or increase bone mass when measured by radiogrametry and single photon absorptiometry. The compound used in some of the studies was norethindrone (Abdalla et al., 1985), albeit in a dose (10 mg/day) far in excess of that found in low-dose OCs.

Although there was some theoretical concern that progestins might counteract the positive effect of estrogens on bone, studies have shown that, if anything, there is actually an additive effect. This was first reported by Christiansen's 1985 study of ten postmenopausal women receiving estradiol, with 1 mg norethindrone acetate per day from day 13 through 22 of the hormone cycle. The addition of norethisterone was associated with increased levels of osteocalcin (BGP) and alkaline phosphatase—markers of new bone formation. More recently, it was reported that a combination of 2 mg estradiol and 1 mg norethisterone acetate (used continuously) increases bone mass; the bone mineral content in the trabecular compartment (distal radius and spine) of the treated group was 8% greater than the placebo-treated subjects after only 1 year. The mean age of these two groups was 64 and 65 years, respectively, ages at which bone is thought by some to be nonresponsive to hormonal manipulation.

Appropriate bone mass measurements to test the bioequivalence of estradiol versus other estrogens have not been published. However, in young surgically menopausal women, Lindsay et al. (1976) demonstrated that 25 μg mestranol per day was effective in reducing bone mineral loss (as compared to nontreated controls) and that this conserving effect continued for 10 to 15 years. More recently, Williams et al. (1990) reported a progressive dose/response of bone mass to ethynyl estradiol/norethindrone acetate, with the lowest positive effect noted at 5 μg ethynyl estradiol/0.5 mg norethindrone, and the maximum increase with 20 μg ethynyl estradiol/1 mg norethindrone.

ORAL CONTRACEPTIVES AND BONE MASS

There is only one published prospective placebo-controlled study evaluating the effect of OCs on bone mass in premenopausal women. Shargil (1985) followed 200 perimenopausal women (mean age = 44 years) for 3 years and compared the bone mineral conservation in 100 triphasic OC-treated women (the OCs contained ethynyl estradiol and levonorgestrel as the progestin) with 100 matched women. The latter group used nonsteroidal forms of contraception. Bone mass was measured by radiographic densitometry. The control group lost 6% of bone mass at the end of the 3-year study, while the OC-treated group maintained their bone mass (Fig. 2). There are some concerns about the study, including the relatively large percentage decrease in bone mineral from cortical bone. All other studies clearly demonstrate that cortical bone is maintained until menopause.

Recker et al. (1992) reported a prospective longitudinal study of 156 college-aged women, seeking to determine whether bone mass increases in healthy nonpregnant white women during early adult life after cessation of linear growth. The study also looked at whether physical activity, nutrient intake, and OC use influence increase in bone mass. A bivariate analysis showed that the use of OCs was associated with a greater gain in total bone mass ($r = .31$, $p = 0.01$).

Using single photon absorptiometry as the biological marker, Goldsmith and Johnson (1975) reported enhanced bone mass in premenopausal women on OCs

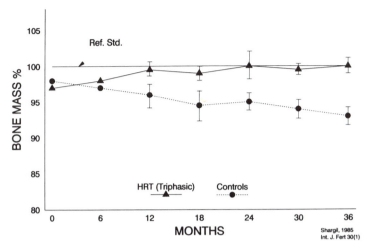

FIG. 2. Previous oral contraceptive use and the bone mineral density of the lumbar spine in premenopausal women.

with an ethynyl estradiol content greater than 50 μg; the same was not seen in younger women (age 20 to 30 years) taking lower-dose OCs (ethynyl estradiol of less than 50 μg.) More recently, Lindsay et al. (1986) reported their retrospective analysis of pre- and postmenopausal women who were either currently taking OCs or had taken them in the past. They were compared with age-matched women who had never used OCs, but were identical in terms of physical characteristics (height and weight), calcium intake, exercise pattern, and family history of osteoporosis. The bone mineral content was measured by dual photon absorptiometry and, in one subset, with single photon absorptiometry as well. Vertebral bone mineral was increased by about 1% per year of OC use. As a group, the bone mineral density of the treated younger women studied (mean age = 42) was 1.17 ± 0.27 g/cm^2 versus 1.08 ± 0.021 g/cm^2 in controls who had never used OCs (P<0.02). On further analysis, it was found that a mean exposure to 7.9 years of OCs resulted in a 12% higher bone mass than in controls (P<0.01) and that 82% of the study group subjects had bone densities in excess of the mean for their normal population.

The objective of premenopausal OC use—as far as its effect on bone mass is concerned—is to prevent peri/postmenopausal osteopenia/osteoporosis. Although Lindsay et al. (1986) demonstrated no significant difference in bone mass in postmenopausal women who had used OCs versus those who had not (1.13 ± 0.04 g/cm^2 versus 1.14 ± 0.03 g/cm^2 respectively), the duration of years since menopause was twice as long in the treated group (3.92 ± 0.8 years versus 1.183 ± 0.4 years, P<0.05). If there was no protective effect, the longer exposure to the physiologic postmenopausal bone loss should have resulted in the treated group having a lower bone mineral density. Indeed, when subgroups of patients with the same duration of menopause were compared, the bone density of the previous OC users was 4.3%

higher than that of the controls. This difference was not statistically significant, but the numbers were small; moreover, this was a cross-sectional retrospective study and the pre-OC use bone mineral data were not known. While clinical experience has demonstrated that estrogen replacement therapy does not increase bone mineral in women with normal bone mass, this does not infer that estrogen replacement therapy is unable to enhance the bone strength of women with normal bone mass. Other variables not measured at present, such as the collagen matrix of bone, may be positively influenced by estrogen replacement therapy—even in "normal" women. A cross-sectional study from the United Kingdom (Stevenson et al., 1989) confirmed that previous OC use did positively influence postmenopausal bone mass. These authors also highlighted the impact of lifestyle factors: whereas exercise in postmenopausal women was associated with increased bone mass in the proximal femur, premenopausal alcohol use significantly decreased bone mass in the hip (Ward's triangle). The same was found for smoking and its detrimental effect on the bone mineral density of the lumbar spine.

Of other published studies, one found no effect of OCs on premenopausal bone mass (Collins et al., 1988), while another found a protective effect on bone density in postmenopausal women who had previously been on previous OCs for 10 or more years (Enzelsberger et al., 1988). The design, numbers of patients involved, and statistical analysis of these two studies preclude meaningful conclusions. More recently, a cross-sectional retrospective study by Kleerekoper et al. (1991) investigated risk factors for low bone mineral density in a group of 2,297 women, 76% of whom were postmenopausal. Thirty percent of the women reported prior OC use, a history that was protective against low bone mineral density (odds ratio = 0.35, 95% confidence intervals 0.23–0.53). Further analysis demonstrated that increasing duration of use offered increasing protection; those who reported OC use for 10 years or more were afforded the greatest protection (odds ratio = 0.23, 95% confidence intervals 0.07–0.73) when compared to those who never used OCs. These results held whether forearm or lumbar spine measurements were made. The mean age of the participants (54 years) indicates that they were probably users of high-dose OCs.

A large community-based sample of older postmenopausal women (239 women aged 55 to 69) also found that OC use for 6 or more years had significantly greater spine and femoral neck bone densities than never-users (Kritz-Silverstein and Barrett-Connor 1993). However, higher bone density was not found in the distal radius. The investigators noted that the association was so strong, when other confounding factors were taken into account, that it was detectable with very small samples (n = 21).

ORAL CONTRACEPTIVE USE IN WOMEN WITH REDUCED BONE MASS

Premenopausal women with reduced bone mass should be prime candidates for treatment with oral contraceptives. Table 1 lists some clinical situations associated with the potential for osteopenia. The need for effective treatment is highlighted by

TABLE 1. *Conditions associated with osteopenia in young women*

Reduced bone density in mother and/or father
Late menarche
Irregular menstruation
Anovulatory menstruation
Exercise-induced oligo/amenorrhea

Eating disorders:	Anorexia nervosa
	Bulimia
Endocrinopathies:	Turners syndrome
	Hyperprolactinemia
	Premature menopause

reports of an irreversible degree of osteopenia following athletic-induced amenorrhea (Drinkwater et al, 1986) and anorexia nervosa (Rigotti et al., 1991). These changes usually affect cancellous bone, but cortical bone is also involved, especially with severe eating disorders.

A number of studies have shown that normal bone density is usually maintained in young women athletes, as long as their menstrual cycles remain regular. In those who develop (or start with) oligomenorrhea or amenorrhea, bone mass is low and may remain at a permanently compromised level, even after resumption of regular menstruation subsequent to the reduction in the intensity of the exercise (Drinkwater et al., 1986). This is especially true in athletes with reduced body weight.

Oral contraceptives may help to restore this lost bone mass. DeCreé et al. (1988) used an antiandrogenic OC containing 2 mg cyproterone acetate and 50 μg ethynyl estradiol to treat seven high-performance athletes with exercise-induced osteopenia. Treatment was for eight cycles and bone density was measured by dual photon absorptiometry of the lumbar vertebrae L2-L4. Four women with similar clinical characteristics served as untreated controls. The bone mineral response of the treated athletes is shown in Fig. 3. All of the women improved their bone densities, with the percentage from baseline varying from 5.6 to 11.9%. The mean improvement in bone mineral density was $9.5 \pm 2.5\%$. Women with the greatest degree of estrogen deficiency showed the best response. Only one control subject improved her bone mass; the percentage change from baseline for the group was a nonsignificant $1.6 \pm 1.9\%$.

Prospective studies using other OCs are obviously needed to confirm the results of this study and to answer additional questions: What is the optimal dose and type of OC?; What is the duration of OC use needed to restore bone density to normal?; Will the bone density return to pretreatment levels on cessation of OC use, as is the case with surgically menopausal women who stop their estrogen replacement?

Osteopenia associated with anorexia nervosa may be more resistant to oral contraceptive use. Rigotti et al. (1991) reported that anorexics treated with OCs or a combination of conjugated equine estrogen and medroxyprogesterone acetate did not show a significant change in cortical bone mass, irrespective of whether withdrawal bleeding occurred.

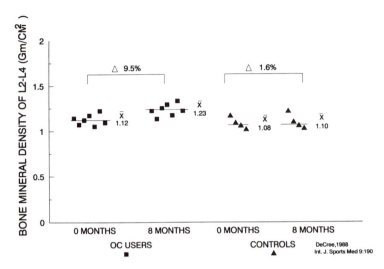

FIG. 3. Change in the bone mineral density of women with athletic amenorrhea using oral contraceptives versus controls. (DeCreé, 1988.)

ORAL CONTRACEPTIVE USE AND STRESS FRACTURES

It has been estimated that over seven million women in the United States participate in vigorous exercise and that about 80% of these women are premenopausal. The intensity of this exercise is directly related to the prevalence of oligomenorrhea and amenorrhea—from an estimate of 5% in sedentary women to 20% in women who exercise intensively and regularly (Speroff, 1982). The oligomenorrhea/amenorrhea is associated with reduced hormonal levels. In one study (Boyden et al., 1983), the plasma estradiol levels in 18 healthy women training for a marathon and who subsequently developed menstrual irregularities fell from a baseline of 70 pg/ml to 54 pg/ml when the women were running 30 miles per week and 34 pg/ml at 50 miles per week. It is not surprising, therefore, that exercise-induced amenorrhea is associated with a 20 to 30% decrease in spinal trabecular bone mass, and a high incidence of running-related fractures (Cann et al, 1984).

Three features discriminate those athletes who injure themselves from those who remain healthy: significantly more injured athletes have lower lumbar and femoral bone mass, menstrual irregularity, and are less likely to be taking OCs. Fig. 4 illustrates the bone mineral density in 25 women with stress fractures and 25 matched control athletes (Myburgh et al., 1990). The respective values for bone mineral density were 1.04 ± 0.142 versus 1.108 ± 0.131 (p<0.02) for the lumbar vertebrae (L2-L4); 0.838 ± 0.09 versus 0.98 ± 0.11 (p<0.005) for the femoral neck; and 0.670 ± 0.11 versus 0.736 ± 0.01 (p<0.01) for Ward's triangle. (Fig. 4) The fractures in the injured athletes occurred in the foot, femoral neck, pubic ramus, tibia, and fibula. None occurred in the lumbar spine, the area where most studies have demonstrated maximal bone mineral loss. Although stress fractures

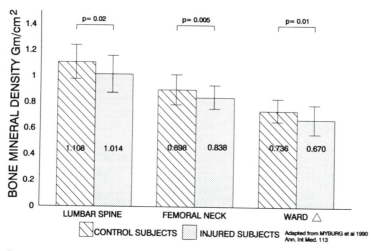

FIG. 4. Bone mineral density in young athletes with and without stress fractures. (Adapted from Myburgh et al., 1990.)

involve factors other than reduced bone mineral, this reduction can certainly be used as an important predictor.

Stress fractures are related to current, but not past, menstrual irregularity (Myburgh et al., 1990). This association, plus the observation that some bone loss in female athletes is reversed when menstruation resumes (Lindberg et al., 1987) suggests that the bone mineral deficiency associated with exercise-related hypoestrogenism is potentially reversible (DeCreé et al., 1988). Exogenous estrogens may also be protective. Two studies have shown that OC use protects against stress fractures. Two out of 80 injured women were on OCs versus 64 of 180 noninjured women running in one study (P<0.001; Lloyd et al., 1986); significantly more control than injured subjects were taking OCs (11 versus 5, respectively; P<0.05) in the other study (Lindberg et al., 1987). A final point linking estrogen/progestin status, osteopenia, and stress fractures is the observation that stress fractures occur more frequently in female than in male athletes (Orava et al., 1978).

SUMMARY

An appropriately designed randomized controlled study linking OC use to bone mineral strength and risk of postmenopausal osteoporosis still needs to be done. However, there are teleologic reasons why OCs may prove to have a bone-preserving effect. Postmenopausal estrogen/progestin therapy is prescribed in doses with lower biologic activity (relative to the OCs) to women with a relatively inert bone remodeling cycle. Yet, the extended use of hormone replacement therapy is clearly associated with improved bone mineral density and a corresponding decrease in osteoporosis related fractures. Younger women with athletic amenorrhea (equivalent hormonally to a premature menopause) do exhibit increased bone mass when placed on OCs, and the use of OC does protect against stress fractures. Although the latter are different in many respects from osteoporotic fractures, there are two similar pathologies: damage to the microarchitecture of the bone and reduced trabecular/cortical bone mineral.

One of the additional confounding issues is whether one can improve normal bone mass and strength by using OCs. Most of the published studies were unable to prove these effects, since they were retrospective analyses, and the pre-OC use bone mineral densities were not known. In the one study where pretreatment bone mineral values were known, subjects with the greater bone mineral density deficiencies improved more than those with higher initial bone mineral values. Thus, it may be that in terms of its potential bone mineral enhancing effect, OCs should be considered specifically for women who, in addition to having a need for contraception, are more likely to have reduced bone mass (e.g., women with a late menarche, irregular menses, anovulatory cycles, athletic amenorrhea, and eating disorders).

REFERENCES

Abdalla JI, Hart DM, Lindsay R, et al. Prevention of bone mineral loss in postmenopausal women by norethisterone. *Obstet Gynecol* 1985;66:789–92.

Barrow G, Saha R. Menstrual irregularity and stress fractures in collegiate female distance runners. *Am J Sports Med* 1988;16:209–16.

Boyden TW, Pamenter RW, Stanforth P, et al. Sex steroids and endurance running in women. *Fertil Steril* 1983;39:629–32.

Cann CE, Martin MC, Gennant HK, Jaffe RB. Decreased spinal mineral content in amenorrheic women. *JAMA* 1984;251:626–9.

Chen TL, Aronow L, Feldman DL. Glucocorticoid receptors and inhibition of bone cell growth in primary culture. *Endocrinology* 1977;100:619–28.

Christensen MS, Hagen C. Christiansen C, Transbol I. Dose-response evaluation of cyclic estrogen/gestagen in post-menopausal women. Placebo controlled trial of 175 gynecologic and metabolic actions. *Am J Obstet Gynecol* 1982;144:873–9.

Christiansen C, Lindsay R. Estrogens, bone loss and preservation. *Osteoporosis Int* 1990;1:7–13.

Christiansen C, Nilas L, Riis BJ, et al. Uncoupling of bone formation and resorption by combined oestrogen and progestogen therapy in postmenopausal osteoporosis. *Lancet* 1985;2:800–1.

Christiansen C, Riis BJ. 17-beta estradiol and continuous norethisterone: a unique treatment for established osteoporosis in elderly women. *J Clin Endocrinol Metab* 1990;71:836–41.

Collins CL, Thomas KA, Harding AF, et al. The effect of oral contraceptives on lumbar bone density in premenopausal women. *J LA State Med Soc* 1988;140:31–9.

Cummings JR, Black DM, Nevitt MC, et al. Appendicular bone density and age predict hip fracture in women. *JAMA* 1990;263:665–8.

DeCreé C. Lewin R, Ostyn M. Suitability of cyproterone acetate in the treatment of osteoporosis associated with athletic amenorrhea. *Int J Sports Med* 1988;9:187–92.

Drinkwater BL, Nilson K, Ott S, Chestnut CH III. Bone mineral density after resumption of menses in amenorrheic women. *JAMA* 1986;256:380–2.

Enzelsberger H, Netka M, Heytmanek G, et al. Influence of oral contraceptive use on bone density in climacteric women. *Maturitas* 1988;9:375–8.

Eriksen EF, Colyard DS, Beret NJ, et al. Evidence of estrogen receptors in normal human osteoblast-like cells. *Science* 1988;241:84–6.

Goldsmith NF, Johnston JO. Bone mineral: effects of oral contraceptives, pregnancy and lactation. *J Bone Joint Surg.* 1975;57A:657–68.

Hui SL, Slemenda CW, Johnston CC Jr. Baseline measurement of bone mass predicts fracture in white women. *Ann Intern Med* 1989;3:355–61.

Kanis JA. Osteoporosis and osteopenia. *J Bone Min Res* 1990;5:209–11.

Kleerekoper M, Brienza RS, Schultz LR, et al: Oral contraceptive use may protect against low bone mass. *Arch Int Med* 1991;151:1971–6.

Kritz-Silverstein D, Barrett-Connor E. Bone mineral density in postmenopausal women as determined by prior oral contraceptive use. *Am J Public Health* 1993;83:100–2.

Lindberg JS, Powell MR, Hunt MM. Increased vertebral bone mineral response to reduced exercise in amenorrheic runners. *West J Med* 1987;146:39–42.

Lindsay R, Aitken JM, Anderson JR, et al. Long-term prevention of postmenopausal osteoporosis by oestrogen. *Lancet* 1976;1:1,038–40.

Lindsay R, Tohme J, Kanders B. The effect of oral contraceptive use on vertebral bone mass in pre- and post-menopausal women. *Contraception* 1986;34:333–40.

Lloyd T, Triantafyllou SJ, Baker ER. Women athletes with menstrual irregularity have increased musculoskeletal injuries. *Med Sci Sports Exerc* 1986;18:374–9.

Marcus R, Cann C, Madvig P, et al. Menstrual functions and bone mass in elite women distance runners: endocrine and metabolic factors. *Ann Intern Med* 1985;102:158–67.

Myburgh KH, Hutchins J, Fataar AB, et al. Low bone density is an etiologic factor for stress fractures in athletes. *Ann Int Med* 1990;113:754–9.

Orava S, Puranen J, Ala-Ketola C. Stress fractures caused by physical exercise. *Acta Orthop Scand* 1978;49:19–47.

Parfitt AM. Bone remodeling and bone loss: understanding the pathophysiology of osteoporosis. *Clin Obstet Gynec* 1987;30:789–811.

Prior JC. Progesterone as a bone-trophic hormone. *Endocrine Rev* 1990;11:386–98.

Recker RR, Davies M, Hinders SM, et al. Bone gain in young adult women. *JAMA* 1992;268:2,403–8.

Rigotti NA, Neer RM, Skates SJ. The clinical course of osteoporosis in anorexia nervosa. *JAMA* 1991; 265:1,133–8.

Rigotti NA, Nussbaum SR, Herzog DB, Neer RM. Osteoporosis in women with anorexia nervosa. *N Eng J Med* 1984;311:1,601–6.

Ross PD, Wasnich RD, Vogel JM. Detection of pre-fracture spinal osteoporosis using bone mineral absorptiometry. *J Bone Min Res* 1988;3:1–11.

Shargil AA. Hormone replacement therapy in perimenopausal women with a triphasic contraceptive compound: a three year prospective study. *Int J Fertil* 1985;30:15–28.

Speroff L. Impact of exercise on menstruation and reproduction. *Contemp Obstet Gynecol* 1982;19:54–78.

Stevonson JE, Lees B, Devenport M, et al. Determinants of bone density in normal women: risk factors for future osteoporosis? *Br Med J* 1989;298:924–8.

Williams SR, Frenchek B, Speroff T, Speroff L. A study of combined continuous ethinyl estradiol and norethisterone acetate for postmenopausal hormone replacement. *Am J Obstet Gynecol* 1990;162:438–46.

Pharmacology of the Contraceptive Steroids,
edited by Joseph W. Goldzieher.
Raven Press, Ltd., New York © 1994.

17

Effects on the Skin

Joseph W. Goldzieher

*Department of Obstetrics and Gynecology, Baylor College of Medicine
Houston, Texas 77030*

The effects of sex steroids on the skin have long been known. Fine wrinkling and the sallow, waxy color due to accumulation of melanoid in the skin of adult hypogonad males are quite characteristic. Atrophic senile skin shows regenerative changes when exposed to estrogen applied topically; the epidermis thickens and there is an increase in collagen fibers but no restoration of elastic fibrils (Goldzieher et al., 1951,1952).

Shakespeare's "mask of pregnancy" is traditional knowledge. This condition, known as melasma or chloasma, is a brown hypermelanosis of the face that has genetic, racial, and endocrine etiologic factors; it is exacerbated by exposure to the ultraviolet rays in sunlight. Histologic studies reveal an increase in the number and activity of type-specific melanocytes, which appear to be engaged in increased formation, melanization, and transfer of pigment granules to the epidermis and dermis (Sanchez et al., 1981). Endogenous or exogenous estrogens stimulate this process in some individuals. The mechanism is not known, but does not involve an increase in pituitary β-MSH secretion (Smith et al., 1977; Perez et al., 1983) as is the case with the quite different melanosis of Addison's disease. A thyroid factor also seems to be at work; 70% of women who developed melasma during pregnancy or oral contraceptive (OC) use displayed evidence of autoimmune thyroid disorders, compared to 39.4% of women with idiopathic melasma (Lutfi et al., 1985).

With the earliest high-dose OCs, as many as 29% of users developed melasma. Histologically, normal numbers of melanocytes were seen, but they were larger and produced more melanin (Resnik, 1967). In two large series consisting of several hundred Puerto Rican and Mexican women, the incidence was about 8% (Cook et al., 1961; Rice-Wray et al., 1962). Differences in incidence were seen between Costa Rican and Trinidadian women (Sanhueza et al., 1979). In a recent study of "complexion changes" in 6,382 U.S. women using a low-dose OC, 89% reported no such changes and three quarters of the rest observed an improvement; the data on the remaining 2.5% who reported worsening did not even address the problem of melasma (Wheeler and Malinak, 1991).

NEOPLASIA OF CUTANEOUS MELANOCYTES

Melanocytic nevi are known risk factors for melanoma. Sex hormones may influence nevus prevalence; however, the evidence for this is purely circumstantial. Pregnancy induces clinical changes in nevi but evidence for associated atypia is controversial (Sanchez et al., 1984; Foucar et al., 1985). The evident proliferation of nevi at puberty also suggests sensitivity to sex hormones. Ellis et al. (1985) have demonstrated estrogen and progesterone receptors in melanocytic lesions and increased ligand binding related to pregnancy or OC use (Ellis and Wheeland, 1986). Other studies of benign nevi have given conflicting results (Chaudhuri et al., 1980; Grill et al., 1982). However, there have been no studies of the receptor status of normal melanocytes. Two studies (MacKie et al., 1985; English et al., 1987), both from Scotland, have shown no statistically significant relationship between nevus counts and OC use. The numbers of nevi were unassociated with duration of use or age at OC initiation.

The incidence of melanoma varies widely, from 40 per 100,000 in Queensland, Australia to 10 and 5 per 100,000 in the U.S. and U.K., respectively (Elwood, 1989). In developing countries, the incidence is up to ten times lower. The sex distribution varies between countries; occurrence is rare before puberty. The sharp increase that has occurred among young and middle-aged white adults in the last few decades may well be caused by excessive ultraviolet exposure early in life, or a relatively short latent period from exposure to diagnosis (Osterlind et al., 1986).

Pregnancy can affect the occurrence or prognosis of melanoma (Holly, 1986), and regression may occur after delivery (Pennington, 1983).

Both case-control and prospective studies have examined the association of OC use and melanoma. The usual problems encountered in epidemiological studies of OC use also affect these case-control investigations; selection, interviewer and recall bias, increased surveillance of OC users, neglect of confounding variables can create problems of interpretation. Greene (1991) has summarized the nine published case-control and two cohort studies. With respect to the former, Greene concluded that the "findings were null." Almost all positive associations with long-term OC use could have been due to chance, and when trends were observed, the data were not internally consistent. In recent British cohort studies, Hannaford et al. (1991) found relative risks whose confidence limits included one in every standardized category in the Royal College data and the same in the Oxford/Family Planning Association study. Given the increasing incidence of melanoma in white populations, it is reassuring to know that OC use plays no part in this phenomenon.

ACNE AND HIRSUTISM

Androgens are known to promote sebum formation and hair growth in susceptible individuals (Uno, 1986). Acne is an inflammatory disease of the pilosebaceous unit, mainly affecting the sites of maximum sebaceous gland density (Lever and Marks, 1990). The effect of steroid contraceptives on the pilosebaceous unit is complex, since these compounds have a direct, dose-related action (Strauss and Kligman, 1960; Pochi and Strauss, 1965). These substances also affect indirectly the estrogenic/androgenic environment by influences on adrenal and ovarian androgen secretion, and on the plasma equilibrium of bound/unbound androgenic and estrogenic steroids via effects on sex-hormone-binding globulin (SHBG).

The bioassay of the androgenic and estrogenic activities of the contraceptive steroids and their interaction when combined are discussed in Chapter 6 (Edgren). Important in this context are studies of the effect of progestational compounds on skin fibroblast 5α-reductase activity, the enzyme system that converts testosterone to the locally active form, dihydrotestosterone. In their *in vitro* system, Dean and Winter (1984) found that progesterone and norethindrone inhibited this enzyme activity in a dose-dependent manner to a maximum of 95% and 50% of basal levels at 10^{-5} M. Similar concentrations of norethynodrel, norgestrel, and levonorgestrel had little or no effect. Cassidenti et al. (1991) found that progesterone, levonorgestrel, and norethindrone demonstrated 97 ± 5.3, 47.9 ± 6.3 and $59 \pm 4.6\%$ inhibition, respectively, at 10^{-4} M, while medroxyprogesterone acetate displayed no activity. Estradiol caused $40.8 \pm 14.2\%$ inhibition, whereas ethynyl estradiol (EE) at concentrations ranging from 10^{-8} to 10^{-4} M, had no inhibitory effect. This suggests that the use of progestins of the 19-nor type might be preferable in the treatment of hirsutism (excepting, of course, those C_{21}-compounds which are specific anti-androgens).

The contributions of adrenal cortex and ovary to plasma androgens are discussed in their respective chapters (10 and 13). We turn now to the technical problem of assaying the biological activity of circulating plasma androgens, and the relationship of such measurements to clinical events. Total plasma testosterone is elevated in perhaps half of women with hirsutism; free (unbound) testosterone estimates correlate somewhat better. Levell et al. (1989) maintain that there is no association of abnormal plasma androgen levels and acne; on the contrary, Palatsi et al. (1984) found abnormal free testosterone and SHBG values in 57% of their acne patients.

The properties of SHBG have been studied in detail (Rosenfield and Moll, 1983), and the effect of various OCs on SHBG levels and the resulting bound/unbound equilibria have been detailed by Cullberg (Ch. 7) and Fotherby (Ch. 24). A study of seven monophasic or triphasic OCs with the same EE content has been carried out by Van der Vange et al. (1990). The various combinations with norethindrone, levonorgestrel, desogestrel, gestodene, and cyproterone acetate showed distinct differences in SHBG and absolute free testosterone values. However, total and free testosterone values decreased with all seven formulations, except for total testosterone during use of the cyproterone acetate OC. This value actually increased— a change not attributable to an increase in SHBG. However, in 6–month studies (Vermeulen and Rubens, 1988) both 35 μg and 50 μg EE/cyproterone acetate 2 mg OCs produced an impressive decrease in free testosterone plasma levels and urinary excretion of androstanediol glucuronide, the metabolite of 5α-dihydrotestosterone. OC-induced changes in plasma levels return to baseline within a month of discontinuation.

Improvement of acne during OC use was observed early on (Mears, 1961; Wansker, 1964) and has been amply documented, together with improvement in hirsutism, since then (Givens et al., 1976; Belisle and Love, 1986; Upton and Corbin, 1989; Lemay et al., 1990). Upton and Corbin (1989) pointed out that OCs with levonorgestrel, which has relatively greater androgenicity than other 19-norsteroids in pure-compound animal assays, nevertheless has high clinical efficacy in acne. Lemay et al. (1990), also using norgestrel, found clinical improvement after the first cycle of use, even though plasma androgen levels were not consistently normalized. Hammerstein et al. reported in 1975 on the use of the antiandrogen, cyproterone acetate, in acne and hirsutism, using a "reverse sequential regimen" consisting of 100 mg cyproterone acetate from cycle day 5 to 14, concomitantly with 50 μg EE from cycle day 5 to 25. It usually required 6 to 9 months for hirsutism to improve or disappear in 60% to 80% of subjects. Alopecia responded in only about 50%. Others have used the standard OC formulations containing this steroid as a treatment (Holdaway et al., 1985; Belisle and Love., 1986) for acne and hirsutism.

Various anecdotal reports of cutaneous effects of OCs have appeared in the literature. Sensitivity to sunlight has been noted in a woman experiencing the same phenomenon with estrogen alone (Erickson and Peterka, 1968). Cutaneous eruptions in women with *in vitro* lymphocyte sensitivity (also produced by estrogen) were reported in 1970 (Savel et al.). Cutaneous porphyria may be estrogen-sensitive, and cases of variegate porphyria and porphyria cutanea tarda appearing with OC use have been published (McKenzie and Acharya, 1972). Alopecia apparently analogous to postpartum telogen effluvium has also been noted (Cormia, 1967). It is noteworthy that all of these events occurred during the use of the earliest, very-high-dose OCs.

REFERENCES

Belisle S, Love EJ. Clinical efficacy and safety of cyproterone acetate in severe hirsutism: results of a multicentered Canadian study. *Fertil Steril* 1986;46:1015–20.

Cassidenti DL, Paulson RJ, Serafini P, et al. Effects of sex steroids on skin 5α-reductase activity in vitro. *Obstet Gynecol* 1991;78:103–7.

Chaudhuri PK, Walker MJ, Briele HA, et al. Incidence of estrogen receptors in benign nevi and human malignant melanoma. *JAMA* 1980;244:791–3.

Cormia FE. Alopecia from oral contraceptives. *JAMA* 1967;201:635–7.

Cook HH, Gamble CJ, Satterthwaite AP. Oral contraception by norethynodrel. *Am J Obstet Gynecol* 1961;82:437.

Dean HJ, Winter JSD. The effect of five synthetic progestational compounds on 5α-reductase activity in genital skin fibroblast monolayers. *Steroids* 1984;43:13–23.

Ellis DL, Wheeland RG. Increased nevus estrogen and progesterone ligand binding related to oral contraceptives or pregnancy. *J Am Acad Dermatol* 1986;14:25–31.

Ellis DL, Wheeland RG, Solomon H. Estrogen and progesterone receptors in melanocytic lesions. *Arch Dermatol* 1985;121:1282–5.

Elwood JM. Trends in incidence and mortality from cutaneous melanoma in England and Wales. *Trans Menz Fndn* 1989;15:135–6.

English JSC, Swerdlow AJ, MacKie RM, et al. Relation between phenotype and banal melanocytic nevi. *Br Med J* 1987;294:152–64.

Erickson LR, Peterka ES. Sunlight sensitivity from oral contraceptives. *JAMA* 1968;203:980–1.

Foucar E, Bentley T, Laube DW, Rosai T. Histopathologic evaluation of nevocellular nevi in pregnancy. *Arch Dermatol* 1985;121:350–4.

Givens JR, Andersen RN, Wiser WL, et al. The effectiveness of two oral contraceptives in suppressing plasma androstenedione, testosterone, LH and FSH, and in stimulating plasma testosterone-binding capacity in hirsute women. *Am J Obstet Gynecol* 1976;124:333–9.

Goldzieher JW, Roberts IS, Rawls WB, Goldzieher MA. Chemical analysis of the intact skin by reflectance spectrophotometry. *Arch Dermatol Syphil* 1951;64:533–8.

Goldzieher JW, Roberts IS, Rawls WB, Goldzieher MA. Local action of steroids on senile human skin. *Arch Dermatol Syphil* 1952;66:304–15.

Green A. Oral contraceptives and skin neoplasia. *Contraception* 1991;43:653–66.

Grill HJ, Benes B, Manz B, et al. Steroid hormone receptor analysis in human melanoma and nonmalignant human skin. *Br J Dermatol* 1982;107[Suppl 23]:64–5.

Hammerstein J, Meckies J, Leo-Rossberg I, et al. Use of cyproterone acetate (CPA) in the treatment of acne, hirsutism and virilism. *J Steroid Biochem* 1975;6:827–36.

Hannaford PC, Villard-Mackintosh L, Vessey MP, et al. Oral contraceptives and malignant melanoma. *Br J Cancer* 1991;63:430–3.

Holdaway IM, Croxson MS, Ibbertson HK, et al. Cyproterone acetate as initial treatment and maintenance therapy for hirsutism. *Acta Endocrinol* 1985;109:522–9.

Holly EA. Melanoma and pregnancy. In: Gallagher RP, ed. *Recent results in cancer research: epidemiology of malignant melanoma*. Berlin: Springer-Verlag; 1986:118–26.

Lemay A, Dewailly SD, Grenier R, et al. Attenuation of mild hyperandrogenic activity in postpubertal acne by a triphasic oral contraceptive containing low doses of ethynyl estradiol and d,1-norgestrel. *J Clin Endocrinol Metab* 1990;71:8–14.

Levell MJ, Cawood ML, Burke B, Cunliffe WJ. Acne is not associated with abnormal plasma androgens. *Br J Dermatol* 1989;120:649–54.

Lever L, Marks R. Current views on the aetiology, pathogenesis and treatment of acne vulgaris. *Drugs* 1990;39:681–92.

Lutfi RJ, Fridmanis M, Misiunas AL, Pafumo O, et al. Association of melasma with thyroid autoimmunity and other thyroidal abnormalities and their relationship to the origin of the melasma. *J Clin Endocrinol Metab* 1985;61:28–31.

MacKie RM, English J, Aitchison TC, et al. The number and distribution of benign pigmented moles (melanocytic naevi) in a healthy British population. *Br J Dermatol* 1985;113:167–74.

McKenzie AW, Acharya U. The oral contraceptive and variegate porphyria. *Br J Dermatol* 1972;86:453–7.

Mears E. Clinical trials of oral contraceptives. *Br Med J* 1961;2:1,179.

Osterlind A, Moller-Jensen O. Trends in incidence of malignant melanoma of the skin in Denmark 1943–1982. In: Gallagher RP, ed. *Recent results in cancer research: epidemiology of malignant melanoma*. Berlin: Springer-Verlag; 1986:8–17.

Palatsi R, Hirvensalo E, Liukko P, et al. Serum total and unbound testosterone and sex hormone binding globulin (SHBG) in female acne patients treated with two different oral contraceptives. *Acta Dermatol Venereol* (Stockholm) 1984;64:517–23.

Perez M, Sanchez JL, Aquilo F. Endocrinologic profile of patients with idiopathic melasma. *J Invest Dermatol* 1983;81:543–5.

Pochi PE, Strauss JS. Lack of androgen effect on human sebaceous glands with low-dosage norethindrone. *Am J Obstet Gynecol* 1965;93:1,002–4.

Resnick S. Melasma induced by oral contraceptive drugs. *JAMA* 1967;199:601–5.

Rice-Wray E, Schult-Contreras M, Guerrero I, Aranda Rosell A. Long-term administration of norethindrone in fertility control. *JAMA* 1962;180:355.

Rosenfield RL, Moll GW Jr. The role of proteins in the distribution of plasma androgens and estradiol. In: Molinatti G, Martini L, James VHT, eds. *Androgenization in women*. New York: Raven Press; 1983:25–45.

Sanchez JL, Figueroa LD, Rodriguez E. Behavior of melanocytic nevi during pregnancy. *Am J Dermatopathol* 1984;6[Suppl 1]:89–91.

Sanchez NP, Pathak MA, Sato S, Fitzpatrick TB, et al. Melasma: a clinical, light microscopic, ultrastructural and immunofluorescence study. *J Am Acad Dermatol* 1981;4:698–710.

Sanhueza H, Sivin I, Kumar S, Kessler M, et al. A randomized double blind study of two oral contraceptives. *Contraception* 1979;20:29–48.

Savel H, Madison JF, Meeker CI. Cutaneous eruptions and in vitro lymphocyte hypersensitivity. *Arch Dermatol* 1970;101:187–190.

Smith AG, Shuster S, Thody AJ, Peberdy M. Chloasma, oral contraceptives and plasma immunoreactive beta-MSH. *J Invest Dermatol* 1977;68:169–1070.

Strauss JS, Kligman AM. Androgenic effects of a progestational compound, 17α-ethynyl-19-nor-testosterone (norlutin), on the human sebaceous gland. *J Clin Endocrinol Metab* 1961;21:215–9.

Uno H. Biology of hair growth. *Sem Reprod Endocrinol* 1986;4:131–41.

Upton GV, Corbin A. The relevance of the pharmacologic properties of a progestational agent to its clinical effects as a combination oral contraceptive. *Yale J Biol Med* 1989;62:445–7.

Van der Vange N, Blankenstein MA, Kloosterboer HJ, et al. Effects of seven low-dose combined oral contraceptives on sex hormone binding globulin, corticosteroid binding globulin, total and free testosterone. *Contraception* 1990;41:345–52.

Vermeulen A, Rubens R. Effects of cyproterone acetate plus ethinyl estradiol low dose on plasma androgens and lipids in mildly hirsute or acneic young women. *Contraception* 1988;38:419–28.

Wansker BA. Norethynodrel with mestranol in the treatment of acne. *South Med J* 1964;57:917–9.

Wheeler JM, Malinak LR. Complexion changes in oral contraceptive users. *J Reprod Med* 1991;36:340–4.

Pharmacology of the Contraceptive Steroids,
edited by Joseph W. Goldzieher.
Raven Press, Ltd., New York © 1994.

18

Skeletal Muscle Function

John C. Wirth

*Department of Physical Education, Wayne State University College of Education,
Detroit, Michigan 48202*

Despite the widespread use of steroid contraceptives and the extensive research conducted into their effects, very little is known regarding their impact on skeletal muscle function. One reason for the lack of research in this area may be that such effects are not perceived as posing a health hazard. Nevertheless, any effects of steroid contraceptives on skeletal muscle function may have significant implications, not only in persons for whom skeletal muscle function is particularly important, but also in the general population whose health status may be significantly affected by these substances in ways still unknown.

SKELETAL MUSCLE FUNCTION AND ENERGY PRODUCTION

A primary function of skeletal muscle tissue is to generate energy in order to enable the muscle to produce force and movement. The reader is referred to any basic exercise physiology text for a more complete discussion of this topic (e.g., Åstrand and Rodahl, 1986; Fox et al., 1988; McArdle et al., 1991). Three metabolic pathways present in skeletal muscle are the major sources of energy production. The first of these is the ATP-PC system, which is composed of two high-energy compounds: adenosine 5'-triphosphate (ATP) and phosphocreatine (PC). The second is anaerobic glycolysis, the breakdown of carbohydrate into lactic acid; energy for ATP regeneration is produced during the process. Since the theoretical framework for investigations into the effect of oral contraceptives (OCs) on energy production in human skeletal muscle has been based on the mechanisms of anaerobic glycolysis, a few of the details of that system bear mentioning. As is the case with most reaction series within the human body, there are a few steps that may be rate limiting for the entire process. The first is the initial reaction—the uncoupling and phosphorylation of one glucose molecule from the branched chain. This reaction is catalyzed by the enzyme glycogen phosphorylase. The second step that may be rate limiting is the phosphorylation of fructose-6-phosphate to fructose-1,6-diphosphate, which is catalyzed by the enzyme phosphofructokinase.

The third pathway for energy production is the aerobic system. The primary rate limiter for aerobic energy production is probably the ability of the cardiorespiratory system to deliver oxygen to the working muscle; however, citric acid cycle enzyme activities may also be rate limiting.

Each of the three systems just discussed provides a unique contribution to the total energy production and, therefore, muscle function. These unique contributions are the result of the differing capabilities of each system. In terms of power (i.e., the ability to produce energy rapidly), the ATP-PC system ranks first, followed by anaerobic glycolysis, followed by the aerobic system. In terms of overall capacity, the rankings are reversed. The implication of these qualities is that short-term, intense efforts are dependent on the anaerobic systems, whereas long-term moderate efforts are dependent upon the aerobic system.

STEROID CONTRACEPTIVES AND ENERGY METABOLISM

In order to discuss such effects in terms of energy production, one must identify the effects of steroid contraceptives on each of the three energy-producing systems. Unfortunately, to date no research has investigated the effects of OCs on the ATP-PC system.

At least one study (McNeil and Mozingo, 1981) has investigated the effects of OCs on aerobic energy production. These researchers reported an increase in metabolic energy production (oxygen consumption) at a submaximal workload. One must recognize, however, that aerobic energy production is a product not only of the ability of the muscle tissue to utilize energy but also of the ability of the cardiorespiratory system to deliver oxygen. Although it appears that the findings of McNeil and Mozingo (1981) may be the result of a shift towards a greater dependence on lipids rather than carbohydrates for energy production, no available data has confirmed this as the causal mechanism. Therefore, it is as yet unclear whether the effect of OCs on aerobic energy metabolism occurs due to some effect on skeletal muscle tissue itself.

The effects of steroid contraceptives on anaerobic glycolysis and the enzymes connected with anaerobic glycolysis have been the subject of a small number of research studies (Wirth and Lohman, 1982; Vijayalakshmi and Bamji, 1987; Vijayalakshmi et al., 1988). The results indicate that OCs may cause a significant decrease in the ability of the muscle to produce force anaerobically, and that this loss of ability is most likely the result of a decrease in the activity of certain glycolytic enzymes. Also, results from these studies indicate that vitamin B-6 may negate these effects.

Several studies have concluded that use of OCs causes abnormalities in the metabolism of tryptophan. In particular, OC users exhibited an increase in the urinary excretion of a tryptophan metabolite, xanthurenic acid following an oral loading dose of tryptophan, as compared to nonusers (Luhby et al., 1971). Such an abnormality was first thought to be the result of a vitamin B-6 deficiency (Linkswiler,

1967), and correctable by the administration of vitamin B-6 (Luhby et al., 1971). (For a detailed discussion, see Chapter 25).

Both Cori and Illingworth (1957) and Illingworth et al. (1958) demonstrated that vitamin B-6 is a constituent of one of the rate-limiting enzymes of anaerobic glycolysis, glycogen phosphorylase. Other research (Illingworth et al., 1960; Graves et al., 1975) indicated that glycogen phosphorylase activity in vitamin B-6 deficient rats was significantly decreased.

It is believed that, under conditions of isometric (static) work, energy production is dependent upon enzyme activity levels rather than substrate availability (Bergstrom et al., 1971; Hultman and Bergstrom, 1973). As stated earlier, the principal regulatory enzyme of anaerobic glycolysis is phosphofructokinase. Phosphofructokinase is not a vitamin B-6 dependent enzyme; however, phosphofructokinase activity is positively related to the level of fructose-6-phosphate (Ui, 1966). Fructose-6-phosphate levels are in equilibrium with glucose-6-phosphate levels which, in turn, are controlled by glycogen phosphorylase activity (Wilson et al., 1967). Therefore, the effect of steroid contraceptives on muscle energy production may occur via changes in vitamin B-6 status which, in turn, affect glycogen phosphorylase activity, glucose-6-phosphate levels, fructose-6-phosphate levels, and, finally, phosphofructokinase activity.

Wirth and Lohman (1982) investigated the effect of OCs and vitamin B-6 status on the ability of human muscle, *in vitro*, to produce force anaerobically. Three groups of female volunteers were examined: 1) those already using OCs; 2) those already using both OCs and a vitamin supplement, including vitamin B-6; and 3) those who were using neither (normals). Variables measured included muscle strength, endurance time, and total force output during the endurance test. Endurance time was measured as the total time for which the subjects could maintain a contraction of 50% ($\pm 5\%$) of their maximal. Force output was the total force output achieved during this period. For the endurance test, circulation to the working muscles (palmar flexors) was occluded by an inflated blood pressure cuff. In general, the flexor muscle groups are composed of a relatively high percentage of white, fast-twitch, muscle fibers. This type of fiber depends mainly on anaerobic sources for energy production. Therefore, because of the muscle fiber type and the fact that circulation was occluded—preventing the delivery of oxygen and the subsequent production of energy aerobically—it was assumed that, for this particular endurance test, anaerobic glycolysis was the major source of energy production, and that the capacity of this system was the major determinant of endurance time and total force output.

No statistically significant ($P > 0.05$) differences among the groups were found for muscle strength. After adjusting for interindividual differences in strength, both endurance time and force output were statistically significantly ($P < 0.05$) greater for the normals than for the combined groups of users of OCs and users of OCs plus vitamin B-6. The values of endurance time and force output for the users of OCs and vitamin B-6 as opposed to those for the users of OCs alone were not statistically significant ($P > 0.05$). The clinical significance of these results is not so easily determined. Both endurance time and force output were approximately 20% less in the group of OC users as compared to the nonusers. Although this is a relatively large difference, caution is recommended in interpreting these results; the design of the study allowed for the groups to be self selected. Unfortunately, the same subjects were not tested under conditions of use and nonuse of OCs. Also, in order to minimize the sources of energy production, a highly artificial task, handgrip endurance with circulation occluded, was chosen. Further research is required before the clinical significance of the effects of OCs on skeletal muscle can be determined.

The second portion of the study examined the subjects during both the administration of vitamin B-6 and the administration of a placebo. This was conducted in a double-blind fashion with the order of the treatments randomized so that half of the subjects in each group received the placebo first and half the vitamin first. No statistically significant effect of vitamin B-6 supplementation was detected. However, the statistical power of this analysis was limited by the small number of subjects used: ten normals, seven users of OCs, and nine users of OCs and vitamin B-6. The researchers did measure urinary 4-pyridoxic acid levels (an indicator of recent vitamin B-6 intake) and post-tryptophan-load urinary xanthurenic acid excretion to monitor vitamin B-6 status. Results of these analyses indicated that the self-reported users of vitamin B-6 did appear to be taking the supplement and that all subjects who were given the vitamin B-6 supplement during the experiment did, indeed, ingest the supplement. However, only two subjects (both of them users of OCs who were not taking vitamin B-6) were labeled as vitamin B-6 deficient according to the standard criteria based on xanthurenic acid excretion (Sauberlich et al., 1972). An analysis of the muscle function data from these two subjects indicated no consistent effect of vitamin B-6 supplementation on muscle function (Wirth and Lohman, 1984).

In summary, the results of this study indicated that users of OCs exhibit significantly lower endurance time and force output than nonusers. Also, vitamin B-6 status may play a role in mitigating this effect, although definitive results substantiating this hypothesis were not obtained. Due to the nature of the muscle task utilized in this study, it was also theorized that the effects of steroid contraceptives were produced by way of alterations in the activity levels of glycogen phosphorylase and/or phosphofructokinase.

Vijayalakshmi et al. (1987) examined several glycolytic enzyme levels in the tissue of sacrificed rats that had been given contraceptive steroids and/or vitamin B-6. Contraceptive steroids caused a decrease in the activity of phosphofructokinase in muscle; however, fructose-6-phosphate levels were not increased. It was theorized that this latter effect was due to other compensatory influences such as an increase in the pentose phosphate pathway or a decrease in glucose uptake. All of these effects of contraceptive steroid administration were reversed by the administration of vitamin B-6.

Vijayalakshmi et al. (1988) studied women who had been using OCs for varying periods of time. The variables measured included erythrocyte phosphofructokinase activity. Women who had been using OCs for more than 1 year showed a significant decrease in erythrocyte phosphofructokinase activity. Also, as was seen in the previous study using rats, F-6-P levels were not increased in this group of subjects. The authors stated that this effect may be preceded by a similar effect in muscle tissue. This study did not examine the effects of vitamin B-6 on any of the measured variables.

SUMMARY

Human muscle force production capacity is lower in users of steroid contraceptives than in nonusers (Wirth and Lohman, 1982). Data from other studies (Vijayalakshmi et al., 1987; Vijayalakshmi et al., 1988) seem to support the hypothesis that this is due to a reduction in phosphofructokinase activity in OC users. Although supported by data from rats, the hypothesis that the effects of OCs on energy metabolism may be mitigated by vitamin B-6 has not been substantiated in humans.

These conclusions are based on a very small body of data. Also, these data have been collected in part using the rat as a model and in part using the human female as a model. Problems in attaching clinical significance to the data collected on humans have been discussed earlier. Further research in this area should collect both enzyme activity data and muscle function data from human females. The research design should include provisions for testing the same subjects under conditions of both OC use and nonuse. Until such data are available, no definitive assessment of the effect of OCs on human muscle function will be possible.

REFERENCES

Åstrand P-O, Rodahl K. In: *Textbook of Work Physiology*. New York: McGraw-Hill; 1986:

Bergstrom J, Harris RC, Hultman E, Nordesjo L-O. Energy rich phosphagens in dynamic and static work. In: Pernow B, Saltin B, eds. *Muscle metabolism during exercise*. New York: Plenum Press; 1971.

Cori CR, and Illingworth B. The prosthetic group of phosphorylase. *Proc Natl Acad Sci* 1957;43:547.

Fox EL, Bowers RW, Foss ML. *The physiological basis of physical education and athletics*. Philadelphia: W. B. Saunders; 1988:

Graves DJ, Carlson GM, Skuster JR, Parrish RF, Carty TJ, Tessmer GW. Pyridoxal phosphate-dependent conformational states of glycogen phosphorylase as proved by interconverting enzymes. *J Biol Chem* 1975;250:2,254.

Hultman E, Bergstrom J. Local energy-supplying substrates as limiting factors in different types of leg muscle work in normal man. In: Keul J, ed. *Limiting factors of physical performance*. Stuttgart: George Thieme; 1973:

Illingworth B, Jansz HS, Brown DH, Cori CF. Observations on the function of pyridoxal-5-phosphate in phosphorylase. *Proc Natl Acad Sci* 1958;44:1,180.

Illingworth B, Kornfeld R, Brown DH. Phosphorylase and uridinediphosphoglucose-glycogen transferase in pyridoxine deficiency. *Biochim Biophys Acta* 1960;48:486.

Linkswiler H. Biochemical and physiological changes in vitamin B-6 deficiency. *Am J Clin Nutr* 1967; 20:547.

Luhby AL, Brin M, Gordon M, Davis P, Murphy M, Spiegel H. Vitamin B-6 metabolism in users of oral contraceptive agents. I. abnormal urinary xanthurenic acid excretion and its correction by pyridoxine. *Am J Clin Nutr* 1971;24:684.

McArdle WD, Katch FI, Katch VL. *Exercise physiology*. Philadelphia: Lea & Febiger; (1991):

McNeil AW, Mozingo E. Changes in the metabolic cost of standardized work associated with the use of an oral contraceptive. *J Sports Med* 1981;21:238.

Sauberlich HE, Canham JE, Baker EM, Raica N, Herman YF. Biochemical assessment of the Nutritional Status of Vitamin B-6 in the Human. *Am J Clin Nutr* 1972;25:629.

Wilson JE, Sacktor B, Tiekert CE. In situ regulation of glycolysis in tetanized cat skeletal muscle. *Arch Biochem Biophys* 1967;120:542.

Vijayalakshmi R, Bamji MS. Altered glucose metabolism in female rats treated with sex steroids: reversal by excess pyridoxine. *Indian J of Biochem Biophys* 1987;24:329.

Vijayalakshmi R, Bamji MS, Ramalakshmi BA. Reduced anaerobic glycolysis in oral contraceptive users. *Contraception* 1988;38(1):91.

Wirth JC, Lohman TG. The relationship of muscle function to the use of oral contraceptives. *Med Sci Sports Exer* 1982. 14(1):16.

Wirth JC, Lohman TG. Vitamin B-6 status and static muscle function: two case reports. *Ann Nutr Metab* 1984;28:240.

Pharmacology of the Contraceptive Steroids,
edited by Joseph W. Goldzieher.
Raven Press, Ltd., New York © 1994.

19

Nervous System

David Keefe

*Department of Obstetrics and Gynecology, Yale School of Medicine,
New Haven, Connecticut 06510*

Great strides made over the past 2 decades towards clarifying cellular and molecular sites of sex steroid action provide a framework for understanding the neuropsychiatric effects of oral contraceptives (OCs). Sex steroid receptors appear in a widespread but characteristic distribution throughout the body, including some phylogenetically ancient parts of the brain (Pfaff and Keiner, 1973; MacLusky et al., 1980; Parsons et al., 1982; Pfaff and Schwartz-Giblin, 1988; Brown et al., 1990; Simerly et al., 1990). Estrogen and progesterone receptors are found in their highest concentrations in parts of the limbic system that are involved in the regulation of mood, behavior, sex drive, and autonomic function, and also in parts of the brain stem, which contain neuronal circuits involved in the regulation of autonomic function. Steroid receptors also appear in some smooth muscle cells located in blood vessels (Harder and Coulson, 1979).

The sex steroids modulate a number of neurotransmitter, neuropeptide, and ion-channel systems involved in the regulation of neural and vascular function in humans. Receptors for these steroids appear in neurons showing immunoreactivity for various neurotransmitters and neuropeptides, including catecholamines, γ-aminobutyric acid (GABA) and endorphins. Thus, estrogens and progestins can influence the turnover of these neurotransmittors, as well as of serotonin and acetylcholine, and alter the number and sensitivity of their receptors (Luine et al., 1977,1983; Kendall et al., 1981; Biegon et al., 1982; Fischette et al., 1984; Casper et al., 1984; Clarke and Maayan, 1990). In addition, neurons with steroid receptors project their axons to many other parts of the brain, so that even neurons lacking steroid receptors may be influenced indirectly by steroid hormones.

Evidence supports the existence of specific binding sites for estrogen and progesterone within cell membranes, while steroid receptors typically are believed to reside within the nucleus. Indeed, even when progesterone is linked to albumin, which prevents its translocalization into the nucleus, it still can influence neuronal function (Dluzen and Ramirez, 1989). Other studies show that cells containing no detectable high-affinity binding nor immunoreactivity for steroid receptors, as determined by a number of specific assays, may still bind fluorescein-conjugated estradiol at extranuclear sites (Keefe et al., 1991). Various molecular mechanisms have been proposed to explain receptor-independent mechanisms of sex steroid action. Some steroid actions appear so rapidly after exposure to the hormone (milliseconds) that there could not be enough time for transcriptional regulation that is the hallmark of steroid receptor action (Pfaff, 1983; Kow and Pfaff, 1984). Estrogens are metabolized to catechol estrogens which, because of their structural similarity to catecholamines, may influence the metabolism and activity of these neurotransmitters (Axelrod and Tomchick, 1958; Ball et al., 1978; MacLusky et al., 1981). A-ring reduced metabolites of progesterone influence the GABA-A-linked chloride ion channel, one of the most ubiquitous ion channels in the brain (Majewski, 1986). The GABA-A receptor is coupled to a chloride channel that allows these ions to cross the membrane and regulate its excitability. A-ring reduced metabolites of progesterone bind to the GABA receptor complex with higher affinity than benzodiazepines. The effect of such metabolites on the GABA receptor provides a hypothetical molecular basis for their well-known sedative-hypnotic activity in humans and experimental animals (Holzbauer, 1959).

However promising these findings may seem, extrapolation of basic mechanisms to predict neuropsychiatric effects of OCs in humans has a number of limitations. Undoubtedly, there are species differences in reactions to sex steroids. First, most basic studies examine the neural effects of individual steroids, whereas most OCs contain both a synthetic estrogen and progestin that in turn give rise to multiple metabolites, many of them biologically active. Second, these steroids and their metabolites have complex actions on different parts of the brain. A particular steroid may even have opposite effects on the same neurotransmitter system in different parts of the brain. This complexity makes it difficult to generalize findings from specific neuronal systems to other systems, or to predict how neural systems interact to regulate behavior. Indeed, with the possible exception of sexual activity in rodents (Pfaff and Schwartz-Giblin, 1988), the neurobiological basis of sex steroid-induced behavior itself remains poorly understood even in laboratory animals. Species differences also limit the clinical extrapolation of basic neurobiological studies of behavior, especially in understanding the physiological basis of higher brain functions, which are so specialized in humans. Moreover, until recently most studies have employed tissues other than brain (e.g., platelets, endometrium) to study basic mechanisms, and assumed that similar effects occur within the CNS (Grant and Pryse-Davies, 1968). Perhaps the most obvious species difference between humans and most laboratory animals used in neuroendocrine research is the highly psychological and social nature of human behavior. Humans are influenced as much by their inner world and social environment as by biological makeup. These factors weigh especially heavily in understanding emotional reactions to OCs, because for many women "the pill" has powerful emotional impact, associated as it is with issues of sexuality and years of coverage in the popular press (Wood et al., 1970; Wood, 1974). These factors necessitate separation of patient and doctor expectations from physiological effects. Prospective, double-blind, randomized, and placebo-controlled studies come the closest to achieving this separation.

Recognizing the limitations of basic studies in understanding the clinical effects of OCs, this review focuses on the clinical literature on neuropsychiatric side effects and complications, and includes some discussion of changes associated with physiologic endocrine states in order to provide perspective.

A number of neurologic complications including migraine, cerebrovascular accidents, movement disorders, exacerbation of seizure disorder, and CNS neoplasms have been associated with OC use.

MIGRAINE HEADACHES

Numerous clinical observations report an association between OCs and exacerbation of migraine headaches (Whitty et al., 1966; Bickerstaff, 1975; Welch et al., 1984). Most migraine attacks occur during the placebo portion of the pack, consistent with an association of hormone withdrawal with the onset of the headache. Most commonly afflicted are individuals with a prior history of migraine headaches. Many women experience increased frequency and intensity of migraines, while others develop prodromal symptoms for the first time while on OCs. Other clinical observations also support the notion of steroid hormone sensitivity of migraine headaches. Women have a threefold higher incidence of migraine headaches than men, and this sex difference does not appear until after puberty (Welch et al., 1984). Exacerbation at the onset of menses occurs in up to 60% of migraine sufferers (Welsh et al., 1984). Estrogen rather than progesterone withdrawal probably contributes to premenstrual migraines, because perimenstrual progesterone administration does not influence migraine frequency (Somerville, 1971), whereas perimenstrual estradiol valerate administration delays the onset of migraines (Somerville, 1972) and administration of estrogen during the follicular phase triggers migraine attacks as the estrogen levels fall (Somerville, 1975). Indeed, estrogen suppression of ovarian cyclicity may alleviate catamenial migraine in some women (Magos et al., 1983), who often find relief during pregnancy (Somerville, 1972).

CEREBROVASCULAR ACCIDENTS

Early in the 1960s anecdotal reports of strokes in young OC users appeared in the British and U.S. literature. Expert committees were appointed by the American Medical Association in 1962 and by the FDA in 1963 to review the evidence. They concluded that no causal relationship between OC use and adverse cardiovascular events could be established by the available data. Because of the rarity of these events, immediate research required the use of case-control studies, and a number of these, as well as the Collaborative Group for the Study of Stroke in Young Women (1973) reported a statistically significant relationship. These epidemiological studies became the focus of lively controversy (Goldzieher and Dozier, 1975). A decade later, Realini and Goldzieher (1985) reexamined the relevant literature. One of four case-control studies suggested an association with subarachnoid hemorrhage. For thrombotic and/or embolic stroke, three studies found an association, one had mixed findings, and two found no significant association. The prospective studies showed a mixed pattern of associations and are difficult to compare because of the different definitions of cerebrovascular disease categories. The studies of Heyman et al. (1969) of the cerebrovascular disease findings at the Mayo Clinic, which essentially monitored the population of Rochester, Minnesota, in the pre- and post-pill era, found no differences in number or types of cerebrovascular events in age-matched women. When the Royal College Study in England came under new management, the confounding factor of smoking was finally addressed and it turned out that the excess cardiovascular mortality was almost entirely among the smokers. Circulatory disease mortality, in general, among nonsmokers at any age was no greater than could be expected in a population of pill nonusers. Specifically, there was no increased risk of stroke among nonsmoking pill users. The updated Oxford study (Vessey et al., 1989) showed only two strokes during 51,524 woman-years of use: one in a smoker and one in a never-user. Among eight cases of subarachnoid hemorrhage five were in smokers, none were current users, and seven were former users. In the Puget Sound study (Porter et al., 1985), seven of the eight cerebrovascular accidents were in nonusers, possibly suggesting a protective effect. In the Walnut Creek study (1981), all four episodes of stroke occurred in nonusers; only in the case of subarachnoid hemorrhage were there more events in users than in nonusers. In the most recent report on the Nurses' Health Study (Colditz et al., 1990), encompassing followup on nearly 122,000 women, there were too few cases of stroke to assess an effect of pill use.

There are at least three possible explanations for the marked difference between the studies from the 1960s to the early 1980s and those published subsequently. First, the initial case control studies may have been so flawed technically and by uncritical data acquisition that the results were incorrect (Goldzieher and Dozier, 1975; Realini and Goldzieher, 1985); subsequent prospective studies using multiple logistic regression and correcting for the smoking factor yielded more accurate results. Second, subsequent to the general alarm raised regarding cardiovascular complications generally, the selection of women who would be offered the pill might have changed; however, there are no studies to document this possibility. Third, lowering the steroid content of the OCs may have reduced the risk of the alleged hazard; however, Sturtevant (1989) has questioned the validity of a dose-relationship. The atherogenic or thrombotic etiologies of vascular disease generally have been discussed in Chapters 21 and 22. A mechanism by which steroid hormones might be involved in subarachnoid hemorrhage is not known.

MOVEMENT DISORDERS

Drug-associated Movement Disorders

Many patients using neuroleptics and tricyclic antidepressants experience akathisia, a subjective sensation of restlessness, and parkinsonism which arise from effects on the extrapyramidal system. Such extrapyramidal reactions are more common in women, and estrogen facilitates their development (Krishnan et al., 1984). This is consistent with animal studies showing that pretreatment with estrogen intensifies the effect of dopaminergic drugs (Chiodo et al., 1981). The effect of OCs on these symptoms has not been well studied.

Tardive Dyskinesia

Tardive dyskinesia is a movement disorder afflicting chronic users of neuroleptic antipsychotic drugs. The leading hypothesis regarding its neurobiologic basis involves supersensitivity of nigrostriatal dopamine receptors. Postmenopausal women on neuroleptic drugs are at increased risk of developing this disorder, and estrogen therapy may decrease the number and severity of abnormal movements both in women (Glazer et al., 1985) and men (Beclard et al., 1977). An effect of OCs in reproductive-age women has not been reported.

Chorea

Chorea refers to nonrhythmic involuntary movement of the extremities and facial muscles, often in association with hypotonia of the involved limbs. Chorea has been reported in association with OC use as well as pregnancy (Zegart and Schwartz, 1968; Wilson and Preece, 1982; Ghanem, 1985). The OC dose does not seem to influence the risk of developing this rare complication (Nausieda et al., 1979). Although the condition resolves promptly after OC discontinuation, afflicted women remain predisposed to chorea gravidarum. Conversely, women who develop chorea gravidarum are at risk of developing chorea if they use OCs (Gamboa et al., 1971). The underlying mechanism remains unclear, although estrogen modulation of nigrostriatal aminergic neurotransmission has been implicated (Beclard, 1977).

NERVOUS SYSTEM NEOPLASMS

Meningioma

Among the most common brain tumors, meningiomas have a marked predilection for women, with female:male sex ratios ranging from 2:1 to 9:1 (Rausing et al., 1970). Their incidence peaks during the reproductive years (Poisson, 1984), and they may grow, at times quite rapidly, during pregnancy and often regress during the puerperium (Bickerstaff et al., 1958; Chaudhuri and Wallenburn, 1980). Both meningiomas and normal meninges contain estrogen as well as progestrone receptors (Poisson, 1984). There are no reports of the effect of OCs on meningioma.

Pituitary Adenomas

The use of OCs may elevate plasma prolactin levels (as do estrogens) in some individuals; when observed this elevation is typically mild and does not signify higher risk of prolactinomas (Pituitary Adenoma Study Group, 1983). At one time the condition of "post-pill amenorrhea" was put forward as an entity, and a possible association with prolactinomas was suggested. This turned out to be a non-disease, originating in the fact that significant numbers of women are prescribed OCs to regulate irregular or infrequent menses. The etiology of the disturbance may in some cases be hyperprolactinemia, with or without a detectable alteration in the appearance of the sella turcica. When these patients discontinued OC use, the underlying pathology reappeared, and was then classified by some unwary individuals as a side-effect of OC use. The Pituitary Adenoma Study Group (1983) settled this issue.

METABOLIC CONDITIONS WITH NEUROLOGIC MANIFESTATIONS

Porphyria

The porphyrias arise from defects in the heme-biosynthetic pathway. Neurologic manifestations include mental status changes, seizures, and sensorimotor and autonomic neuropathies. Oral contraceptives may precipitate attacks, perhaps by inducing aminolevulinic acid synthase, the rate-limiting enzyme in the heme synthesis pathway. The sex-steroid sensitivity of acute intermittent porphyria has made possible, in some women, successful treatment with a long-acting gonadotropin-releasing hormone (GnRH) agonist, which suppresses the pituitary-ovarian axis by down-regulating pituitary GnRH receptors (Anderson et al., 1984).

SEIZURE DISORDERS

In experimental animals, estrogen lowers the seizure threshold induced by electroshock, pentylene tetrazol, and kainic acid. Progesterone decreases spontaneous and induced epileptiform discharges (Herzog, 1990). The combination of estrogen and progesterone lowers the threshold to picrotoxin-induced seizures in the rat (Schwartz-Giblin and Pfaff, 1990). Sex steroids also influence human electrical brain wave activity and epilepsy. Oral estrogen activates epileptiform discharges and seizure activity (Cogothetis et al., 1959), while progesterone decreases interictal spike frequency in women (Backstrom et al., 1984). The occasional exacerbation of epilepsy during certain phases of the menstrual cycle furnishes further evidence of the steroid sensitivity of CNS excitability. Exacerbation of seizure activity in relation to the menstrual cycle occurs in up to 75% of women with epilepsy. Most report increased seizure activity during the late luteal phase, while others find the greatest risk of seizures at midcycle. Late luteal exacerbation has been attributed to epileptogenic effects of progesterone withdrawal, while midcycle worsening may arise from the preovulatory surge of estrogen unaccompanied by a rise in the progesterone level (Laidlaw, 1965; Backstrom, 1976). Sex steroids, including OCs, may influence seizure frequency by inducing hepatic microsomal enzymes responsible for the metabolism of antiseizure medications (Shavit et al., 1984; Roscizewska et al., 1986). (See also Chapters 15,28.)

MOOD AND BEHAVIOR

Users of OCs may complain of mood and behavior alterations, which they attribute to these agents (Carranza-Acevedo, 1967; Branham, 1970; Andrews, 1978; Fleming and Seager, 1978). Depression is the most commonly reported mood change (Grant and Mears, 1967; Herzberg et al., 1970; Adams et al., 1971; Kutner and Brown, 1972; Leeton, 1973). This mood change can signify a broad range of states, from minor unease to psychotic states requiring hospitalization. Although early studies rarely made such distinctions, OCs at one time or another have been alleged to cause or worsen all of them. Most studies suggest the most common reaction is a mild dysphoria. Of course, even minor effects may be of clinical significance by influencing patient compliance.

Despite the frequency of these complaints, little consensus exists about their actual relationship to OC use, and to what extent such complaints arise from pharmacological effects versus user expectations or artifact from reporting bias. Although scores of studies have addressed this issue, those supporting such an association suffer from a number of methodological weaknesses (Blumenthal and Nadelson, 1988), including: 1) imprecise definition and inadequate quantification of moods and behaviors; 2) failure to determine the temporal relationship between the onset of mood change and the beginning of OC use; 3) failure to control for placebo effects; 4) failure to relate specific hormonal changes to specific moods or behaviors; and 5) inadequate sample size to interpret negative results.

Since suffering is intensely personal and its measurement depends on the subjects' willingness and ability to reveal their pain to the investigator, it is not surprising that the problem of quantifiability plagues psychiatric research. Current rating scales and psychological instruments facilitate reliable measurement of symptoms, but few studies used them. Until recently, most instruments were designed to measure symptoms of classical psychiatric syndromes, not steroid-related manifestations, thus undoubtedly decreasing their sensitivity for the detection of OC-related effects.

Many studies rely on retrospective reports, which increase the chances of recall bias, and hence the likelihood of making spurious associations between OC use and adverse moods or behaviors. Conversely, an association may be missed if the link between disrupted mood and OC use does not occur to the patient or the clinician at the time of the study (Ananth and Ghadirian, 1980). Retrospective studies make it difficult to determine whether altered mood results from effects of OCs themselves or from particular characteristics of the OC choosers. For example, OC users exhibit greater orientation toward future goals compared to users of other contraceptives, perhaps explaining their choice of "safe" contraceptives such as OCs (Harvey, 1976). Such personality characteristics could predispose OC users to depression independent of any direct OC effect. Prospective design and randomization are the optimal methods to minimize such confounding variables.

In some individuals, even inert placebos can bring about depression (Beecher, 1955), suggesting that drug-related depressions may be affected by individual expectations. Oral contraceptives can induce mood changes by placebo effect, in some women given an inert placebo thought to be an OC, 29% reported decreased libido, 16% reported headaches, and 6% reported nervousness (Aznar-Ramos et al., 1969). Such findings suggest that some individuals use OCs as a scapegoat to explain their preexisting symptomatology (Bakker and Dightman, 1966).

A related problem in interpreting existing studies on OCs and mood is that subjects often harbor strong and conflicting feelings about "the pill" (Bakker and Dightman, 1966). For example, some early studies suggested that many women experience guilt over the delay in starting a family that OC use represents (Lidz, 1969; Fortin et al., 1972). While the meaning of OC use may change with time, the popular press, word of mouth, and even professional opinions based on older, poorly controlled studies have raised expectations of adverse outcomes. Because of the controversial societal position of OCs today, our judgment of their psychological effects must depend heavily on double-blind protocols for the sorting out of objective and attributed effects.

The doses in current OCs differ greatly from those in older preparations, making it difficult to generalize results to formulations used today. Studies must also take into account the baseline endocrine status of the subjects, since steroids might have variable, even opposite effects depending on whether the subjects have high or low baseline hormone levels.

Depression has been reported to be increased (Kane, 1968; Grant and Pryse-Davies, 1968; Herzberg et al., 1971), decreased (Ziegler et al., 1968), or unaffected (Bakker and Dightman, 1961; Zell and Crisp, 1964; Murawski et al., 1968; Goldzieher et al., 1971; Kutner and Brown, 1972) by OC use. Reports of the incidence of depression range from 6% (Nilsson et al., 1967; Grant and Pryce-Davies, 1968; Lewis and Hoghughi, 1969; Grounds et al., 1970; Herzberg et al., 1970) to 34% (Kane, 1968). Methodological problems limit the interpretation of these retrospective, cross-sectional studies. For example, the latter study overestimates the incidence of depression by recruiting subjects who report psychological effects with prior OC use (Kane, 1967).

A number of studies feature double-blind, placebo-controlled, randomized design, and two studies included crossover (Goldzieher et al., 1971; Leeton, 1973). A double-blind, placebo-controlled, randomized study reported the incidence of depression in the OC group as 15% compared to 0% when they were crossed over to placebo (Leeton, 1973). Another randomized double-blind study (Cullberg, 1972) and a prospective cohort study (Royal College of General Practitioners, 1974) reported a 10% to 15% increase in the incidence of depression. The prospective design of two studies (Herzberg et al., 1971; Cullberg, 1972) established that OC use preceded the onset of depression, an important criterion to establish causality.

One randomized, prospective, placebo-controlled, double-blind cross-over study showed no increase in depression during the OC arm compared to the placebo arm (Goldzieher et al., 1971). An increase in anxiety occurred in early cycles of the high estrogen preparation protocols, but the effect did not persist after crossover to another OC, diminishing the significance of the results. The size of this study (N = 398) did not confer sufficient power to rule out an effect of OCs on depression, but made a large effect unlikely. One study reported less depression, as measured by the Hopkins Symptom Checklist, in OC or estrogen users compared to those who had taken placebo or progestins for 6 months (Rickels et al., 1976). The differences among these treatment groups were not significant at 3 months. Other studies suggest that OCs might improve the users' sense of well-being. Patients taking an estrogen-progestin preparation, estrogen alone, or placebo were asked which compound they preferred. Twenty of 27 women (74%) preferred taking either the estrogen/progestin compound or the estrogen, while only three (11%) preferred the placebo (Bakke, 1965).

Women who are affected negatively by OC use differ in a number of ways from those who are affected positively or unaffected. They more often reported a history of premenstrual mood disturbance, engaged less frequently in sexual intercourse, and experienced less frequent orgasm compared to women who did not report adverse symptoms during OC use (Kane et al., 1967). Furthermore, women starting on OCs more often reported adverse effects on mood if they used triphasic as compared to monophasic OCs (Bancroft et al., 1987), and if they used a high estrogen pill, a pharmacologically inconsistent observation.

Some evidence suggests that the depressive reaction relates to the progestin (Kane et al., 1967; McGregor, 1967). Recent studies on the effects of progestins on hypogonadal women receiving hormone replacement therapy corroborate a usually mild, but consistent effect of progestins on mood (Siddle et al., 1984; Holst et al., 1989).

Large doses of oral conjugated estrogen (Premarin) administered to severely depressed, inpatient premenopausal and postmenopausal women in a double-blind study significantly reduced Hamilton depression ratings (Klaiber et al., 1979), suggesting that estrogens may improve mood, at least in women suffering from major depression who are estrogen-deficient.

PSYCHOTIC REACTIONS

Reports of psychosis in association with OC use are limited to anecdotal cases or small series, and almost all patients who developed psychosis while on OCs had preexistent major psychiatric disorders (Idestrom,1966; Kane,1968; Sturgis,1968). A number of women developed psychotic episodes upon withdrawal of the OC, and three of four cases in one series had a history of postpartum mood disturbance (Kane,1968; Kane et al., 1969). These reports suggest that, while psychotic reactions in OC users are extremely rare, some women may be especially sensitive to fluctuating levels of sex steroids.

An alternative hypothesis is that psychiatric illness itself nonspecifically predisposes the OC user to exaggerated psychological reactions. However, evidence against this hypothesis is provided by a study of the psychological response to OC use of 11 psychiatric inpatients with diverse diagnoses of major psychiatric disorders. Clinical interviews and personality tests yielded a mixed response: some patients reported reduced, while others reported increased psychological symptoms (Kane, 1968).

LIBIDO

OCs have been reported to decrease (Grant and Pryse-Davies, 1968), increase (Ringrose, 1965) or not affect (Bakker and Dightmann, 1966; Udry and Morris, 1970; Cullberg, 1972) sex drive. One major study showing adverse effects of OCs on libido studied some subjects during the puerperium, so the decreased libido reported in that study may have reflected the influence of recent childbirth rather than that of OCs themselves. A broad array of factors, including psychological, social, and endocrine influences could affect an individual woman's sexual response. In humans and experimental animals, androgens and sex drive appear to be closely linked (Bancroft et al., 1983). Although most circulating androgens are bound to sex-hormone-binding globulin (SHBG), only the small unbound fraction maintains biological activity. By elevating levels of SHBG, OCs might be expected to reduce the androgenic environment. Indeed, OC use has been associated with lower anger and hostility scores on psychometric tests, two effects that are also correlated with androgenicity (Worsley and Chang, 1978). Other studies using the free association test found that subjects on norethynodrel/mestranol experienced increased "hostility outward" (Silbergeld et al., 1971). These contrasting results may be explained by different individual emotional responses and perhaps by variation in the androgenic potency of OCs.

OCs may increase sexual drive in some women by relieving them of anxiety over the possibility of unwanted pregnancy. To make matters even more complex, different women experience the same OC-related effects on sex drive in different ways. For example, of 12 women who experienced increased sexual drive in association with OC use, six rated this change as favorable, while another six women stopped their OC use because this reaction was regarded unfavorably (Bakke, 1965).

PREMENSTRUAL SYNDROME

A wide variety of somatic, psychological, and affective symptoms change in concert with the ovarian cycle, even in women whose uteri are surgically absent;

this suggests an effect of sex steroids on these symptoms, a phenomenon that has been termed the premenstrual syndrome (PMS) (Dennerstein and Burrows, 1979; DeJong et al., 1985). These symptoms usually abate at the time of natural, surgical, or medical menopause, lending further credence to steroid influence (Muse et al., 1984). Such observations have been invoked to suggest that OCs might alleviate premenstrual mood changes by decreasing or eliminating the magnitude of fluctuations in endogenous hormones. In support of the hypothesis that OCs improve global functioning and mood during the menstrual cycle are studies demonstrating that users show fewer peaks and troughs in their moods throughout the month. The reduction in mood cyclicity was most obvious with monophasic and less so with triphasic formulations, possibly due to different degrees of gonadotropin suppression (Glick and Bennett, 1982; Warner and Bancroft, 1988; Walker and Bancroft, 1990). However, OCs do not consistently relieve PMS, and may even exacerbate it in some patients (O'Brien, 1987). In fact, some studies show that OCs have minimal effects on premenstrual symptoms in long-term users. When levels of breast tenderness, mood, irritability, energy, tension, bloating, and sexual interest were compared among long-term users of monophasic OCs and triphasic OCs, as well as nonusers, differences were found among the groups only in the level of breast tenderness. Another study carried out retrospectively using the Premenstrual Assessment Form found little difference in premenstrual symptomatology between women taking low-dose OCs and nonusers (Yuk et al., 1991). Even a prospective cohort study found no significant differences between users and nonusers on the Moos Menstrual Distress Questionnaire (MDQ) for specific symptoms or for the total score (Marriott and Faragher, 1986). This study may have missed an effect on PMS; it was not randomized and the women had used OCs for at least 6 months, so it excluded women who would have discontinued use because of prior mood or behaviorally related side effects.

Women with PMS are said to be more likely to develop adverse mental reactions to OCs (Cullberg, 1972; Kutner and Brown, 1972; Forrest, 1979), suggesting that some women may have a diathesis toward steroid-related mood disturbance. A genetic basis for such sensitivity remains speculative at this time (Kendler et al., 1988). In a study of genetic factors in OC-related mood disturbance in 715 monozygotic and 416 dizygotic twin pairs, the tendency to develop OC-related depression was shared much more by monozygotic than by dizygotic twins. Similar, although less robust concordance appeared with OC-related irritability. A limitation of this study is that twins share many traits that are not necessarily genetic (e.g., preferences for clothes and hair styles) but rather arise from their shared upbringing, so that a higher concordance rate for OC-related mood disturbance among monozygotic as opposed to dizygotic twins does not establish its genetic basis. Furthermore, the study depended on the subjects' ability to recall and self-report their symptoms. Twins, especially identical twins, would be expected to share many things in their lives, including selective recall of OC effects. Future studies should examine OC-related mood changes in twins reared apart, to separate biological from familial and social factors. Finally, since the subjects were all volunteers, the sample probably tended to overrepresent those suffering from OC-related side effects.

Despite the controversy about the incidence and etiology of OC-related mood changes, a number of conclusions are inescapable. First, for most women, OCs have minimal impact on their psychological and neurological well-being. Second, a subset of women develop psychological reactions in association with OC use, the most common being mild depression. While this may prompt discontinuation, it rarely triggers major depressive episodes, even in predisposed individuals (Orchard, 1969). Third, women on OCs who have a predisposition toward depression, based on their family history and/or past personal history, may be more likely to develop depression. Fourth, the mechanisms underlying OC-related psychological changes probably involve a complex integration of user expectation (Orchard, 1969) and direct action on steroid-sensitive circuits within the CNS.

REFERENCES

Ananth J, Ghadirian AM. Drug-induced mood disorders. *Int Pharmacopsychiatr* 1980;15:59–73.

Anderson K, Spitz I, Sassa S, et al. Prevention of cyclical attacks of acute intermittent porphyria with a long-acting agonist of luteinizing hormone-releasing hormone. *N Engl J Med* 1984;311:643–5.

Andrews WC. Oral contraception physiologic and pathologic effects. *Obstet Gynecol Annu* 1978;7:325–51.

Anon. The pill and porphyria. *Br Med J* 1972;3:603–4.

Axelrod J, Tomchick R. Enzymatic *o*-methylation of epinephrine and other catechols. *J Biol Chem* 1958;233:702–5.

Aznar-Ramos R, Giner-Velasquez J, Lara-Ricalde R, Martinez-Manautou J. Incidence of side effects with contraceptive placebo. *Am J Obstet Gynecol* 1969;105:1,144.

Backstrom T. Epileptic seizures in women related to plasma estrogen and progesterone during the menstrual cycle. *Acta Neurol Scand* 1976;54:321–47.

Backstrom T, Zetterlund B, Blum S, and Romano M. Effects of IV progesterone infusion on the epileptic discharge frequency in women with partial epilepsy. *Acta Neurol Scand* 1984;69:240–8.

Bakker CB, Dightman CR. Side effects of oral contraceptives. *Obstet Gynecol* 1966;28:373–9.

Ball P, Haupt M, Knuppen R. Comparative studies on the metabolism of oestradiol in the brain, the pituitary and the liver of the rat. *Acta Endocrinol* 1978;87:1–11.

Bancroft J, Sanders D, Davidson D, Warner P. Mood, sexuality, hormones and the menstrual cycle. III. Sexuality and the role of androgens. *Psychosom Med* 1983;45:509–16.

Bancroft J, Sanders D, Warner P, Loudon N. The effect of oral contraceptives on mood and sexuality: a comparison of triphasic and combined preparation. *J Psychosom Obstet Gynecol* 1987;7:1–8.

Bedard P, Langelier P, Villeneuve A. Oestrogens and extrapyramidal system. *Lancet* 1977;1,367–8.

Beecher HK. The powerful placebo. *JAMA* 1955;159:1,602–6.

Bickerstaff E, Small J, Guest I. The relapsing course of certain meningiomas in relation to pregnancy and menstruation. *J Neurol Neurosurg Psychiatry* 1958;21:89–91.

Biegon A, Reches A, Snyder L, McEwen B. Serotonergic and noradrenergic receptors in the rat brain: modulation by chronic exposure to ovarian hormones. *Life Sci* 1982;32:2,015–1.

Blumenthal SJ, Nadelson CC. Mood changes associated with reproductive life events: an overview of research and treatment strategies. *J Clin Psychiatry* 1988;49:466–8.

Branham J. Oral contraceptive and depression. *Br Med J* 1970;1:237.

Brown TJ, MacLusky NJ, Toran-Allerand D, et al. Characterization of 11β-methoxy-16α-(^{125}I) iodoestradiol binding: neuronal localization of estrogen-bound sites in the developing rat brain. *Endocrinology* 1990;124:2,074–88.

Carranza-Acevedo J. Oral contraceptive and depression. *Lancet* 1967;2:104.

Casper RF, Bhanot R, Wilkinson M. Prolonged elevation of hypothalamic opioid peptide activity in women taking oral contraceptives. *J Clin Endocrinol Metab* 1984:58:582–4.

Chaudhuri P, Wallenburn H. Brain tumors and pregnancy. *Eur J Obstet Gynecol Reprod Biol* 1980;11:109–14.

Chiodo LA, Caggiula AR, Saller CF. Estrogen potentiates the stereotypy induced by dopamine agonists in the rat. *Life Sci* 1981;28:827–35.

Clarke WP, Maayani S. Estrogen effects on 5–HTIA receptors in hippocampal membranes from ovariectomized rats: functional and binding studies. *Brain Res* 1990;518:287–91.

Clarkson TB, Adams MR, et al. From menarche to menopause: coronary atherosclerosis and protection in cynomolgus monkeys. *Am J Obstet Gynecol* 1989;160:1,280.

Colditz et al. *Curr Probl Obstet Gynecol Fertil* 1990;13:130.

Cogothetis J, Harner R, Morrell F, Torres F. The role of estrogens in catamenial exacerbation of epilepsy. *Neurology* 1959;9:352–60.

Collaborative Group for the Study of Stroke in Young Women. Oral contraception and increased risk of cerebral ischemia or thrombosis. *N Engl J Med* 1973;288:871–8.

Croft P, Hannaford PC. *Br Med J* 1989;198;165.

Cullberg J. Mood changes and menstrual symptoms, with different gestagen/estrogen combinations: a double blind comparison with a placebo. *Acta Psychiatr Scand* 1972; [Suppl 236]:

DeGennes P, et al. *Diabetes Metab* 1976;2:81.

DeJong R, Rubinow DR, Roy-Byrne P, Hoban MC, et al. Premenstrual mood disorder and psychiatric illness. *Am J Psychiatry* 1985;142:1,359–61.

Dennerstein L, Burrows G. Affect and the menstrual cycle. *J Affect Disorders* 1979;1:77–92.

Dluzen DE, Ramirez VD. Progesterone effects upon dopamine release from the corpus striatum of female rats. II. Evidence for a membrane site of action and the role of albumin. *Brain Res* 1989; 476:338–44.

Fischette CT, Biegon A, McEwen BS. Sex steroid modulation of the serotonin behavioral syndrome. *Life Sci* 1984;35:1,197–1206.

Fleming O, Seager CP. Incidence of depressive symptoms in users of oral contraceptives. *Br J Psychiatry* 1978;32:431–40.

Forrest ARW. Variations in mood in normal women taking oral contraceptives. *Br Med J* 1979;2:1 403–8.

Fortin JN, Wittkower ED, Paiement J, Tetreault L. Side effects of oral contraceptive medication: a psychosomatic problem. *Can Psychiatr Assoc J* 1972;17:3–10.

Gamboa E, Isaacs G, Harter D. Chorea associated with oral contraceptive therapy. *Arch Neurol* 1971; 25:112–4.

Ghanem Q. Recurrent chorea gravidarum in four pregnancies. *Can J Neurol Sci* 1985;12:136–8.

Glazer WM, Naftolin F, Morgenstein H, Barnea ER, et al. Estrogen replacement and tardive dyskinesia. *Psychoneuroendocrin* 1985;10:345–50.

Glick I, Bennett SE. Oral contraceptives and the menstrual cycle. In: Friedman RC, ed. *Behavior and the menstrual cycle.* New York: Marcel Dekker; 1982:345–65.

Glick I, Bennett SE. Psychiatric complications of progesterone and oral contraceptives. *J Clin Psychopharmacol* 1981;1:350–67.

Goldzieher JW, Brody SA. Pharmacokinetics of ethinyl estradiol and mestranol. *Am J Obstet Gynecol* 1990;163:2,114–9.

Goldzieher JW, Dozier TS. Oral contraceptives and thromboembolism: a reassessment. *Am J Obstet Gynecol* 1975;123:878–914.

Goldzieher JW, Moses LE, Averkin E, Scheel C, et al. Nervousness and depression attributed to oral contraceptives: a double-blind, placebo-controlled study. *Am J Obstet Gynecol* 1971;111:1,013–20.

Grant ECG, Mears E. Mental effects of oral contraceptives. *Lancet* 1967;2:945.

Grant ECG, Pryse-Davies J. Effect of oral contraceptives on depressive mood changes and on endometrial monoamine oxidase and phosphatases. *Br Med J* 1968;3:777–80.

Grounds D, Davies B, Mowbray R. The contraceptive pill, side effects and personality: report of a controlled double blind trial. *Br J Psychiatry* 1970;116:169–72.

Harder DR, Coulson PB. Estrogen receptors and effects of estrogen on membrane electrical properties of coronary vascular smooth muscle. *J Cell Physiol* 1979;100:375–82.

Harvey AL. Risky and safe contraceptors: some personality factors. *J Psychol* 1976;92:109–12.

Herzberg BN, Johnson AL, Brown S. Depressive symptoms and oral contraceptives. *Br Med J* 1970; 4:142–3.

Herzberg BN, Johnson AL, Nichol GC, Draper KC. Oral contraceptives, depression and libido. *Br Med J* 1971;111:495.

Herzog N. Cerebral excitability and ovarian secretions In Naftolin F, DeCherney AH, Gutmann J et al., eds. *Ovarian secretions and cardiovascular and neurological function.* New York: Raven Press; 1990:179–97.

Heyman A, Arons M, et al. *Neurology* 1969;18:519.

Holst J, Backstrom T, Hammarback S, von Schoultz B. Progestogen addition during oestrogen replacement therapy-effects on vasomotor symptoms and mood. *Maturitas* 1989;11:13–20.

Holzbauer M. Physiological aspects of steroids with anesthetic properties. *Med Biol* 1959;54:227–42.

Kane FF. Evaluation of emotional reactions to oral contraceptive use. *Am J Obstet Gynecol* 1976; 126:968–72.

Kane FJ. Psychiatric reactions to oral contraceptives. *Am J Obstet Gynecol* 1968;102:1,053–63.

Kane FJ, Daly RJ, Ewing JA, Keller MH. Mood and behavioral changes with progestational agents. *Br J Psychiatry* 1967;113:265.

Kane FJ, Treadway R, Ewing F. Emotional changes associated with oral contraceptives in female psychiatric patients. *Compr Psychiatry* 1969;10:16–30.

Keefe DL, Michelson D, Lee SH, Naftolin F. Astrocytes within the hypothalamic arcuate nucleus contain estrogen-sensitive peroxidase, bind fluorescein-conjugated estradiol and may mediate synaptic plasticity in the rat. *Am J Obstet Gynecol* 1991;164:959–66.

Kendall DA, Stancel GM, Enna SJ. Imipramine: effect of ovarian steroids on modifications in serotonin receptor binding. *Science* 1981;211:1,183–5.

Kendler S, Martin N, Heath AC, et al. A twin study of the psychiatric side effects of oral contraceptives. *J Nervous Mental Dis* 1988;176:153–160.

Klaiber EL, Broverman DM, Vogel W, et al. Estrogen therapy for severe persistent depression in women. *Arch Gen Psychiatry* 1979;

Kow L-M, Pfaff DW. Suprachiasmatic neurons in tissue slices from ovariectomized rats: electrophysiological and neuropharmacological characterization and the effects of estrogen treatment. *Brain Res* 1984;297:275–86.

Krishnan KR, France RD, Ellinwood EH. Tricyclic-induced akathisia in patients taking conjugated estrogens. *Am J Psychiatry* 1984;141:696–697.

Kutner SJ, Brown WL. History of depression as a risk factor for depression with oral contraceptives. *J Nerv Mental Dis* 1972a;155:163–169.

Kutner SJ, Brown WL. Types of oral contraceptives, depression and premenstrual symptoms. *J Nerv Mental Dis* 1972b;155:153–162.

Laidlaw J. Catamenial epilepsy. *Lancet* 1956;271:1,235–37.

Leeton J. The relationship of oral contraception to depressive symptoms. *Aust NZ J Obstet Gynaecol* 1973;13:115–20.

Lewis A, Hoghughi M. An evaluation of depression as a side effect of oral contraceptives. *Br J Psychiatry* 1969;115:697.

Lidz RW. Emotional factors in the success of contraception. *Fertil Steril* 1969;20:761–71.

Luine VN, McEwen BS, Black IB. Effect of 17β-estradiol on hypothalamic tyrosine hydroxylase activity. *Brain Res* 1977;120:188–92.

Luine VN, Rhodes JC. Gonadal hormone regulation of MAO and other enzymes in hypothalamic areas. *Neuroendocrinol* 1983;36:235–41.

MacLusky NJ, Liederberg I, Krey LC, et al. Progesterone receptors in the brain and pituitary of a primate, the bonnet monkey (Macaca radiata). *Endocrinol* 1880;106:185.

MacLusky NJ, Naftolin F, Krey LC, et al. The catechol estrogens. *J Steroid Biochem* 1981;15:111–24.

Magos A, Zilkha K, Studd J. Treatment of menstrual migraine by estradiol implants. *J Neurol Neurosurg Psychiatry* 1983;46:1,044–6.

Majewska, MD. Steroid hormone metabolites are barbiturate-like modulators of the GABA receptor. *Science* 1986;232:1,004.

Marriott A, Faragher EB. An assessment of psychological states associated with the menstrual cycle in users of oral contraception. *J Psychosom Res* 1986;30:41–7.

Murawski BJ, Sapir PE, Shulman N, et al. An investigation of mood states in women taking oral contraceptives. *Fertil Steril* 1968;19:50–63.

Muse KN, Cetel NS, Futterman LA, et al. The premenstrual syndrome: effects of medical ovariectomy. *N Engl J Med* 1984;311:1,345–9.

Nausieda P, Koller W, Weiner W, et al. Chorea induced by oral contraceptives. *Neurology* 1979; 29:1,605–9.

Nilsson A, Jacobson L, Ingemanson CA. Side effects of an oral contraceptive with particular attention to mental and sexual adaptation. *Acta Obstet Gynecol Scand* 1967;46:537–56.

O'Brien PMS. Hormonal therapy and hormone antagonists. In: O'Brien PMS, ed. *Premenstrual syndrome*. Boston: Blackwell; 1987:148–77.

Orchard WH. Psychiatric aspects of oral contraceptives. *Med J Austral* 1969;1:872–6.

Parsons B, Rainbow TC, MacLusky N, et al. Progestin receptor levels in rat hypothalamic and limbic nuclei. *J Neurosci* 1982;2:1,446.

Pfaff DW. Impact of estrogens on hypothalamic nerve cells: ultrastructural, chemical, and electrical effects. *Recent Progress Horm Res* 1983;39:127–79.

Pfaff DW, Keiner M. Atlas of estradiol-concentrating cells in the central nervous system of the female rat. *J Comp Neurol* 1973;151:121–58.

Pfaff DW, Schwartz-Giblin S. Cellular mechanisms of female reproductive behaviors. In: Knobil E, Neill J, eds. *The physiology of reproduction*. New York: Raven Press; 1988:1,487–1568.

Pituitary Adenoma Study Group: Pituitary adenomas and oral contraceptives: a multicenter case-control study. *Fertil Steril* 1983;39:753–60.

Poisson M. Steroid receptors in human meningiomas. *Clin Neuropharmacol* 1984;7:320–4.

Porter JB, Jick H, et al. *Obstet Gynecol* 1985;66:1.

Ramcharan S, Pellegrin FA, Ray R, et al. The Walnut Creek contraceptive drug study. NIH Publication No. 81–564;1981.

Rausing A, Ybo W, Stenflo J. Intracranial meningioma: a population study of ten years. *Acta Neurol Scand* 1970;46:102–10.

Realini JP, Goldzieher JW. Oral contraceptives and cardiovascular disease: A critique of the epidemiological studies. *Am J Obstet Gynecol* 1985;152:729.

Rickels K, Garcia CR, Lipman RS, et al. The Hopkins Symptom Checklist. *Prim Care* 1976;3:751–64.

Ringrose CAD. The emotional responses of married women receiving oral contraceptives. *Can Med Assoc J* 1965;92:1,207.

Roscizewska D, Buntner B, Guz I, et al. Ovarian hormones, anticonvulsant drugs and seizures during the menstrual cycle in women with epilepsy. *J Neurol Neurosurg Psychiatry* 1986;49:47–51.

Schwartz-Giblin S, Pfaff D. Sensorimotor actions of ovarian steroid hormones on spinal cord and brainstem function. In Naftolin F, DeCherney AH, Gutmann J, Sarrel PM, eds. *Ovarian secretions and cardiovascular and neurological function*. New York: Raven Press; 1990:179–97.

Shavit G, Lerman P, Korezyn AD, et al. Phenytoin pharmacokinetics in catamenial epilepsy. *Neurology* 1984:34:959–61.

Siddle N, Williams V, Young O, et al. Psychological effects of progestogens on oestrogen-treated postmenopausal women. *Maturitas* 1984;6:183–4.

Silbergeld S, Brast N, Noble E. The menstrual cycle: a double-blind study of symptoms, mood and behavior, and biochemical variables using Enovid and placebo. *Psychosom Med* 1971;33:411–28.

Simerly RB, Chang C, Muramatsu M, et al. Distribution of androgen and estrogen receptor mRNA-containing cells in the rat brain: an in situ hybridization study. *J Comp Neurol* 1990;294:76–95.

Somerville B. Estrogen withdrawal migraine. II. Attempted prophylaxis by continuous estradiol administration. *Neurology* 1975;25:245–50.

Somerville B: The role of estradiol withdrawal in the etiology of menstrual migraine. *Neurology* 1972b: 22:355–65.

Somerville B. The role of progesterone in menstrual migraine. *Neurology* 1971;21:853–9.

Somerville B. A study of migraine in pregnancy. *Neurology* 1972;22:824–9.

Sturtevant FM. Special report: safety of oral contraceptives related to steroid content: a critical review. *Int J Fertil* 1989;34:323–32.

Tietze C, Lewit S. Use-effectiveness of oral and intrauterine contraception. *Fertil Steril* 1971;22:508–13.

Urdry R, Morris NM. Effect of contraceptive pills on the distribution of sexual activity in the menstrual cycle. *Nature* 1970;27:502–3.

Vessey M, et al. *Br Med J* 1989;289:1,487.

Walker A, Bancroft J. Relationship between premenstrual symptoms and oral contraceptive use: a controlled study. *Psychosom Med* 1990;52:86–96.

Warner P, Bancroft J. Mood, sexuality, oral contraceptives and the menstrual cycle. *J Psychosom Res* 1988;32:417–27.

Welch K, Darnley D, Simkins R. The role of estrogen in migraine: a review and hypothesis. *Cephalalgia* 1984;4:227–36.

Westoff CF, Bumpass L, Ryder NB. Oral contraception, coital pregnancy and the time required to conceive. *Soc Biol* 1969;16:1–10.

Whitty C, Hockaday J, Whitty M. The effects of oral contraceptives on migraine. *Lancet* 1966;1:856–9.

Wilson P, Preece A. Chorea gravidarum: a statistical study of 951 collected cases, 846 from the literature and 105 previously unreported. *Arch Intern Med* 1932;49:471–533.

Wood C. A study of attitudes to contraceptives in a middle-class group of women. *Med J Austral* 1974;1:659–60.

Wood C, Leeton J, Downing B. Emotional attitudes to contraceptive methods. *Contraception* 1970;2:2–3.

Worsley A. A prospective study of the effects of the progestogen content of oral contraceptives on measures of affect, automatization, and perceptual restructuring ability. *Psychopharmacol* 1980; 67:289–96.

Worsley A, Chang A. Oral contraceptives and emotional state. *J Psychosom Res* 1978;22:13–6.

Yuk VJ, Cumming CE, Fox EE, et al. Frequency and severity of premenstrual symptoms in women taking birth control pills. *Gynecol Obstet Invest* 1991;31:42–5.

Zegart K, Schwartz R. Chorea gravidarum. *Obstet Gynecol* 1968;32:24–7.

Zell JR, Crisp WE. A psychiatric evaluation of the use of oral contraceptives. *Obstet Gynecol* 1964; 28:373.

Ziegler FJ, Rodgers DA, Kriegsman SA, et al. *JAMA* 1968;204:849.

Pharmacology of the Contraceptive Steroids,
edited by Joseph W. Goldzieher.
Raven Press, Ltd., New York © 1994.

20

Cardiovascular System: Blood Pressure

Robert Fraser and Ronald J. Weir

MRC Blood Pressure Unit, Medical Research Council, Glasgow, G11 6NT, Scotland

Among the earliest side effects of oral contraceptive (OC) use to be noted was a rise in blood pressure (Brownrigg, 1962). This chapter considers the causes of this rise. More detailed reviews on aspects of this subject are available (Weinberger and Weir, 1983; Woods, 1988).

Combined estrogen/progestin OCs, especially the original high dosage types, have been reported to produce a rise in blood pressure (Kunin et al., 1969; Clezy et al., 1972; Spellacy and Birk, 1972; Royal College of General Practitioners (RCGP) 1974; Weir et al., 1974; Fisch and Frank, 1977; Meade et al., 1977; Wallace et al., 1982; Khaw and Peart, 1982; Wilson et al., 1984; Cook et al., 1985; Tsai et al., 1985). This has been observed in developing as well as developed countries (Task Force on Oral Contraceptives, 1989). The reported mean changes have ranged from 3.6 to 16.2 mmHg (average 3 to 4 mmHg) systolic and 1.0 to 10.2 mm Hg diastolic. The rise in blood pressure, especially systolic pressure, is usually seen within the first 6 months. In most women, it seems to remain level after 1 to 2 years, whereas in others it may continue to rise. In most cases, the blood pressure returns to previous levels within a few months after the OC is stopped, but this may take as long as 1 year (Woods, 1967; Laragh et al., 1967; Weinberger et al., 1969, Weir et al., 1974; Brown et al., 1978; Weir, 1982). In a few cases, particularly in older women, the blood pressure may not return to pre-OC-use levels. Similar residual blood pressure effects have been noted after treatment of other specific types of hypertension such as renovascular hypertension (Ramsay and Waller, 1990) and Conn's syndrome (Ferriss et al., 1978), and have been attributed to pressure-induced changes such as vascular hypertrophy in the resistance vessels (Folkow et al., 1973; Lever, 1986).

Analysis of the extensive prospective observations just listed shows a prevalence of hypertension (defined by a blood pressure of 140/90 mm Hg) of 4% to 5%. In large, prospective studies in initially normotensive women conducted in both the U.S. and U.K., the frequency of frank hypertension after 3 to 5 years of using OCs containing 50 to 100 µg estrogen and 1 to 4 mg progestin was 2.6 to 5 times higher than in nonusers. This estimate may be too low, however, since the arbitrary levels of 140/90 are based on epidemiological and actuarial data that may not be specifically applicable to young women under the age of 25 years, in whom much lower levels of blood pressure are usually observed.

Occasionally severe hypertension may occur in OC users, and this can develop into malignant (accelerated) phase hypertension and possibly renal failure (Harris, 1969; Wallace, 1971; Dunn et al., 1975; Hodsman et al., 1982; Petitti and Klatsky, 1983; Lim et al., 1987). This hypertension can occur within 4 months after starting OCs in previously normotensive women. It is less likely to be associated with underlying renal disease than malignant hypertension in nonusers. After withdrawal of the OC, the blood pressure may not return to normal but these women usually require less antihypertensive therapy than nonusers (Lim et al., 1987).

EFFECT OF ESTROGEN AND PROGESTIN DOSE

Earlier studies of blood pressure changes associated with OCs were based mainly on combinations containing 50 to 100 μg estrogen and 1 to 4 mg progestin. The effect of lower doses is less well defined. One cross-sectional population study claimed that the blood pressure was higher in women taking pills containing 30 μg estrogen than in those taking 50 μg estrogen combinations (Meade et al., 1977).

Another trial using a low-dose OC showed no significant blood pressure change in 36 women after 1 year, nor in 10 women after 2 years (Rudel et al., 1978).

In a standardized prospective study (Wilson et al., 1984), 64 women taking 30 μg ethynylestradiol (EE) plus 150 μg levonorgestrel (LNG) for 2 years showed mean increases of 7.0 mm Hg (P< 0.02) and 3.2 mm Hg systolic and diastolic, respectively. Sixty-eight women taking 30 μg EE plus 2 mg ethynodiol diacetate had a mean increase of 7.2 mm Hg systolic (P<0.01) and 3.0 mm Hg diastolic (P<0.05). No significant change in pressure occurred in women taking 500 μg ethynodiol diacetate, 350 μg norethisterone, or 75 μg norgestrel progestin-only OCs, nor in a control group using intrauterine devices or barrier methods.

The WHO Task Force on Oral Contraceptives reported the results of a randomized double blind trial of 680 women using contraceptives containing either 50 or 30 μg EE combined with 250 μg LNG (1989). There was no significant difference in the changes in blood pressure between the higher- and lower-dose estrogen groups.

Even with the use of lower-dose estrogen/progestin combinations, malignant phase hypertension can still rarely occur (Hodsman et al., 1982; Lim et al., 1987).

It seems likely that the estrogen component is the major factor causing the rise in blood pressure, as there is no evidence that progestins alone have this effect (MacKay et al., 1971; Spellacy and Birk, 1972; Hawkins and Benster, 1977; Wilson et al., 1984). However, there is some evidence that the progestin may contribute to the hypertensive effect of the combined preparation (Khaw and Peart 1982); since it has no independent action, some form of interaction with the estrogen must be assumed. To date, there are no adequate data to suggest that this effect is more likely to occur with one type of progestin than another.

SUSCEPTIBILITY AND CARDIOVASCULAR RISKS

Several studies have shown that women who have high blood pressure when taking combined OCs may well be those who would be likely to develop hypertension spontaneously. Among these candidates are women who are older, heavier, or have a family history of hypertension and cardiovascular disease (Spellacy and Birk, 1972; Clezy et al., 1972; Fisch et al., 1972; RCGP, 1974; Fisch and Frank, 1977; Khaw and Peart, 1982). However, this development was not found in the WHO Task Force Study (1989). Women with preexisting hypertension do not appear to be more susceptible (Spellacy and Birk, 1974). Some reports have suggested that women with previous pregnancy-induced hypertension are more likely to develop hypertension while taking OCs, but other workers have not confirmed this (Spellacy and Birk, 1972; Clezy et al., 1972; Smith, 1972; Pritchard and Pritchard, 1977; Khaw and Peart, 1982; Task Force on Oral Contraceptives, 1989).

No evidence suggests that a rise in blood pressure is associated with a concurrent gain in weight, fluid retention, or cigarette smoking, or with social class (Weir et al., 1974). No significant change in mean blood pressure was found in a group of 2,000 black women taking OCs for up to 2 years in the U.S. (Blumstein et al., 1980), but in a U.K. study black women had a rise in blood pressure similar to white women (Khaw and Peart, 1982). The current evidence, therefore, indicates that a high-risk group, likely to develop OC hypertension, cannot easily be identified. However, there are characteristics known to increase the risk of cardiovascular diseases in OC users, including cigarette smoking, diabetes mellitus, and hyperlipidemia (Kannel, 1977; Meade, 1988).

It is widely believed that the cardiovascular risks attributed to OCs have been substantially reduced by the use of lower-dose combinations containing 20 to 35 μg estrogen and 75 μg to 2 mg progestin (Porter et al., 1987; Meade, 1988; Mishell, 1988). Also, past users of OCs do not appear to be at greater risk of cardiovascular or cerebrovascular disease than women who have never taken these agents (Stampfer et al., 1988).

MECHANISMS OF ACTION OF ORAL CONTRACEPTIVES ON BLOOD PRESSURE

The Determinants of Systemic Blood Pressure

Blood pressure is the result of cardiac output, which depends on heart rate, stroke volume, venous return, and total peripheral resistance (TPR) (which is inversely related to the diameter of the resistance vessels). The lumen diameter depends on vascular smooth muscle mass, tone, and elasticity. Blood viscosity will also affect resistance. An uncompensated effect on any of these components could result in altered blood pressure. The major controlling factors are neurotransmitters such as noradrenaline and acetylcholine, and a wide range of endocrine and paracrine systems with either vasoconstricting (e.g., angiotensin II) or vasorelaxing (e.g., some prostaglandins) action (see Benjamin and Vallance, 1991).

It is probably fair to state that the precise mechanisms of OC effects on blood pressure are not yet known. However, there is some information on their actions on a number of aspects of blood pressure control; this provides a basis on which to speculate. The OCs may act by either promoting pressor systems or inhibiting depressor systems.

EFFECTS ON CARDIAC FUNCTION

Estradiol administration to guinea pigs over a period of weeks raised cardiac output, whereas progesterone did not (Hart et al., 1985; Veille et al., 1986). Heart rate remained unchanged but stroke volume increased. Since no change in blood pressure occurred over this period, TPR must have fallen. Thus, it is difficult to say whether the change in cardiac output was the primary estrogen effect or whether it was a secondary response to reduced TPR. Similar results have been reported in sheep (Lumbers, 1990) and in women taking combined OCs (Lim et al., 1970).

The mechanism of these changes is not known. It is of interest that the large blood vessels and the heart have well-characterized estrogen receptors, making some direct cardiovascular action a possibility. Alternatively, estrogens may act centrally, since the brain possesses receptors (e.g., Peck et al., 1979). It is only possible to speculate on the relevance of these changes to the rise in blood pressure. However, it is known that certain types of hormone excess may affect blood pressure at first by raising cardiac output; this elevation may then return to normal, but the pressure is maintained by a subsequent rise in TPR (Wenting et al., 1982; Scoggins et al., 1984).

CHANGES IN ELECTROLYTE AND FLUID BALANCE

As Weinberger and Weir (1983) point out, edema may occur during OC use, suggesting a positive sodium balance with associated fluid retention. This edema would tend to raise blood pressure, in part because of increased intravascular volume and secondly because sodium retention increases pressor sensitivity. However, when measured directly, total body sodium in a small group of OC users with raised blood pressure during use was not different from a matched group with essential hypertension (McAreavy et al., 1983). In this group and another study, total body sodium was within a previously published normal range (Beretta-Piccoli et al., 1981). McAreavy et al. (1983) also found no OC-related changes in total body potassium or plasma electrolyte concentrations.

CHANGES IN PRESSOR HORMONE LEVELS
AND PRESSOR SENSITIVITY

Hormones such as angiotensin II, noradrenaline, and vasopressin raise blood pressure by direct action on the smooth muscle of the vessel wall. Sensitivity of the vascular wall to these agonists can vary (e.g., due to body electrolyte status (see previous section), agonist receptor numbers or affinity, cell electrolyte content, vessel wall structure, and many other variables).

Angiotensin II is an octapeptide released in the circulation: 1) from an α_2 globulin substrate, plasma renin substrate, or angiotensinogen; and 2) by the successive actions of the renal enzyme renin, and a converting enzyme located in blood and tissues. Plasma renin substrate concentrations are rate-limiting in humans (Gordon, 1983). Levels are invariably raised during OC use; the rise is large but not correlated with changes in blood pressure. Angiotensin II concentration may be raised (see McAreavey et al., 1983; Kotchen et al., 1979; Leenen et al., 1980), but the change is proportionately smaller because plasma renin concentration may fall. No useful data on catecholamines or vasopressin are available; evidence of a causal relationship between blood pressure and these changes is therefore lacking.

It is also possible that the response to a given quantity of an agonist is increased. For example, high sodium intake increases pressor sensitivity to angiotensin II (Fraser et al., 1969) and glucocorticoid excess elicits the same effect with respect to noradrenaline (Russo et al., 1990). Are OC users sensitized to pressor agents? This possibility, raised by McAreavy et al. (1983), has recently received some corroboration by experiments in sheep (Lumbers, 1990). Although EE caused a small fall in basal blood pressure, subsequent responses to angiotensin II were greater than those of control animals. No other pressor agents were tested, so that the specificity of this effect is unknown. However, no such sensitization resulted from progestin treatment.

POSSIBLE MECHANISMS OF INCREASED PRESSOR SENSITIVITY

The control of contractility of vascular smooth muscle is complex (see Stull et al., 1991) and, as stated earlier, changes in its responsiveness to pressor agonists might result from several separate and/or interacting processes. Some pressor hormones are also thought to act as vascular smooth muscle growth factors. Continuous infusion of initially subpressor doses of angiotensin II into rats slowly raises blood pressure over a period of weeks, and this is accompanied by an increase in sensitivity to acutely administered angiotensin II (Brown et al., 1983; Lever, 1986; Griffin et al., 1991). Angiotensin II stimulates vascular smooth muscle growth rate *in vitro* (Lyall et al., 1988). The small increases in plasma angiotensin II concentration reported during OC treatment might possibly act in this way. Insulin may have a similar action (Lever and Harrap, 1991).

Increased wall:lumen ratio should increase pressor sensitivity. Another mechanism may be a change in the responsiveness of individual cells. There appears to be no relevant information on the effect of OC treatment on the characteristics of vascular smooth muscle pressor agonist receptors. However, there is evidence that cell electrolyte status and plasma membrane characteristics are changed.

Cell electrolytes such as sodium, calcium, and magnesium, as well as intracellular pH are correlated with blood pressure (see Resnick et al., 1991) and specific changes in the Na^+/H^+ exchange process, with accompanying changes in cell volume, have been reported in both hypertensive rats and human subjects with essential hypertension (see Wehling et al., 1991). Oral contraceptives cause changes in red blood cell sodium flux rates (Smith et al., 1986). Similarly, changes in physical characteristics of cell membranes may alter their contractility. Thus, in certain types of genetically hypertensive rat, the viscosity of the cell membrane is increased (Gleason et al., 1991; Quan Sang et al., 1991; Dominiczak et al., 1991). Viscosity changes with lipid content and there are changes in lipid and lipoprotein metabolism with the use of some OCs (e.g., Ylikorkala et al., 1987, Bagdade and Subbaiah, 1988). However, white blood cell membrane viscosity is reported to be reduced (Bagdade and Subbaiah, 1988).

Finally, increased pressor response could occur if the synthesis of a compensating vasorelaxing factor is impaired. One such factor is prostaglandin.

OTHER RELEVANT HORMONAL CHANGES

Hypertension is a common feature of non-insulin-dependent diabetes mellitus and obesity, both of which are characterized by insulin resistance and reduced glucose tolerance. The relationship of insulin resistance and blood pressure has recently been reviewed by Rocchini (1991). Related changes in intracellular calcium, magnesium, and pH have been studied by Resnick et al. (1991). A similar resistance, albeit smaller and readily reversible, has frequently been noted in OC users (Tsibris et al., 1980; Skouby et al., 1987; Kasdorf and Kalkoff, 1988). The progestin component may at least contribute to this phenomenon; in the isolated perfused rat hind limb, Hager and Kalkoff (1991) report an impairment of insulin's action on glucose uptake by norethindrone but not LNG. Earlier studies suggest that increased insulin levels stimulate arterial cholesterol synthesis (Stout, 1969), which might increase cell membrane viscosity.

Prostaglandin (PGI_2) infusion attenuates the pressor action of angiotensin II (Broughton-Pipkin et al., 1989), and antiprogestins stimulate PGI_2 release from some types of tissue *in vitro* (Kelly et al., 1986; Smith and Kelly, 1987). Prostaglandin production is positively correlated with circulating lipoprotein levels that may be altered during OC-use. However, available evidence suggests that some progestins may also increase PGI_2 release, thus tending to reduce blood pressure (Ylikorkala et al., 1987). In recent years, OCs have been discussed briefly by Nawroth and Ziegler (1991) but no direct information on endothelial hormones is yet available.

There is some evidence that the clearance rate of synthetic glucocorticoids such as prednisolone is reduced by OCs (Frey and Frey, 1985; Gustavson et al., 1986). Very small increases in the circulating levels of glucocorticoids can cause significant increases in blood pressure (Tonolo et al., 1988). However, whether this increase provides a pressor mechanism in women taking OCs remains to be determined.

Finally, Scoggins et al. (1984) have postulated on the basis of experiments in sheep that some steroids may have a direct effect on blood pressure. It is of interest that two such components were derivatives of progesterone.

SUMMARY

Oral contraceptives raise blood pressure to a small extent on the average; in some women with other factors or life styles predisposing them to hypertension and cardiovascular disease this elevation may reach the level of clinical significance. The risks in terms of increased morbidity and mortality of rises in blood pressure of this small magnitude have been evaluated (Isles et al., 1986; Stokes et al., 1989).

It is likely that the estrogenic component is largely responsible for the changes in blood pressure; any such risk may be reduced by using lower-dose OCs (however, see Hodsman et al., 1982). It is possible that the progestin may also contribute. OCs have many diverse metabolic and endocrine repercussions, several of which could affect blood pressure. However, the precise mechanism of action in this respect remains unknown.

REFERENCES

Bagdade JD, Subbaiah PV. Influence of low-estrogen-containing oral contraceptives on lipoprotein phospholipid composition and mononuclear cell membrane fluidity. *J Clin Endocrinol Metab* 1988; 66:857–61.

Beretta-Piccoli C, Davies DL, Boddy K, et al. Relation of arterial pressure with body sodium, body potassium and plasma potassium in essential hypertension. *Clin Sci* 1981;76:529–34.

Blumstein BA, Douglas MB, Hall WD. Blood pressure changes and oral contraceptive use: a study of 2,676 black women in the South-Eastern United States. *Am J Epidemiol* 1980;112:529–32.

Broughton-Pipkin F, Morrison R, O'Brien PMS: Prostacyclin attenuates both the pressor and adrenocortical response to angiotensin II in human pregnancy. *Clin Sci* 1989;76:529–34.

Brown AJ, Clark SA, Lever AF. Slow rise and diurnal change of blood pressure with saralasin and angiotensin II in rats. *Am J Physiol* 1983;244:F84–8.

Brown JJ, Cumming AMM, Lever AF, et al. Hypertension in coronary artery heart disease in young women. In Oliver MF, ed. *Coronary heart disease in young women*. Edinburgh: Churchill-Livingstone; 1978: 162–72.

Brownrigg GM. Toxemia in hormone-induced pseudopregnancy. *Can Med Assoc J* 1962;87:408–9.

Clezy TM, Foy BM, Hodge RL, Lumbers ER. Oral Contraceptives and hypertension: an epidemiological survey. *Br Heart J* 1972;34:1,238–43.

Cook NR, Scherr PA, Evans DA, et al. Regression analysis of changes in blood pressure with oral contraceptive use. *Am J Epidemiol* 1985;121:530–40.

Crane MG, Harris JJ, Winsor W. Hypertension, oral contraceptive agents and conjugated estrogens. *Ann Intern Med* 1971;74:13–21.

Dominiczak AF, Lazar DF, Das AK, Bohr DF. The lipid layer in genetic hypertension. *Hypertension* [*in press*].

Dunn FG, Jones JV, Fife R. Malignant hypertension associated with the use of oral contraceptives. *Br Heart J* 1975;37:336–8.

Elkik F, Basdevant A, Jackanicz TM, et al. Contraception in hypertensive women using a vaginal ring delivering estradiol and levonorgestrel. *J Clin Endocrinol Metab* 1986;63:29–35.

Faraci FM, Heistad DD. Regulation of cerebral blood vessels by humoral and endothelium-dependent mechanisms. Update on humoral regulation of vascular tone. *Hypertension* 1991;17:917–22.

Ferriss JB, Beevers DG, Brown JJ, et al. Clinical, biochemical and pathological features of low-renin (primary) hyperaldosteronism. *Am Heart J* 1978;95:375–88.

Fisch LR, Freedman SH, Myatt AV. Oral contraceptives, pregnancy and blood pressure. *JAMA* 1972; 22:1,507–10.

Fisch LR, Frank J. Oral contraceptives and blood pressure. *JAMA* 1977;237;2,499–503.

Folkow B, Hallback M , Lundgren Y, et al. Importance of adaptive changes in vascular design for establishment of primary hypertension, studied in man and in spontaneously hypertensive rats. *Circulation Res* 1973;32[Suppl 1]:2–16.

Fraser R, Brown JJ, Chinn R, et al. The control of aldosterone secretion and its relationship to the diagnosis of hyperaldosteronism. *Scot Med J* 1969;14:420–40.

Frey BM, Frey FJ. The effect of altered prednisolone kinetics in patients with the nephrotic syndrome and in women taking oral contraceptive steroids on human mixed lymphocyte cultures. *J Clin Endocrinol Metab* 1985;60:361–9.

Gleason MM, Medow MS, Tulenko TN. Excess membrane cholesterol alters calcium movements, cytosolic calcium levels and membrane fluidity in arterial smooth muscle cells. *Circulation Res* 1991; 69:216–27.

Gordon DB. The role of renin substrate in hypertension. *Hypertension* 1983;5:353–62.

Griffin SA, Brown WC, McPherson F, et al. Angiotensin II causes vascular hypertrophy in part by a nonpressor mechanism. *Hypertension* 1991;17:626–35.

Gustavson LE, Legler UF, Benet LZ. Impairment of prednisolone disposition in women taking oral contraceptives or conjugated estrogens. *J Clin Endocrinol Metab* 1986;62:234–7.

Hager SR, Kalkhoff RK. Levonorgestrel and norethindrone alter insulin action on skeletal muscle of the female rat. *Horm Metab Res* 1991;22:265–8.

Harris PWR. Malignant hypertension with oral contraceptives. *Lancet* 1969;2:466–7.

Hart MV, Hosenpud JD, Hohimes AR, Morton MJ. Haemodynamics during pregnancy and sex steroid administration in guinea pigs. *Am J Physiol* 1985;249:R179–85.

Hawkins DF, Benster B. A comparative study of three low dose progestogens, chlormadinone acetate, megestrol acetate and norethisterone as oral contraceptives. *Br J Obstet Gynaecol* 1977;84:708–13.

Hodsman GP, Robertson JIS, Semple PF, McKay A. Malignant hypertension and oral contraceptives: four cases with two due to 30 μg oestrogen pill. *Europ Heart J* 1982;3:255–9.

Isles CG, Walker LM, Beevers GD, et al. Mortality in patients of the Glasgow Blood Pressure Clinic. *J Hypertension* 1986;4:141–156.

Kannel WB. Cardiovascular hazards of oral contraceptive use. *JAMA* 1977;237:2,530.

Kasdorf G, Kalkhoff RK. Prospective studies of insulin sensitivity in normal women receiving oral contraceptive agents. *J Clin Endocrinol Metab* 1988;66:846–52.

Kelly RW, Healy DL, Cameron MJ, et al. The stimulation of prostaglandin production by two antiprogesterone steroids in human endometrial cells. *J Clin Endocrinol Metab* 1986;62:1,116–1,123.

Khaw KT, Peart WS. Blood pressure and contraceptive use. *Br Med J* 1982;285:403–7.

Kotchen TA, Kotchen JM, Guthrie G, Cottrill CM. Plasma renin activity, reactivity, concentration and substrate following hypertension during pregnancy. Effect of oral contraceptive agents. *Hypertension* 1979;1:355–61.

Kunin CM, McCormack RC, Abernathy JR. Oral contraceptives and blood pressure. *Arch Intern Med* 1969;123:363–5.

Laragh JH, Sealey JE, Ledingham JGG, Newton MA. Oral contraceptives: renin, aldosterone and high blood pressure. *JAMA* 1967;201:918–22.

Leenen FHH, Boer P, Mees EJD. Oral contraceptives and responsiveness of plasma renin activity and blood pressure in normotensive women. *Clin Exp Hypertension* 1980;A2:197–211.

Lever AF. Slow pressor mechanisms in hypertension: a role for hypertrophy of resistance vessels. *J Hypertension* 1986;4:515–24.

Lever AF, Harrap SB. Essential hypotension: a disorder of growth with origins in childhood. *J Hypertension* 1992;10:101–20.

Lim KG, Isles CG, Hodsman GP, et al. Malignant hypertension in women of childbearing age and its relation to the contraceptive pill. *Br Med J* 1987;294:1,057–9.

Lim YL, Lumbers ER, Walters WAW, Whelan RF. Effect of oestrogen on the human circulation. *Br J Obstet Gynaecol* 1970;77:349–55.

Lumbers ER. Effects on sheep blood pressure of treatment with angiotensin, steroids and salt. *Clin Exp Pharmacol Physiol* 1990;17:315–9.

Lyall F, Morton JJ, Lever AF, Cragoe EJ. Angiotensin II activates Na^+/H^+ exchange and stimulates growth in cultured vascular smooth muscle cells. *J Hypertension* 1988;6[Suppl 4]:S438–41.

McAreavey D, Cumming AMM, Boddy K, et al. The renin-angiotensin system and total body sodium and potassium in hypertensive women taking oestrogen-progestogen oral contraceptives. *Clin Endocrinol* 1983;18:111–8.

MacKay EV, Khoo SH, Adam R. Contraception with a six-monthly injection of progestogen. 1. Effects on blood pressure, body weight, and uterine bleeding pattern, side effects, efficacy and acceptability. *Austral N Zeal J Obstet Gynaecol* 1971;11:148–55.

Meade TW, Haines AP, North WRS, et al. Haemostatic, lipid, and blood pressure profiles of women on oral contraceptives containing 50 μg and 30 μg oestrogen. *Lancet* 1977;2:948-51.

Mishell DR. Contraception. *N Engl J Med* 1989;320:777–87.

Nawroth PP, Ziegler R. Die antibaby-pille als risikfaktor einer thrombose: sind molekulare mechanismen bekannt? *Klin Wchschr* 1991;69:335–9.

Peck EJ, Miller AL, Kener KL. Estrogen receptors and the activation of RNA polymerases by estrogens in the central nervous system. In: Hamilton, TH, Clark JH, Sadler WA, eds. *Ontogeny of receptors and reproductive hormone action.* New York: Raven Press; pp 1979:403–10.

Petitti DB, Klatsky AK. Malignant hypertension in women aged 15 to 44 years and its relation to cigarette smoking and oral contraceptives. *Am J Cardiol* 1983;52:297–8.

Porter JB, Jick H, Walker AM. Mortality among oral contraceptives users. *Obstet Gynecol* 1987;70:29–32.

Pritchard JA, Pritchard SA. Blood pressure response to estrogen-progestagen oral contraceptives after pregnancy-induced hypertension. *Am J Obstet Gynecol* 1977;129:733–9.

Quan Sang KH, Montenau-Garestier T, Devynck MA. Alterations of platelet membrane viscosity in essential hypertension. *Clin Sci* 1991;80:205–11.

Ramsay LE, Waller PC. Blood pressure response to percutaneous transluminal angioplasty for reno-vascular hypertension: an overview of published series. *Br Med J* 1990;300:560–72.

Resnick LM, Gupta RK, Bhargava KK, et al. Cellular ions in hypertension, diabetes and obesity. A nuclear magnetic resonance spectroscopy study. *Hypertension* 1991;17:951–7.

Rocchini AP. Insulin resistance and blood pressure. Regulation in obese and non-obese subjects. *Hypertension* 1991;17:837–42.

Royal College of General Practitioners. *Oral contraceptives and health.* New York: Pitman; 1974:37–42.

Royal College of General Practitioners. Further analyses of mortality in oral contraceptive users. *Lancet* 1981;1:541–6.

Rudel HN, Maqueo M, Calderon J, et al. Safety and effectiveness of a new low dose oral contraceptive: a three year study of 1000 women. *J Reprod Med* 1978;21:79.

Russo D, Fraser R, Kenyon CJ. Increased sensitivity to noradrenaline in glucocorticoid-treated rats: the effects of indomethacin and desipramine. *J Hypertension* 1990;8:827–33.

Scoggins BA, Coghlan JP, Denton DA, Whitworth JA. ACTH-dependent hypertension. *Clin Exp Hypertension* 1984;A6:599–646.

Shaw RW. Adverse long-term effects of oral contraceptives. *Br J Obstet Gynaecol* 1987;94:724–30.

Skouby SO, Andersen O, Saubrey N, Kuhl C. Oral contraception and insulin sensitivity in vivo: assessment in normal women and women with previous gestational diabetes. *J Clin Endocrinol Metab* 1987; 64:519–23.

Smith RW. Hypertension and oral contraceptives. *Am J Obstet Gynecol* 1972;113:482–7.

Smith JB, Wade MB, Fineberg NS, Weinberger MH. Sodium pump parameters of blood cells in men, women and women taking oral contraceptives. *Clin Exp Hypertension* 1986;A8:1,189–1,209.

Smith SK, Kelly RW. The effect of the antiprogestins RU486 and ZK98734 on the synthesis of prostaglandins F_{2a} and E_2 in separated cells from early human decidua. *J Clin Endocrinol Metab* 1987; 65:527–34.

Spellacy WN, Birk SA. The effect of intrauterine devices, oral contraceptives and progestogens on blood pressure. *Am J Obstet Gynecol* 1972;112:912–9.

Spellacy WN, Birk JA. The effects of mechanical and steroid contraceptive methods on blood pressure in hypertensive women. *Fertil Steril* 1974;25:467.

Stampfer MJ, Willett WC, Colditz GA, et al. A prospective study of past use of oral contraceptive agents and risk of cardiovascular disease. *N Engl J Med* 1988;319:1,313–7.

Stokes J, Kannel WB, Wolf PA, et al. Blood pressure as a risk factor for cardiovascular disease. The Framingham Study - 30 years of follow up. *Hypertension* 1989;13[Suppl1]: I-13–8.

Stout RW. Insulin stimulation of cholesterol synthesis by arterial tissue. *Lancet* 1969;2:467–8.

Stull JT, Gallagher PJ, Herring BP, Kamm KE. Vascular smooth muscle contractile elements. Cellular regulation. *Hypertension* 1991;17:723–32.

Task Force on Oral Contraceptives. The WHO Multicentre Trial of the vasopressor effects of combined oral contraceptives: 1. Comparisons with IUD. *Contraception* 1989;40:129–45.

Tolins JP, Shultz PJ, Raij L. Role of endothelium-derived relaxing factor in regulating of vascular tone and remodelling. Update humoral regulation of vascular tone. *Hypertension* 1991;17:909–17.

Tonolo G, Fraser R, Connell JMC, Kenyon CJK. Chronic low-dose infusion of dexamethasone in rats: effects on blood pressure, body weight and plasma atrial natriuretic peptide. *J Hypertension* 1988; 6:25–31.

Tsai CC, Williamson HO, Kirkland BH, et al. Low dose oral contraceptives and blood pressure in women with a past history of elevated blood pressure. *Am J Obstet Gynecol* 1985;151:28–32.

Tsibris JCM, Raynor LO, Buhl WC, et al. Insulin receptors in circulating erythrocytes and monocytes from women on oral contraceptives or pregnancy women near term. *J Clin Endocrinol Metab* 1980; 51:711–7.

Veille JC, Morton MJ, Burry K, et al. Estradiol and hemodynamics during ovulation induction. *J Clin Endocrinol Metab* 1986;63:721–4.

Wallace MR. Oral contraceptives and severe hypertension. *Austral N Zeal J Med* 1971;1:49–52.

Wallace RB, Barrett-Connor E, Criqui M, et al. Alteration in blood pressures associated with combined alcohol and oral contraceptives use - the Lipid Research Clinics Prevalence Study. *J Chron Dis* 1982; 35:251–7.

Wehling M, Käsmayr J, Theisen K. The Na + H + exchanger is stimulated and cell volume increased in lymphocytes from patients with essential hypertension. *J Hypertension* 1991;9:519–24.

Weinberger MH, Collins RD, Dowdy AJ, et al. Hypertension induced by oral contraceptives containing estrogen and gestagen: effects on plasma renin activity and aldosterone excretion. *Ann Intern Med* 1969;71:891–902.

Weinberger MH, Weir RJ. Oral contraceptives and hypertension. In: Robertson JIS, ed. *Handbook of Hypertension*, vol. 2. Amsterdam: Elsevier; 1983:196–207.

Weir RJ. Effect on blood pressure of changing from high to low dose steroid preparations in women with oral contraceptive-induced hypertension. *Scott Med J* 1982;27:212–5.

Weir RJ, Briggs E, Mack A, et al. Blood pressure in women taking oral contraceptives. *Br Med J* 1974;1:533–5.

Weir RJ, Fraser R, McElwee G, et al. The effect of oestrogen-progestogen oral contraceptives on blood pressure and on the renin-angiotensin-aldosterone system. In: Fregly MJ, Fregly MS, eds. *Oral contraception and high blood pressure*. Gainesville: Dolphin Press; 1974:68–81.

Wenting GJ, Man in't Veld AJ, Derkx FHM, Schalekamp MADH. Recurrence of hypertension in primary aldosteronism after discontinuation of spironolactone. Time course of changes in cardiac output and body fluid volumes. *Clin Exp Hypertension* 1982;A4:1,727–48.

Wilson ESB, Cruikshank J, McMaster M, Weir RJ. A prospective controlled study of the effect on blood pressure of contraceptive preparations containing different types and dosages of progestogen. *Br J Obstet Gynaecol* 1984;91:1,254–60.

Woods JW. Oral contraceptives and hypertension. *Lancet* 1967;2:653–4.

Woods JW. Oral contraceptives and hypertension. *Hypertension* 1988;[Suppl 2]:II-ll–5.

Ylikorkala O, Kuusi T, Tikkanen MJ, Viinikka L. Desogestrel- and levonorgestrel-containing oral contraceptives have different effects on urinary excretion of prostacyclin metabolites and serum high density lipoproteins. *J Clin Endocrinol Metab* 1987;65:1,238–42.

Pharmacology of the Contraceptive Steroids,
edited by Joseph W. Goldzieher.
Raven Press, Ltd., New York © 1994.

21

Cardiovascular System: Coagulation, Thrombosis, and Contraceptive Steroids— Is There a Link?

Fritz K. Beller

Department of Obstetrics and Gynecology, University of Iowa College of Medicine, Iowa City, Iowa 52242

The history of epidemiological studies relevant to this issue was recently summarized by Realini and Goldzieher (1985) and Sturtevant (1991). The coagulation story began when anecdotal reports of thrombosis in the *British Medical Journal* in 1961 prompted a group in Oslo to study in a randomized fashion the levels of blood coagulation factors during the use of oral contraceptives (OC)s. Although the number of subjects studied was small, a trend to increased concentrations was noted (Egeberg and Owren, 1963). In a study in which individuals were treated for endometriosis with increasing doses of Enovid (150 μg mestranol/10 mg norethynodrel per tablet, up to 1000 μg per day), it was noted that the increase in certain coagulation factors (I, II, VII, X, plasminogen) was dose-related (Beller and Porges, 1967). The various reports from the Royal College of General Practitioners' study and the British Committee on Safety of Drugs, as well as other reports (Vessey, 1968; Inman and Vessey, 1968; Vessey and Doll, 1968), stimulated a large-scale investigation of the relationship between OCs and blood coagulation. This investigation provided little insight into the development of thromboembolism, but it supported many research laboratories in dealing with blood coagulation worldwide.

PHYSIOLOGY OF BLOOD COAGULATION AND FIBRINOLYSIS

Details of the coagulation cascade belongs to basic physiology and will not be reiterated here. The coagulation factors are procoagulants, a form in which they are inactive. This applies to all coagulation factors, regardless of their production site (Fig. 1). Activation requires a complicated system whereby the cascade is activated step by step, requiring calcium ions. The activated factor is given the affix "a"

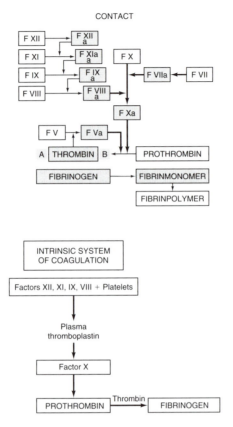

FIG. 1. Coagulation cascade a) intrinsic b) extrinsic system

whether activated by the intrinsic system or via tissue thromboplastin from damaged cells (the extrinsic system). Factor VII is activated to factor VIIa, X to Xa, and so on. The intrinsic pathway is initiated by contact activation of a variety of biological surfaces: long-chain fatty acids and lipopolysaccharin and vascular membranes are only a few. Factor XII is required.

Factor VIII is a complex consisting of VIII:c and VIII:R CoF. Hemophiliacs are deficient in Factor v.WF:C. Von Willebrands's disease results from a deficiency in Factor VIII:RCoF. Also involved is the kinin system. The short-lived activation products make assaying of activation steps of the coagulation cascade difficult. After formation, these products are immediately attacked by a variety of inhibitors, of which the inhibitor against factor Xa is presumably the most important in the prevention of thrombotic episodes. If the cascade has been activated and thrombin has been formed as an end product, it will be attacked by antithrombin (AT). Since thrombin is the activated enzyme, it explains the significance of this inhibitor. (AT III is presumably consumed during its interactions with thrombin.) AT III (belonging to the group of inhibitors that includes alpha one trypsin, alpha two antiplasmin,

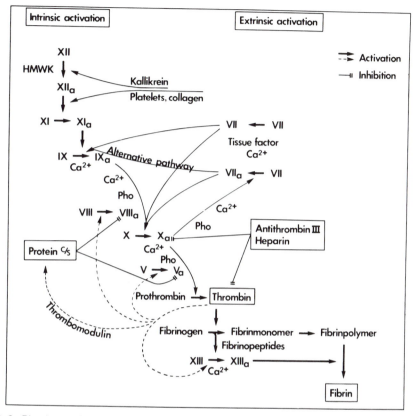

FIG. 2. Blood coagulation activation (From Jespersen et al., 1991, with permission)

and Cl-esterase inhibitor) is the principal inhibitor of thrombin and factor Xa, but also of Factors IXa, XIa, plasmin, and kallikrein.

Platelets are an additional requirement for fibrin formation in the circulation. The interaction with subendothelial collagens requires the Von Willebrand factor (adhesion). Aggregation requires the release of adenosine diphosphate (ADP), platelet factors 3 and 4, serotonin, and thromboxane A_2 (T_xA_2). The surrounding endothelium releases endothelium-derived relaxing factors (EDRF) and prostacyclin. Fibronectin is known to be a marker for the endothelial reaction.

Prostacyclin (prostaglandin I-2, PGI-2) is therefore synthesized in the endothelial lining. It is an antiplatelet aggregator and vasodilator. Platelet membrane, on the other hand, produces thromboxane A-2, which is a powerful platelet aggregator.

Protein C and S are Vitamin-K-dependent plasma proteins. Protein Ca inactivates factor Va and VIIIa, and destroys PA t-l. Protein S serves as a cofactor for the activated C (Fig. 2). If fibrin is formed by the activation of thrombin, it will be

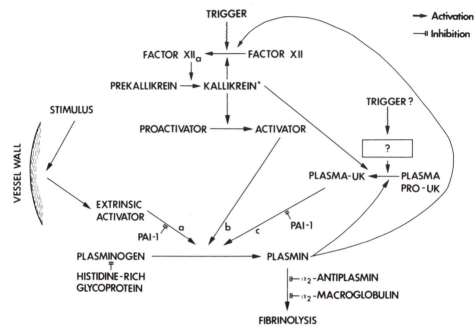

FIG. 3. The fibrinolytic activation (From Jespersen et al., 1990, with permission)

attacked by the fibrinolytic enzyme system. Presumably a predominantly localized phenomenon, the activator substance tPA is present in cells and released in a hypoxic state by a complicated mechanism. The activator diffuses in a given fibrin structure. As a biological phenomenon, the inactive precursor of plasminogen is adherent to fibrinogen. The formation of a fibrin plug thus provides the proenzyme plasminogen, which is activated to plasmin by activator substances. The breakdown of a fibrin clot (a thrombus) releases fibrin breakdown products. Fibrin dimers are the markers for this reaction. In the absence of fibrin, tPA has only a low affinity to plasminogen (Fig. 3).

CRITICAL VALUES

In biology, whenever an enzyme system supports preservation for life or reproduction, the system components are present in excessive amounts. Examples in the field of reproduction are overproduction of sperm and loss of 70% of fertilized eggs. The same applies for the coagulation system as a lifesaving system essential for preserving the integrity of the organism (Table 1). The concentration of factor VIII normally ranges from 60% to 200%. Hemostasis in a hemophiliac is accomplished if a level of 25% is reached. The plasma fibrinogen concentration is normally in the

TABLE 1. *Range of coagulation factors*

Moiety	Normal range	Lowest range
Fibrinogen	250 to 350 mg%	<100
Platelets	200,000 mm^3	<70,000
Factor VIII	90% to 120%	<25%
AT III	90% to 120%	<50%
Factor VII/X	80% to 120%	?

250 to 350 mg/dl range, and blood fails to clot only if the concentration drops to less than 100 mg/dl. Occasionally high fibrinogen concentrations are related to thromboembolic disease. Platelet number in a normal individual is around 200,000/mm^3. But bleeding time is prolonged only when there is less than 75,000/mm^3 available, and patients with thrombocytopenia can support a normal bleeding time with 20,000/mm^3. It is assumed that after clotting, only 11% of prothrombin is converted to thrombin (Table 1).

As first described by Egeberg and Owren (1963), a congenitally low AT III concentration may be associated with frequent episodes of thromboembolic disease. Only if the normal level of 100% drops to less than 50% may some (not all) members of an afflicted family experience thromboembolic episodes. Similar relationships are known for protein C and S deficiencies. Heterozygous deficiency of proteins may be related to venous thrombosis (homozygous deficiency is incompatible with life). Protein S deficiency has also been associated with thrombosis (Comp and Esmon, 1984). The incidence of congenital AT III deficiency is in the magnitude of 1:5,000, and that of protein C is even greater (Winkler et al., 1989).

It is therefore apparent that in order for the system to get biologically out of hand in either the extreme thrombosis or bleeding diathesis, the changes have to be large. Variations within the normal range are of no significance.

HYPERCOAGULABILITY AND THROMBOPHILIC STATE

Terminology

Egeberg and Owren (1963) were most likely the first to use the term "hypercoagulability" in reference to an increase in coagulation factors induced by OCs. The term hypercoagulability had been used improperly for decades to indicate a change in the biochemistry of the coagulation system as a precursor of thrombosis, DIC (disseminated intravascular coagulation) and thrombophlebitis. However, Mammen (1982) pointed out, "If one were to use this word accurately, then consumption coagulopathy, or disseminated intravascular coagulation (DIC) would be the only disease entities that would qualify to be associated with hypercoagulability. Under these circumstances, the patient is truly clotting intravascularly, and this process can be identified by laboratory procedures." Unfortunately, a large number of investigators failed to recognize this basic understanding. Clinically, the term

TABLE 2. *Features of hypercoagulability in blood*

Elevated levels of activated coagulation factors or derivatives:
  F. XIIa, XIa, IXa, Va, Xa
  Thrombin
  Fibrinopeptide A
  Fibrinmonomer
Reduced levels of inhibitors of coagulation:
  Antithrombin III
Accelerated fibrinogen turnover
Platelet release products
  β-Thromboglobulin
  Platelet factor 4
  Circulating platelet aggregates
  Accelerated platelet turnover
Fibrinolytic system:
  Increased titer of plasmin-antiplasmin complexes
  FDP

(According to H Graeff, 1973.)

hypercoagulability was widely used when the clotting mechanism was altered in some way that contributed to thrombosis. But no two clinicians agree on the definition. Stewart (1977) indicated that it is doubtful that an increased level of individual clotting factors would contribute to thrombosis; thus a causal relationship between the level of any factors and thrombosis cannot be established. In Europe the term "thrombophilic" was used to mean that it was a precursor state for thromboembolism. Indeed, there are four pathophysiologically distinct disease entities that are grouped in the category of thromboembolic disease: 1) disseminated intravascular coagulation; 2) thromboembolic disease; 3) thrombophlebitis; and 4) atheromatous disease.

When the coagulation system is triggered *in vitro*, disseminated intravascular coagulation results. This ends in capillary thrombosis of the microcirculation. Trigger systems were identified as: immune complexes; endotoxin (e.g., as in gram-negative septic shock) snake poisons; possibly pregnancy-induced hypertension; and many others (McKay, 1964). The coagulation system in the circulation behaves similarly to the clotting of blood in a test tube; when coagulation factors are assayed in the resulting serum, a variety of coagulation factors have decreased to low values because they were consumed. This behavior is characteristic of plasma fibrinogen and platelets (Fig. 3). It is generally accepted that a decrease in plasma fibrinogen concentration and platelet number relevant to febrile conditions demonstrates a slow, steady development of DIC, but there is no precursor state known.

Thromboembolic disease circumscribes a disease state whereby a thrombus is formed in a given venous channel, usually in the lower extremity. Fragmentation of the red apposition thrombus may lead to pulmonary embolism with survival or death. There is no increase in the concentration of various coagulation factors preceding a thromboembolic episode, as indicated in countless papers.

Although thrombophlebitis is the most frequently acquired disease in this group, the etiology is poorly understood. Some investigators believe that the local phlebitis of a superficial vein is related to inflammatory processes (as in pelvic vein thrombosis). Other authors refer to an immunologic etiology. Regardless of the origin, activation of the coagulation cascade is not an etiologic event. Only if a given thrombus extends into the deep venous system may phlebothrombosis be the final stage.

Atheromatous disease is related to the arterial vascular tree and is secondary to an altered fat metabolism, ending in atheromatous plaques that may lead to myocardial infarction. However, there are no coagulation changes that may predict myocardial disease. This also applies to changes in fat metabolism.

At present, there is controversy about the classification of cerebral vascular accidents in this grouping.

None of the four phenomena interrelate; thromboembolism is almost never associated with DIC, and vice versa. There is also no relationship between thromboembolism and cardiovascular disease. Numerous investigators have tried to construct a laboratory definition for the term hypercoagulability. This was summarized by Kitchens (1985), who concluded in his review that it is "naive to expect that any test or series of tests could detect all processes that result in an increased tendency to thrombosis."

The most frequent use of the term hypercoagulability applies to pregnancy.

Hypercoagulable State in Pregnancy

Various coagulation problems in pregnancy, which are explained by acute or chronic DIC, toxemia, premature separation of the placenta, and the dead fetus syndrome (and many others) were described before the physiology of the coagulation system in pregnancy was clarified. The first reports by Beller (1958) indicated an increase in coagulation factors (Fig. 4). Some coagulation times were observed to be shorter for women in the nonpregnant state (e.g., bleeding time and plasma coagulation time).

It is said that thromboembolic episodes are approximately 10 times more frequent in the puerperal phase. However, all publications failed to evaluate what cesarean section as a surgical procedure contributed to the higher incidence in the puerperium (Beller et al., unpublished). Considering the presence of all factors of Virchow's Triad in pregnancy, thromboembolism in pregnancy is rather rare, with the exception of thrombophlebitis. To bridge the difference between assumption and facts, researchers frequently use the phrase, "The hypercoagulability in pregnancy is balanced." At present it is unknown why the various coagulation factors are increased. A variety of etiologic explanations were proposed:

a) increased protein production by estrogens
b) rebound relevant to chronic consumption or low-grade DIC (McKay, 1982)
c) altered turnover (especially platelets and fibrinogen)
d) altered function of the RES in pregnancy

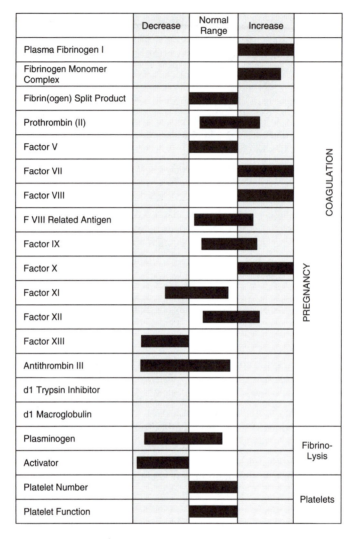

FIG. 4. Changes of the coagulation and fibrinolytic system in pregnancy (semischematic). (From Beller and Ebert, 1984, with permission.)

Since the increase of coagulation proteins is speculative and may be multifactorial, the comparison between the increase in coagulation factors in pregnancy and those in OCs is at present an analogy at best.

NORMAL CYCLE AND AGE CHANGES

The older literature reflects an increase in platelet number at ovulation time. Coagulation factors varied slightly with the cycle but not significantly (Ambrus et al., 1972; Beller et al., 1968; Jespersen et al., 1983; Lebech et al., 1990; Siegbahn and Odlind, 1992). According to Ygge (1969), variation within the cycle was smaller than variation between individuals during the menstrual cycle. Mandalaki et al. (1980) found an increase in factor VIII from day 15 to 21.

The literature indicates an age-related increase in plasmatic components without an increase in thrombosis (Mammen, 1990). However, investigators have used women in specific age groups and compared them with general data. Gram et al. (1990) concluded that "healthy women older than 30 years who use oral contraceptives containing 30 to 50 mcg of EE have an enhanced generation and resolution of fibrin." There were, however, no age-specific controls to support this statement. This applies also to the assumption of Siegbahn and Ruusuvara (1988). When an age-controlled study employing modern technology was performed, in a group of women age 15 to 25 versus age 35 to 45, there was no difference in coagulation and fat metabolism data (Beller and Mantman, unpublished).

INFLUENCE OF STEROIDS ON COAGULATION FACTORS

Animal Experimentation

The small number of animal experiments using estrogens and progesterone is remarkable. The classic animal experiment for DIC is the generalized Schwarzman reaction. In this experiment, rabbits experience clotting in their microcirculation after two intravenous injections of lipopolysaccharide spaced 24 hours apart (McKay, 1964). However, DIC can be elicited in all species if the endotoxin is infused over several hours (Beller and Graeff, 1967). In term pregnancy, less endotoxin is required in comparison to the nonpregnant state to elicit an identical phenomenon (Beller et al., 1983). When rabbits, rats, and guinea pigs were prepared with estrogens and progestational agents, the potentiating activity so effective in pregnancy failed to appear (Beller and Schoendorff, 1976). Similarly, in a few experiments Wessler's group did not see thrombosis in his activated factor X model in rabbits, although some changes were obvious. A thrombogenic stimulus was needed in order to elicit thrombosis (Gitel et al., 1978). Kobayashi and Takeda (1977) found a decrease in AT III in dogs after intramuscular injection of two excessive doses of estrogen 8 hours apart, corresponding to a thousandfold overdose compared with those used in human beings.

Receptors

Recently, estrogen and progesterone receptors in vascular channels were related to thromboembolic events. These data were derived almost exclusively from endometrial tissue. Immunocytochemical studies revealed the presence of estrogen and progesterone receptors in smooth muscle walls of uterine arteries (Perrot-Applaud et al., 1988), while others were unable to confirm this study (Press and Greene, 1988; Jordan et al., 1990). Vascular endothelium does not contain steroid receptors;

it is therefore uncertain whether steroid hormones have a direct action on blood vessels (Sheppard, 1991). It is purely speculative to relate microthrombosis in capillaries of the endometrium under OC use to the etiology of thrombosis in general (Song et al., 1970). Endometrial tissue differs from all other functional linings in that it exerts coagulation properties unique in the human body.

Progesterone, Progestational Agents

Medroxyprogesterone Acetate (MPA)

A number of authors have demonstrated that there is little or no effect on blood coagulation after use of MPA (Passo et al., 1982; Stangel et al., 1977; Poller et al., 1969, 1971, 1977; Coope and Poller, 1977; Astedt et al., 1972). This applies also to MPA when given in injected doses of 150 mg every 3 months (Weenick et al., 1984). Very small changes were noted in women taking progestin-only OCs (Ball et al., 1991). Depo provera did not induce changes in the coagulation and fibrinolytic enzyme systems (Fahmy et al., 1991; Ibrahim et al., 1988; Schwallie and Assenzo, 1973; Tsakok et al., 1980; Whigham et al., 1979). A slight decrease in AT III was found after 15 months of use (Fahmy et al., 1991), but no change was seen in soluble fibrin monomers. When MPA was used in a very high dosage of 800 mg/day for treatment of breast cancer, only variations within the normal range were found, except for an increase in AT III (Ganzina and Robuscelli, 1982). Astedt et al. (1972) failed to find changes in the tissue activator of the fibrinolytic enzyme system after use of MPA.

Other Progestins

Little change was found after use of norgestrenone except in cases of high doses (350 mg), when AT III was affected (Conrad et al., 1991). Poller et al. (1972) found a reduced tendency of coagulability with 0.35 mg norethindrone after 6 months of use. After depot norethisterone was given for 2 years, factor X was reduced from 90.3% to 78.7%. After 5 years of use it was significantly higher than in the controls (McEwan and Griffin, 1991). After injectable NET acetate/ estradiol valerate was given, no changes were found (Meng et al., 1990). The new progestational device Norplant produced a decrease in coagulation factors after 2 years (Prasad et al., 1989), but no change was noted after 5 years (Singh et al., 1992). No decrease was noted when chlormadinone acetate was given in daily doses of 0.5 mg (Nilson et al., 1970). Also, nomegestrol (a 19-norprogesterone derivative) did not change coagulation parameters in a dose of 5 mg/day.

Cyproterone Acetate (CPA)

This potent progestational agent was also found to be coagulation inert (Hirvonen et al., 1988; Jamin and Aiach, 1987).

Recently a new steroid, OD14, that is structurally related to norethynodrel has been introduced. It has very mild estrogenic, androgenic, and progestational activity. It is supposed to be used in premenopausal women. Factor I, VII, and VIII dropped slightly in the normal range and platelets increased as a reflection of a hematopoetic effect (Walker et al., 1985; Parkin et al., 1987; Cortes-Pietro, 1987).

It should be especially noted that the lack of change in the coagulation system or even reduced concentration of factors concurs with the total lack of evidence of thrombotic phenomena of any kind in the international literature on progestins. The progestins used in recently developed combination OCs (desogestrel, gestodene, norgestimate) have not been studied without estrogens added.

A "trend toward hypercoagulability" was also noted during the use of MPA: the partial thromboplastin time was "activated," but no other change in coagulation factors was present (Baele et al.,). Blombäck (1991) stated that "newer markers can determine whether hypercoagulation is present instead of guessing about it on the basis of increased levels of coagulation factors or decreased levels of inhibitors." Perhaps the most bewildering statements in this regard come from Oriental authors. Although a decrease (and not an increase) of nearly all coagulation factors and an increase (and not a decrease) of AT III was noted 2 years after Norplant insertion, the authors state that "the acceptors have an increased predisposition to thrombosis" (Prasad et al., 1989). It has to be noted that no epidemiological data relate thromboembolism to progestational agents. The frequently quoted incidence of around 1.5% (Bastert and Michel, 1983) relates to cancer therapy, and was seen only when used in a thousandfold increase of dose in a nonrandomized study. When MPA was given orally in amounts of 800 mg/day for 6 months, the authors noted: 1) a decrease in factor VII and fibrinogen; 2) an increase in AT III, plasminogen, and alpha 2-plasmin inhibitor complex; and 3) a decrease in fibrin degradation products. They believe that "these results indicate that MPA may induce hypercoagulability, but this state does not directly lead to the development of thrombosis" (Yamamoto et al., 1991).

Estrogens

Research on pure estrogen preparations is related to menopausal replacement therapy except in some "morning after" pills that use high doses of estrogens. The study of Weenick et al. (1984) did not reveal dramatic changes with this high-dose, short application. The so-called "natural" estrogens rather than mestranol or ethynyl estradiol (EE) are used in the menopause. However, it should be remembered that the activity of a given estrogen can be increased by increasing the dose. Beller et al. (1978) have shown that 80 μg mestranol, which in activity corresponds to approximately 50 μg EE changed the coagulation system similar to the OC. The data of Poller et al. (1977) are difficult to interpret, since they did not differentiate between 0.625 mg and 1.25 mg equine estrogens (Premarin), although the latter is already a dose producing a high estrogen activity. Astedt (1977) found no signs of "ongoing intravascular coagulation" exemplified by platelet count, fibrinogen, activity of AT

III, and other inhibitors when 0.625 mg or 1.25 mg Premarin was given for 21 of 28 days and MPA added (10 mg for 7 of 28 days). Similar data were reported by Hunter et al. (1979) and Notelovitz, (1977). The application of estradiol via patch produced only minimal or no changes in AT III and tissue plasminogen activator (TPA) (Alkjaersig et al., 1988; Lindoff et al., 1988).

Conjugated estrogens and estradiol implants of 50 to 100 mg in the forearm given in 3 to 4 monthly applications decreased AT III and protein S but not prothrombin fragment 1 + 2 (see later section) (Rugman et al., 1991). Although postmenopausal estrogen replacement therapy is not associated with a higher incidence of thromboembolism, the authors state that their finding may "predispose to thrombosis." However, Young et al. (1991), reviewing the world literature, have concluded that there is no evidence that estrogen replacement therapy is conducive to venous thrombosis.

Tamoxifen is a weak estrogen/antiestrogen frequently used for treatment of breast cancer. Jordan et al. (1987) did not find any changes of the coagulation system after use of this compound.

The Effect of Combination OCs on Coagulation

The effect of OCs on blood coagulation have been summarized in various publications in the mid 1980s (Jespersen, 1988; Notelovitz, 1985). In our own review (Beller and Ebert, 1986), the data from studies with OCs with 50 or more μg EE were used. Three patterns emerged Fig. 5:

1. The increase in Factors I (fibrinogen), VII/X and plasminogen were congruent;
2. The changes were very similar to those found physiologically in pregnancy;
3. The extreme variation in results between various groups of investigators reflected the low comparability of various techniques used.

Meade et al. (1976) listed the following factors to explain the confusing picture of the outcome of OC studies:

a) the small groups of women studied
b) wide variations in individuals' biological clotting factor levels, so that real differences between groups may be missed unless fairly large numbers are studied
c) the fact that women using or not using OCs have rarely been drawn from the same defined population and may differ in various respects
d) differences in laboratory methods and the large laboratory error in many of the biological assays used

These reviews referred to OCs with an EE component of ≥50 μg. In the meantime, preparations were studied with 35 μg and even 20 μg EE. For the data on higher dose EE, the reader is referred to the reviews mentioned. Regardless of dose, no change was seen in the contact activation system (i.e., factor XII and prekallekrein levels (Gordon et al., 1983; Winkler et al., 1989). Sabra and Bonnar

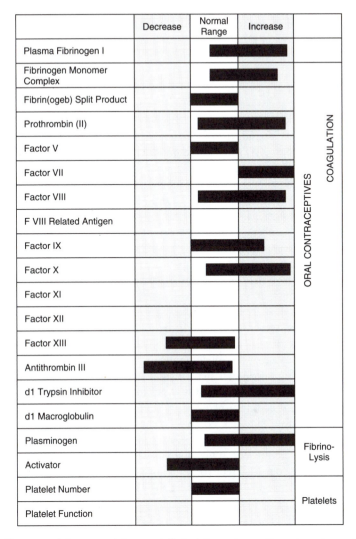

FIG. 5. Changes of the coagulation and fibrinolytic system with oral contraception (semi-schematic). (From Beller and Ebert, 1984, with permission.)

(1983) compared a 50 μg against a 30 μg dose and found a lower increase of factors with the lower dose. Using low EE in combination with a variety of progestins, fibrinogen and the coagulation factors VII and X varied within the normal range or not at all (Jespersen, 1983; Prasad et al., 1989; Winkler et al., 1991), Meade and Thompson, (1980) indicated that EE in a dose of 30 μg together with desogestrel seemed "virtually to eliminate the effect of OCs on hemostasis." This finding contradicts the opinion that the new low estrogen/progestin OCs induce major changes in the fibrinolytic and coagulation systems as claimed by Sabra and Bonnar (1983). Very little change was found when 30 μg EE were combined with the new progestational agents gestodene and desogestrel (Abatter et al., 1990; Becker, 1990; Daume, 1990; Gevers-Leuven et al., 1987; Robinson et al., 1991; Notelovitz et al., 1992). This lack of change was evident whether monophasic or triphasic combinations were used (Ball et al., 1990; Bonnar et al., 1987; Cohen et al., 1988; Conrad et al., 1991; Notelovitz et al., 1992).

Such minimal changes were also observed after 35 μg EE combined with CPA, a combination not marketed in the U.S. (Bruno et al., 1987; Hirvonen et al., 1988). Winkler et al. (1991) found, using the same drug, an increase in fibrinogen and D dimer but not in factor XII, AT III, and protein S and C. von Kaulla and von Kaulla (1973) observed a decrease of AT III in serum by a technique that has been abandoned; newer methodology revealed unchanged values (Abdelmonen et al., 1988; Jespersen et al., 1983; Notelovitz and Craig, 1976) or increased values (Abatter et al., 1990; Fagerhol et al., 1970; Gram et al., 1990; Walters and Lim, 1970; Weenik et al., 1984). The number of authors observing a decrease was small (Poller et al., 1990). However, regardless of the change up or down, it was found to be in the ± 10% range of variation. No investigator claimed a decrease in the range below 50% of normal, which may occur in individuals genetically predisposed to thromboembolism. Weenick et al. (1990) explained a possible slight decrease by hemodilution during the menstrual cycle. They specifically stated, "If low dose pills are thrombogenic, mass screening for AT III deficiency will not identify those at risk." Weiner and Brandt (1980) concluded "that a decrease in AT III of [that little] magnitude cannot be a cause of thromboembolic disease." When Blombäck (1991) gave tall girls the very high dose of 1 mg EE, a decrease from 100% to 88% was seen. Finally, Wessler (1980) claimed that it is not the decrease of AT III that results in thrombosis; rather, it is diminished plasma Xa inhibitory activity.

Recently, data from the Task Force on coagulation and the pill from WHO was published. The baseline of four different centers—Dublin, Salvadore, Santiago, and Singapore—were present in the first paper (Bocaz et al., 1986). Women were then given OCs of four different formulations: 1) 2 or 5 mg levonogestrel (LNG) plus 50 μg EE (Formula F 1); 2 or 5 mg LNG plus 30 μg EE (F 2); 1 or 5 mg LNG plus 30 μg EE (F 3); and 4) norethisterone acetate (NEA) plus 50 μg EE (F 4). Thomson et al. (1991) stated in an additional report that there was increase of the accelerated prothrombin time, and an increase in factor X and fibrinogen in the pill users. Formula 4 containing NEA also increased factor VIIc, and reduced AT III and alpha 2 antiplasmin. A third paper from this group (Leck et al., 1991) stated that the various coagulation factors differed after the intake of the different formulas in different cities. Although the same data were used in all three papers, the baseline values for the different coagulation factors differed from each other in every paper. Even more intriguing are the actual differences. For instance, Factor X varied in the centers as follows: 91.6(17.9) for Salvador, 70.0(13.0.) for Santiago, 72.2(12.8) for Singapore and, 96.8(19.1) for Dublin. The initial values before drugs were given as 82.(12.3) (before F1), 80.0(10.6) (F2), 81.8(9,8)(F3) and 80.1(12.5.) (F4). These findings contrast with the value of the factor X given in the paper of Leck et al. (1991) as 77 % for all centers. Differences of the same magnitude were present in all other data comparing the three papers. Under these conditions it is noteworthy that the increase in factor X after 12 months is not more than 1 second, and that the decrease of AT III by immune technique is of the order of 1%, and by functional methods 1.5%!

It is obvious that the interlaboratory variation was larger than the marginal changes that are within the normal range. Even more important is that these small changes were not larger in the formulas containing 50 μg EE. The authors believe that these data support their assumption that thromboembolism differs in different parts of the world. But they use for support of this statement the original epidemiological data of Inman et al. from 1970. These papers have only historical interest and have been corrected in many papers since.

Fibrinopeptide A (FPA) emerged as one of the markers for a possible activation of the coagulation cascade. Abbater et al. (1990) observed normal factor VIIc/VIII ratios and FPA during use of low-dose combination pills, and normal FPA patterns were found under the low-estrogen pills by Singh et al. (1980) and Prasad et al. (1989). In some papers the intrinsic variation of the FPA assay was not taken into consideration, making these small changes biologically meaningless. Any discussion regarding hypercoagulability in this context should have terminated when Nossel et al. (1973), who developed the assay, stated that "FPA is not specific for diagnosing thromboembolic disease."

The study of protein C and S under low-EE OCs revealed unchanged or slightly increased values (Gilabert et al., 1987; Huisveld et al., 1987; Jespersen, 1983; Malm et al., 1988; Meade et al., 1985). Data on protein S were conflicting (Boerger et al., 1987; Conrad et al., 1991; Farag et al., 1988; Gilabert et al., 1987; Huisveld et al., 1987; Malm et al., 1988; Meade et al., 1985; Melissari and Kakkar, 1988), and Jespersen and Nielsen (1989) failed to find an increase with improved technology. Total protein S decreased but the ranges of total protein did not differ (Jespersen et al., 1990). The significance of prothrombin fragment 1 + 2 is not clear as yet, but it has already been claimed that this may explain a "hypercoagulable state" (Gevers-Leuven et al., 1987, 1991). "F 1 + 2 is useful in the diagnosis of the prethrombotic state, i.e. a procoagulant imbalance between the producer and the inhibitor of enzyme activity in the coagulation pathway short of fibrin deposition" (Mannuci et al., 1991). This claim belongs to those statements not supported by facts. Recently Saleh et al. (1992), based on data from Mammen's laboratory in Detroit, were unable to find differences.

Disruption of vascular endothelium may be of significance for the development of thrombosis. Vascular endothelial injury is at least partly responsible for the hemostatic changes associated with preeclampsia. Fibronectin, a marker for endothelial injury, was more closely related to pregnancy-induced hypertension (PIH) than any other coagulation factor, indicating that coagulation has been triggered (Saleh et al., 1987). Taylor (1974) speculated that vascular tissue may react to endogenous (pregnancy) or exogenous (sex steroids) causes in some patients in an idiosyncratic fashion. Some investigators described a vascular lesion that they attributed to OC use (Irey and Norris, 1973; Osterholzer et al., 1977), but the reproducibility and specificity remains in doubt. Another marker for interaction with platelet and endothelium fibronectin was found to be unchanged under OCs (Farag et al., 1988).

Oral contraceptives were studied in regard to thrombogenesis induced by vascular subendothelium of rabbit aortas exposed to flowing human blood (Inauen et al. 1987). Increased deposition of fibrin and platelet thrombi were observed in women using OCs with high EE content but not with low-dose pills (Inauen et al., 1987, 1989; Stocker and Inauen, 1991). However, the meaning of these highly experimental data are difficult to ascertain, since the plasma fibrinogen concentration varied in both groups. There were no controls with increased fibrinogen levels due to agents other than OCs.

The fibrinolytic enzyme system is believed to keep the coagulation system in balance. This statement is imprecise since the fibrinolytic enzyme acts predominantly when there is a substrate, fibrin. A change in coagulation factors caused by increasing synthesis is not counterbalanced by fibrinolysis except when the factors of this system are estrogen-stimulated proteins. The most sensitive proteins in this regard are plasma-fibrinogen, factors VII/X, and plasminogen. In order to measure the influence on production rate, it is sufficient to measure one of these factors. Until recently, the methodology for studying fibrinolytic enzyme factors was inadequate because of poor reproducibility and lack of standards. Astedt (1971) was the first to observe a decreased tissue activator concentration in vascular channels during OC use. Jespersen et al. (1990) concluded that, up to now, changes have been associated only with the extrinsic or tissue plasminogen activator (TPA) system, which forms the relationship between TPA and its fast-acting plasminogen activator inhibitor type 1 (PAI-l). Recent studies found TPA activity increased and inhibition decreased (Gevers-Leuven et al., 1987; Jespersen et al., 1986). Jespersen and Kluft (1982) found an increased euglobulin fibrinolytic potential during OC use. The lack of significance of the euglobulin lysis time was observed in two age groups by Meade et al. (1976).

A strong marker for the action of the fibrinolytic system on fibrin is found in fibrinogen and fibrin breakdown products (e.g., split products, fibrin monomers, D-dimers). Investigators who have focused on breakdown products failed to find an increase under low-dose EE OCs (Notelovitz et al., 1981; Farag et al., 1988; Gram et al., 1990). However, others did note an increase (Winkler et al., 1989).

Discontinuing OCs Before Elective Surgery

Researchers mostly in the U. K. claimed that estrogens increase women's risk of postoperative thromboembolism, advocating the discontinuation of OCs 30 days before and 14 days after elective surgery (Guillebaud, 1985,1988; Bonnar, 1985). This group was joined by von Hugo (1987) in Germany and the advisory boards of the German Bundesärztekammer from 1970, and the advisory board of the Swedish National Board of Health and Welfare (Astedt) advised withdrawal. Vessey (1992) supported this concept only for major surgery with extended immobilization. There are no data regarding the low-dose estrogen pill.

The basis for advising discontinuation of the OC was the hematological changes induced by OCs, although these changes were not present after surgery. Epidemiologically, an increase in risk caused by OCs and surgery has not been demonstrated. The suggestion was based on two axioms which then in turn were accepted as facts: 1) surgery induces thrombosis, and 2) oral contraceptives induce thrombosis. Therefore, taking these two axioms together; estrogens and surgery must induce more thrombosis. Scientifically, this is not a very convincing reasoning; moreover, Realini and Goldzieher (1985) believe that there is absolutely no evidence for an increased incidence of thromboembolism after OCs. They are joined in their opinion by Notelovitz and Beller. These authors all concluded that it makes much more sense to advocate low-dose prophylactic heparin after major surgery, which may be followed by anticoagulation with a coumarin-type drug in case of longstanding immobilization (e.g., after cancer surgery or orthopedic surgery). Data suggest that low-dose heparin reduces postoperative thromboembolism. Niedner and Beller (1989) have indicated that the pill can be used in patients using anticoagulation. The concept then to advocate prophylactic heparin for extended surgery without discontinuation of the pill seems to be logical, both biologically and in a litigation context. Discontinuation of the pill may end in unwanted pregnancies and abortion, adding to the risk of the surgery itself. The suggestion to change to Depo-Provera (Guillebaud) seems much too complicated to be practical.

Oral-contraceptive manufacturers recommend stopping the pill preoperatively but it is not stated for what type of surgical procedure. In addition, it is added "if feasible." (Physicians Desk Reference, 1991). This addendum is the result of the revision labeling by the FDA in 1988. Corfman (1992) from the FDA is quoted as saying "We agree that the risk of thromboembolism with today's OCs is practically nonexistent. . . .We consider this a relatively minor issue. We're considering omitting it in the next revision of the labeling."

Smoking and OCs

Epidemiological studies indicate strongly that, for thromboembolism, smoking is the most dangerous risk factor. However, smoking influenced coagulation data very little when studied with respect to OCs (Balleisen et al., 1985; Costongs et al., 1985; Meade and Thomson, 1980; von Hugo et al., 1990).

NEW MARKERS OF COAGULATION ACTIVATION

It is obvious from the previous discussion that the measurement of coagulation factors that most likely reflect an increase in synthesis to predict a prethrombotic state has not been substantiated. Modern methodology has provided a battery of methods that may indicate that the coagulation system was activated. Markers for such an activation of hemostasis are: 1) platelet factor 4 and beta thromboglobulin released from platelets; 2) prothrombin fragment 1 + 2; 3) B-β peptides from fibrinogen; and 4) interaction products such as thrombin-antithrombin III (TAT) complexes and plasmin antiplasmin complexes. In a recent study by Mammen's group in Detroit, it was found that these markers were unchanged under a variety of OCs, which fails to indicate an activation of coagulation. The authors specifically deny the notion of a "hypercoagulable state." The three hemostatic parameters that counteract clotting—prekallikrein, plasminogen, and protein C—were significantly higher in pill users (Farag et al., 1988). However, these new techniques are easily influenced by poor blood drawing and handling techniques. Also, an activation of the hemostatic system by trauma or surgery will increase the levels of hemostatic parameters. This applies, for instance, to the placement of a Swan-Ganz catheter (Saleh et al., 1992). These pitfalls may explain the large variation in data, especially regarding fibrin degradation products. Similar techniques with similar reagents do not exclude these factors.

CONCLUSION

Coagulation researchers have tried to prove the validity of epidemiological studies by their data, and vice versa. To demonstrate a prethrombotic state when there never was a clinical risk or the risk had decreased epidemiologically indicates a misunderstanding of epidemiological data. This is true also for the epidemiologist who uses results to "disprove" coagulation data (Lawson et al., 1977).

At present, the spontaneous rate of thromboembolic disease is unknown and the time has come to disengage from costly studies that do not add to our understanding. It remains doubtful that the most valuable way to study the possible risks of thrombosis is investigation of the changes induced in the hemostatic system as indicated by Bonnar and Sabra (1986). The advice for a government agency still interested in such data for whatever reasons would be to set up the study with a single reference laboratory. This type of study might reduce interlaboratory variations which are obvious in the WHO study (Bocaz et al., 1986).

Obviously, statistical differences in the normal variation are without biological or pathophysiological significance. A slight increase of a given coagulation factor within the normal variance does not expose an individual to a risk of thrombosis. A decrease in components of the fibrinolytic system also pose no risk. Vice versa, an increase in the fibrinolytic system or a decrease of coagulation factors is not beneficial for the individual, as frequently stated. Statements of this kind are without scientific merit (Beller, 1987). Clinicians are advised to examine such data most critically. The "prospective approach" has so far failed to explain a risk of thromboembolism by differences in coagulation changes. Winkler et al. (1991) refer to a dynamic balance of hemostasis, a concept going back to the hypothesis that the integrity of the vasculature is supported by a continuous, slow-going intravascular coagulation process. They suggest that OCs may induce a higher threshold, but not thrombosis. However, the data are not sufficient to support such a concept and must be considered speculative at best. A similar conclusion was reached by Ludwig already in 1965.

Researchers in the coagulation field have failed to notice that epidemiologists have changed their interpretation of data drastically (see especially the Task Force study of WHO). While OCs were at first related to a risk of cardiovascular disease, especially myocardial infarction, it is now obvious that they are rather protective. But it was not the critique of data by Goldzieher and his group (Goldzieher and Dozier, 1975; Realini and Goldzieher, 1985) that changed the interpretation, but the outcome of newer epidemiological studies which in turn confirmed the critique of Goldzieher et al. Sturtevant's (1991) survey of the epidemiological literature led him to conclude that there is no relationship (dose-related or otherwise) and never has been between OCs and thromboembolic disease. Thus the question is raised: what were the coagulationists hunting for? Biochemists should be very careful not to overinterpret their data and explain epidemiological phenomena that are questionable at best.

Coagulation studies may be of significance in a special group of women having a history of thromboembolism or DIC. For instance, Abdelmonen et al. (1988) observed that antithrombin levels were significantly lower among pill users with a family history of thromboembolism. Therefore, when a patient is at special risk, an investigation to identify such a risk factor may be appropriate—and preferable to the screening of large numbers of women with an inadequate methodology and inexact definitions.

REFERENCES

Abbater SC, Pinto S, Rostagno C, et al. Effects of long term gestodene-containing oral contraceptive administration in hemostasis. *Am J Obstet Gynecol* 1990;163:424–9.

Abdelmonen MF, Bottoms SF, Mammen EF. Oral contraceptives and the hemostatic system. *Obstet Gynecol* 1988;71:584–7.

Adama A, Alberta A, Boulanger J, et al. Influence of oral contraceptives and pregnancy constituents of the kallekrein-kininogen system in plasma. *Clin Chem* 1985;31:1533–6.

Alkjaersig N, Fletcher A, Burstein R. Association between oral contraceptive use and thromboembolism: a new approach to its investigation based on plasma fibrinogen chromatography. *Am J Obstet Gynecol* 1975;122:199–211.

Alkjaersig N, Fletcher A, De Ziegler D, et al. Blood coagulation in postmenopausal women given estrogen treatment: comparison of transdermal and oral administration. *J Lab Clin Med* 1988;111:224–8.

Ambrus JL, Ambrus CM, Lillie MA, et al. Effect of various estrogen treatment schedules on antithrombin levels. *Res Common Chem Path Pharm Col* 1976;14;543–7.

Ambrus JL, Niswander, KR, Courey NG, et al. Progestational agents and blood coagulation: 3 menstrual cycle effects. *J Reprod Med* 1971;6:110–5.

Astedt B. Does estrogen replacement therapy predispose to thrombosis? *Acta Obstet Gynecol Scand* 1985;130 [Suppl]:71–4.

Astedt B. Oral contraception and some debatable side effects. *Acta Obstet Gynecol Scand* 1982;105 [Suppl]:17–9.

Astedt B. Low fibrinolytic activity of veins during treatment with ethinyl estradiol. *Acta Obstet Gynecol Scand* 1971;50:279–83.

Astedt B, Jeppson S, Pandolf M. Fibrinolytic activity of veins during treatment with medroxyprogesterone acetate. *Acta Obstet Gynecol Scand* 1972;51:283–6.

Ball M, Ashwell E, Gillmer M. Progestagen only contraceptives: comparison of the levonogestrel and norethisterone. *Contraception* 1991;44:223–33.

Ball MJ, Ashwell E, Jackson M, et al. Comparison of two triphasic contraceptives with different progestogens: effect on metabolism and coagulation proteins. *Contraception* 1990;41:363–76.

Balleisen L, Bailey J, Epping PH, et al. Epidemiological study on Factor VII, Factor VIII and fibrinogen in an industrial population. *Thromb Haemost* 1985;54:475–9.

Basdevant A, Pelissier C, Conrad J, et al. Effects of nomegestrol acetate (5 mg/d) on hormonal metabolic and hemostatic parameters in premenopausal women. *Contraception* 1991;44:589–99.

Bastert G, Michel R. Hochdosierte gestagen therapie mit MPA beim metastasierenden mamma karzinom. *Med Welt* 1983;34:378–82.

Becker H. Supportive European data on a new oral contraceptive containing norgestimate. *Acta Obstet Gynecol Scand* 1990;152 [Suppl]:33–9.

Beller FK. *Die gerinnungsverhältnisse bei der schwangeren und beim neugeborenen.* Bart, Leipzig, 1958, pp 11–27.

Beller FK. Thromboembolie und Pille - sinn und unsinn von analogieschlüssen. In: Beller FK, Giesing M, Graeff H, eds. *Hormonale kontrazeption und herzkreislauf.* Gräfelfing: Wiss Verlagsgesellsch; 1987:ll–27.

Beller FK, Ebert CH. Effects of oral contraceptives on blood coagulation: A review. *Obstet Gynecol Survey* 1985;40:425–36.

Beller FK, Ebert CH. The coagulation and fibrinolytic system in pregnancy and the puerperium. *Europ J Obstet Gynecol Reprod Med* 1982;13:171–5.

Beller FK, Goebelsmann V, Douglas CW, et al. The fibrinolytic system during the menstrual cycle. *Obstet Gynecol* 1964;23:12–5.

Beller FK, Graeff H. Deposition of glomerular fibrin in the rabbit after infusion with endotoxin. *Nature* 1967;215:295–6.

Beller FK, Nachtigall L, Rosenberg M. Coagulation studies of menopausal women taking estrogen replacement therapy. *Obstet Gynecol* 1972;39:775–8.

Beller FK, Porges RF. Blood coagulation and fibrinolytic enzyme studies during cyclic and continuous application of progestational agents. *Am J Obstet Gynecol* 1967;87:448–59.

Beller FK, Schoendorf TH. Augmentation of endotoxin induced fibrin deposits by pregnancy and estrogen-progesterone treatment. *Gynecol Invest* 1976;3:176–83.

Blömback M. Changes in blood coagulation and fibrinolysis during pregnancy and the menstrual cycle. *Adv Contraception* 1991;7[Suppl 3]:285–9.

Blömback M, Hall K, Ritzen H. Estrogen treatment of tall girls: risk of thrombosis. *Pediatrics* 1983;72:416–8.

Bocaz JA, Barjar P, Bonnar J, et al. Differences in coagulation and hemostatic parameters in normal women of child bearing age from different ethnic groups and geographical locations. *Thromb Haemost* 1986;55:390–5.

Boerger LM, Morris PC, Thurneau GR. Oral contraceptives and gender effect on protein S status. *Blood* 1987;69:692–8.

Bonnar J. Coagulation effects and oral contraceptives. *Adv Contraception* 1987;7[Suppl 3].

Bonnar J. *Effects of synthetic and natural estrogen on the coagulation systems in postmenopausal women.* Lancaster: MT Press; 1989:321–9.

Bonnar J, Daly L, Carolle. Blood coagulation with a combination pill containing gestodene and ethinyl estradiol. *Int J Fert* 1987;32[Suppl]:21–8.

Bonnar J, Sabra AM. Oral contraception and blood coagulation. *J Reprod Med* 1986;31[Suppl]:551–5.

Bruno V, Rosaki D, Bucciantini S. Platelet and coagulation functions during the triphasic estrogen-progestogen treatment. *Contraception* 1986;31:39–46.

Bruno V, Rosaki D, Bucciantini S, et al. Wirkungen eines antiandrogenen kombinations präparates auf das hämostatische system. *Fortschr Med* 1987;105:55–8.

Cohen H, Mackie I, Walsh K, et al. A comparison of the effects of two triphasic oral contraceptives on hemostasis. *Br J Haematol* 1988;69:259–263.

Comp PC, Esmon CT. Recurrent venous thromboembolism in patients with a partial deficiency of proteins. *N Engl J Med* 1984;311:1525–33.

Conrad J, Serfaty D, Bauen K, et al. Prothrombin in fragment 1+2 in women treated with oral contraceptives containing estradiol and gestodene. *Thromb Haemost* 1991;65:1520–1522.

Conrad JB, Cazenave M, Samama, et al. AT III content and antithrombin activity in oestrogen-progesterone and progestogen only treated women. *Thromb Res* 1980;18:675–81.

Coope J, Thomson JM, Poller L. Effects of "natural oestrogen" replacement therapy on menopausal symptoms and blood clotting. *Br Med J* 1975;4:139–43.

Corfman P. Experts debate discontinuing OCs before elective surgery. *Contraception Technol* 1992; 13:57–68.

Cortes-Pietro J. Coagulation and fibrinolysis in postmenopausal women treated with OD 14. *Maturitas* 1987;4[Suppl]:67–72.

Costongs GM, Bas BM, Janson PS, et al. Short term and long term individual variations and critical differences of coagulation parameters. *J Clin Chem Clin Biochem* 1985;23:405–10.

Dallback B. Protein S and C4 binding protein. *Thromb Haemost* 1991;66:49–61.

Daume E. Influence of modern low dose oral contraceptives on hemostasis. *Adv Contraception* 1990; 6[Suppl]:51–7.

Drill VA, Calhoun DW. Oral contraceptives and thromboembolic diseases. *JAMA* 1968;206:77–83.

Deutsch Aerztebl 1984;43:3,170. Editorial.

Egeberg O. Inherited antithrombin deficiency causing thrombophilia. *Thromb Diath Haem* 1965; 13:516–20.

Egeberg O, Owren PA. Oral contraception and blood coagulability. *Br Med J* 1963;1:26–7.

Fagerhol MK, Albidgaard V, Berjo P, et al. Oral contraceptives and low antithrombin III concentration. *Lancet* 1970;2:1175.

Fahmy K, Khairy M, Allam A, et al. Effect of depo-medroxy progesterone acetate on coagulation factors and serum lipids in Egyptian women. *Contraception* 1991;44:431–45.

Farag A, Bottoms SF, Mammen EF, et al. Oral contraceptives and the hemostatic system. *Obstet Gynecol* 1988;71:584–8.

Fawer R, Dettling A, Weihs D. Effect of the menstrual cycle, oral contraception, and pregnancy on forearm blood flow. *Europ J Clin Pharmacol* 1978;13:251–7.

Ganzina F, Robuscelli DC. Adverse events during high dose on medroxyprogesterone acetate for therapy of endocrine tumors. In: Cavalli F, et al. eds. *Proc Int Sympos MPA*. Amsterdam: Excerpta Medica; 1982:158–66.

Gevers-Leuven JA, Kluft C, et al. Effects of two low dose oral contraceptives on circulating components of the coagulation and fibrinolytic system. *J Lab Clin Med* 1987;109:631–6.

Gevers-Leuven JA, Kluft C, Dersjant-Rooda MC, et al. Difference in effect of two oral contraceptives on arterial coagulation risk factors. *Thromb Haemost* 1991;65:358–62.

Gilabert J, Fernandez JA, Espana F, et al. Physiological coagulation inhibitors (protein S, protein C and AT III) in severe preeclamptic states and users of oral contraceptives. *Thromb Res* 1987;49:319–29.

Gitel SN, Stephenson RC, Wessler S. The activated factor X antithrombin III reaction rate: a measure of the increased thrombotic tendency induced by estrogen-containing oral contraceptives in rabbits. *Hemostasis* 1978;7:10–8.

Goldzieher JW. Hormonal contraception. Benefits versus risks. *Am J Obstet Gynecol* 1987;157:1,023–8.

Gordon EM, Douglas J, Ratnoff OB. Influence of augmented Hageman factor (factor XII) titers on the cytoactivation of plasma prorenin on women using oral contraceptives. *J Clin Invest* 1983;72:1,833–8.

Gordon EM, Williams SR, Frenchek CA, et al. Dose dependent effects of postmenopausal estrogen and progestin on AT III and Factor XII. *J Lab Clin Med* 1988;111:52–6.

Graeff H. Hypercoagulable states in thromboembolic disorders. In: Van de Loo J, Prentice CR, Beller FK, eds. Stuttgart: Schattauer; 1973:91–7.

Gram J, Munkvad S, Jespersen J. Enhanced generation and resolution of fibrinogen in women above the age of 30 years using oral contraceptives low in estrogen. *Am J Obst Gynecol* 1990;163:438–42.

Guaueu W, Baumgarten HR, Haebeoli A, et al. Excessive deposition of fibrin, platelets and platelet thrombi on vascular subendothelium during contraceptive drug treatment. *Thromb Haemost* 1987; 57:306–9.

Guaueu W, Stocker G, Baumgarten HR, et al. Effects of low and high dose oral contraceptives on plasma estrogen levels, blood coagulation and fibrinolysis, and thrombogenesis induced by vascular subendothelium. *Thromb Haemost* 1989;62:557–61.

Guillebaud J. Should the pill be stopped preoperatively? *Br Med J* 1988;296:786–7.

Guillebaud J. Surgery and the pill. *Br Med J* 1985;291:498–9.

Hirvonen E, Stenman UH, Malkonen, et al. New estradiol/cyproterone acetate oral contraceptive for premenopausal women. *Maturitas* 1988;10:201–13.

Hunter DJS, Anderson AB, Haddon M. Changes in coagulation factors in postmenopausal women on ethinyl estradiol. *Br J Obstet Gynecol* 1979;86:488–91.

Huisveld IA, Hospers JE, Meijers JC, et al. Oral contraceptives reduce total protein S but not free protein S. *Thromb Res* 1987;45:109–14.

Ibrahim NM, Hassan MI, Abd El-Megeed SF, et al. Effect of injectable contraceptive on coagulation profile and lipid pattern in Egyptian women. *Egypt J Biochem* 1988;6:21–38.

Inauen W, Baumgarten HR, Haeberli A, et al. Excessive deposition of fibrin, platelets and platelet thrombin on vascular subendothelium during contraceptive drug treatment. *Thromb Haemost* 1987; 57:306–7.

Inauen WG, Stocker G, Baumgartner HR, et al. Effects of low and high dose oral contraceptives on plasma estrogen levels, blood coagulation and fibrinolysis, and thrombogenesis induced by vascular subendothelium. *Thromb Haemost* 1989;63:552–7.

Inman WHW, Vessey MP, Westerholm B, et al. Thromboembolic disease and the steroidal content of oral contraceptives: a report to the Committee on the Safety of Drugs. *Br Med J* 1970;2:203.

Irey NS, Horris HJ. Individual vascular lesions associated with female reproductive steroids. *Arch Path* 1973;96:227–34.

Jamin C, Aiach H. Effect de l'association acetate de cyproterone-estradiol par voie cutanee sur l'anti-thrombine III. *Presse Med* 1987;16:1007.

Jespersen J. Pathophysiology and clinical aspects of fibrinolysis and inhibition of coagulation. Experimental and clinical studies with special reference to women on oral contraceptives. *Dan Med Bull* 1988;35;1–33.

Jespersen J, Gevers-Leuven JA, Kluft C. Variations of levels in plasma of tissue type plasminogen activator (tPA) and inhibition of tPA in women using oral contraceptives (OC). *Fibrinolysis* 1986; [Suppl]:184–6.

Jespersen J, Ingeberg S, Bach E. Antithrombin and platelets during the normal menstrual cycle and in women receiving oral contraceptives low in estrogen. *Gynecol Invest* 1983;15:153–62.

Jespersen J, Ingeberg S, Bach E. Antithrombin III and platelets during the menstrual cycle and in women receiving oral contraceptives low in estrogen. *Gynecol Invest* 1983;15:153–62.

Jespersen J, Kluft C. Individual levels of plasma histidine glycoprotein (HRG) during the normal menstrual cycle and in women on oral contraceptives low in oestrogen. *Scand J Clin Lab Invest* 1982; 42:563–6.

Jespersen JR, Kresten SO, Skouby S. Effects of newer oral contraceptives on the inhibition of coagulation and fibrinolysis in relation to dosage and type of steroid. *Am J Obstet Gynecol* 1990;163:396–403.

Jespersen J, Nielsen MT. Levels of protein S during the normal menstrual cycle and in women on oral contraception low in estrogen. *Gynecol Invest* 1989;28:82–6.

Jespersen J, Petersen KR, Skouby S. Coagulation and fibrinolysis comparative study of two low dose oral contraceptives. *Adv Contraception* 1991;7[Suppl 3]:392–6.

Jordan VC, Fritz NF, Tormey DC. Long term adjuvant therapy with tamoxifen; effects on sex hormone binding and antithrombin III. *Cancer Res* 1987;47:4517–9.

Jordan M, Sheppard BC, Bonnar J, et al. Immunochemistry of oestrogen and progesterone receptors in the uterus of women with normal and excessive menstrual bleeding. *Irish J Med Sci* 1990;159:52–3.

Kitchens CS. Concept of hypercoagulability: a review of its development, clinical application and recent progress. *Sem Thromb Hemost* 1985;2:293–315.

Kluft C. Disorders of the hemostatic system and the rise of the development of thrombotic and cardiovascular diseases: limitation and laboratory diagnosis. *Am J Obstet Gynecol* 1990;163:305–12.

Kobayashi N, Takeda Y. Effects of a large dose of estradiol on antithrombin III metabolism in male and female dogs. *Europ J Clin Invest* 1977;7:373–81.

Kovacs IB, Chandana P, Ratnatunga P, et al. Is elevated plasma fibrinogen a causative factor in arterial thrombosis? XIII Cong Intern Soc Thromb Haemost, June 1991. *Thromb Haemost* 1991;65:10(abst).

Kullander S, Svanberg L, Astedt B. Coagulative and fibrinolytic studies on postmenopausal women treated with a new nonsteroidal estrogen. *Acta Obstet Gynecol Scand* 1977;56:371–4.

Largelius A, Lunell NO, Blomback M. Natural estrogens in the female climacteric: influence on blood coagulation and fibrinolysis. *Thromb Haemost* 1978;40:532–41.

Lawson DM, Davidson JF, Jick H. Oral contraceptive use and venous thromboembolism: absence of the effect of smoking. *Br Med J* 1977;2:729.

Antithrombin. *Lancet* 1976;2:1333. Leading article.

Lebech AM, Lebech PE. Metabolic changes during the normal menstrual cycle: a longitudinal study. *Am J Obstet Gynecol* 1990;163:414–6.

Lebech AM, Kjaer KA. Lipid metabolism and coagulation during the normal menstrual cycle. *Horm Metab Res* 1989;21:445–8.

Leck I, Thompson JM, Bocaz JA, et al. A multicenter study of coagulation and haemostatic variables during oral contraceptives. Variations with geographical location and ethnicity. *Int J Epidemiol* 1991; 20:913–20.

Lindoff C, Petersson F, Astedt B. Fibrinolytic components during transdermal estrogen replacement therapy. *J North Am Menopausal Soc*, Montreal, 1991.

Ludwig H. Hämatologische und hämostaseologische befunde bei der ovulationshemmung durch oestrogen-gestagen kombination. *Fortschr Geburtsh Gynäk* 1965;21:198–214.

Malm J, Laurell MA, Dahlback B. Changes in the plasma levels of vitamin K-dependent proteins C and S and C4b-binding protein during pregnancy and oral contraceptives. *Br J Haematol* 1988;68:437–44.

Mammen E. Altersabhängige veränderungen der blutgerrinung. In: Beller FK. *(Hrsg) Hormon Anwendung beider Frau über 40.* Berlin: Grosse; 1990:85.

Mammen EF. Oral contraceptives and blood coagulation: a critical review. *Am J Obstet Gynecol* 1982;142:781–90.

Mandalaki T, Louizoo C, Dimitriadou C, et al. Variations in factor VIII during the menstrual cycle in normal women. *N Engl J Med* 1980;302:1093–6.

Mannuci PM, Bottaso B, Tripodi A. Prothrombin fragment 1 2 and intensity of treatment with oral anticoagulants. *Thromb Haemost* 1991;66:741–5.

McEwan JA, Griffin M. Long-term use of depot norethisterone enanthate: effect on blood coagulation factors and menstrual bleeding patterns. *Contraception* 1991;94:639–49.

McKay DG. Chronic intravascular coagulation in normal pregnancy and preeclampsia. *Contrib Nephrol* 1982;25:108–28.

McKay DG. *Disseminated intravascular coagulation.* New York: Hoeber; 1964:

Meade TW, Brozovic M, Chakraborti, et al. An epidemiological study of the hemostasis and other effects after oral contraception. *Br J Haematol* 1976;34:353–64.

Meade TW, Stirling H, Wilkens S., et al. Effects of oral contraceptives and obesity on protein C antigen. *Thromb Haemost* 1985;53:198–9.

Meade TW, Thompson SG. Progestogens and cardiovascular reactions associated with oral contraceptives and a comparison of the safety of 50 and 30 mcg estrogen preparations. *Br Med J* 1980;1:1,157–9.

Melis GB, Fruzetti F, Paoletti AM, et al. Fibrinopeptide in plasma levels during low estrogen oral contraceptive treatment. *Contraception* 1984;30:575–8.

Melis GR, Fruzetti F, Ricci C, et al. Oral contraceptives and venous thromboembolic disease: the effect of the estrogen dose. *Maturitas* 1988;[Suppl 1]:131–9.

Melissari E, Kakkar W. The effects of estrogen administration of plasma free protein S and C4b-binding protein. *Thromb Res* 1988;49:489–95.

Meng YX, Jiang HY, Chen AJ, et al. Hemostatic drugs in women using a monthly injectable contraceptive. *Contraception* 1990;42:455–66.

Meng YX, Jiang HY, Lu FY. The effects of long-term using once a monthly injectable contraceptive. *Thromb Haemost* 1990;28:548–9.

Mink IB, Corvey MG, Moore MA, et al. Progestational agents and blood coagulation induced by progestogen alone. *Am J Obstet Gynecol* 1972;113:739–43.

Niedner W, Beller FK. Hormonale kontrazeption und gerinnungshemmende behandlung. In: Beller FK, Giesing M, Graeff H, eds. *Hormonale kontrazeption und herzkreislauf.* Gräfelfing: SMV Verlagsgesellschaft; 1989:209.

Nilsson IM, Kullander S, Astedt BA. Coagulation and fibrinolytic studies during continuous use of low-dose gestagen. *Acta Endocrinol* 1970;65:111–6.

Nossel HL, Buther VP, Canfield RE, et al. Potential use of fibrinopeptide A measurements in the diagnosis and measurement of thrombosis. *Thromb Diath Haemorrh* 1973;33:426–34.

Notelovitz M. Coagulation, estrogen, and the menopause. *Clin Obstet Gynecol* 1977;4:107–11.

Notelovitz M. Oral contraception and coagulation. *Clin Obstet Gynecol* 1985;28:73–83.

Notelovitz M, Craig HBW. Natural estrogen and antithrombin III activity in postmenopausal women *J Reprod Med* 1976;16:87–90.

Notelovitz M, Kitchens CS, Coone L, et al. Low dose oral contraceptive usage and coagulation. *Am J Obstet Gynecol* 1981;141:71–5.

Notelovitz M, Kitchens CS, Khan FY. Changes in coagulation and anticoagulation in women taking low dose triphasic oral contraceptives: a controlled comparative 12 month clinical trial. *Am J Obstet Gynecol* 1992;167:1255–61.

Omsj IH, Oian P, Maltau VM. Effects of two triphasic oral contraceptives containing ethinyl-estradiol plus levonogestrel or gestodene on blood coagulation and fibrinolysis. *Acta Obstet Gynecol Scand* 1989;68:27–30.

Osterholzer HO, Girillo D, Kruger PS, et al. The effect of oral contraceptives steroids on branches of the uterine artery. *Obstet Gynecol* 1977;49:227–32.

Parkin DE, Smith DM, Azzawi F. Effects of long-term OD 14 administration on blood coagulation in climacteric women. *Maturitas* 1987;9:95–101.

Passo R, Boccardo F, Canobbio L, et al. Effects of high dose medroxyprogesterone acetate on blood clotting factors and platelet function. In: Cavelle F, ed. *Proc Symp MPA* Amsterdam: Excerpta Med; 1982:151–7.

Perrot-Applaud M, Groyer-Picard MT, Garcia E, et al. Immunocytological demonstration of estrogen and progesterone receptors in muscle cells in uterine arteries in rabbits and humans. *Endocrinol* 1988;123:1,511–9.

Physicians Desk Reference. (1991) Oradell, New Jersey: Medical Economics; 1991.

Poller L. Oral contraceptives, blood clotting, and thrombosis. *Br Med J* 1978;34:151.

Poller L, Thomsen JM, Coope J. Conjugated equine estrogens and blood clotting: a follow-up report. *Br Med J* 1977;1:935–6.

Poller L, Thomsen JM, Tabiowo A, et al. Progesterone oral contraception and blood coagulation. *Br Med J* 1969;1:554–6.

Poller L, Thomsen JM, Thomas PW. Effects of oral contraception with norethisterone on blood clotting and platelets. *Br Med J* 1972;2:391–3.

Poller L, Thomsen JM, Thomas W, et al. Blood clotting and platelet aggregation during oral progestogen contraception: a follow-up study. *Br Med J* 1971;1:705–8.

Prasad RN, Koh S, Ratnam SS. Effects of three types of combined OC pills on blood coagulation, fibrinolysis and platelet function. *Contraception* 1989;39:369–83.

Press MF, Greene GL. Localization of progesterone receptor with monoclonal antibodies to the human progestin receptor. *Endocrinology* 1988;122:1,165–1,175.

Rakoczi I, Gero G, Demeter J, et al. Comparative metabolic effects of oral contraceptive preparations containing different progestins. *Arznei Mittel Forsch* 1985;35:630–3.

Ramcharan S, Pellegrini FA, Ray RM, et al. Walnut Creek Contraceptive Study. *J Reprod Med* 1980; 25[Suppl]:346–50.

Realini JP, Goldzieher JW. Oral contraceptives and cardiovascular disease: a critique of the epidemiological studies. *Am J Obstet Gynecol* 1985;152:729–92.

Robinson GE, Burrent T, Mackie IU, et al. Changes in hemostasis after stopping the combined contraceptive pill: implications of major surgery. *Br Med J* 1991;302:269–71.

Royal College of General Practitioners. Oral contraception and thromboembolic disease. *J Coll Gen Pract* 1967;13:267.

Rugman FP, Hay CRM, Yoong A. Evidence of prethrombotic state in postmenopausal women with depo + hormonal replacement therapy. *Thromb Haemost* 1991;65:1,522–8.

Sabra A, Bonnar J. Haemostatic system changes induced by 50 mcg and 30 mcg estrogen/progesterone oral contraceptives. *J Reprod Med* 1983;28:85–91.

Saleh AA, Bottoms SF, Welch RA, et al. Preeclampsia, delivery, and the hemostatic system. *Am J Obst Gynecol* 1987;157:331–6.

Saleh AA, Brockbank N, Dorey LG, et al. TAT complexes and prothrombin fragment 1 2 in oral contraceptive users. *Thromb Res [in press].*

Sartwell PE, Stolley PD, Tonascia JA, et al. Overview: pulmonary embolism mortality in relation to oral contraceptive use. *Prev Med* 1976;5:15–9.

Schwallie PC, Assenzo JR. Contraceptive efficacy study utilizing medroxyprogesterone acetate. *Fertil Steril* 1973;24:331–9.

Sheppard BL. Cellular processes and oral contraception. *Adv Contraception* 1991;7[Suppl 3]:331–6.

Siegbahn A, Odlind V, Hedner U, et al. Coagulation and fibrinolysis during the menstrual cycle. *Uppsala J Med Sci* 1989;94:137–40.

Siegbahn A, Ruusavaava L. Age dependence of blood fibrinolytic components and the effect of low-dose oral contraceptives on coagulation and fibrinolysis in teenagers. *Thromb Haemost* 1988;60:361–4.

Singh K, Viegas OAC, Koh SCL. Effects of longterm use of Norplant implants on haemostatic function. *Contraception* 1992;45:203–7.

Sitruk-Ware R, De Palacios I. Estrogen replacement therapy in cardiovascular disease in postmenopausal women. *Maturitas* 1989;11:259–74.

Solash J, Perez R, Keates JS, et al. Hormonal steroids: effects on vascular system. *Gynaecol Invest* 1974;6:329–36.

Song J, Mark MS, Lawler MP. Endometrial changes in women receiving oral contraceptives. *Am J Obstet Gynecol* 1970;107:717–28.

Stangel J, Inner J, Reyniak V, et al. The effect of conjugated estrogens on coagulability in menopausal women. *Obstet Gynecol* 1977;49:314–16.

Stewart GV. The intravascular generation of fibrinogen derivatives and the blood vessel wall in venous thrombosis and DIC. *Thromb Haemost* 1977;38:831–41.

Stocker G, Inauen N. Thrombogenesis on vascular subendothelium dose-dependent effects of oral contraceptives. *Adv Contraception* 1991;7[Suppl 3]:302–8.

Sturtevant FM. Cardiovascular safety of oral contraceptives: a critical commentary. *Int J Fertil* 1991; 36[Suppl 3]:32–36.

Sturtevant FM. Special report: safety of oral contraceptives related to steroid content. A critical review. *Int J Fertil* 1989;34:323–6.

Swyer GIM. Oral contraceptives, thrombosis, and cyclical factors affecting veins. *Br Med J* 1966;1:355.

Taylor E. *Obstet Gynec Survey* 1974;29:181. Editorial.

Thomson JM, Poller L, et al. A multicenter study of coagulation and hemostatic variables during oral contraception. Variations with four formulations. *Br J Obstet Gynecol* 1991;98:1117–28.

Tsakok FH, Koh S, Yuen R, et al. Coagulation studies in Asian women using injectable progestogen contraception. *Int J Gynecol Obstet* 1980;81:105–8.

Vessey M. Experts debate discontinuing OCs before elective surgery. *Contrapt Techn* 1992;13:57–68.

Vessey MP. Venous thromboembolic disease and the use of oral contraceptives. *Lancet* 1968;1:94–6.

Vessey MP, Doll R. Investigation of relations between use of oral contraceptives and thromboembolic disease. *Br Med J* 1968;2:199–205.

von Hugo RV. Vor operation pille absetzen? *Med Trib* 1987;21:27.

von Hugo RV, Briel RC, Schindler AE. Wirkung oraler kontrazeptiva auf die blutgerinnung bei rauchenden und nichtrauchenden probandinnen. *Akta Endocr Stoffw* 1989;10:6–12.

von Kaulla E, Droegemuller W, von Kaulla WN. Conjugated estrogens and hypercoagulatbility. *Am J Obstet Gynecol* 1973;122:888–92.

von Kaulla E, von Kaulla WN. Oral contraceptives and low antithrombin III activity. *Lancet* 1970;1:36.

Wakefield AJ, Sawyer AM, Hudson M. Smoking, the oral contraceptive pill and Crohn's disease. *Digest Dis Sci* 1991;36:1147–50.

Walker ID, Davidson JF, Richards F, et al. The effect of the synthetic steroid org OD 14 on fibrinolysis and blood lipids in menopausal women. *Thromb Haemost* 1985;53:303–5.

Walters W, Aw Lim YL. Hemodynamic changes in women taking oral contraceptives. *J Obstet Gynecol Br Commonw* 1970;77:1,007–11.

Weenik GH, Kahle LH, Lamping RJ, et al. Antithrombin III in oral contraceptive users and during pregnancy. *Acta Obstet Gynecol Scand* 1984;63:57–61.

Weiner CP, Brandt J. Plasma antithrombin III activity in normal pregnancy. *Obstet Gynecol* 1980; 56:601–3.

Wessler ST. Thrombosis and sex hormones: a perplexing liaison. *J Lab Clin Med* 1980;96:757–62.

Wessler ST, Citel N, Wan LS, et al. Estrogen containing oral contraceptives. *JAMA* 1976;236:2,179–82.

Whigham KE, Howie PN, Mack A. The effect of an injectable progestogen contraceptive on blood coagulation and fibrinolysis. *Br J Obstet Gynecol* 1979;86:806–9.

Winkler VH, Buhler K, Schindler AE. The dynamic balance of hemostasis: implications for the risk of oral contraceptive use. In: Runnebaum B, Rabe E, Kiesel L, eds. *Female contraception and male fertility regulation*. Park Ridge: Parthenon Publishing Group; 1991:

Winkler UH, Koslowski C, Oberhoff C, et al. Changes in the dynamic equilibrium of hemostatis associated with the use of low dose oral contraceptives. *Adv Contraception* 1991;7[Suppl 3]:273.

Winkler VH, Koslowski S, Schindler AE. PAI activity is reduced in users of oral contraceptives. *Thromb Haemost* 1989;62:394.

Yamamoto H, Noguchi S, Miyauchi K, et al. Changes in hematologic parameters during treatment with medroxyprogesterone acetate for breast cancer. *Jap J Cancer Res* 1991;82:425.

Ygge J. Variation in the individual subject of some parameters in blood coagulation and fibrinolysis. A longitudinal study in young healthy women. *Scand J Haematol* 1969;6:343–6.

Young RL, Goepfert AR, Goldzieher JW. Estrogen replacement therapy is not conducive of venous thromboembolism. *Maturitas* 1991;13:189–92.

Zhu P, Luo H, Shi W, et al. Observation of the activity of factor VIII in the endometrium of women pre and post insertion of three types of IUDs. *Contraception* 1991;44:367–85.

Pharmacology of the Contraceptive Steroids,
edited by Joseph W. Goldzieher.
Raven Press, Ltd., New York © 1994.

22

Cardiovascular System: Contraceptive Steroids, Plasma Lipoprotein Levels, and Coronary Artery Atherosclerosis

*†Scott A. Washburn, †Janice D. Wagner, †Michael R. Adams, and †Thomas B. Clarkson

Department of Obstetrics and Gynecology, †Department of Comparative Medicine and Comparative Medicine Clinical Research Center, Bowman Gray School of Medicine of Wake Forest University, Winston-Salem, North Carolina 27157

The past two decades have seen an intense interest in elucidating the effects of exogenous sex steroids, especially oral contraceptives (OCs), on cardiovascular risk factors and risk of coronary heart disease in women. There has been no reliable means of measuring the extent of atherosclerotic plaque in women except at autopsy. This has limited the scope of investigation largely to effects on lipid and lipoprotein metabolism, and effects on risk of certain clinical endpoints, such as myocardial infarction or angina pectoris. We describe here the accumulated data on effects of contraceptive steroids on lipoprotein metabolism and risk of coronary heart disease in women, as well as their effects on coronary artery atherosclerosis in a nonhuman primate model.

EFFECTS OF CONTRACEPTIVE STEROIDS ON PLASMA LIPOPROTEINS OF WOMEN

Increased risk of coronary heart disease (CHD) is associated epidemiologically with elevated concentrations of total plasma cholesterol (TPC) and low-density lipoprotein cholesterol (LDL), and decreased plasma concentrations of high-density lipoprotein cholesterol (HDL). Because of this relationship, and because clinical studies have shown that estrogens and progestins influence lipoprotein metabolism, many investigators have studied the effects of combination OCs on plasma lipid and lipoprotein levels in large cohorts of women (Bradley et al., 1978; Knopp et al., 1981; Wahl et al., 1983). These data have demonstrated that plasma concentrations of triglycerides and HDL are increased and LDL concentrations decreased in direct relationship to the dose and potency of the estrogen component of the OC. Also, HDL, particularly the HDL2 subfraction, is decreased and LDL is increased in

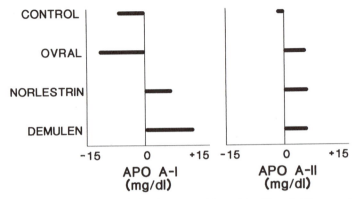

FIG. 1. Approximate change (in %) in plasma apolipoprotein AI and AII concentrations in women taking three oral contraceptive formulations (Ovral, Norlestrin, and Demulen) versus controls. (Modified from Lipson et al., 1986.)

relation to the androgenic potency and dose of the progestin component. The findings of these cohort studies have been confirmed in numerous randomized prospective trials.

Oral contraceptive formulations have changed markedly over the past 30 years. As the doses of both estrogen and progestin components have decreased and triphasic preparations have evolved, the plasma lipid and lipoprotein effects of the various combination OCs have proved to be much less pronounced than in the earlier studies of "high-dose" preparations (van der Vange et al., 1987; Notelovitz et al., 1989; Godsland et al., 1990). The recently developed contraceptive progestins norgestimate, desogestrel, and gestodene, although chemically related to levonorgestrel, have been shown to have little or no effect on plasma lipid and lipoprotein levels (van der Vange et al., 1987; Godsland et al., 1990; Chez, 1989). Furthermore, the lipoprotein effects of combination contraceptives containing either desogestrel or gestodene are "estrogenic"; that is, they result in increased levels of HDL and apoprotein A1 (apo A1) and decreased levels of LDL and apoprotein B (apo B) (van der Vange et al., 1987; Godsland et al., 1990; Kloosterboer et al., 1986; Gevers-Leuven et al., 1990).

As will be discussed in succeeding sections, the clinical relevance of plasma lipid and lipoprotein changes associated with OC use is suspect, since there is no evidence of an association between OC-induced alterations in plasma lipoproteins and increased risk of coronary heart disease. Furthermore, most studies of OCs have addressed only effects on plasma TPC, LDL, and HDL, and have neglected potentially important effects on lipoprotein size and compositional heterogeneity. For example, the studies of Lipson et al., (1986) and others (Burkman et al., 1988; Notelovitz et al., 1989) have shown that some OCs have divergent effects on plasma HDL, apo A1, and apo A2 concentrations; while HDL levels are decreased or unaffected, apo A1 and apo A2 levels are often increased (Fig. 1). Since apo A1 and apo A2 seem to be important determinants of the mechanism by which HDL is

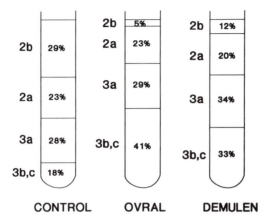

FIG. 2. Changes in HDL subfractions induced by Ovral and Demulen in treated female cynomolgus monkeys versus controls. (Modified from Adams et al., 1987.)

protective against atherosclerosis (Babiak and Rudel, 1987), it is possible that the functional capacity of HDL is unaffected, or perhaps even enhanced, by OC treatment.

EFFECTS ON PLASMA LIPOPROTEIN CONCENTRATIONS IN CYNOMOLGUS MACAQUES

The change in plasma lipoprotein profile induced by older high-dose combination OC treatment in cynomolgus macaques is very similar to that observed in women. Plasma TPC, LDL, and triglyceride concentrations are increased, and plasma HDL concentrations are decreased (Adams et al., 1987; Parks et al., 1989). In addition, we have found evidence for marked effects of OCs on the subfractional heterogeneity of plasma LDL and HDL cholesterol (Parks et al., 1989). The average molecular weight of plasma LDL is decreased by treatment with the OC Demulen ($p<0.05$) but not Ovral ($p>0.10$). Furthermore, these OCs have marked effects on the heterogeneity of HDL subfractions. The marked decrease in plasma HDL levels associated with OC treatment is accounted for by marked decreases in the levels of the HDL2B subfraction (Fig. 2).

EFFECTS ON CORONARY ARTERY ATHEROSCLEROSIS IN WOMEN

While there have been numerous epidemiologic studies of the effects of OCs on the relative risk of certain clinical cardiovascular endpoints such as myocardial infarction or angina pectoris, no studies have addressed directly the effects of OCs on the atherosclerotic process. Indirect evidence that OCs do not worsen atherosclerosis is provided by studies of premenopausal women undergoing coronary an-

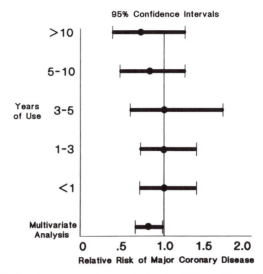

FIG. 3. Relative risk of major coronary disease (+/− the 95% confidence interval) among oral contraceptive users and nonusers from the Nurses' Health Study. (Modified from Stampfer et al., 1990.)

giography for the diagnosis of myocardial infarction (Engel et al., 1983; Jugdutt et al., 1983). In contrast with nonusers, OC users had little or no angiographic evidence of coronary atherosclerosis. These studies indicate that, whereas OC use might predispose to coronary thrombosis, it does not lead to worsened atherosclerosis and may, in fact, inhibit atherosclerosis.

The hypothesis that OCs do not hasten the development of atherosclerosis is supported further by the epidemiologic observation that CHD risk is not increased in past users of OCs (Stampfer et al., 1990), regardless of duration of use (Fig. 3). Furthermore, among current users, there is no association between duration of use and risk (Mishell, 1988). The results of experimental studies of the effects of OCs on atherosclerosis in animal models also support this hypothesis. This will be discussed in the succeeding section.

Although there is no apparent increase in CHD risk in past OC users, there seems to be evidence of increased risk of thrombotic cardiovascular disease in certain groups of current OC users (i.e., OC users with other CHD risk factors). Case-control and cohort studies in the U.S. and U.K. have consistently found that current OC users over 35 years of age who also smoke cigarettes heavily have a two- to eightfold increase in risk of CHD (Stampfer et al., 1988; Thorneycroft, 1990; Thorogood and Vessey, 1990; Realini and Goldzieher, 1985), an effect that is independent of duration of use. The increased risk of CHD in current OC users seems to be confined largely to this group.

Continued evaluation of the Royal College of General Practitioners Study, Oxford/FPA, and the Nurses Health Study cohorts has revealed a decreasing rate of

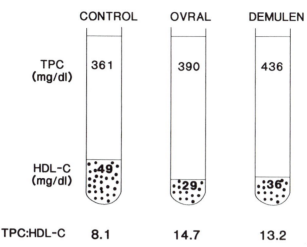

FIG. 4. Effect of Ovral and Demulen on total plasma cholesterol (TPC), HDL concentrations (HDL-C), and the overall proportion of HDL in plasma (TPC:HDL-C) in premenopausal cynomolgus monkeys. (Modified from Clarkson et al., 1990.)

cardiovascular risk in all groups (Thorogood and Vessey, 1990; Stampfer et al., 1990). This finding has been attributed both to the decreased dose of the estrogenic component of the OC as well as the avoidance of OCs as a means of contraception in high-risk groups.

In conclusion, there is no evidence that OCs increase the risk of atherosclerosis-related CHD in women.

EFFECTS ON CORONARY ARTERY ATHEROSCLEROSIS IN CYNOMOLGUS MACAQUES

We summarize here the results of a large study in which we determined the effects of the combination OCs Ovral and Demulen on diet-induced atherosclerosis in cynomolgus macaques (Clarkson et al., 1990). These OC combinations contain equivalent amounts of ethynyl estradiol (50 μg) but structurally and pharmacologically different progestins, norgestrel and ethynodiol diacetate. Effects on the plasma lipoprotein profiles are summarized in Figs. 4 and 5. Despite the marked decrease in plasma HDL and HDL2B levels (Fig. 2) and marked increases in TPC:HDL cholesterol ratio, the extent of coronary artery atherosclerosis was *decreased by* both OCs. This effect was especially marked among females at highest risk due to their plasma lipid profiles (Fig. 6).

Multiple regression analysis was used to estimate the predicted effects of OCs based on altered plasma lipoprotein profiles. When all subjects were considered, an approximate doubling of atherosclerosis extent was predicted, whereas atherosclerosis actually decreased by 50% to 75%. Among high-risk individuals, the contrast

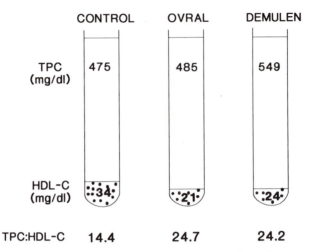

FIG. 5. Effect of Ovral and Demulen on TPC and HDL concentrations of premenopausal cynomolgus monkeys at high risk (pretreatment TPC:HDL-C ratio >4.5) for coronary artery atherosclerosis. (Modified from Clarkson et al., 1990.)

is even more striking: a doubling of atherosclerosis extent was again predicted, whereas a 75% to 85% *decrease* was observed.

The finding of a large inhibitory influence of OC treatment on initiation and progression of atherosclerosis was surprising and indicates that, in terms of their atherogenicity, steroid-induced changes in plasma lipid concentrations are not the same as changes induced by diet. We hypothesize that this atherosclerosis-inhibiting effect is due to the ethynyl estradiol component of the OCs. There is consider-

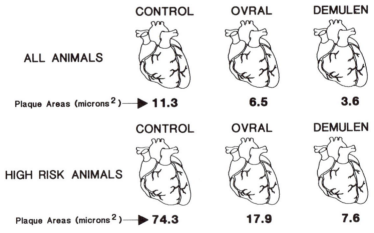

FIG. 6. Effect of oral contraceptives on coronary artery atherosclerosis plaque size in all subjects and the subset of high risk (pretreatment TPC:HDL-C ratio >4.5) premenopausal cynomolgus macaques versus controls. (Modified from Clarkson et al., 1990.)

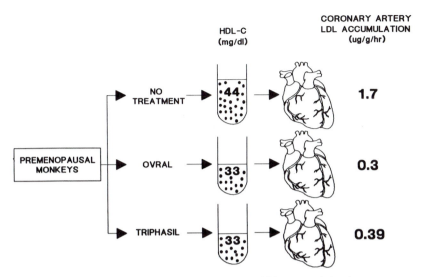

FIG. 7. Mean HDL-C concentrations and coronary artery LDL accumulation in premenopausal cynomolgus females treated with either Ovral or Triphasil versus controls. (Modified from Wagner et al., 1993.)

able evidence to suggest that estrogen affects atherogenesis independent of its effects on plasma lipoproteins. Estrogen and progestin receptors have been identified in arterial endothelial and smooth-muscle cells of several species, most recently in coronary arteries of humans (Ingegno et al., 1988) and nonhuman primates (Lin et al., 1986). Other experimental studies have shown that estrogen treatment results in 1) reduced lipoprotein-induced arterial smooth-muscle cell proliferation (Fischer-Dzoga et al., 1983); 2) inhibition of the myointimal proliferation associated with mechanical endothelial injury (Rhee et al., 1978; Weigensberg et al., 1984), reduced cholesterol ester influx and hydrolysis (Hough and Zilversmit, 1986); 3) inhibition of platelet aggregation (Johnson et al., 1977); 4) increased prostacyclin production (Chang et al., 1980); and 5) decreased collagen and elastin production (Fischer, 1972; Fischer and Swain, 1977; Wolinsky, 1972) by arterial smooth-muscle cells. These findings provide further evidence that vascular estrogen receptors are physiologically functional and that estrogen may directly influence the atherosclerotic process.

In seeking the mechanism that could account for the protective effect of ethynyl estradiol, we used radiolabeled LDL coupled with tyramine cellobiose, a residualizing label, to measure intracellular accumulation of LDL and LDL degradation products in arteries of female cynomolgus monkeys. The animals were fed a moderately atherogenic diet and treated with an OC for 16 weeks (Wagner et al., 1993). The results of these studies are summarized in Fig. 7. The OCs Ovral and Triphasil both induced a more atherogenic lipid profile than diet alone, yet the accumulation of LDL degradation products in the coronary arteries was significantly reduced. This finding is consistent with the findings of Haarbo et al. (1991), who studied the effects of exogenous estrogen and estrogen-progestin combinations on arterial cholesterol accumulation in rabbits fed an atherogenic diet. In these studies, arterial cholesterol accumulation was reduced by one third in rabbits treated with 17β-estradiol, given either alone or in combination with norethisterone or levonorgestrel. This effect was not explained by variation in plasma lipoprotein levels.

Taken together, the evidence from these studies of monkeys and rabbits suggests a mechanism by which an antiatherogenic effect of combination OCs may be mediated. The accumulation of cholesterol is a central characteristic of the development of atherosclerotic plaque (Steinberg et al., 1989). Since plasma LDL is the major source of this cholesterol (Steinberg et al., 1989), factors that inhibit the uptake and degradation of LDL by the arterial wall can be assumed to result in inhibition of atherosclerosis.

Regardless of the mechanism, we conclude from our findings that contraceptive progestin-induced lowering of HDL is not atherogenic if a sufficiently potent estrogen is coadministered. The striking difference between the expected and observed outcome suggests a beneficial effect of ethynyl estradiol on the artery wall.

REFERENCES

Adams MR, Clarkson TB, Koritnik DR, Nash HA. Contraceptive steroids and coronary artery atherosclerosis in cynomolgus macaques. *Fertil Steril* 1987;47:1010.

Babiak J, Rudel LL. Lipoproteins and atherosclerosis. In: Shepherd J, ed. Clinical endocrinology and metabolism. London: Bailliere Tindall; 1987:515–50.

Bradley DD, Wingerd J, Pettiti DB, et al. Serum high-density lipoprotein cholesterol in women using oral contraceptives, estrogens and progestins. *N Engl J Med* 1978;299:17.

Burkman RT, Robinson JC, Kruszon-Moran D, et al. Lipid and lipoprotein changes associated with oral contraceptive use: a randomized clinical trial. *Obstet Gynecol* 1988;71:33.

Chang W-C, Nakao J, Orimo H, Murota S-I. Stimulation of prostacyclin activity by estradiol in rat aorta smooth muscle cell in culture. *Biochim Biophys Acta* 1980;619:107.

Chez RA. Clinical aspects of three new progestogens: desogestrel, gestodene, and norgestimate. *Am J Obstet Gynecol* 1989;160:1296.

Clarkson TB, Shively CA, Morgan TM, et al. Oral contraceptives and coronary artery atherosclerosis of cynomolgus monkeys. *Obstet Gynecol* 1990;75:217.

Engel HJ, Engel E, Lichtlen PR. Coronary atherosclerosis and myocardial infarction in young women—role of oral contraceptives. *Eur Heart J* 1983;4:1.

Fischer GM, Swain ML. Effect of sex hormones on blood pressure and vascular connective tissue in castrated and noncastrated male rats. *Am J Physiol* 1977;232:H617.

Fischer GM. In vivo effects of estradiol on collagen and elastin dynamics in rat aorta. *Endocrinology* 1972;91:1,227.

Fischer-Dzoga K, Wissler RW, Vesselinovitch D. The effect of estradiol on the proliferation of rabbit aorta medial tissue culture cells induced by hyperlipemic serum. *Exp Mol Pathol* 1983;39:355.

Gevers-Leuven JA, Dersjant-Roorda MC, Helmerhorst FM, et al. Estrogenic effect of gestodene- or desogestrel-containing oral contraceptives on lipoprotein metabolism. *Am J Obstet Gynecol* 1990;163:358.

Godsland IF, Crook D, Simpson R, et al. The effects of different formulations of oral contraceptive agents on lipid and carbohydrate metabolism. *N Engl J Med* 1990;323:1,375.

Haarbo J, Leth-Espensen P, Stender S, Christiansen C. Estrogen monotherapy and combined estrogen-progestogen replacement therapy attenuate aortic accumulation of cholesterol in ovariectomized cholesterol-fed rabbits. *J Clin Invest* 1991;87:1,274.

Hough JL, Zilversmit DB. Effect of 17-beta estradiol on aortic cholesterol content and metabolism in cholesterol-fed rabbits. *Arteriosclerosis* 1986;6:57.

Ingegno MD, Money SR, Thelmo W, et al. Progesterone receptors in the human heart and great vessels. *Lab Invest* 1988;59:353.

Johnson M, Ramey E, Ramwell PW. Androgen-mediated sensitivity in platelet aggregation. *Am J Physiol* 1977;232:H381.

Jugdutt BI, Stevens GF, Zacks DJ, et al. Myocardial infarction, oral contraception, cigarette smoking, and coronary artery spasm in young women. *Am Heart J* 1983;106:757.

Kloosterboer HJ, van Wayjen RGA, van den Ende A. Comparative effects of monophasic desogestrel plus ethinyl estradiol and triphasic levonorgestrel plus ethinyl estradiol on lipid metabolism. *Contraception* 1986;34:135.

Knopp RH, Walden CE, Wahl PW, et al. Oral contraceptive and postmenopausal estrogen effects on lipoprotein triglyceride and cholesterol in an adult female population: relationships to estrogen and progestin potency. *J Clin Endocrinol Metab* 1981;53:1123.

Lin AL, Gonzalez R Jr, Carey KD, et al. Estradiol-17 beta affects estrogen receptor distribution and elevates progesterone receptor content in baboon aorta. *Arteriosclerosis* 1986;6:495.

Lipson A, Stoy DB, LaRosa JC, et al. Progestins and oral contraceptive-induced lipoprotein changes: a prospective study. *Contraception* 1986;34:121.

Mishell DR Jr. Use of oral contraceptives in women of older reproductive age. *Am J Obstet Gynecol* 1988;158:1,652.

Notelovitz M, Feldman EB, Gillespy M, et al. Lipid and lipoprotein changes in women taking low-dose, triphasic oral contraceptives: a controlled, comparative, 12-month clinical trial. *Am J Obstet Gynecol* 1989;160:1,269.

Parks JS, Pelkey SJ, Babiak J, et al. Contraceptive steroid effects on lipids and lipoproteins in cynomolgus monkeys. *Arteriosclerosis* 1989;9:261.

Realini JP, Goldzieher JW. Oral contraceptives and cardiovascular disease: a critique of the epidemiologic studies. *Amer J Obstet Gynec* 1985;152:729:798.

Rhee CY, Drouet RO, Spaet YH, Geiger CH. Growth inhibition of cultured vascular smooth muscle cells by estradiol. *Fed Proc* 1978;37:474.

Stampfer MJ, Willett WC, Colditz GA, et al. Past use of oral contraceptives and cardiovascular disease: a meta-analysis in the context of the Nurses' Health Study. *Am J Obstet Gynecol* 1990;163:285.

Stampfer MJ, Willett WC, Colditz GA, et al. A prospective study of past use of oral contraceptive agents and risk of cardiovascular disease. *N Engl J Med* 1988;319:1,313.

Steinberg D, Parthasarathy S, Carew TE, et al. Beyond cholesterol. Modifications of low-density lipoprotein that increase its atherogenicity. *N Engl J Med* 1989;320:915.

Thorneycroft IH. Oral contraceptives and myocardial infarction. *Am J Obstet Gynecol* 1990;163:1,393.

Thorogood M, Vessey MP. An epidemiologic survey of cardiovascular disease in women taking oral contraceptives. *Am J Obstet Gynecol* 1990;163:274.

van der Vange N, Kloosterboer HJ, Haspels AA. Effects of seven low dose combined oral contraceptives on high density lipoprotein subfractions. *Br J Obstet Gynaecol* 1987;94:559.

Wagner JD, Adams MR, Schwenke DC, et al. Oral contraceptive treatment decreases arterial low density lipoprotein degradation in female cynomolgus monkeys. *Circ Res* 1993;72:1300–1307.

Wahl P, Walden C, Knopp R, et al. Effect of estrogen/progestin potency on lipid/lipoprotein cholesterol. *N Engl J Med* 1983;308:862.

Weigensberg BI, Lough H, More RH, et al. Effects of estradiol on myointimal thickenings from catheter injury and on organizing white mural non-occlusive thrombi. *Atherosclerosis* 1984;52:253.

Wolinsky H. Effects of estrogen and progesterone treatment on the response of the aorta of male rats to hypertension. *Circ Res* 1972;30:341.

Pharmacology of the Contraceptive Steroids,
edited by Joseph W. Goldzieher.
Raven Press, Ltd., New York © 1994.

23

Metabolism: Carbohydrate Metabolism

*Karen Elkind-Hirsch and †Joseph W. Goldzieher

*Internal Medicine Specialty Laboratories, Houston, Texas 77054 and
†Department of Obstetrics and Gynecology,
Baylor College of Medicine, Houston, Texas 77030

As early as 1963, there were reports of alterations of carbohydrate metabolism from the use of one of the first oral contraceptives (OCs), which contained 150 μg mestranol and 10 mg norethynodrel. Since then, there have been innumerable studies of the effects of synthetic estrogens and progestins, alone and in combination, on carbohydrate metabolism. The various investigations into the effects of combined OCs are difficult to compare because of the number of different steroids available, the great variety of contraceptive formulations in clinical use, and the frequent changes in dosage. Very few investigators have included simultaneous, comparable control groups not receiving steroids; moreover, most of them tended to use cross-sectional rather than prospective data. The experiments themselves frequently are disparate in study design and test protocols, and analyze different types of women (e.g., obese versus nonobese). An added complication is the well-known within-individual variability in the oral glucose tolerance test (OGTT); this mandates large sample sizes. Greater numbers of abnormal responses have been associated with OGT tests than with the intravenous procedure. Reportedly, more insulin is released in the oral than in the intravenous test, probably because gut factors, in addition to the glucose itself, stimulate the beta cells in the oral test. Nevertheless, in earlier studies, a consistent impairment of glucose tolerance was demonstrated by increases in fasting glucose and insulin levels, and the response of these parameters to a glucose challenge. With changes in the OC formulations, particularly lowering the dose of each component, elevations in insulin and glucose levels have been minimized or eliminated entirely. Recent studies by van der Vange et al. (1987) of women using seven different monophasic or multiphasic preparations consisting of a constant dose of ethynyl estradiol plus levonorgestrel, norethindrone, or one of the newer progestins (gestodene or desogestrel) showed no clinically significant change in glucose tolerance after 6 months of use. In short, as the progestin component was reduced in low-estrogen formulations, there was a concomitant reduction in alterations of carbohydrate parameters.

Although glucose metabolism may be altered in women by OC use, the observed changes in tolerance are related not only to the combination of steroids employed, but also to the ability of the individual user's pancreas to increase insulin production in the face of a hyperglycemic challenge. A confounding problem in understanding the metabolic derangements of carbohydrate metabolism has been the lack of consensus on what is meant by the term "insulin resistance" and its importance relative to altered beta cell function in the progression from a normal state to one of impaired glucose tolerance. In obese nondiabetic subjects, tissue sensitivity to insulin is markedly reduced, yet oral glucose tolerance is little affected because of the beta cells' ability to augment insulin secretion that thereby offsets the defect in insulin action. Even with progression to impaired glucose tolerance and further reduction in insulin-mediated glucose disposal, postprandial glucose levels might only be modestly elevated because of the capacity of the beta cells to meet the extra demand for insulin. Another factor contributing to development of fasting hyperglycemia is excessive hepatic glucose production, but this defect becomes particularly noticeable only when individuals shift from impaired glucose tolerance to frank diabetes mellitus. In general, it would appear that normal glucose levels may be maintained in OC users at the expense of increased insulin levels. Such observations suggest an increased peripheral resistance to the action of insulin during OC use.

Interpretation of contraceptive steroid studies has been further clouded by the tendency to ascribe observed metabolic changes to birth control pills in general, without any attempt to identify the contribution of each steroid in the formulation under study. The individual components have been reported variously to improve carbohydrate tolerance, reduce it, or leave it unaffected. Greater numbers of abnormal responses have been associated with the use of combination-type preparations than with sequential or multiphasic types. In this review, we shall address the unique metabolic effects of each class of contraceptive steroid (synthetic estrogens, 19-norprogestins, and acetoxyprogestins) on glucose tolerance, and on basal and glucose-stimulated peripheral insulin concentrations. While the metabolic effects of OCs superficially resemble changes that occur during pregnancy, it must be realized that the actions of natural and synthetic steroids often differ greatly.

A wide variety of synthetic estrogens has been studied with regard to their effect on carbohydrate metabolism. Comparative studies in rhesus monkeys (Beck, 1969) of various estrogenic compounds showed mestranol to have more pronounced or even exclusively adverse effects on carbohydrate metabolism as compared with ethynyl estradiol. Mestranol not only antagonized the peripheral hypoglycemic action of insulin but also enhanced the plasma response to a glucose stimulus. These results are most surprising since mestranol, estrogenically inactive in itself, is a prodrug for ethynyl estradiol. Some early clinical studies (Di Paolo et al., 1968, 1970) confirmed this exclusive role of mestranol as compared with ethynyl estradiol in humans by using prednisone tolerance tests to study carbohydrate metabolism. In contrast, Leis and coworkers (1977) found no observable differences between the effects of ethynyl estradiol and mestranol on glucose tolerance. As shown by Spellacy and coworkers (1972a, 1978, 1982), conjugated estrogens, mestranol, and ethynyl estradiol had little or no effect on fasting or post-glucose challenge levels of glucose or insulin in normal women after 6 months of use. This was true whether the dosage was equivalent to that used in "high-dose" OC agents (50 μg/day) or was ten times larger. Goldzieher et al. (1978) also found no effect of ethynyl estradiol or mestranol in humans, whereas baboons and beagles yielded opposite changes in glucose disposal rate. Buchler and Warren (1966) noted no effect of diethylstilbestrol on intravenous glucose tolerance. Most recent studies appear to support the hypothesis that the lower estrogenic dose in current OCs (about 30 μg) is not responsible for any impairment of carbohydrate metabolism.

Numerous studies have also examined the effect of progestins on glucose tolerance. High progesterone levels during the luteal phase (Jarrett and Graver, 1968; Roy et al., 1971; Peppler et al., 1978) or exogenously administered progesterone (Kalkhoff et al., 1970) have been associated with a deterioration of glucose tolerance and a decrease in insulin sensitivity as measured by oral and intravenous glucose tolerance tests, as well as when measured by the glucose clamp technique (Valdes and Elkind-Hirsch, 1992; Diamond et al., 1989). Beck (1969) observed that rhesus monkeys treated with large doses of progesterone for 3 weeks exhibited a much slower glucose disappearance rate after exogenous insulin administration; this effect could be overcome by increasing the dose of insulin. He postulated that progesterone produced a mild but significant peripheral resistance to the hypoglycemic effect of insulin. Increased fasting plasma insulin concentrations and plasma insulin responses to oral glucose or intravenous tolbutamide have been observed by Kalkhoff, Jacobson, and Lemper (1970) in women after administration of intramuscular progesterone daily for 6 days, and by Costrini and Kalkhoff (1971) in rats after 21 days of subcutaneous progesterone treatment.

The progesterone-IUD releases some steroid into the circulation; however, Spellacy et al. (1979) found glucose levels remained virtually unchanged whereas plasma insulin values were increased in the fasting, 30-minute, and 3-hour OGTT samples at the 1-year test. These data suggest a decrease in peripheral tissue receptor sites, causing a need for higher levels of insulin in order to maintain glucose homeostasis.

Unlike OCs and injectable progestins, where the dose may range from 150 μg to 2 mg/day, Norplant releases about 60 μg/day of levonorgestrel for the first year, with declining release thereafter. Konje et al. (1992) found alterations in carbohydrate metabolism occurring as early as 1 month after insertion but most markedly after 6 months. As with other progestin-only contraceptives, none of the glucose tolerance curves were either diabetic or suggestive of impaired glucose tolerance in these normal women. In another study, Konje et al. (1992) showed that changes in carbohydrate metabolism revert to normal once the implants are removed. The reversion in blood glucose was apparent at testing 1 month after removal; the insulin values had also dropped 1 month after Norplant removal but were slower to return to preimplant values.

Whereas oral administration of 17-acetoxyprogestins produced no changes in insulin production (Beck, 1970; Larsson-Cohn et al., 1969; Vermeulen et al., 1970; Spellacy et al., 1973b), several investigators have observed a modest increase in circulating insulin after parenteral administration of depot medroxyprogesterone acetate to human subjects (Tuttle and Turkington, 1974; Spellacy et al., 1970a). Spellacy et al. (1970a) found a slight deterioration in glucose tolerance, with concurrent increases in plasma insulin concentrations in 33 of 37 women after 1 year of using DMPA. Beck (1977) observed a similar discrepancy in the effects of short-term orally administered versus parenterally administered 17-acetoxyprogesterone derivatives on insulin production in rhesus monkeys. A number of studies by Spellacy and coworkers (1972a, 1972b, 1975, 1976, 1981, 1982), in which a variety of OCs were employed, have shown the following effects: 1) ethynodiol diacetate caused an elevation of glucose levels and insulin concentration; 2) norethindrone did not alter glucose levels but caused an elevation of insulin concentration, suggesting increased resistance of peripheral tissues with this formulation. Norgestrel administration resulted in an elevation of both glucose and insulin levels and caused the greatest changes in parameters of carbohydrate metabolism during an OGTT. Spellacy et al. suggested that peripheral resistance to the action of insulin increased during OC use, and that higher levels of insulin secretion were needed in order to maintain glucose homeostasis. Oral contraceptives containing 19-norprogestins appeared to be more diabetogenic than other contraceptive preparations in normal women. Spellacy et al. (1972b) observed deterioration of oral glucose tolerance in 13% of normal women after 6 months' use of ethynodiol diacetate (without estrogen). Additionally, the mean plasma insulin concentrations (before and after glucose ingestion) were increased. Wynn and Godsland (1986) compared two types of combination OCs taken over 3 years and showed that the norgestrel formulation produced a larger percentage change in glucose tolerance, with inappropriately low insulin secretion, than an OC containing norethindrone. A recent study by Luyckx and coworkers (1986) compared the effects of a low-dose triphasic norgestrel-containing OC to one containing desogestrel; they found a slight but significant deterioration in glucose tolerance with the former after 6 months, as assessed by the area under the curve during glucose tolerance testing. The trend noted for desogestrel was similar, but did not reach statistical significance.

Clearly, the type of progestin, its dosage, and the frequency and duration of its administration affect the findings, as noted in the differences between different OC preparations containing the same type and dose of estrogen but different progestins.

Synthetic estrogens may modify the effect of progesterone on insulin production. Kalkhoff and colleagues (1970) have shown that concurrent estradiol plus progesterone treatment increases pancreatic islet diameter and isolated islet insulin secretion, and increases fasting plasma insulin concentrations in the rat to a greater extent than does progesterone treatment alone (Costrini and Kalkhoff, 1971; Matute and Kalkhoff, 1973). In rhesus monkeys, concurrent treatment with norethindrone plus mestranol or ethynyl estradiol produced a greater fasting serum insulin concentration and response after intravenous glucose administration than did treatment with any of these three synthetic steroids alone (Beck, 1977). Furthermore, mestranol appears to potentiate the hyperglycemic effect of 19-norprogestins. Spellacy et al. (1970b) reported that women who had been long-term users of norethindrone/mestranol had a much higher incidence of altered carbohydrate tolerance than women using chlormadinone acetate/mestranol. The norethindrone/mestranol group had a 40% incidence of abnormal oral glucose tolerance tests, and an equal number of women were borderline abnormal. By contrast, the women who had received chlormadinone acetate/mestranol sequentially for 6 years had a much lower incidence of carbohydrate intolerance. Similar data were reported in prospective studies. Normal women using OCs that contained a 19-norprogestin for 1 year developed a greater incidence of deterioration of carbohydrate tolerance than women using agents that contained a 17-acetoxyprogestin (Spellacy et al., 1971a, 1971b). Goldman et al. (1969) found a significant deterioration of intravenous glucose tolerance in normal women treated with norethynodrel/mestranol for 3 months, whereas neither Starup et al. (1968) nor Vermeulen and associates (1970) found any significant change in glucose utilization in women treated with megestrol acetate plus either mestranol or ethynyl estradiol. (These studies all used monophasic regimens, thereby eliminating the confounding effect of a sequential regimen.) This finding confirms the conclusion that the dose and type of progestin component are the major influences on carbohydrate metabolism.

Concern about the metabolic effects of OCs led to a continued reduction in steroid dosage, as well as development of triphasic regimens. Rabe and Runnebaum (1986) recommended the use of such formulations to minimize alterations in carbohydrate metabolism. A prospective 2-year study by Spellacy et al. (1990) confirmed data presented in isolated short-term studies (Spellacy et al., 1988, 1989). These data showed that the levonorgestrel preparation was associated with a significant elevation of the plasma glucose and fasting insulin value during an oral glucose tolerance test, whereas minimal alterations were detected in the norethindrone OC users. In contrast, van der Vange et al. (1987) compared seven low-dose monophasic or triphasic OCs, some of which were identical with those used in the studies of Spellacy and others, and did not detect any significant differences in insulin or glucose responses to an oral glucose tolerance test. More recent work reported by Gillespy et al. (1991) also showed no clinically significant effect of two triphasic OCs using levonorgestrel or norethindrone on carbohydrate metabolism.

Recently, Godsland et al. (1991) investigated OC users' carbohydrate metabolism changes by computer modeling of I.V. glucose tolerance test responses of glucose, insulin, and C-peptide concentrations. Insulin resistance, secretion, and metabolism were evaluated in 296 OC users and 95 nonusers. Four combined OCs with similar estrogen level but different progestins and one progestin-only formulation were studied. Incremental glucose, insulin, and C-peptide areas were increased by the levonorgestrel combinations. The desogestrel combination raised incremental glucose and insulin areas to a lesser extent, and the norethindrone combination affected only the incremental glucose area. The glucose elimination constant (k) was reduced by all combinations, the least with the desogestrel formulation; k was unaffected by the norethindrone-only regimen. Combined formulations reduced insulin sensitivity by 30% to 40%; the progestin-only regimen had no effect. Glucose-dependent glucose disposal was not affected by any of the regimens. Insulin concentrations were significantly higher with the desogestrel combination compared to levonorgestrel from 3 to 10 min, and significantly lower from 60 to 90 min. The desogestrel monophasic increased first-phase insulin responsiveness by 39% and reduced the insulin elimination constant by 22%, while the levonorgestrel combination did not affect parameters of the posthepatic insulin delivery model. The desogestrel combination did not affect pancreatic insulin secretion during the intravenous GTT, whereas levonorgestrel combinations increased incremental pancreatic insulin secretion by 23% to 31%; this was due to a 60%-to-90% increase in second-phase secretion. The hepatic insulin throughput index was unaffected by any formulation. The desogestrel monophasic reduced the elimination constants of insulin and C-peptide, increasing their half-lives by 24% and 14%, respectively, while levonorgestrel formulations did not affect insulin or C-peptide elimination. Godsland et al. (1991) concluded that the various combined agents, all containing a similar amount of estrogen, caused similar degrees of insulin resistance, whereas the progestin-only formulation had no effect. They therefore inferred that the estrogenic component was primarily responsible for the insulin resistance, with the progestin modifying this effect, presumably by a progestin-associated difference in insulin half-life (as already noted in 1975 with a norethindrone combination by Srivastava et al.). While the substantial numbers of subjects allow for discernment of statistically significant differences, it should be pointed out that the range of OC users' values is almost invariably within 1 SD of the mean of the controls for the various parameters of posthepatic insulin delivery and pancreatic insulin secretion. Thus, while the frequency distribution of these parameters is shifted in the direction of decreased insulin sensitivity, the values themselves lie within the normal range. Another difficulty with this study is that the control female mean insulin sensitivity index (S_i) of 3.07 is significantly lower than the S_i of 6.2 ± 0.91 reported for normally cycling women during the follicular phase, and is comparable to the decreased mean S_i of 3.2 ± 0.25 found during the luteal phase of the same patients (Valdes and Elkind-Hirsch, 1992).

The minimal model has been used to assess the S_i in various physiological and pathophysiological states. S_i varied from a high of 7.6×10^{-4} min/μU/ml in young whites to 2.3×10^{-4} in obese nondiabetic subjects; in all of the nondiabetic subjects, S_i was normal (Bergman, 1989). The use of norgestrel-containing OCs has been reported to reduce S_i in young women from 5.6 to 2.4×10^{-4} min/μU/ml (Watanabe et al., 1988), similar in degree to insulin resistance seen in obesity.

Early reports of high-dose OC use in women with prior gestational diabetes mellitus showed marked deterioration in glucose tolerance (Beck and Wells, 1969). On the other hand, a high-estrogen sequential formulation given for 2 years to 26 women with a family history of diabetes, of whom half showed an abnormal OGTT, resulted in a shift toward normal carbohydrate metabolism (Moses and Goldzieher, 1970). A study with monophasic OCs containing different doses of levonorgestrel indicated that the dose of progestin determined the degree of carbohydrate disturbance (Briggs, 1979). While Kung et al. (1987) demonstrated an increase in glucose and insulin levels with low-dose OCs in women with prior gestational diabetes mellitus, Skouby and colleagues (1985, 1987) reported that low-dose levorgestrel/ethynyl estradiol may be administered to women with previously impaired glucose tolerance during pregnancy without any deterioration of the glucose metabolism postpartum. Other recent studies on the short-term use of low-dose OCs in women with prior gestational diabetes mellitus also did not show any adverse effect on carbohydrate metabolism (Kjos et al., 1990). Both OC and nonuser groups showed a significant and similar deterioration in glucose tolerance 6 to 13 months postpartum, with an overall prevalence of 14% impaired glucose tolerance and 17% diabetes mellitus.

Clearly, the cause of the deterioration in glucose tolerance in women using OCs is uncertain. Variations in sex hormone levels have been increasingly implicated in alterations of insulin and glucose metabolism. One theory is that this effect may be similar to the effect of luteal phase progesterone, namely an impairment of binding of insulin to its receptor. Investigations of the action of insulin at the cellular level suggest such a relationship; insulin binding has been found to decrease with increasing estradiol and progesterone levels (de Pirro et al., 1978, 1981; Moore et al., 1981; Tsibris et al., 1980). Early reports showed that insulin binding was decreased during OC administration as compared to the normal follicular phase (Beck-Nielsen et al., 1979). Subsequently, de Pirro et al. (1981) confirmed these observations and specifically noted a reduction in receptor concentration during progestin-only OC use. Other possible mechanisms by which OCs might alter carbohydrate metabolism are by: 1) increase in insulin-antagonistic hormones such as cortisol, growth hormone, or glucagon; 2) alteration in liver morphologic characteristics and function; 3) alteration of the GI tract (absorption and/or gut-insulin release factors); and 4) increase in peripheral insulin resistance. As just outlined, the differences in glucose and insulin profiles during the OGTT in OC users have been interpreted by a number of investigators as the result of oral-steroid-induced insulin resistance and hypersecretion of insulin by the pancreas. To eliminate the possibility that OC steroids elevate insulin levels by reducing the rate of insulin clearance, Wynn and Godsland (1986) measured plasma C-peptide as a measure of insulin secretion that is relatively unconfounded by the effects of clearance. These studies supported the interpretation that hyperinsulinemia in OC users results from an increased pancreatic beta-cell response to the glucose load. This interpretation is consistent with the demonstrated action of progesterone in potentiating beta-cell insulin secretion (Howell et al., 1977). However, Kasdorf and Kalkhoff (1988) found no consistent relationship between total plasma insulin responses during OGTT and the insulin sensitivity results of the euglycemic clamp technique. They concluded that administration of 30 μg ethynyl estradiol/150 μg levonorgestrel induces a mild state of insulin resistance due to an altered peripheral tissue sensitivity to the hormones, and may diminish with time. This effect did not correlate consistently with the total plasma insulin responses during OGTTs, nor was it associated with elevations of plasma androgen levels. In other recent studies examining the metabolic effects of low-dose OCs, no impairment of glucose tolerance was found in nondiabetic women or women with gestational diabetes given low-dose triphasic OCs (Skouby et al., 1985). Using the euglycemic clamp technique, Skouby and colleagues (1987) further assessed sensitivity to insulin in normal women and women with gestational diabetes, before and twice during administration of triphasic low-dose OCs. While the increased insulin resistance during OC use was more apparent in previous gestational diabetic women, the decrease in insulin sensitivity was not sufficient to alter glucose tolerance in either group. The results of this study point to a postreceptor defect such as abnormal coupling between the insulin-receptor complexes and the glucose transport system, or an intracellular enzymatic defect induced by the contraceptive steroids (Skouby et al., 1987).

Alterations in glucose and insulin levels per se are thought by some to increase cardiovascular risk (Haffner et al., 1990); consequently, any lessening of the carbohydrate and lipid metabolic effects of OCs is a prudent goal to pursue, and this has driven the engine of change toward lower dosage and more "metabolically neutral" progestational compounds in the latest generation of OCs. However, formulation of the concept in these terms sidesteps the issue of how much change is of pathogenetic importance, considering the fluctuations that occur in the course of normal existence. Moreover, the basis for cardiovascular concerns relies in large part on epidemiological studies carried out almost exclusively in males and to a minimal extent, if at all, in young women with a full complement of endogenous reproductive hormones. The cardioprotective effect of estrogens is now well established by epidemiological and experimental investigation, as well as by primate studies (see Chapter 22). It may be timely to rethink the alleged hazards of contraceptive-steroid-induced changes in carbohydrate metabolism in this perspective.

While studies of the effect of OCs on carbohydrate metabolism have been for 3 decades a well-funded, thriving industry generating scores if not hundreds of publications, reports of the clinical consequences of these alterations are most notable for their scarcity. The absence of an atherogenic effect of long-term (mostly high-dose) OC use is now well documented (e.g., Stampfer et al., see Chapter 22) as is the overriding of the potentially harmful effects of "adverse" lipid changes by estrogen in OC formulations. From a practical point of view, both the Royal College of General Practitioners and the Oxford FPA prospective studies examined the incidence of first occurrences of diabetes mellitus in high-dose OC users prior to 1979. No differences were found among nonusers, past OC users, and current OC users. The large study of Duffy and Ray (1984) followed a subset of 593 women (out of a cohort of 8,652 healthy women) who failed a 1-hour OGTT, for a mean of 8.55 years from 1969 through 1978 (again, high-dose OC use). No permanent change in glucose status as a result of OC use was found in an analysis for impaired glucose tolerance, diabetes mellitus, diabetic symptoms, or the use of oral anti-diabetic agents and/or insulin.

Radberg et al. (1982) studied the effect of two types of OC in 25 diabetic women. In those taking a combination of 50 μg ethynyl estradiol/2.5mg lyndiol, 13 of 23 (57%) had their mean insulin requirement raised by 7% (3.5 units); "no dramatic deterioration of the diabetes control was experienced...it is our impression that changes in diabetes control...are so small that they cannot account for any increased risk of aggravation of the diabetes" (Radberg et al., 1982). A 5-year prospective study of nearly 1,000 diabetic women (Klein et al., 1990) concluded that "neither current or past use nor number of years of use of oral contraceptives was associated with severity of retinopathy, hypertension, or current glycosylated hemoglobin." Finally, one of us (Goldzieher) has, over the past 20 years, made a specific point of inquiring on the subject of OCs at the end of any lecture given or session attended, whether anyone in the (clinical) audience had personally witnessed the control of an overt diabetic worsen or a subclinical diabetic become an overt diabetic as a consequence of OC initiation or use; to date there has not been a single report of a positive response.

It may be time to conclude that the mechanism of the effect of contraceptive steroids on carbohydrate metabolism remains to be fully elucidated, but that, in any event, the findings will not be of clinical or prognostic significance. More important is the point that it has been common to withhold prescription of OCs to women with impaired carbohydrate tolerance. Since pregnancy (wanted or unwanted) in diabetic women is a life-threatening risk to both mother and fetus, it would seem that avoidance of one of the most effective contraceptive modalities at our disposal approaches the ultimate in counterproductive decision-making.

REFERENCES

Beck P. Comparison of the metabolic effects of chlormadinone acetate and conventional contraceptive steroids in man. *J Clin Endocrinol Metab* 1970;30:785–91.

Beck P. Effect of progestin on glucose and lipid metabolism. *Ann NY Acad Sci* 1977;286:434–45.

Beck P. Effects of gonadal hormones and contraceptive steroids on glucose and insulin metabolism. In: *Metabolic effects of gonadal hormones and contraceptive steroids.* New York: Plenum Press; 1969:

Beck P, Wells SA. Comparison of the mechanisms underlying carbohydrate intolerance in subclinical diabetic women during pregnancy and during postpartum oral contraceptive steroid treatment. *J Clin Endocrinol Metab* 1969;29:807–18.

Beck-Nielsen H, Kuhl C, Pederson O, et al. Decreased insulin binding to monocytes from normal pregnant women. *J Clin Endocrinol Metab* 1979;49:810.

Bergman RN. Toward physiological understanding of glucose tolerance. Minimal model approach. *Diabetes* 1989;38:1512–27.

Bertoli A, De Pirro R, Fusco A, et al. Differences in insulin receptors between men and menstruating women and influence of sex hormones on insulin binding during the menstrual cycle. *J Clin Endocrinol Metab* 1980;50:246–50.

Briggs MH. Biochemical basis for the selection of oral contraceptives. *Internat J Gynaecol Obstet* 1979;16:509–17.

Buchler D, Warren JC. Effects of estrogen on glucose tolerance. *Am J Obstet Gynecol* 1966;95:479–83.

Costrini NV, Kalkhoff RK. Relative effects of pregnancy, estradiol and progesterone on plasma insulin and pancreatic islet insulin secretion. *J Clin Endocrinol Metab* 1971;50:992–9.

De Pirro R, Forte F, Bertoli A, et al. Changes in insulin receptors during oral contraception. *J Clin Endocrinol Metab* 1981;52:29–33.

De Pirro R, Fusco A, Bertoli A, et al. Insulin receptors during the menstrual cycle in normal women. *J Clin Endocrinol Metab* 1978;47:1,387–90.

Diamond MP, Simonson DC, DeFronzo RA. Menstrual cyclicity has a profound effect on glucose homeostasis. *Fertil Steril* 1989;52:204–8.

DiPaola G, Puchulu F, Robin M, et al. Oral contraceptives and carbohydrate metabolism. *Am J Obstet Gynecol* 1968;101:206–16.

DiPaola G, Robin M, Nicholson R. Estrogen therapy and glucose tolerance test. *Am J Obstet Gynecol* 1970;107:124–32.

Duffy TJ, Ray R. Oral contraceptive use: prospective followup of women with suspected glucose intolerance. *Contraception* 1984;30:197–208.

Gillespy M, Notelovitz M, Ellingson AB, Khan YF. Effect of long-term triphasic oral contraceptive use on glucose tolerance and insulin secretion. *Obstet Gynecol* 1991;78:108–14.

Godsland IF, Walton C, Felton C, et al. Insulin resistance, secretion, and metabolism in users of oral contraceptives. *J Clin Endocrinol Metab* 1991;74:64–70.

Goldman JA, Ovadia JL, Eckerling B. The effect of pseudopregnancy by ovulatory suppressants on the glucose tolerance in women. *Fertil Steril* 1969;20:393.

Goldzieher JW, Chenault CB, de la Pena A, et al. Comparative studies of the ethynyl estrogens used in oral contraceptives VI. Effects with and without progestational agents on carbohydrate metabolism in humans, baboons and beagles. *Fertil Steril* 1978;30:146–52.

Haffner SM, Stern MP, Hazuda HP, et al. Cardiovascular risk factors in confirmed prediabetic individuals. *JAMA* 1990;263:2,893–8.

Howell SL, Tyhurst M, Green I. Direct effects of progesterone on rat islets of Langerhans in vivo and in tissue culture. *Diabetologia* 1977;13:579–83.

Jarrett RJ, Graver HJ. Changes in oral glucose tolerance during the menstrual cycle. *Br Med J* 1968; 2:528–9.

Kalkhoff RK, Jacobson M, Lemper D. Progesterone, pregnancy and the augmented plasma insulin response. *J Clin Endocrinol Metab* 1970;31:24–8.

Kasdorf G, Kalkhoff RK. Prospective studies of insulin sensitivity in normal women receiving oral contraceptive agents. *J Clin Endocrinol Metab* 1988;66:846–852.

Kjos SL, Shoupe D, Douyan S, et al. Effect of low dose oral contraceptives on carbohydrate and lipid metabolism in women with recent gestational diabetes: results of a controlled, randomized, prospective study. *Am J Obstet Gynecol* 1990;163;1,822–7.

Klein BEK, Moss SE, Klein R. Oral contraceptives in women with diabetes. *Diabetes Care* 1990;13: 895.

Konje JC, Otolorin EO, Ladipo OA. The effect of continuous subdermal levonorgestrel (Norplant) on carbohydrate metabolism. *Am J Obstet Gynecol* 1992;166:15–9.

Kung AW, Ma JT, Wong VC, et al. Glucose and lipid metabolism with triphasic oral contraceptives in women with history of gestational diabetes. *Contraception* 1987;35:257–69.

Larsson-Cohn U, Tengstrom B, Wide L. Glucose tolerance and insulin response during daily continuous low dose oral contraceptive treatment. *Acta Endocrinol* 1969;62:242–50.

Leis D, Bottermann P, Roswitha E, Udo M. Comparison of ethinylestradiol and mestranol in sequential type oral contraceptives in their effect on blood glucose and serum insulin in oral glucose tolerance tests. *Fertil Steril* 1977;28:737–40.

Luyckx AS, Gaspard UJ, Romus MA, et al. Carbohydrate metabolism in women who used oral contraceptives containing levonorgestrel or desogestrel: a 6 months' prospective study. *Fertil Steril* 1986;45: 635.

Matute M, Kalkhoff R. Sex steroid influence on hepatic gluconeogenesis and glycogen formation. *Endocrinol* 1973;92:762–8.

Moore P, Kolterman O, Weyant J, Olefsky JM. Insulin binding in human pregnancy: comparisons to the postpartum, luteal, and follicular states. *J Clin Endocrinol Metab* 1981;52:937–41.

Moses LE, Goldzieher JW. The influence of a sequential oral contraceptive on the carbohydrate metabolism of diabetics and prediabetics. *Advanced planned parenthood*. In: Proceedings of the VIII Annual Meeting of the AAPPP. Boston: Exc Medical International Congress Series 224. 1970:

Peppler U, Thefeld W, Wincenty U. Oraler glukosetoleranztest bei frauen in abhangigkeit vom menstruationszyklus. *Klin Wochenschr* 1978;56:659–62.

Phillips N, Duffy T. One hour glucose tolerance in relation to use of oral contraceptive drugs. *Am J Obstet Gynecol* 1973;116:91–100.

Rabe T, Runnebaum B. Progestins and carbohydrate metabolism. *Internat J Fertil* 1986;31:31–45.

Radberg T, Gustafson A, Skryten A, Karlsson K. Oral contraception in diabetic women. *Horm Metab Res* 1982;14:61–5.

Roy SK, Ghosh BP, Bhattacharjee SK. Changes in oral glucose tolerance during normal menstrual cycle. *J Indian Med Assoc* 1971;57:201–4.

Skouby SO, Anderson O, Saurbrey N, Kuhl C. Oral contraception and insulin sensitivity: in vivo assessment in normal women and women with previous gestational diabetes. *J Clin Endocrinol Metab* 1987;64:519–23.

Skouby SO, Kuhl C, Molsted-Pederson L. Triphasic oral contraception: metabolic effects in normal women and those with previous gestational diabetes. *Am J Obstet Gynecol* 1985;153:495–500.

Skouby SO, Mosted-Pederson L, Kuhl C. Low dosage oral contraception in women with previous gestational diabetes. *Obstet Gynecol* 1982;59:325–328.

Spellacy WN. Carbohydrate metabolism during treatment with estrogen, progestogen and low dose oral contraceptives. *Am J Obstet Gynecol* 1982;142;732.

Spellacy WN, Buhi WC, Birk SA. Carbohydrate and lipid metabolic studies before and after one year of treatment with ethynodiol diacetate in "normal" women. *Fertil Steril* 1976;27:900.

Spellacy WN, Buhi WC, Birk S. Carbohydrate and lipid studies in women using the progesterone intrauterine device for one year. *Fertil Steril* 1979;31:381–4.

Spellacy WN, Buhi WC, Birk SA. The effect of estrogen on carbohydrate metabolism: glucose, insulin and growth hormone studies on 170 women ingesting Premarin, mestranol, and ethinyl estradiol for 6 months. *Am J Obstet Gynecol* 1972a;114:378–92.

Spellacy WN, Buhi WC, Birk SA. Effect of estrogen treatment for 1 year on carbohydrate and lipid metabolism in women with normal and abnormal glucose tolerance tests. *Am J Obstet Gynecol* 1978; 131:87.

Spellacy WN, Buhi WC, Birk SA. The effect of the progestin ethynodiol diacetate on glucose, insulin and growth hormone after 6 months' treatment. *Acta Endocrinol* 1972b;70;373.

Spellacy WN, Buhi WC, Birk SA. The effect of two years of mestranol treatment on carbohydrate metabolism. *Metabolism* 1982;31:1,006.

Spellacy WN, Buhi WC, Birk SA. Effects of norethindrone on carbohydrate and lipid metabolism. *Obstet Gynecol* 1975;46:560.

Spellacy WN, Buhi WC, Birk SA. The effects of norgestrel on carbohydrate and lipid metabolism over one year. *Am J Obstet Gynecol* 1976;125:984.

Spellacy WN, Buhi WC, Birk SA. Prospective studies of carbohydrate metabolism in "normal" women using norgestrel for 18 months. *Fertil Steril* 1981;35:167.

Spellacy WN, Buhi WC, Birk SA, McCreary SA. Metabolic studies in women taking norethindrone for 6 months' time (measurement of blood glucose, insulin, and triglyceride concentrations). *Fertil Steril* 1973a;24:419–25.

Spellacy WN, Buhi WC, Birk SA, McCreary SA. Studies of chlormadinone acetate and mestranol on blood glucose and insulin II. Twelfth month oral glucose tolerance test. *Fertil Steril* 1971b;4:224.

Spellacy WN, Buhi WC, Birk SA, McCreary SA. Studies of ethynodiol diacetate and mestranol on blood glucose and plasma insulin. *Contraception* 1971a;3:185.

Spellacy WN, Buhi WC, Spellacy CE, et al. Glucose, insulin and growth hormone studies in long-term users of oral contraceptives. *Am J Obstet Gynec* 1970b;106:173.

Spellacy WN, Ellingson AB, Kotlik A, Tsibris JCM. Glucose and insulin levels after 6 months' treatment with a triphasic oral contraceptive containing ethinyl estradiol and norethindrone. *J Reprod Med* 1989;34:540–2.

Spellacy WN, Ellingson AB, Kotlik A, Tsibris JCM. Prospective study of carbohydrate metabolism in women using a triphasic oral contraceptive containing norethindrone and ethinyl estradiol for 3 months. *Am J Obstet Gynecol* 1988;159:877–9.

Spellacy WN, Ellingson AB, Tsibris JCM. Two year carbohydrate metabolism studies in women using a norethindrone or levonorgestrel triphasic oral contraceptive. *Adv Contraception* 1990;6:185–91.

Spellacy WN, Newton RE, Buhi WC, Birk SA. Carbohydrate and lipid studies during 6 months treatment with megestrol acetate. *Am J Obstet Gynecol* 1973b;116:1,074–8.

Spellacy WN, McLeod AGW, Buhi WC, et al. Medroxyprogesterone acetate and carbohydrate metabolism: measurement of glucose, insulin, and growth hormone during 6 months' time. *Fertil Steril* 1970a;21:457.

Starup J, Date J, Deckert T. Serum insulin and intravenous glucose tolerance in oral contraception. *Acta Endocrinol* 1968;58:537–44.

Tsibris JC, Raynor LO, Buhi WC, et al. Insulin receptors in circulating erythrocytes and monocytes from women on oral contraceptives or pregnant women near term. *J Clin Endocrinol Metab* 1980;51: 711–7.

Tuttle S, Turkington VE. Effects of medroxyprogesterone acetate on carbohydrate metabolism. *Obstet Gynecol* 1974;43:685–92.

Valdes CT, Elkind-Hirsch KE. IVGTT-derived insulin sensitivity changes during the menstrual cycle. *J Clin Endocrinol Metab* 1991;72:642–6.

Van der Vange N, Kloosterboer HJ, Haspels AA. Effect of seven low dose combined oral contraceptive preparations on carbohydrate metabolism. *Am J Obstet Gynecol* 1987;156:918–22.

Vermeulen A, Daneels R, Thiery M. Effects of oral contraceptives on carbohydrate metabolism. *Diabetologia* 1970;6:519–23.

Watanabe R, Bergman RN, Roy S. Application of the minimal model method to the evaluation of metabolic changes during oral contraceptive therapy. In: *Proceedings of the Society Gynecologic Investigation.* Baltimore: 1988:1(abst).

Wynn V, Godsland I. Effects of oral contraceptives on carbohydrate metabolism. *J Reprod Med* 1986; 31:892–7

Pharmacology of the Contraceptive Steroids,
edited by Joseph W. Goldzieher.
Raven Press, Ltd., New York © 1994.

24

Metabolism: Contraceptive Steroids and Some Plasma Proteins

Göran Cullberg

Department of Obstetrics and Gynecology, University of Goathenburg S-43362, Sweden

In 1968 it was shown (Laurell et al.) that combined estrogen-progestin oral contraceptives induced several changes in the plasma protein pattern in humans. A thorough study on 25 known sex steroid-reacting plasma proteins was reported in 1979 by Laurell and Kullander, who compared the effects of pregnancy against hypoestrogenicity in amenorrheic women versus the effect of danocrine as an androgenic/anabolic substance.

The possibility of using plasma proteins as indicators of the metabolic effects of contraceptives has been extensively discussed, especially concerning androgenicity of progestational compounds (Cullberg et al., 1985).

The intent of this chapter is:

1. To establish patterns to characterize oral contraceptive (OC) steroids by their effect on plasma proteins in man.
2. To describe plasma protein changes observed with some of the progestational compounds used in OCs.
3. To discuss the possible clinical implications of these changes.

The proteins involved in blood coagulation and lipoproteins are discussed in other chapters.

ESTROGENS

Nonalkylated "natural" estrogens (estradiol, estrone, and estriol) have rather limited plasma protein effects when given in low to moderate dosages. The use of estradiol and estriol in OCs has had very limited clinical trial. Subnormal levels of estradiol (e.g., in amenorrhea or menopause) produce very small changes in the estrogen-sensitive plasma proteins (Laurell and Rannevik, 1979).

Alkylated estrogens are protected against rapid metabolic degradation and have strong effects on the liver. Mestranol, used early on for OCs, was shown to be metabolized to ethynyl estradiol (EE), and EE is now generally used in the range of 20 to 50 μg. It has a dose-dependent effect over the range from 10 to 70 μg on many plasma proteins. After oral or sublingual intake (Mattson et al., 1983) there is increased synthesis of sex-hormone-binding globulin (SHBG), cortisol-binding globulin (CBG), thyroxine-binding globulin (TBG) and ceruloplasmin (CP) (Laurell et al., 1968). Pregnancy-zone protein (PZ) is another sensitive estrogen responder (Damber et al., 1979). Some other plasma proteins such as albumin and orosomucoid decrease in concentration, probably due to dilution in an increased plasma volume (Laurell et al., 1968).

PROGESTINS

Progestins are by definition substances with a high affinity for the progesterone receptor, but they can also have estrogenic or androgenic/anabolic effects.

Progesterone in its micronized form has been shown to have little, if any, estrogen-counteracting effect on plasma protein changes (Ottoson, 1984).

The synthetic *17α-hydroxyprogestins* such as medroxyprogesterone acetate have little effect on SHBG capacity (Victor and Johansson, 1977) unless given in very high doses (van Kammen et al., 1975). Megestrol acetate given alone even induces an estrogen-like increase in SHBG capacity (el Makhzangy et al., 1979).

The *19-norprogestins*, when given alone, suppress the synthesis of SHBG (Laurell and Rannevik, 1979; Cullberg, 1984; Si et al., 1989) and increase the synthesis of prealbumin (PA), a property that seems to be linked with androgenicity or 17α-alkylation (Laurell and Rannevik, 1979; Cullberg, 1984). Changes in endogenous estrogen levels due to hypothalamic effects of the steroid seem to mean little in this context, since low SHBG levels have been found in spite of normal estradiol levels (Laurell and Rannevik, 1979; Cullberg, 1984) and vice versa.

When given together with EE, these progestins have varying and sometimes dose-dependent effects that abolish the estrogen-induced increase in SHBG and TBG, for example (Cullberg et al., 1985; Si et al., 1989; Barbosa et al., 1971). The variation between the different 19-norprogestins has been discussed by some researchers (Laurell and Rannevik, 1979; Cullberg et al., 1985; el Makhzangy et al., 1979; Barbosa et al., 1971) as a sign of varying intrinsic androgenic effects, and by others as antiestrogenic effects (Cullberg, 1984; Fotherby, 1988).

The subgroup of norethindrone and its analogues includes lynestrenol, which is a prodrug that is converted by oxidation in the liver into norethindrone, the active substance. This group of progestins generally has a dose-dependent, estrogen-counteracting effect (Cullberg et al., 1985; el Makhzangy et al., 1979; Cullberg, 1984) that permits SHBG increases when 1 mg norethindrone or less is combined with 30 to 50 μg EE. When 5 mg lynestrenol is given alone it elevates PA levels as a measure of androgenicity, but TBG is not changed (Cullberg, 1984).

The gonane group includes levonorgestrel (LNG), desogestrel (DSG), gestodene

TABLE 1. *Sex-steroid-induced changes in some plasma proteins*

	Ethynyl. estrog.	17α-OH- prog.	19-nor- prog.	Comb. OC:s
PZ	+	0	0	+
CP	+	0	0, – ?	+
CBG	+	0	0	+
SHBG	+	+,0, –	–	+,0, –
TBG	+	0	0, –	+,0 –
PA	–	0	+	–,0

+ —denoting increasing concentrations
0—no change
– —decreasing concentrations
Based on references given in text.

(GSD), and norgestimate (NGM). Desogestrel is, like lynestrenol, a prodrug with 3-keto-desogestrel as active metabolite. Since metabolization is easy and plasma protein effects are equal (unpublished data), in the text that follows DSG and 3-keto-DSG are used synonymously.

When 0.15 mg LNG is given alone, it has a moderate CP-lowering effect (Fotherby, 1988) that may be taken as an antiestrogenic effect. This, however, is the only observation of its kind. DSG alone in dosages from 0.125 to 0.5 mg (Cullberg, 1984) does not affect the levels of CBG, CP, and TBG, but SHBG is dose-dependently suppressed. Prealbumin was not influenced.

The more remarkable androgenic/antiestrogenic effect of LNG is apparent as an annihilation of SHBG changes at dosages of 0.15 mg in combination with 30 μg EE (Cullberg et al., 1985; Fotherby, 1988). Increases in SHBG are very slight and, in some cases, SHBG concentrations are even decreasing. In this context, androgenic side effects (acne, weight gain, hirsutism) have been observed (Cullberg et al., 1985). It has been debated whether these androgenic side effects depend on increasing nonbound (free) testosterone displaced from SHBG, or if the LNG itself has enough androgenicity to induce them (Laurell and Rannevik, 1979; Cullberg et al., 1985; Victor and Johansson, 1977; Fotherby, 1988). However, simultaneously there is also a decrease in total testosterone of some 30% to 50%, and several studies have shown unchanged percentages of free testosterone (Bergink et al., 1981; Hammond et al., 1984; Janaud et al., 1992) after treatment with both monophasic and triphasic combinations. Another study shows a 50% reduction in absolute free testosterone (van der Vange et al., 1990).

In contrast, SHBG concentrations increase 200% to 300% with the other gonanes when combined with EE (Cullberg et al., 1985; van der Vange et al., 1990; Corson, 1990), and absolute free testosterone is reduced by 50%. The level is doubled in 7 to 8 days, with maximal levels obtained after 15 to 18 days (Fotherby, 1988; Cullberg et al., 1982). Ceruloplasmin, CBG, and TBG are increased to the same degree with all gonanes combined with EE. These findings are summarized in Table 1. The last row gives the effect of EE + a progestin in combination.

ANTIESTROGENICITY

The androgen-like effect of LNG on SHBG has been termed antiestrogenic. Certainly this is an estrogen-counteracting effect, but similar effects are induced by androgens (Laurell and Rannevik, 1979; Barbosa et al., 1971).The term antiestrogenicity has been used in animal assays for the progesterone effect on estrogen-primed vaginal mucosa with decreased karyopyknotic index as a result (Allen-Doisy test) (Cullberg, 1984). Such effects have been shown for all progestins in their initial testing. A "true antiestrogenicity" ought to mean a block also on estrogen-only induced changes (e.g., in CP and CBG). Such reports are very scarce; there is only one (Si et al., 1989), with a 35% suppression of CP after long-term treatment with LNG. When EE is added, no such effects can be seen. It is thus more appropriate to speak of androgenicity rather than antiestrogenicity of LNG in terms of its effect on plasma proteins.

CONCLUSIONS

Plasma protein changes can be used as measures of estrogenic and androgenic/anabolic effects with characteristic patterns. The changes can be used to compare potency of estrogens as well as progestins, since many changes are dose-dependent. The norethindrone group and LNG suppress dose-dependently the EE-induced SHBG increases; the other gonanes have no such effect. The only change that might be of clinical importance is the decrease in SHBG, which can cause androgenic side effects in women with initially low SHBG levels and thus high free testosterone. Increased TBG and CBG levels do not change the levels of free thyroxine or cortisol.

REFERENCES

Barbosa J, Ulysses SS, Doe RP. Effects of anabolic steroids on hormone-binding proteins, serum cortisol and serum non-bound cortisol. *J Clin Endocrinol* 1971;32:232.

Bergink EW, Holma P, Pyörälä T. Effects of oral contraceptive combinations containing levonorgestrel or desogestrel on serum proteins and androgen binding. *Scand J Clin Lab Invest* 1981;41:663.

Corson SL. Efficacy and clinical profile of a new oral contraceptive containing norgestimate. *Acta Obstet Gynecol Scand* 1990;152 [Suppl]:25.

Cullberg G. Androgenic, anabolic, estrogenic and antiestrogenic effects of desogestrel and lynestrenol: effects on serum protein and vaginal cytology. *Contraception* 1984;30:73.

Cullberg G, Dovre PA, Lindstedt G, Steffensen K. On the use of plasma proteins as indicators of the metabolic effects of combined oral contraceptives. *Acta Obstet Gynecol Scand* 1985;111 [Suppl]:29.

Cullberg G, Knutsson F, Lindstedt G, Mattsson LÅ, Steffensen K. Ethinylestradiol and a new progestogen (desogestrel) in a low-dose combination. *Acta Obstet Gynecol Scand* 1982;111 [Suppl]:29.

Damber MG, Sandström B, von Schoultz B, Stigbrand T. A new and sensitive method to quantify and compare the biological potency of various estrogens in man. *Acta Obstet Gynecol Scand* 1979;58:527.

el Makhzangy MN, Wynn V, Lawrence M. Sex hormone binding globulin capacity as an index of oestrogenicity or androgenicity in women on oral contraceptive steroids. *Clin Endocrinol* 1979;10:39.

Fotherby K. Interactions with contraceptive steroids with binding proteins and the clinical implications. *Ann NY Acad Sci* 1988;538:313.

Hammond GL, Langley MS, Robinson PA, Nummi S, Lund S. Serum steroid binding concentrations, distribution of progestogens and bioavailability of testosterone during treatment with contraceptives containing desogestrel or levonorgestrel. *Fertil Steril* 1984;42:44.

Janaud A et al. A comparison study of lipid and androgen metabolism with triphasic oral contraceptive formulations containing norgestimate or levonorgestrel. *Acta Obstet Scand* 1992;156 [Suppl]:33–8.

Laurell CB, Kullander S, Thorell J. Effect of administration of a combined estrogen-progestin contraceptive on the level of individual plasma proteins. *Scand J Clin Lab Invest* 1968;21:337.

Laurell CB, Rannevik G. A comparison of plasma protein changes induced by danazol, pregnancy, and estrogens. *J Clin Endocrinol Metab* 1979;49:719.

Mattson LÅ, Cullberg G, Lindstedt G. Ethinylestradiol administered by oral and sublingual routes: a comparative study in ovarectomised women. *Horm Metab Res* 1983;15:36.

Ottoson UB. Oral progesterone and estrogen-progestogen therapy. *Acta Obstet Gynecol Scand* 1984;127 [Suppl]:26.

Si S, Jun-Kang C, Mei-Li H, Fotherby K. Effect of some oral contraceptives on serum concentrations of sex hormone binding globulin and ceruloplasmin. *Contraception* 1989;39:385.

van der Vange N, Blankenstein MA, Klosterboer HJ, Haspels AA, Thijssen JHH. Effects of seven low-dose combined oral contraceptives on sex hormone binding globulin, corticosteroid binding globulin, total and free testosterone. *Contraception* 1990;41:345.

van Kammen E, Thijssen JHH, Rademaker B, Schwartz F. The influence of hormonal contraceptives on sex hormone binding globulin (SHBG) capacity. *Contraception* 1975;11:53.

Victor A, Johansson EDB. Effects of d-norgestrel induced decreases in sex hormone binding globulin capacity on the d-norgestrel levels in plasma. *Contraception* 1977;16:115.

Pharmacology of the Contraceptive Steroids,
edited by Joseph W. Goldzieher.
Raven Press, Ltd., New York © 1994.

25

Metabolism: Vitamins and Trace Elements

Kosin Amatayakul

Department of Obstetrics and Gynecology, Faculty of Medicine and Research Institute for Health Sciences, Chiang Mai University, Chiang Mai 50002, Thailand

Studies in several developed countries have suggested that oral contraceptives (OCs) may hasten the onset of signs of vitamin B deficiency. Prasad et al. (1975) indicated that the prevalence of such signs tended to increase in lower socio-economic groups. Other studies suggest that some side effects of OCs may be attributable to a deficiency particularly of vitamin B-6, and that supplementation with pyridoxine reversed certain of these symptoms (Adams et al., 1973; Larsson-Cohn, 1975; Coelingh-Bennink and Schreurs, 1975; Spellacy, Buhi, and Birk, 1972; and Amatayakul, 1979a). A report of the WHO Task Force on Oral Contraceptives (1985) found no further changes in the biochemical indices of vitamins in women already deficient. This raises questions as to whether the woman who is already grossly deficient is resistant to any further deficiency, and whether resistance to further biochemical deterioration is also true for the clinical signs (Prasad et al., 1975). Bamji and Prema (1978a) found that women with evidence of deficiency and with poor nutritional status who used OCs often showed no clinical signs or symptoms of vitamin deficiencies.

Under WHO's Special Programme for Research, Development, and Research Training in Human Reproduction auspices, a study using standardized procedures for assessment of clinical symptomatologies together with biochemical vitamin assays with good quality control assessment was undertaken on 2,001 rural northern Thai women of active reproductive ages—499 on OCs, 500 on depot-medroxy-progesterone acetate (DMPA), 501 not on hormonal contraceptives, and an additional 501 pregnant subjects not on routine supplement with vitamins and minerals. The overall objective was to document whether prevalence of signs of vitamin deficiency were greater in women on OCs with poor nutrition. (Identical protocols of these studies were also being carried out in India (Bombay and Hyderabad), Mexico, South Korea, Australia and Great Britain.) Great emphasis was placed on standardization of the working definition of clinical symptomatology of vitamin deficiency, with standardization and quality control of clinical assessments employing color photographs and slides.

TABLE 1. *Contraceptive steroids and vitamin A*

Contraceptives	Months of treatment				ANOVA
	0	1	6	12	
OC + Vit.Suppl	100 ± 26*	143 ± 38	150 ± 30	147 ± 31	<0.01
OC	100 ± 29	150 ± 37	160 ± 34	155 ± 37	<0.01
IUCD	100 ± 30	117 ± 17	123 ± 40	117 ± 33	NS
DMPA	100 ± 15	100 ± 17	100 ± 28	89 ± 24	NS
NET-EN	100 ± 30	96 ± 24	93 ± 19	85 ± 15	NS

* = $\overline{X}$ ± SD expressed as per cent changes from 0-month.
AC—activation coefficient
ANOVA—analysis of variance
DMPA—depot-medroxyprogesterone acetate
ETK—erythrocyte transketolase
IUCD—intrauterine contraceptive device
NET-EN—norethindrone enanthate
OC—oral contraceptive

Results obtained from Chiang Mai indicated that prevalence of clinical signs and symptoms of vitamin deficiencies were not different in OC users, those who used nonhormonal methods, those who were pregnant, and those who used DMPA.

VITAMIN A

The suspicion that contraceptive steroid hormones might affect vitamin A status arose from the analogy drawn with the state of pregnancy, so that Gal, Parkinson, and Craft (1971) were able to report that the plasma concentration of vitamin A was considerably higher than in non-OC users. This finding has been confirmed by the author and other workers (Task Force on Oral Contraceptives, 1985; Amatayakul, 1978a). The increase ranged between 40% and 55% above normal, and, as indicated in Table 1, was evident even after the first few cycles of OC use (Gal, Parkinson, and Craft, 1971; Ahmed, Bamji, and Iyengar, 1975; Yeung and Chan, 1975; and Amatayakul, 1984a). The elevated level remained more or less constant throughout 3 years of observation (Singkamani et al., 1991). It has also been demonstrated that retinol-binding protein (RBP), the specific transport protein to which most of the plasma retinol is bound, also undergoes marked increase (Yeung and Chan, 1975; Supapark and Olson, 1974). The estrogenic component is responsible for the changes, whether they occur naturally (i.e., in pregnancy) or during treatment (i.e., estrogen given during reproductive life or after menopause), or even in males (Vahquist, Johnson and Nygren, 1979). Progestin administration alone, as oral norethindrone 350 μg daily (Yeung and Chan, 1975; Cumming, 1981), injectable (200 mg in oil) every 8 to 12 weeks (Amatayakul, 1984a), norgestrel (Amatayakul, 1985; Cumming, 1981), or DMPA (Amatayakul, 1979b) did not increase plasma concentration of either RBP or vitamin A (see Table 3).

The estrogenic agent stimulates hepatic synthesis and release of RBP, to some extent in a dose-dependent manner (Horwitt, Harvey, and Dahum, 1975). Data from Chiang Mai showed a highly significant rise of RBP of about 80%, from 1.79 + 0.43(SD) to 3.19 + 0.29 mmol/L (P<0.01) after 13 cycles of low-dose OC use.

Despite this elevation, the molar ratios remained unchanged at an average of 64% to 74% saturation of the total circulating carrier protein (Amatayakul et al., 1989). Elevation of the vitamin A level appears to be secondary to this change (Supapark and Olson, 1974; Vahquist, Johnson, and Nygren, 1979). The significance of altered vitamin A status has caused some concern, as it has been shown to be toxic to fetal rats *in utero* (Moore, 1967). There appears to be little justification for any concern, since the degree of elevation is not large and most of circulating retinol is in fact bound to RBP and other plasma proteins, and should not be able to pass through the placental barrier. Contrary to popular belief, supplementation of vitamin A to OC users does not further increase its plasma concentration (Amatayakul et al., 1984b; Bamji et al., 1985). This is probably because most if not all of the binding sites on the circulating transport proteins have already been occupied by increased mobilization of vitamin from liver storage. Several workers have also suggested that increased plasma vitamin A may occur at the expense of liver vitamin A storage, and may therefore hasten storage depletion (Gal, 1975; Bamji, 1978b). Our study of liver vitamin A storage in 33 Thai women of low socioeconomic status in Chiang Mai who had used OCs for 13 cycles showed adequate liver vitamin A reserve that was sufficient to maintain blood concentration (Amatayakul et al., 1989).

VITAMIN B_1

Thiamin or vitamin B_1 functions in the body as a coenzyme, thiamin pyrophosphate, to catalyze energy metabolism reactions. Its requirement therefore is related to energy expenditure (Task Force on Oral Contraceptives, 1985). In addition, thiamin is also required for the activation of transketolase, an enzyme involved in the formation of ribose in the pentose-phosphate pathway. Measurement of erythrocytic transketolase (ETK) and its *in vitro* stimulated activities has been used as an indirect assessment of vitamin B_1 status. Other tests that include 24-hour urinary excretion of thiamin and its load test, and blood thiamin levels are not much in use generally (Sauberlich, 1984). Vitamin B_1 status had been reported to deteriorate slightly with OC usage in both normal and 6-weeks postpartum women (Prasad et al., 1975a). Subsequent studies carried out by both the author and others have not shown an adverse association (Bamji and Prema, 1978a; Ahmed, Bamji, and Iyengar, 1975; Amatayakul, 1984a; Joshi et al, 1975; Egoramaiphol et al., 1975; Egoramaiphol, Migasena, and Supawan, 1985), despite the fact that the study population came almost exclusively from a low socioeconomic background and was on OCs for 1 year (or 13 cycles) prior to final reassessment. They were judged to be either on the borderline or marginally deficient with respect to vitamin B_2 and B_6, though not to thiamin, viewed either as individuals or as a group. Supplementation with vitamin B_1

TABLE 2. *Contraceptive steroids and vitamin B-1*
[ETK-ACs]

| Contraceptives | Months of treatment | | | | ANOVA |
	0	1	6	12	
OC + Vit.Suppl	$100 \pm 10^*$	95 ± 4	95 ± 3	95 ± 3	<0.01
OC	100 ± 10	96 ± 5	101 ± 5	100 ± 5	NS
IUCD	100 ± 5	99 ± 4	103 ± 6	102 ± 5	NS
DMPA	100 ± 6	99 ± 5	100 ± 4	101 ± 5	NS
NET-EN	100 ± 4	97 ± 7	104 ± 3	98 ± 5	NS

$^* = \overline{X} \pm SD$ expressed as per cent changes from 0-month.
AC—activation coefficient
ANOVA—analysis of variance
DMPA—depot-medroxyprogesterone acetate
ETK—erythrocyte trans-ketolase
IUCD—intrauterine contraceptive device
NET-EN—norethindrone enanthate
OC—oral contraceptive

during OC use, however, significantly improved their vitamin status. This finding suggests that thiamin nutritional status is either marginally or not at all affected by combined low-dose OC (see Table 2).

VITAMIN B$_2$

Early studies from Chiang Mai by Sanpitak and Chayutimonkul (1974) and several others (Ahmed, Bamji, and Iyengar, 1975; Newman et al., 1978) suggested that vitamin B$_2$ status (as assessed by erythrocyte glutatthione reductase activity) was adversely affected by OCs, even with low-dose types, although progestins administered parenterally did not result in such effects (Amatayakul, 1984; Amatayakul, Sivasomboon, and Thanangkul, 1978b). The frequency of depletion was reported to be higher in those who had taken the pill over a period of at least 3 years (Newman et al., 1978). This finding may have importance for individuals with glucose-6-phosphate dehydrogenase deficiency. In this genetically determined metabolic derangement, the life span and integrity of the red blood cells appear to be maintained within the normal range by a compensatory increase in the intracellular glutathione reductase activity. Therefore, a further lowering of this enzyme activity in the red blood cells by an OC may represent a health hazard, especially for borderline or deficient individuals who are relatively common in this part of the world.

We did not find any significant changes of riboflavin, either during or at the end of 1 year's use of OCs in Chiang Mai women. This finding was similar to previous reports by Prasad et al. (1975), Amatayakul et al. (1984b), and Bamji et al. (1985). (See Table 3.)

Our previous WHO collaborative study suggested that it might not be possible to demonstrate deterioration, as a further reduction of an already low erythrocytic glutathione reductase activity (EGR) may not be discernible by this test (Prasad et

TABLE 3. *Contraceptive steroids and vitamin B-2*
[EGR-ACs]

| Contraceptives | Months of treatment | | | | ANOVA |
	0	1	6	12	
OC + Vit.Suppl	100 ± 35*	73 ± 9	77 ± 16	74 ± 10	<0.01
OC	100 ± 24	97 ± 2	97 ± 19	101 ± 25	NS
IUCD	100 ± 28	94 ± 24	102 ± 26	106 ± 30	NS
DMPA	100 ± 17	109 ± 19	99 ± 17	101 ± 21	NS
NET-EN	100 ± 18	95 ± 27	93 ± 21	101 ± 21	NS

* = $\overline{X}$ ± SD expressed as per cent changes from 0-month.
AC—activation coefficient
ANOVA—analysis of variance
DMPA—depot-medroxyprogesterone acetate
EGR—erythrocyte glutathione reductase
IUCD—intrauterine contraceptive device
NET-EN—norethindrone enanthate
OC—oral contraceptive

al., 1975; Bamji and Prema, 1978a). Therefore a recalculation was made with data from 12 of our Chiang Mai subjects who had a normal pretreatment EGR activation coefficient (AC), to see whether or not their status worsened with OC use. The mean pre-OC value of ACs of $1.17 + 0.12$ (SD) remained unchanged at $1.23 + 0.15$ after one full year of OC use (P<0.2) (Amatayakul et al., 1984b). Bamji et al. (1986) also reported nondeviation of maternal riboflavin and milk status from that of controls. It can be concluded at least that OCs with low estrogen content (30 μg) do not exert a significant adverse effect on riboflavin status.

VITAMIN B_6

It has been shown that tryptophan metabolism appears to be abnormal in women taking OCs, similar to women deficient in pyridoxine; administration of a loading dose of tryptophan further amplifies already altered patterns of excretion of certain intermediate metabolites when vitamin B_6 is limiting. It was further demonstrated that deficiency of vitamin B_6 induced by OCs interfered with certain vitamin-independent enzymatic functions (Mason and Gluckson, 1960; Miller, 1985). In the case of the kynurenase reaction of tryptophan metabolism, excessive excretion of tryptophan intermediate metabolites such as xanthurenic acid, distal from this enzyme blockage, can readily be demonstrated (see Fig. 1). An abnormally large amount of this amino acid is shunted into the metabolic pathways due to an OC-increased induction of liver tryptophan oxygenase by the pill. The physiological implication of this is a marked reduction of free tryptophan available for serotonin (5-hydroxytryptamine) synthesis. This interference with serotonin synthesis has been linked to depression, headache, loss of libido, and other affective disorders (Adams et al., 1973; Medical Research Council, 1972). The administration of either 5-hydroxytryptamine or tryptophan has been reported to be effective in the treat-

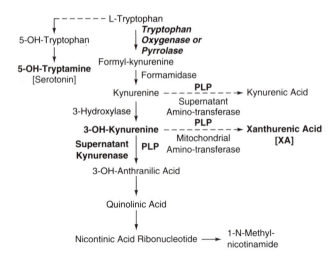

FIG. 1. Tryptophan—niacin metabolic pathway

ment of these conditions (Baumblatt and Winston, 1970). A more recent self-rating study of symptoms in women on OCs showed no difference between pyridoxine or placebo (Doll et al., 1989). Excessive formation of tryptophan intermediate metabolites has been implicated in the abnormal carbohydrate metabolism commonly seen in these subjects (Kotake and Murakami, 1968; Kotake et al., 1968), and excessive urinary XA excretion can lead to bladder carcinoma in rats (Brown et al., 1960). Treatment with large doses of vitamin B_6 has been reported to correct the abnormality (Bamji and Prema, 1978; Ahmed, Bamji, and Iyengar, 1975; Horwitt, Harvey, and Dahum, 1975; Amatayakul et al., 1984; Joshi et al., 1975; Price, Thornton, and Mueller, 1967; Green et al., 1978).

Another and perhaps better means by which this vitamin can be assessed is through measurement of the activity of erythrocyte enzymes dependent on the coenzyme form of the vitamin, such as erythrocytic aspartate aminotransferase (EAspat) activities. In vitamin B_6 deficiency, activity of enzyme can be markedly stimulated by the *in vitro* addition of pyridoxal-5-phosphate (PLP) (Sauberlich, 1984). Use of

TABLE 4. *Contraceptive steroids and vitamin B-6*
[Tryptophan load test—urinary XA excretion]

| Contraceptives | months of treatment | | | | ANOVA |
	0	1	6	12	
OC + Vit.Suppl	100 ± 122*	103 ± 163	147 ± 176	115 ± 97	NS
OC	100 ± 138	291 ± 228	294 ± 224	300 ± 217	<0.01
IUCD	100 ± 94	114 ± 80	146 ± 106	144 ± 132	NS
DMPA	100 ± 3	138 ± 48	118 ± 22	122 ± 81	NS
NET-EN	100 ± 53	135 ± 61	144 ± 95	128 ± 78	NS

* = $\overline{X} \pm SD$ expressed as per cent changes from 0-month.

TABLE 5. *Contraceptive steroids and vitamin B-6*
[EAsp at.-ACs]

| Contraceptives | Months of treatment | | | | ANOVA |
	0	1	6	12	
OC + Vit.Suppl	100 ± 12*	82 ± 8	84 ± 11	83 ± 8	<0.01
OC	100 ± 9	97 ± 11	95 ± 9	96 ± 10	NS
IUCD	100 ± 10	98 ± 7	98 ± 10	94 ± 10	NS
DMPA	100 ± 8	94 ± 6	98 ± 6	105 ± 8	NS
NET-EN	100 ± 12	98 ± 7	99 ± 9	100 ± 12	NS

* = $\overline{X}$ ± SD expressed as per cent changes from 0-month.
AC—activation coefficient
ANOVA—analysis of variance
DMPA—depot-medroxyprogesterone acetate
IUCD—intrauterine contraceptive device
NET-EN—norethindrone enanthate
OC—oral contraceptive
XA—xanthurenic acid

this method confirmed the results that we and others had obtained in an earlier study (Amatayakul, 1979). The altered excretion of tryptophan metabolites was prevented by a daily dose of 10 mg pyridoxine hydrochloride (see Table 5).

The alteration in the tryptophan-niacin metabolic pathway (see Fig. 1) seen in OC users has been linked to increased hepatic synthesis and release of tryptophan oxygenase, which shunts more of the available tryptophan into the pathway. In addition, the metabolism of tryptophan is partially or almost completely blocked by the metabolic products of estrogen, which interferes with the binding of vitamin B_6 coenzyme to the B_6-dependent apoenzyme systems (Mason and Gluckson, 1960). This interference further increases the requirement of pyridoxine or PLP for the normal metabolism of tryptophan. Thus, it can be seen that abnormal XA excretion in OC users is based on a different mechanism from that seen in pyridoxine-deficient individuals: a competitive blocking by estrogen or its metabolic products, rather than a true deficiency of PLP. Since OC users still possess adequate amount of PLP, and considering the inability of estrogen metabolic products to enter intact cells, it was not surprising to see that EAspat (Amatayakul et al., 1984) or erythrocytic glutamate oxaloacetate transaminase activities [EGOT], and also normal plasma PLP concentration (Van der Vange et al., 1989) in the red cell hemolysate, were not in any way impaired [see Table 5].

We conclude that vitamin B_6 itself, like thiamin and riboflavin, is not adversely affected by OC usage. Similar conclusions were also reached by Tyrer (1984) and Leklem (1986).

FOLATE AND VITAMIN B_{12}

A potential problem of OC use is concerned with hematopoiesis through interference with hematinic vitamin B_{12} and folate metabolism. The first report that serum folic acid levels were reduced in OC users was that of Shojania et al. (1968).

TABLE 6. *Contraceptive steroids and plasma folate*
[ng/ml]

| Contraceptives | Months of treatment | | | | ANOVA |
	0	1	6	12	
OC + Vit.Suppl	100 ± 37*	154 ± 41	155 ± 41	158 ± 48	<0.01
OC	100 ± 34	123 ± 38	125 ± 42	129 ± 46	<0.01
IUCD	100 ± 37	108 ± 50	111 ± 42	120 ± 45	NS
DMPA	100 ± 37	92 ± 25	100 ± 38	88 ± 28	NS
NET-EN	100 ± 34	97 ± 19	87 ± 26	102 ± 30	NS

* = $\overline{X}$ ± SD expressed as per cent changes from 0-month.
ANOVA—analysis of variance
DMPA—depot-medroxyprogesterone acetate
IUCD—intrauterine contraceptive device
NET-EN—norethindrone enanthate
OC—oral contraceptive

However, this was not confirmed (Spray, 1968). Anecdotal reports of megaloblastic anemia responsive to folic acid treatment in some OC users appeared (Gaafar et al., 1973; Ryser, Farquet, and Hozayen, 1973; Toghill and Smith, 1971; Johnson et al., 1973); in many of these subjects the anemia recurred in the absence of OC use. In other reports, megaloblastic changes were observed in the erythrocytic precursors, and also in the cervical epithelium. However, Ross et al. (1976) studied serum folate, hematology, and cervical cytology simultaneously in 116 women and found no significant differences between OC users and nonusers. Depressed serum folate levels were detected by some (Lawrence and Smith, 1974; Smith, Goldsmith, and Lawrence, 1975; Davis and Smith, 1973; Westalix et al., 1971; Alperin, 1973; Shojania, Hornady, and Barnes, 1969; Shojania, Hornady, and Scaletta, 1975) but not by others (Prasad et al., 1975; Amatayakul, Sivasomboon, and Thanangkul, 1984; Areekul et al., 1977; Manniego-Bantista and Bazzano, 1969; Karlin, Dumont, and Long, 1977; Mountifield, 1986).

Our own results showed a slight but significant increase in both the serum and red

TABLE 7. *Contraceptive steroids and RBC folate*
[ng/ml]

| Contraceptives | Months of treatment | | | | ANOVA |
	0	1	6	12	
OC + Vit.Suppl	100 ± 28*	134 ± 31	136 ± 29	145 ± 32	<0.01
OC	100 ± 28	113 ± 27	115 ± 30	126 ± 34	<0.01
IUCD	100 ± 20	107 ± 25	108 ± 29	142 ± 28	NS
DMPA	100 ± 26	109 ± 32	102 ± 23	103 ± 15	NS
NET-EN	100 ± 23	100 ± 23	93 ± 16	99 ± 19	NS

* = $\overline{X}$ ± SD expressed as per cent changes from 0-month.
ANOVA—analysis of variance
DMPA—depot-medroxyprogesterone acetate
IUCD—intrauterine contraceptive device
NET-EN—norethindrone enanthate
OC—oral contraceptive

TABLE 8. *Contraceptive steroids and vitamin B-12*
[pg/ml]

Contraceptives	Months of treatment 0	1	6	12	ANOVA
OC + Vit.Suppl	100 ± 44*	77 ± 26	85 ± 28	85 ± 28	NS
OC	100 ± 37	66 ± 21	65 ± 21	71 ± 23	<0.01
IUCD	100 ± 31	89 ± 30	91 ± 28	83 ± 25	NS
DMPA	100 ± 26	109 ± 32	102 ± 23	103 ± 15	NS
NET-EN	100 ± 34	82 ± 25	81 ± 27	88 ± 25	NS

* = $\bar{X}$ ± SD expressed as per cent changes from 0-month.
ANOVA—analysis of variance
DMPA—depot-medroxyprogesterone acetate
IUCD—intrauterine contraceptive device
NET-EN—norethindrone enanthate
OC—oral contraceptive

cell folate after 1 year of OC use (see Tables 6, 7, and 8). Similar results were also reported from India by Bamji and Prema (1978). Serum cyanocobalamine, on the other hand, was reduced by almost 30%, from about 1,000 to 710 pg/ml, possibly as a result of the decrease of vitamin B_{12} binding capacity (Hjelt et al., 1985). In any event, the reduced concentration is still considerably above the deficiency level and is not significant clinically. This conclusion was also reached by Larsson-Cohn (1975) and Hjelt et al. (1985).

VITAMIN E

An initial study carried out in rats indicated that plasma vitamin E levels were lowered when OCs were administered. This was believed to be the result of OC-induced reduction of the lipoprotein carrier in plasma (Aftergood and Alfin-Slater, 1974). A slight reduction of about 20% was also observed in humans, though there was an apparent ethnic difference (Aftergood, Alexander, and Alfin-Slater, 1975). Later studies failed to show this effect (Horwitt, Harvey, and Dahum, 1975; Smith, Goldsmith, and Lawrence, 1975; Yeung, 1976), even when individual tocopherols (i.e., α- ,β- and γ-) were measured separately (Tangney and Driskell, 1978). Further study carried out by the writer in subjects with OCs containing low estrogen dosage showed no significant change in the level of α-tocopherol, either with or without simultaneous multivitamin supplementation of A, B-1, B-2, B-6, C, niacin, folic acid, and cyanocobalamin (see Table 9).

VITAMIN C

Studies in both animals (Clemetson, 1968; Saroja, Mallikerjuneswara, and Clemetson, 1971) and women (Harris, Hartley, and Moore, 1973; Rivers, 1975) indicated some reduction, but values were still well above those found in clinically

TABLE 9. *Contraceptive steroids and vitamin E*
[mg/100 ml]

Contraceptives	Months of treatment			12	ANOVA
	0	1	6		
OC + Vit.Suppl	100 ± 51*	92 ± 38	92 ± 40	89 ± 43	NS
OC	100 ± 51	104 ± 51	114 ± 47	98 ± 45	NS
IUCD	100 ± 61	83 ± 41	94r ± 39	104 ± 33	NS
DMPA	100 ± 50	106 ± 40	97 ± 43	113 ± 62	NS

* = $\overline{X} \pm$ SD expressed as per cent changes from 0-month.
ANOVA—analysis of variance
DMPA—depot-medroxyprogesterone acetate
IUCD—intrauterine contraceptive device
OC—oral contraceptive

scorbutic individuals. These findings suggest increased utilization (Wynn, 1975), although the exact mechanisms that bring about these changes and their clinical significance are not at present established. Alternatively, these changes may also be related to increased ceruloplasmin, which does have strong ascorbate-oxidase activity (Saroja, Mallikarjuneswara, and Clemetson, 1971). Depot medroxyprogesterone acetate and oral progestins appeared to be without any effect.

VITAMIN D

There are few studies of the effect of OCs on vitamin D. Evaluation of vitamin status has relied on somewhat nonspecific indirect measurements such as serum alkaline phosphatase, calcium, and phosphate levels (Sauberlich, 1984). Simpson and Dale (1972) are apparently alone in reporting that serum calcium and phosphate decreased in OC users. Depot medroxyprogesterone acetate has no effect (Amatayakul, Sivasomboon, and Thanangkul, 1978). On the other hand, bone mineral concentrations have been shown to be higher in estrogen-treated individuals (Goldsmith and Johnson, 1975).

VITAMIN K

Vitamin K is needed in the synthesis of clotting factors II, IV, IX, and X (Suttie, 1976). Reduction of plasma prothrombin (factor II) may therefore lead to a prolonged prothrombin time. This reaction has been employed as an indirect assessment for vitamin K (Sauberlich, Skala, and Dowdy, 1974). The exact mechanism whereby these changes are brought about is not well understood, but believed to be related to the process of carboxylation conversion of the precursor protein produced by liver into prothrombin (Suttie, 1976).

NIACIN AND PANTOTHENIC ACID

The rare occurrence of niacin deficiency was established by Goldberger as far back as 1914 (Darby, McNutt, and Todhunter, 1976) due to predominant consumption of corn; although present in some quantity, niacin is not biologically available in corn as it is in the protein-bound form, niacytin (Hansen et al., 1975). It can be synthesized *in vivo* from tryptophan (Sarett and Goldsmith, 1975), but very little tryptophan is present in corn (Hansen et al., 1975).

It is difficult to produce overt symptoms of pantothenic acid deficiency without giving an antagonist (Hodges et al., 1959), as pantothenic acid is present in a wide variety of foods. Only a limited number of OC studies have been undertaken, and they reported little or no significant changes in niacin or pantothenic acid (Lewis and King, 1980).

TRACE ELEMENTS

Advanced technologies, especially those based on atomic absorption and plasma emission spectroscopies, have made trace mineral analysis more accessible. Iron, copper, and zinc have been the most studied and appear to be affected by combined OCs but not by progestin-only agents.

Iron

The importance of iron deficiency in anemia is so well-known that it needs no elaboration. Since this deficiency is common, and heavy physical work is the general pattern in the Third World, additional undesirable impact should be studied and understood. Iron status is significantly improved in the majority of OC users (Webb, 1980), probably as a result of decreased menstrual blood loss and increases in iron absorption from the GI tract (Tyrer, 1984). An increase in serum concentrations of transferrin and TIBC (Sondheimer, 1981; Prasad et al., 1975) are ascribed to the estrogen component of the OCs. Progestin-only contraceptives do not produce the latter effect (Amatayakul, Sivasomboon, and Thanangkul, 1978). With these agents, menstrual blood loss may be increased or decreased to the point of amenorrhea. Thus, OCs tend to improve iron status and reduce the high prevalence of iron deficiency anemia endemic in many parts of the world.

Copper

Estrogen-containing OCs increase serum copper consistently in all studies (Mendenhall, 1970; Prasad et al., 1975; Margen and King, 1975; Prema, Ramalakshmi, and Babu, 1980; Crews, Taper, and Ritchey, 1980; Sondheimer, 1981; Amatayakul, 1981). The magnitude of increase, however, is greater than that noted for iron, to the extent that fear of copper toxicity was expressed. However, ceruloplasmin, a specific copper-binding protein, also increases concomitantly and proportionately (Amatayakul, 1981). The increase in serum copper is due almost entirely to the increase of bound material; thus, there can be no toxicity since ceruloplasmin-bound copper is biologically inert. The increased synthesis and release of ceruloplasmin is induced by the estrogenic component; progestins have little effect on ceruloplasmin and therefore do not affect copper concentration in the blood.

Zinc

Zinc is associated with more than 100 enzymes involved in a wide range of functions such as DNA metabolism, hormone production, growth and sexual development, immune function, and wound healing (Sandstead, 1984). Disagreement exists regarding the effect of OCs, although reports have indicated a reduction in the plasma zinc level (Halsted, Hackley, and Smith, 1968; Crews, Taper and Ritchey, 1980; Prema, Ramalakshmi, and Babu, 1980). Several explanations have been put forward, including decreased absorption and increased urinary excretion. However, perhaps the most likely cause is decreased serum levels of albumin, a major zinc carrier (Mendenhall, 1970; Amatayakul et al., 1992), since careful studies have shown no effect on zinc absorption and excretion. None of these changes were noted in Thai subjects on progestin-only injectable contraceptives (Amatayakul et al., 1978); however, Prema et al. (1980) reported decreased serum zinc in both DMPA and norethindrone enanthate (NET-EN) users in India.

Normal content of calcium, magnesium, copper, zinc, and iron has been found in colostrum and more mature milk in long-term OC users who stopped OC use prior to conception (Kirksey et al., 1979).

REFERENCES

Adams PW, Rose DP, Folkard J, Wynn V, Seed M, Strong R. Effect of pyridoxine hydrochloride (vitamin B-6) upon depression associated with oral contraception. *Lancet* 1973;1:897.

Aftergood L, Alfin-Slater RB. Oral contraceptive—α-tocopherol interrelationship. *Lipids* 1974;9:91.

Aftergood L, Alexander AR, Alfin-Slater RB. Effect of oral contraceptives on plasma lipoproteins, cholesterol and α-tocopherol levels in young women. *Contraception* 1975;11[4]:295.

Ahmed F, Bamji MS, and Iyengar L. Effects of oral contraceptive agents on vitamin nutritional status. *Am J Clin Nutr* 1975;28:606.

Alperin JB. Folate metabolism in women using oral contraceptive agents. *Am J Clin Nutr* 1973;26: 19(abst).

Amatayakul K. The effects of depo-provera on carbohydrate, lipids and vitamins metabolism. *J Steroid Biochem* 1979b;11:475.

Amatayakul K. Effects of hormonal contraceptives on copper binding protein. In: *Eighteenth scientific meeting of the Thai society of obstetricians and gynecologists*. Khon Kean: 1981:

Amatayakul K. Metabolic effects of DMPA and NET-EN. In: Proceeding of the symposium on the present status of long-acting progestogen contraception. Organized by Department of Maternal and Child Health, Ministry of Public Health of Thailand. Pattaya, Thailand: 1984:51–70.

Amatayakul K. In: McDaniel E, ed. The metabolic effects of hormonal contraceptives. *Proceedings of the second Asian regional workshop on injectable contraceptives.* World Neighbors; 1978:25–8.

Amatayakul K. Viewpoint from Thailand. *Med Progress* 1979a;6:14.

Amatayakul K. Vitamin B-6 nutritional status in hormonal contraceptive users. In: Thailand's Ministry of Public Health. Proceedings in Norplant introduction meeting. Pattaya, Thailand: 1985:11–29.

Amatayakul K, Laokuldilok K, Kootthatep S, Dejsarai W, Rapamontol T, Srirak K, Uttaravichai C. The effect of oral contraceptives on protein metabolism (In: preparation)..1992;

Amatayakul K, Sivasomboon B, Thanangkul O. Vitamin and trace mineral metabolism in medroxy-progesterone acetate users. *Contraception* 1978;18(3):253.

Amatayakul K, Underwood BA, Ruckphaopunt S, Singkamani R, Limpisarn S, Leelapat P, Thanangkul O. Oral contraceptives: effect of long-term use on liver vitamin A storage assessed by the relative dose responses test. *Am J Clin Nutr* 1989;49:845.

Amatayakul K, Uttaravichai C, Singkamani R, Ruckphaopunt S. Vitamin metabolism and the effects of multivitamin supplementation in oral contraceptive users. *Contraception* 1984;30:179.

Areekul S, Panatampon P, Doungbarn J, Yamenat P, Vongynthitum M. Serum vitamin B-12, serum and red cell folates, vitamin B-12 and folic acid binding proteins in women taking oral contraceptives. *Southeast Asian J Trop Med Pub Hlth* 1977;8(4):480.

Bamji MS. Implication of oral contraceptive use on vitamin nutritional status. *Indian J Med Res* 1978;68[Supp]:80.

Bamji MS, Prema K. Oral contraceptive use and vitamin nutritional status of malnourished women—effects of continuous and intermittent vitamin supplements. *J Steroid Biochem* 1978;11:487.

Bamji MS, Prema K, Jacob CM, Ramalakshmi BA, Madhavapeddi R. Relationship between maternal vitamin B2 and B6 status and the levels of these vitamins in milk at different stages of lactation. A study in a low-income group of Indian women. *Hum Nutr Clin Nutr* 1986;40:119.

Bamji MS, Prema K, Jacob CM, Rani M, Samyukta D. Vitamin supplement to Indian women using low dose oral contraceptives. *Contraception* 1985;32:405.

Basnayake S, de Silva SV, Millen PC, Rogers S. A trial of daily vitamin supplementation as a means of reducing oral contraceptive side-effects and discontinuation in Sri Lanka. *Contraception* 1983;27:465.

Baumblatt MJ, Winston F. Pyridoxine and the pill. *Lancet* 1972;1:832.

Brown RR, Price JM, Satter ET, Wear JB. The metabolism of tryptophan in patients with bladder cancer. *Acta Un Int Cancer* 1960;16:299.

Coelingh-Bennink HJT, Schreurs WHP. Improvement of oral glucose tolerance in gestational diabetes by pyridoxine. *Br Med J* 1975;3:1.

Crews MG, Taper LJ, Ritchey SD. Effect of oral contraceptive agents on copper and zinc balance in young women. *Am J Clin Nutr* 1980;33:1,940.

Cumming FJ. Effect of oral contraceptive use on ascorbic acid and vitamin A in lactation. *J Hum Nutr* 1981;35(4):249.

Davis RE, Smith BK. Pyridoxine and depression associated with oral contraception. *Lancet* 1973;1:1,245.

Doll H, Brown S, Thurston, Vessey M. Pyridoxine (vitamin B6) and the premenstrual syndrome: a randomized crossover trial. *J Royal Coll Gen Pract* 1989;39(326):364.

Egoramaiphol S, Migasena P, Supawan V. Effects of oral contraceptive agents on thiamine status. *J Med Assoc Thailand* 1985;68:19.

Gaafar A, Toppozada HK, Hozayen A, Abdel-Malek AT, Moghazy M, Yuossef M. Study of folate status in long-term Egyptian users of oral contraceptive pills. *Contraception* 1973;8:43.

Gal I. Steroidal contraceptive therapy: hepatoma and vitamin A. *Lancet* 1975;1:684.

Gal I , Parkinson C, Craft I. Effects of oral contraceptives on human plasma vitamin A levels. *Br Med J* 1971;2:436.

Green AR, Bloomfield MR, Woods HF, Seed M. Metabolism of an oral tryptophan load by women and evidence against the induction of tryptophan pyrrolase by oral contraceptives. *Br J Clin Pharmacol* 1978;5:233.

Hjelt K, Brynskov J, Hippe E, Lundstrom P, Munck O. Oral contraceptives and the cobalamin (vitamin B12) metabolism. *Acta Obstet Gynecol Scand* 1985;64(1):59.

Horwitt MK, Harvey CC, Dahum CH. Relationship between levels of blood lipids, vitamin C, A and E, serum copper compounds, and urinary excretion of tryptophan metabolites in women taking oral contraceptive therapy. *Am J Clin Nutr* 1975;28:403.

Huber DH, Khan AM, Pitt L. *Bangladesh fertility research programme:4th contributors' conference.* Decca, Bangladesh;1979:75–93.

Johnson GK, Greennan JE, Hensley GT, Soergel K. Small intestinal disease, folate deficiency anaemia, and oral contraceptive agents. *Am J Dig Dis* 1973;18:185.

Joshi UM, Lahiri A, Kora S, Djkshit SS, Virkar K. Short term effect of ovral and norgestrel on vitamin B-6 and B-1 status of women. *Contraception* 1975;12:425.

Karlin R, Dumont M, Long B. Etude des faux sanguins d'acide folique an cours des traitements oestro-progestatifs. *J Gynecol Obstet Biol Reprod* 1977;6:489.

Kirksey A, Ernst JA, Roepke JL, Tsai TL. Influence of mineral intake and use of oral contraceptives before pregnancy on the mineral content of human colostrum and of more mature milk. *Am J Clin Nutr* 1979;32:30

Kotake Y, Murakami E. Studies on the xanthurenic acid-insulin complex: I. Preparation and properties. *J Biochem (Tokyo)* 1968;63:573

Kotake Y, Sotakawa Y, Murakami E, Hisatake A, Abe M, Ikeda Y. Studies on the xanthurenic acid-insulin complex: II. Physiological activities. *J Biochem (Tokyo)* 1968;63:578.

Larsson-Cohn U. Oral contraceptives and vitamins: a review. *Am J Obstet Gynecol* 1975;121:84.

Lawrence JD, Smith JL. Effects of oral contraceptive steroids on nutritional status of low income women. *Federal Proceedings* 1974;33:698(abst).

Leklem JE. Vitamin B-6 requirements and oral contraceptive use—a concern? *J Nutr* 1986;116(3):475.

Magen S, King JC. Effect of OC agents on the metabolism of some trace minerals. *Am J Clin Nutr* 1975;28:392.

Maniego-Bantista LP, Bazzano G. Effects of oral contraceptives on serum folates and lipids levels. *J Lab Clin Med* 1969;74:988.

Mason M, Gluckson EH. Estrogen-enzyme interaction: inhibition and protection of kynurenase trans-aminase by the sulphate esters of diethyl stillbestrol, estradiol, and estrone. *J Biol Chem* 235(5):1,312.

Medical Research Council, Brain Metabolism Unit. Modified amine hypothesis for the aetiology of affective illness. *Lancet* 1972;2:573.

Mendenhall HW. Effect of oral contraceptives on serum protein concentration *Am J Obstet Gynecol* 1970;106:750.

Miller LT. Oral contraceptives and vitamin B-6 metabolism. In: Reynolds RD, Leklem JE, eds. *Vitamin B-6 : its role in health and diseases.* New York: Alan R. Liss, Inc.; 1985:243–55.

Moore T. In: Sebrell WH, Harris RS, eds. *The vitamins.* New York: Academic Press Inc.; 1978:280.

Mountifield JA. Serum vitamin B12 and folate levels in women taking oral contraceptives. *Can Fam Physician* 1986;32:862.

Newman LJ, Lopez R, Cole NS, Boria MC, Cooperman JM. Riboflavine deficiency in women taking oral contraceptive agents. *Am J Clin Nutr* 1978;31:247.

Prasad AS, Lei KY, Oberleas D, Moghissi KS, and Stryker JC. Effect of oral contraceptive agents on nutrients: II. Vitamins. *Am J Clin Nutr* 1975a;28:385.

Prasad AS, Oberleas D, Lei KY, Moghissi KS, Stryker JC. Effect of oral contraceptive agents on nutrients: I. Minerals. *Am J Clin Nutr* 1975b;28:377.

Price JM, Thornton MJ, Mueller LM. Tryptophan metabolism in women using steroid hormones for ovulation control. *Am J Clin Nutr* 1967;20:452.

Rose DP. The influence of oestrogen on tryptophan metabolism in man. *Clin Sci* 1966;31:265.

Ross CE, Stone MK, Reegan JW, Wentz WB, Kellermeyer RW. Lack of influence of OC on serum folate, haematologic values and uterine cervical cytology. *Sem Hematol* 1976;13:233.

Rugpao S, Sanmanechai M, Koonlertgij S, Amatayakul K. Study on the prevalence of signs of vitamin deficiency in association with oral contraception. *Chiang Mai Med Bull* 1982;21:219.

Ryser JE, Farquet JJ, and Petite J. Megaloblastic anaemia due to folic acid deficiency in a young woman on oral contraceptives. *Acta Haematol (Basal)* 1971;45:319.

Sanpitak N, Chayutimonkol L. Oral contraceptives and riboflavine nutrition. *Lancet* 1974;1:836.

Sanstead HH. Trace metals in human nutrition in the 20th century. In: Winick M, ed. *Volume 13 of current concepts in nutrition.* New York: John Wiley and Sons, Inc.; 1984.

Sanstead HH. Zinc. In: Hegsted DM, ed. *Nutrition reviews—present knowledge in nutrition, 4th ed.* New York/Washington, D.C.: The Nutrition Foundation Inc.; 1976.

Sauberlich HE. Implications of nutritional status on human biochemistry, physiology and health. *Clin Biochem* 1984;17:132.

Shojania AM, Hornady GT, Barnes PM. Oral contraceptives and folate metabolism. *Lancet* 1:886.

Shojania AM, Hornady G, Barnes PH. Oral contraceptives and serum folate level. *Lancet* 1968;1:1376.

Shojania AM, Hornady GT, Scaletta D. The effect of oral contraceptives on folate metabolism; III. Plasma clearance and urinary folate excretion. *J Lab Clin Med* 1975;85:185.

Singkamanee R, Ruckphaopunt S, Suwanarach CC, Wichajarn M, Dejsarai W. Effect of more than three years' use of oral contraceptives fat soluble vitamins. *Ninth annual health sciences meeting, Research Institute for Health Sciences, University of Chiang Mai.* Chiang Mai, Thailand: 1991;17(abst).

Smith JL, Goldsmith GA, Lawrence JD. Effects of oral contraceptive steroid on vitamin and lipid levels in serum. *Am J Clin Nutr* 1975;28:371.

Sondheimer S. Metabolic effects of the birth control pill. *Clin Obstet Gynecol* 1981;124:927.

Spellacy WN, Buhi WC, Birk SA. The effects of vitamin B-6 on carbohydrate metabolism in women taking steroid contraceptives. Preliminary report. *Contraception* 1972;6:265.

Spray, GH. Oral contraceptives and serum folate level. *Lancet* 1968;2:110.

Supapark W, Olson JA. Effect of ovral, a combination type of oral contraceptive agent on vitamin A metabolism in rats. *Int J Vitam Nutr Res* 1974;45:113.

Tangney CC, Driskell JA. Vitamin E status of young women on combined-type of oral contraceptives. *Contraception* 1978;17:499.

Task Force on Oral Contraceptives, Special Programme of Research, Development and Research Training in Human Reproduction, World Health Organization. Impact of hormonal contraceptives vis-a-vis non-hormonal factors on the vitamin status of malnourished women in India and Thailand. *Hum Nutr Clin Nutr* 1985;40C:205.

Toghill PJ, Smith PG. Folate deficiency and the pill. *Br Med J* 1971;1:608.

Tyrer LB. Nutrition and the pill. *J Reprod Med* 1984;29(Suppl 7):547.

Vahquist A, Johnson A, Nygren KG. Vitamin A transport plasma protein and female sex steroid. *Am J Clin Nutr* 32:1,433.

Van der Vange N, Van der Berg H, Kloosterboer HJ, Haspels AA. Effects of seven low-dose combined contraceptives on vitamin B-6 status. *Contraception* 1989;40:377.

Westalix LF, Metz EM, LoBuglio AF, Balcerzak SP. Decreased serum B-12 levels secondary to oral contraceptive agents. *Am J Clin Nutr* 1971;24:603.

Yeung DL. Relationships between cigarette smoking, oral contraceptives, and plasma vitamins A, E, C and plasma triglycerides and cholesterol. *Am J Clin Nutr* 1976;29:1,216.

Yeung DL, Chan PL. Effects of a progestogen and a sequential type of oral contraceptive on plasma vitamin A, vitamin E, cholesterol and triglycerides. *Am J Clin Nutr* 1975;28:686.

Pharmacology of the Contraceptive Steroids,
edited by Joseph W. Goldzieher.
Raven Press, Ltd., New York © 1994.

26

Immunologic Effects of Estrogens, Progestins, and Estrogen-Progestin Combinations

*A. H. W. M. Schuurs, *T. B. P. Geurts, *E. M. Goorissen, †J. M. W. Hazes, and *H. A. M. Verheul

Organon Scientific Development Group, 5340 BH Oss, The Netherlands; †Department of Rheumatology, University Hospital Leiden, 2300RC Leiden, The Netherlands

EFFECTS OF GENDER AND PHYSIOLOGICAL HORMONAL CHANGES ON IMMUNE RESPONSES

There is a general notion that, independent of species, females show stronger immune responses than males (Grossman, 1984; Ansar Ahmed et al., 1985; Mooradian et al., 1987; Schuurs and Verheul, 1990). Thus, females would usually be better protected from infectious diseases and, possibly, from neoplasms. On the other hand, females have a higher chance of getting autoimmune disease (AID). In allergic diseases, sexual dimorphism is either not present or variable, and dependent on the particular type of hyperreactivity or age of the patient (Schlumberger, 1987).

Wherever sexual dimorphism occurs, sex hormones are likely to play a role, as is illustrated by observations in humans and experimental animals. Some examples follow:

1. Female ICR Swiss mice infected with the diabetogenic D variant of encephalomyocarditis virus are diabetes-resistant while males are not (Giron and Patterson, 1982). The difference is probably caused by an earlier and stronger rise in interferon-gamma (IFN-gamma) and Interleukin 2 (IL-2) production, and Ia antigens (mouse histocompatibility antigens) expression in the spleen of the female (Huygen and Palfliet, 1984; McFarland and Bigley, 1989). Investigations by Flynn (1986) and Fox et al. (1991) are in support of a relationship with (exogenous) estrogen and/or progestin.
2. The cellular immune response to Candida albicans was found to vary during the menstrual cycle, with the lowest response during the luteal phase. This variation in immune response to Candida was of much lesser magnitude in oral contracep-

tive (OC) users, which suggests that the fluctuation in progesterone or estradiol levels during the menstrual cycle influences the changes in the immune response to Candida albicans (Kalo-Klein and Witkin, 1989).

3. In both males and females, the thymus involutes at puberty and following treatment with androgens, estrogens, or gonadotropins; hypertrophy of thymus, spleen, and lymph nodes is caused by gonadectomy, the effect being counteracted by sex hormones but not by gonadotropins.

4. Skin allograft rejection times are shorter and antibody formation is often higher in female and castrated male animals than in intact males (Graff et al., 1969; Eidinger and Garrett, 1972; Castro, 1978). Ovariectomy seems to stimulate cell-mediated immunity (CMI) (Kittas and Henry, 1979), but to diminish antibody-producing cells after immunization with killed E. coli (Kenny, 1976).

5. In humans and certain animal models, AID may exacerbate or subside by spontaneous or induced hormonal changes, puberty, menstrual cycle, pregnancy and puerperium, menopause, gonadectomy, and administration of steroid hormones.

EFFECTS OF ESTROGENS ON IMMUNE RESPONSES

In comparison with progestogens and androgens, estrogens affect target organs at very low concentrations and have high specific activities. High doses of estrogen resulting in plasma levels well above those naturally found during pregnancy may give rise to toxic effects, particularly in young animals (e.g., Heywood and Wadsworth, 1980). These features are insufficiently appreciated in studies of the effects of estrogens on the immune system. Consequently, in the discussions that follow, the studies in which supraphysiological doses of estrogen have been used will be omitted. Sex hormones have extraordinarily strong effects on fetuses and neonates. Therefore, effects on the immune system of animals surviving such an early exposure are considered of little relevance for the present survey. In addition, data on nonsteroidal estrogens will be disregarded.

Estrogen Receptors in Lymphoid Tissues

High-affinity, low-capacity estrogen receptors (ERs) have been found in the bursa of Fabricius, in the reticuloendothelial cells of the thymus, in thymocytes, and in peripheral lymphoid cells of various species, as well as in CD8 + but not CD4 + cells (reviewed by Grossman, 1984, and Schuurs and Verheul, 1990). In some instances, ERs were only detectable by using strongly radiolabeled ligands (Weusten et al., 1986). Gulsham et al. (1990) detected ERs in rat peritoneal macrophages and the human monocyte line J111. Danel et al. (1985) found ERs in lymphoid and hemopoietic cell lines, but only in discrete maturation stages. The varying results could be explained by the comment made by Sarvetnick and Fox (1990) that only resting lymphocytes have been investigated, and that activated cells may well ex-press ERs while resting cells do not. Tabibzadeh and Satyaswaroop (1989) found ERs in lymphoid aggregates in human endometrium.

Animal-experimental Data on Estrogens

Phagocytic activity of the reticulo-endothelial system (RES) in rats and mice varies at various stages of the estrous cycle and pregnancy, the activity being greatest after periods of increased endogenous estrogen production. In addition, after administration of estrogen, the phagocytic activity of the RES appears to be increased in these species (Nicol et al., 1964). Estrogens enhance clearance of antibody-coated cells in guinea pigs at high physiological (as during pregnancy) and supraphysiological doses; their estrogenic activity (E2 estradiol >>estriol (E3)>> 16β-E2) does not correlate with their effects on clearance (Friedman et al., 1985; Schreiber et al., 1988). Expression of Ia antigens and production of Interleukin-1 (IL-1) by murine macrophages are increased by E2 (Flynn, 1986). Macrophages of mature female rats produce more IL-1 than those of mature males or immature females; ovariectomy causes a reduction in IL-1 production, which is reversed by E2 (Hu et al., 1988).

E2 is generally considered to stimulate the humoral immune response (reviewed by Grossman, 1984; Ansar Ahmed et al., 1985; Schuurs and Verheul, 1990). Erbach and Bahr (1988) compared the effects of chronic and cyclic administration of physiological doses of E2 to ovariectomized rats. Remarkably, cyclic exposure mimicking the estrous cycle did not lower thymus weight but gave the highest stimulating effect on antibody response, while a constant physiological level of E2 maintained by an implant caused a 35% decrease in thymus weight and lower antibody production. The stimulating effect of (cyclic) E2 is in line with the negative effect of ovariectomy on the humoral response (Aycock, 1936; Kenny and Gray, 1971). Wira and Sandoe (1980) found increased IgA and IgG levels in uterine secretions from ovariectomized rats subjected to 2 to 3 days treatment with E2; long-term exposure (6 to 14 days) caused much lower Ig levels. The effects of estrogen on CMI are variable: higher and lower responses have been described. Apart from the use of supraphysiological doses, great differences in experimental design may explain this confusing situation.

The role of estrogens in AID models is perhaps not as clear as sometimes suggested in the literature. For instance, in the NZB/NZW F1 (NZB/W) mouse model for autoimmune lupus and sialoadenitis, deteriorating effects by estrogen have been reported (Roubinian et al., 1978). In these studies E2 was administered by silastic tubing while neither hormone levels in plasma nor hormone effects on body and target organ weights or on estrous cycle were recorded. Therefore, it is not unlikely that a supraphysiological estrogen plasma level has prevailed. This assumption is in line with a report by Melez et al. (1978–79) stating that even the smallest E2-containing silastic tubing caused lymphoid atrophy and accelerated death. In our laboratory, we found no evidence for disease-promoting effects of physiological levels of ethynyl estradiol (EE) in NZB/W mice (Verheul et al., unpublished). Keisler et al. (1991) and Walker et al. (1991) showed that estrogen toxicity rather than lupus was the major cause of accelerated death of NZB/W mice; the animals died before elevated anti-DNA titers and glomerulonephritis developed. The finding that ovariectomy barely affects the AID process does not suggest an important role for estrogen either, but here the difference between cyclic and continuous exposure (vide supra) is also of importance.

The role of E2 in collagen type II (CII)-induced arthritis (CIA), a model for rheumatoid arthritis (RA), is very interesting. Female DBA/1 mice injected with CII had a lower disease incidence than males; this incidence was increased by ovariectomy and decreased again by administration of estrogen (Jansson et al., 1990, and cited literature). Remarkably, in some rat strains an opposite sex dimorphism is found (Holmdahl et al., 1989). One could, of course, question the relevance of these animal models for human disease, but the examples given do illustrate that one should be cautious in making generalizations about the role of estrogen in AID.

Human Data on Estrogens

A deficiency of E2 caused by premature ovarian failure, gonadal dysgenesis, or hypothalamic-pituitary failure is a likely cause for high lymphocyte and CD8 + cell counts (Ho et al., 1988, 1991).

In vitro, 10^{-10}–10^{-9} mol/L E2 causes a rise in IL-1 production by monocytes, and 10^{-8}–10^{-6} mol/L inhibits the production (Polan et al., 1988). Meanwhile, 10^{-12}–10^{-6} mol/L E2 inhibits the release of Tumor Necrosis Factor (TNF) by unstimulated peripheral blood mononuclear cells from postmenopausal women with osteoporosis; this effect was not seen with mononuclear cells from men or premenopausal women (Ralston et al., 1990). Treatment of postmenopausal women with conjugated estrogen causes a reduction of *ex vivo* spontaneous IL-1 release by monocytes (Stock et al., 1989). After ovariectomy of healthy premenopausal women, Pacifici et al. (1991) found a steep rise in the spontaneous secretion of IL-1, TNF, and GM-CSF by unstimulated monocytes, which was counteracted by oral conjugated estrogen. These data may explain the inhibition of bone resorption by estrogen, since both IL-1 and TNF are known to stimulate resorption. *In vitro*, E2 stimulates the IL-1-induced production of IL-6 by human chondrocytes (Guerne et al., 1990). It inhibits IL-6 production by endometrial stromal cells (Tabibzadeh et al., 1989).

Sera from postmenopausal women treated with estrogens inhibit the mixed lymphocyte reaction (MLR) dose-dependently (Helgason and von Schoultz, 1981).

Physiological concentrations of E2 during incubation of human peripheral blood mononuclear cells with pokeweed mitogen stimulate the formation of plasma blasts, mainly synthesizing and secreting IgM, and of plaque-forming cells (PFC), whereas they do not affect thymidine incorporation. Cell fractionation studies suggest that this effect is caused by inhibition of T suppressor (Ts) cells. High E2 concentrations tend to give opposite effects (Paavonen et al., 1981). In addition, granulocyte-macrophage colony formation is stimulated by E2 (Maoz et al., 1985; Barak et al., 1986).

Evidence for a role of estrogen in AID is circumstantial:

1. Rheumatoid arthritis and systemic lupus erythematosus (SLE) occur in women more frequently during and shortly after reproductive life, but SLE occurs earlier than RA.
2. Pregnancy often ameliorates RA, Graves', and Hashimoto's disease, and this could be caused by the high estrogen and/or progesterone levels; for SLE no consistent clinical improvement has been found.
3. The frequent exacerbations of RA, SLE, and thyroid AID postpartum could be due to "withdrawal" of estrogen and/or P.
4. Estrogens are reputedly unfavorable in SLE.

EFFECTS OF PROGESTINS ON IMMUNE RESPONSES

In assessing effects of progestins on immune responses, one has to bear in mind that the two classes can be distinguished; they may influence the immune system differently, irrespective of their progestational potencies. Estrane-based progestins may show weak androgenic or estrogenic, and pregnane-based compounds may show weak corticosteroidal activities, which may be responsible for certain effects, particularly if they are used in high doses or concentrations (cf. Neumann, 1978). Like the other sex hormones, progestins inhibit gonadotropin production so that effects obtained in intact animals cannot always be interpreted unambiguously.

Progesterone Receptors in Lymphoid Tissues

Progesterone receptors have been described in rat thymus, chicken bursa of Fabricius (Pearce et al., 1983; Sullivan and Wira, 1979), and human lymphocytes (Szekeres-Bartho et al., 1990).

Animal-experimental Data on Progestins

Progesterone has little or no effect on the weights of thymus (Luster et al., 1984) and bursa of Fabricius (Verheul et al., 1986c), whereas various estrane-based progestins have variable effects on bursa weights that are not correlated with their progestational potencies (Verheul et al., 1986c).

Corticosteroid-resistant thymocytes and pre-T cells from bone marrow or fetal liver contain 20α-hydroxysteroid dehydrogenase (20α-SDH), which converts progesterone to 20α-hydroxypregn-4-en-3-one (20α-OHP). Castration of mice causes a decrease in 20α-SDH and in splenic Ts cells; testosterone causes an increase that might be related to its protective effect in AID models (Weinstein and Berkovich, 1981). The role of 20α-SDH and its product 20α-OHP in this context is unclear.

Treatment of mice with progesterone does not affect the *ex vivo* mitogen-stimulated lymphocyte proliferation (Luster et al., 1984).

Concanavalin A (Con A)-stimulated formation of suppressor activity is significantly inhibited by progesterone (Holdstock et al., 1982).

Expression of Ia antigens and production of IL-1 by murine macrophages is increased by progesterone and ethisterone (Flynn, 1986). In contrast to E2, progesterone inhibits clearance of IgG-coated erythrocytes (Schreiber et al., 1988).

Mouse spleen cells incubated with progesterone in concentrations found during pregnancy produce a factor—"soluble immune response suppressor"—that inhibits the IgM PFC response, the mixed lymphocyte reaction, and the generation of cytotoxic T-cell response (Kita et al., 1990).

Lynestrenol and ethylestrenol inhibit the development of lupus and sialoadenitis in NZB/W mice while desogestrel has no effect (Verheul et al., 1986a, 1968b). Norethindrone and norgestrel delay the rise in anti-DNA titers in NZB/W mice; medroxyprogesterone acetate has no such effect (Keisler et al., 1991).

Various progestins have been reported to prolong skin graft survival (Kincl and Ciaccio, 1980, and cited literature). Progesterone inhibits the growth inhibition of tumor cells by spleen cells from rats with regressed tumor (Sekiya et al., 1975).

Progesterone administered to ovariectomized rats causes a decrease in cervicovaginal IgA and secretory component (Wira and Sullivan, 1985), but antagonizes estrogen-stimulated IgA and IgG levels in the uterus (Wira and Sandoe, 1980).

Human Data on Progestins

In vitro, progesterone slightly stimulates Con A-stimulated suppressor activity (Holdstock et al., 1982); stimulation of lymphocytes by phytohemagglutinin (PHA) is inhibited by progesterone but only at concentrations above those found in the circulation during pregnancy (Mori et al., 1977). PHA-induced lymphocyte transformation was reduced in women taking 350 mg norethisterone daily; this effect was not seen in women taking an EE/norethisterone or EE/norgestrel combination (Tezabwala et al., 1983).

In healthy men and women, plasma levels of progesterone and antibodies to Candida albicans are positively correlated (Mathur et al., 1978).

For therapeutic purposes progesterone has been used in premenstrual exacerbations of asthma (Beynon et al., 1988) and, intraarticularly, in RA (Cuchacovich et al., 1988). Recent data from Cuchacovich et al. (1991) suggest that progesterone exerts its antiinflammatory effect through local glucocorticoid receptors. Norethynodrel has been used systemically in RA (Blais and Demers, 1962).

EFFECTS OF ESTROGEN-PROGESTIN COMBINATIONS (ORAL CONTRACEPTIVES) ON IMMUNE RESPONSES

Effects of OCs on the immune system have quite often been described without specification of the nature and dosages of the progestin and estrogen, and of the type of OC: mono-, bi-, or triphasic, or sequential.

Changes in OC compositions over time have been important: 1) about ten progestins have been in vogue or are being used, each with its own spectrum of estrogenic, androgenic, and progestational (anti-estrogenic) properties (Neumann, 1978); and 2) two estrogens, mestranol and EE, have been used in daily dosages from 150 μg during the 1960s down to 20 μg in recent years (Piper and Kennedy 1987; Thorogood and Vessey, 1990).

There are also important differences between OCs used in various countries (e.g., during the last 10 years norethindrone and norgestrel have been used in 56% to 61% and 30% to 38% of OCs in the U.S., respectively, while in the U.K. and France the figures were 15% to 25% and 50% to 75%, respectively. The percentage of OCs with less than 50 μg estrogen was 38% to 50% in the U.S., and 54% to 69% in the U.K. and France. In this period, two other progestins, desogestrel and gestodene, were introduced in various European countries, which further widened the gap in OC use between the U.S. and Europe. To the authors' knowledge, no appropriate studies have appeared on triphasic preparations, combinations with less than 50 μg estrogen, and combinations containing gestodene or desogestrel. In conclusion, generalizations and extrapolations, if at all possible, have to be made with great caution.

Oral Contraceptives and Humoral Immunity

Immunoglobulins (Igs) have been measured in several studies in OC users. An increase of IgG and a decrease of IgA were reported in some older studies, but more recent studies do not show statistically significant changes (Horne et al., 1970; Chandra, 1972; Dotchev et al., 1973; Fassati et al., 1983; Bissett and Griffin, 1988a, 1988b).

Various studies (Shahani and Tezabwala, 1982; Delage et al., 1987; Kvist Poulsen, 1988) suggest that the use of OCs does not induce clinically significant changes in serum complement activity. This finding is reassuring in view of the important role of complement in combating infection.

Data obtained by Petermann et al. (1982) suggest that OC use does not induce the formation of circulating immune complexes.

Oral Contraceptives and Cell-mediated Immunity

Cellular immune function has been investigated in OC users by measuring the lymphocyte reaction *in vitro* to several mitogens (PHA, Con A), and *in vivo* to the contact allergen dinitrochlorobenzene (DNCB). In early studies, the PHA-induced response was found to be impaired in OC users (Hagen and Fröland, 1972; Irvine et al., 1974; Keller et al., 1977) and in women using hormone replacement therapy (Morishima and Henrich, 1974). With regard to duration of use, dose, and type of progestin, contradictory results have been obtained. In the study by Irvine et al. (1974), there were no differences between progestins; nor was there any correlation with duration of use. In the study by Keller et al. (1977), depressed PHA-induced lymphocyte transformation responses were observed in OC users as compared with controls, and the magnitude of depression was correlated with duration of OC use; norethindrone- and lynestrenol-containing OCs induced a stronger depression than levonorgestrel-containing OCs. A similar depression of lymphocyte response to PHA has been reported during pregnancy (Purtilo et al., 1972). Other studies, however, showed no statistically significant changes in PHA- or Con A-induced responses in OC users (Dwyer et al., 1975; Gerretsen et al., 1980; Tezabwala et al., 1983; Baker and Thomas, 1984).

A significant suppression of CMI was observed in undernourished progestin-only pill users (Tezabwala et al., 1983; Majumder et al., 1987). On the other hand, enhancement of DNCB-induced skin sensitization in OC users was reported by Gerretsen et al. (1979). According to the authors, this enhanced reaction might be due to differences in type of progestin. Also, the differences in duration of use, dose of progestin, preexisting immune status, and nutritional status should be taken into account.

Oral contraceptives have been reported to stimulate both reticulo-endothelial phagocytic activity (Baar et al., 1974) and polymorphonuclear leukocyte chemotaxis (Nilsson et al., 1980). Use of OCs prevented the decrease in natural killer-cell activity in the periovulatory period that occurred in nonusers (Sulke et al., 1985; Stratton et al., 1986).

Furthermore, the use of low-dose OCs induced no statistically significant changes in levels of T-helper and T-suppressor lymphocytes (Nilsson et al., 1980; Baker et al., 1985). In contrast to the findings by Sulke et al. (1985) and Stratton et al. (1986), Baker et al. (1985) found no statistically significant changes in natural killer-cell activity between OC users and controls.

Oral Contraceptives and Infections

In various studies of the effects of OCs on prevalence and course of infections, confounding factors such as type, duration, and dose of OC have not been taken into account; cohorts have rarely been stratified with respect to age, marital status, nutritional status, and other factors. Use of OCs may imply more frequent medical examinations (increasing detection rate), and different hygienic factors and sexual behavior that render firm conclusions impossible.

Viral Infections

Various reports suggest an increased incidence of certain (mainly sexually transmitted) viral infections among OC users, whereas other studies showed no influence of OCs. Cytomegalovirus (CMV) seropositivity has been correlated with indices of sexual activity among pregnant women and women attending clinics for sexually transmitted diseases (STD), but the importance of sexual transmission is controversial since transmission by nonsexual routes also occurs and in certain populations infection before sexual debut is common (Collier et al., 1990). Although an early study reported a statistically significant increase in CMV infection in OC users (Willmott, 1975), two recent controlled studies showed no increase (Collier et al., 1990; Pereira et al., 1990). The latter finding is supported by a study showing that E2 and progesterone have no stimulating effect on CMV replication *in vitro* (Mackowiak et al., 1987).

Use of OCs did not give statistically significant increases of infection with Epstein-Barr or Herpes Zoster virus, nor was the risk of attaining hepatitis B increased (Royal College of General Practitioners, 1974). No differences in severity or recurrences of hepatitis B were found in a prospective study comparing OC users and nonusers (Schweitzer et al., 1975). Although early studies have shown that OC users had a statistically significantly higher incidence of infection with herpes simplex virus (HSV) (Royal College of General Practitioners, 1974; Willmott and Mair, 1978), a recent controlled study shows absence of such an effect and even a trend to a decreased incidence of HSV infection among ever-OC users (Kjaer et al., 1990).

With respect to infection with the human immunodeficiency virus (HIV), several studies may be of relevance, in spite of the fact that they were not designed to answer questions on OC use and HIV infection. A study of Nairobi prostitutes revealed a positive association between OC use and HIV infection (Simonsen et al., 1990), but the findings are confounded by the protective effect of barrier contraceptives. On the other hand, a study on the risk of transmission from HIV-positive hemophiliacs to their partners demonstrated no association with method of contraception (Goedert et al., 1988). Similarly, no relationship between OC use and HIV infection was observed in a group of American prostitutes (Darrow et al., 1988). In an Italian study, a suggestion of a protective effect of OC use against HIV transmission in female partners of HIV-infected men was found (Musicco, 1990). A multicenter European WHO study showed no statistically significant increase in risk of male-to-female transmission of HIV infection in women using OCs (European Study Group, 1989).

In the Royal College of General Practitioners Study (1974), OC use was not found statistically significantly associated with human papilloma virus infection. In two recent studies there was a trend of increased risk with longer duration of OC use (Daling et al., 1986; Kjaer et al., 1990). Finally, OC users were reported to have an increased risk of attaining rubella and varicella virus infections (Royal College, 1974).

Bacterial Infections

Genital infections with Chlamydia trachomatis are increasing (Thompson and Washington, 1983). In many Western countries this infection appears to be the most prevalent STD. A number of case-control studies have shown an increased risk of Chlamydia infection among OC users with a relative risk of approximately 2, representing a rather modest influence, with 95% confidence intervals (in most of the studies) extending close to 1 (e.g., Shafer et al., 1984). A recent large-scale prospective study (n = 1,000) showed no increased prevalence (Kovacs et al., 1987). Use of OCs does not increase the risk of infection with Neisseria gonorrheae (Bhattacharyya and Jephcott, 1976; Kinghorn and Waugh, 1981; Shafer et al., 1985). In two recent large-scale case-control studies among women whose partners had gonococcal urethritis, no differences in gonorrhea infection rates were seen between women who used either OCs, IUDs, or no contraception at all (McCormack and Reynolds, 1982; Griffiths and Hindley, 1985). There is good evidence that OC users have a reduced risk of pelvic inflammatory disease (PID) caused by Neisseria gonorrheae (Rubin et al., 1982; Washington et al., 1985; Wölner-Hanssen et al., 1985). As PID can be regarded as one of the leading causes of female infertility, this finding is important, especially for young women who have a relatively large number of potentially fertile years ahead.

The use of OCs did not induce increases in genital infection rates with group B Streptococci, Lactobacilli, Staphylococcus aureus, Mycoplasma, Ureaplasma urealyticum, and Gardnerella vaginalis (Shafer et al., 1985; Staerfelt et al., 1983).

In an Indian study, antibody response to tetanus toxoid was found to be considerably lower in OC users than in control women (Joshi et al., 1971). In another study, however, there was no impairment of tetanus toxoid-induced Ig production (Bray, 1976).

Fungal Infections

Early reports suggest an increased risk of infection with Candida albicans among OC users (Oriel et al., 1972; Bramley and Kinghorn, 1979; Staerfelt et al., 1983). This would be due to OC-induced decrease of the glycogen content of vaginal epithelial cells, analogous to the effect of pregnancy (Catterall, 1966; 1971). However, such an effect could not be confirmed in recent large studies with low-dose OCs (Goldacre et al., 1979; Davidson and Oates, 1985; Barbone et al., 1990). Even a decreased relative risk and a higher antibody response to Candida albicans, both statistically significant, have been found (Mathur et al., 1978; Reed et al., 1989).

Protozoal Infections

In Rhesus monkeys, a difference in response was found between two OC regimens; after infection with malaria parasites, the norethindrone-containing OC induced increased parasitemia, as was previously found with progesterone and E2

(Dutta and Kamboj, 1984; Dutta et al., 1984), whereas the norgestrel-containing OC induced decreased parasitemia. No marked differences in antibody levels were observed (Collins et al., 1984).

A recent large-scale case-control WHO study revealed no higher prevalence of parasitemia in users of levonorgestrel-containing OCs when compared with non-users or pregnant women, the severity of parasitemia also being much lower. Larger clinical trials in holoendemic areas are needed to confirm these protective effects (Mati et al., 1986).

Oral contraceptives have no influence on immune function, PHA and purified protein derivative (PPD) response, and antibody levels in malaria patients (Dutta et al., 1984; Collins et al., 1984; Bray, 1976).

Some studies from developing countries reported an increased incidence of Trichomonas vaginalis infection in OC users (El-Boulaqi et al., 1984; Pillay and Yap, 1979). In contrast, studies from Western countries reported no change (Burns et al., 1975; Shafer et al., 1985), or even a decreased incidence (Bramley and Kinghorn, 1979; Kinghorn and Waugh, 1981; Staerfelt et al., 1983).

In a small Indian study, the use of low-dose OCs was not associated with an increased incidence of Giardiasis infection (Guha Mazumder et al., 1990).

Other Infections

Little information exists on the effects of OCs on incidence of or susceptibility to infection with nematodes, cestodes, or trematodes. In mice, rats, and schistosomiasis patients, the use of OCs did not adversely influence the course of the disease, which particularly referred to the course of the schistosomiasis-induced hepatic damage (El Allawy et al., 1977; Shaaban et al., 1982; Sabet El Shammah et al., 1974; Bussolati et al., 1967).

In patients with Opisthorchis viverrini (liver fluke) infection, the use of OCs did not adversely influence liver function parameters (Chulacharit et al., 1972).

Oral Contraceptives and Autoimmune Disease

It is in particular for SLE and RA that the role of OCs has been studied; various relevant data will now be discussed.

Systemic Lupus Erythematosus

Several clinical observations suggest that estrogen can precipitate or aggravate SLE. After the first report by Pimstone (1966) on manifestation of SLE during OC use, the condition has been reported to occur in connection with a variety of estrogen-containing OCs. From the literature we collected some 60 cases with OC-associated SLE: 35 women had a past history predisposing for the disease; 30 had latent or manifest SLE; and five had a history of rheumatic symptoms (Geurts and Goorissen, unpublished review). In the relatively large study by Jungers et al. (1982), it was shown that switching from an estrogen-containing OC to a progestin-only type resulted in remission. Mintz et al. (1984) treated patients with inactive disease with a progestin-only OC; this did not lead to recrudescence of active lupus. These data suggest a negative effect of the estrogen component. During pregnancy, however, the risk for exacerbation of SLE was found not to be increased (Lockshin et al., 1989).

In both male and female SLE patients, an elevated conversion of E2 to 16α-hydroxylated metabolites has been demonstrated (Lahita et al., 1979, 1981, 1985; Stern et al., 1979; Inman et al., 1979). Bucala et al. (1982) found significantly higher levels of 16α-hydroxyestrone in patients with serologically and clinically active disease than in patients with inactive disease. This metabolite can form addition products with proteins, which were found to occur on the membranes of erythrocytes and lymphocytes of SLE patients (Bucala et al., 1984, 1985). Bucala et al. (1987) also reported the presence of antibodies to estrogen in these patients, whereas antibodies were also found in healthy women who had used OCs.

Rheumatoid Arthritis

The ameliorating effect of pregnancy on the course of RA has been well established (Persellin, 1977; Cecere and Persellin, 1981; Klipple and Cecere, 1989). In addition, several early studies have reported a beneficial effect of female sex hormones on the disease course (Kuipers, 1935; Touw and Kuipers, 1938; Blais and Demers, 1962; Gilbert et al., 1964; Demers et al., 1966). Together, these results have been the biological background of the many studies on the association between OCs and the development of RA. Since the Royal College of General Practitioners' oral contraception study provided the first evidence for a protection against RA among OC users (Wingrave and Kay, 1978), many studies have been conducted on this topic. Unfortunately, the results are not conclusive; to date, seven studies have shown a reduction of RA by OC use of about 50% (Wingrave and Kay, 1978; Vandenbroucke et al., 1982;1986; Hazes et al., 1990a;1990b; Spector et al., 1990; Koepsell et al., 1989), five studies reported no effect of OC use on the development of RA (Linos et al., 1983; Del Junco et al., 1985; Vessey et al., 1987; Hernandez-Avila et al., 1990; Hannaford et al., 1990), and one study was inconclusive (Allebeck et al., 1984).

Pooling the relative risks of RA for ever users of OCs of all known studies yielded a slight protective effect of OC use on the onset of RA, with a pooled relative risk of 0.73 and 95% confidence interval, 0.61–0.85 (Spector and Hochberg, 1990). Pooling all results, however, did not solve the problem of the clear discrepancies between the individual studies. Meta-analyses on the various OC studies provided some possible explanations for the divergent results. Vandenbroucke et al. (1989) found a sizable protection against RA among OC users in the pooled European studies and no effect in those originating from the U.S. A possible explanation of this finding may be found in different formulations of OCs across the continents. There are, however, other explanations too. Spector and Hochberg (1990) compared the hospital-based studies with the population-based studies and found a substantial protection of OC use against RA needing specialist attention, as distinct from the absence of an effect of OCs on RA occurring in the population. At close view this finding is not so different from the "great transatlantic divide" (Vandenbroucke et al., 1989), as most of the European studies were hospital-based. This suggests that OC use probably prevents only the more severe forms of RA. Support for this hypothesis was found after a follow-up of the cases of the latest Dutch case-control study (van Zeben et al., 1990); the protective effect of OC use before symptom onset was limited to the most severely affected RA patients.

Accepting a preventive effect of OC use against the development of the more severe forms of RA, we are still left with the biological explanation of this association. In this context, it is impossible to tell which specific influence of "the pill" is involved. In addition to the varying composition (different doses of EE and progestin), OCs contain various progestins that differ in their hormonal profiles. As a result, the balance between estrogenic, androgenic, and glucocorticoid properties may vary considerably, and consequently so will the OC-induced immunological effects. Of further importance is that all studies but one (Spector et al., 1990) failed to find a dose-effect relation, whereas the therapeutic use of OCs in established RA has revealed no or only little beneficial effect on the course of the disease (Hazes et al., 1989; Bijlsma et al., 1987). In addition, contradictory findings have been made with regard to the use of noncontraceptive hormones, in particular estrogens, and the development of RA; one study reported a protective effect (Vandenbroucke et al., 1986), whereas three studies showed negative results (Hernandez-Avila et al., 1990; Carette et al., 1989; Spector et al., 1991).

Studies associating OC use with diseases have to be interpreted cautiously, as there are many possible confounding factors and alternative explanations related to contraceptive behavior that might be important in the risk of developing the disease in question (Hazes and van Zeben, 1991).

CONCLUSIONS

Although many data on immunologic effects of estrogens and progestins are available, it is impossible to draw a coherent picture of the immunomodulating properties of these contraceptive steroids. This is *a fortiori* the case for OCs, since their immunologic effects, if present, could be ascribed to the estrogenic or progestational component, or to antagonistic, additive, or even synergistic activities of both steroids.

Despite the limitations of our knowledge, it seems unlikely that estrogens or progestins in the doses used in OCs have negative effects on the immune system (with the possible exception of application of estrogens in patients with SLE, for whom the progestin-only types seem better suited).

Epidemiologic evidence suggests that OC use may protect against severe forms of RA. Data suggesting a protective effect of estrogens in perimenopausal women were not confirmed, so the role of estrogens in RA remains uncertain. The progestational component, usually a 19-nortestosterone derivative, could just as well be the protective factor in view of their favorable effects in various animal models for autoimmune diseases.

An interesting facet of the various immunomodulating effects of these steroids in experimental animals is that they do not correlate with "classical" estrogenic or progestational activities. As far as such data may be extrapolated to humans, they imply that possible immunomodulating effects of contraceptive steroids cannot be deduced from their estrogenic or progestational potencies.

REFERENCES

Allebeck P, Ahlbom A, Ljungstrom K, Allender E. Do oral contraceptives reduce the incidence of rheumatoid arthritis? *Scand J Rheumatol* 1984;13:140–6.

Ansar Ahmed S, Penhale WJ, Talal N. Sex hormones, immune responses, and autoimmune disease. *Am J Pathol* 1985;121:531–51.

Aycock WL. Alterations in autarceologic susceptibility to experimental poliomyelitis. *Proc Soc Exp Biol Med* 1936;34:573–4.

Baar EH, Hepp H, Köhnlein HE. Die wirkung verschiedener hormonaler antikonzeptiva auf die phagozytosefähigkeit des reticuloendothelialen systems (effect of various hormonal contraceptives on the phagocytic capacity of the reticuloendothelial system). *Arch Gynäkol* 1974;216:257–71.

Baker DA, Hameed C, Tejani N, Milch P, Thomas J, Monheit AG, et al. Lymphocyte subsets in women on low dose oral contraceptives. *Contraception* 1985;32:377–82.

Baker DA, Thomas J. The effect of low dose oral contraceptives on the initial immune response to infection. *Contraception* 1984;29:519–25.

Barak V, Shoshana B, Halimi M, Treves AJ. The effect of estradiol on human myelomonocytic cells. II. Mechanism of enhancing activity of colony formation. *J Reprod Immunol* 1986;9:355–63.

Barbone F, Austin H, Louv WC, Alexander WJ. A follow-up of methods of contraception, sexual activity, and rates of trichomoniasis, candidiasis, and bacterial vaginosis. *Am J Obstet Gynecol* 1990; 163:510–4.

Beynon HLC, Garbett ND, Barnes PJ. Severe premenstrual exacerbations of asthma: effects of intramuscular progesterone. *Lancet* 1988;2:370–2.

Bhattacharyya MN, Jephcott AE. Diagnosis of gonorrhea in women—influence of the contraceptive pill. *J Am Vener Dis Assoc* 1976;2:21–4.

Bijlsma JWJ, Huber-Bruning O, Thijssen JHH. The effect of oestrogen treatment on the clinical and laboratory manifestations of rheumatoid arthritis. *Ann Rheum Dis* 1987;46:779–9.

Bisset LR, Griffin JFT. Humoral immunity in oral contraceptive users. I. Plasma immunoglobulin levels. *Contraception* 1988a;38:567–72.

Bisset LR, Griffin JFT. Humoral immunity in oral contraceptive users. II. In vitro immunoglobulin production. *Contraception* 1988b;38:573–8.

Blais JA, Demers R. The use of norethynodrel (Enovid) in the treatment of rheumatoid arthritis (preliminary report). *Arthritis Rheum* 1962;5:284.

Bramley M, Kinghorn G. Do oral contraceptives inhibit Trichomonas vaginalis? *Sex Transm Dis* 1979; 6:261–3.

Bray RS. Some immune responses of Gambian women taking the combined oral contraceptive pill. *Contraception* 1976;13:417–25.

Bucala R, Fishman J, Cerami A. The reaction of 16alpha-hydroxyestrone with erythrocytes in vitro and in vivo. *Eur J Biochem* 1984;140:593.

Bucala R, Lahita RG, Fishman J, Cerami A. Anti-oestrogen antibodies in users of oral contraceptives and in patients with systemic lupus erythematosus. *Clin Exp Immunol* 1987;65:167–75.

Bucala R, Lahita RG, Fishman J, Cerami A. Increased levels of 16alpha-hydroxyestrone-modified proteins in pregnancy and in systemic lupus erythematosus. *J Clin Endocrinol Metab* 1985;60:841.

Burns DCM, Darougar S, Thin RN, Lothian L, Nicol CS. Isolation of chlamydia from women attending a clinic for sexually transmitted diseases. *Br J Vener Dis* 1975;51:314–8.

Bussolati C, de Carneri I, Castellino S, Marinoni V, Sperzani GL. Treatment of experimental and clinical schistosomiasis with hormonal inhibitors of ovulation. *Am J Trop Med Hyg* 1967;16:497–9.

Carette S, Marcoux S, Gingras S. Postmenopausal hormones and the incidence of rheumatoid arthritis. *J Rheumatol* 1989;16:911–3.

Castro JE. Immunological effects of hormones: a review. *J Roy Soc Med* 1978;71:123–5.

Catterall RD. Candida albicans and the contraceptive pill. *Lancet* 1966;2:30–1.

Catterall RD. Influence of gestogenic contraceptive pills on vaginal candidosis. *Br J Vener Dis* 1971; 47:45–7.

Cecere FA, Persellin RH. The interaction of pregnancy and the rheumatic diseases. *Clin Rheum Dis* 1981;7:747–68.

Chandra RK. Serum levels of IgG and alpha-macroglobulin and incidence of cryofibrinogenaemia in women taking oral contraceptives. *J Reprod Fertil* 1972;28:463–4.

Chulacharit E, Petchakit V, Rosenfield AG. Oral contraception and liver fluke disease. *J Obstet Gynaecol Br Commonwlth* 1972;79:657–60.

Collier AC, Handsfield HH, Roberts PL, Derouen T, Meyers JD, Leach L, et al. Cytomegalovirus infection in women attending a sexually transmitted disease clinic. *J Infect Dis* 1990;162:46–51.

Collins WE, Campbell CC, Barber A, Skinner JC, Huong AY. The effect of oral contraceptives in malaria infections in Rhesus monkeys. *Bull WHO* 1984;62:627–37.

Cuchacovich M, Tchernitchin A, Gatica H, Wurgaft R, Valenzuela C, Cornejo E. Intraarticular progesterone: effects of a local treatment for rheumatoid arthritis. *J Rheumatol* 1988;15:561–5.

Cuchacovich M, Wurgaft R, Mena MA, Valenzuela C, Gatica H, Tchernitchin A. Intraarticular progesterone inhibits ^{3}H-dexamethasone binding to synovial cells from patients with rheumatoid arthritis. A study by dry autoradiographic technique. *J Rheumatol* 1991;18:962–7.

Daling JR, Sherman KJ, Weiss NS. Risk factors for Condyloma acuminatum in women. *Sex Transm Dis* 1986;13:16–8.

Danel L, Menouni M, Cohen JHM, Magaud J-P, Lenoir G, Revillard J-P, Saez S. Distribution of androgen and estrogen receptors among lymphoid and haemopoietic cell lines. *Leukemia Res* 1985;9: 1,373–8.

Darrow WW, Bigler W, Deppe D, et al. HIV antibody in 640 U.S. prostitutes with no evidence of intravenous (IV)-drug abuse. *Fourth International Conference on AIDS.* Stockholm: 1988:4,054 (abst).

Davidson F, Oates JK. The pill does not cause "thrush." *Br J Obstet Gynacol* 1985;92:1,265–6.

Del Junco DJ, Annegers JF, Luthtra HS, Coulam CB, Kurland LT. Do oral contraceptives prevent rheumatoid arthritis? *JAMA* 1985;254:1,938–41.

Delâge JM, Lehner-Netsch G, Brisson J. The classical and alternate pathways of complement in oral contraceptive users. *Contraception* 1987;36:627–32.

Demers R, Blais JA, Pretty H. Arthrite rheumatoide traitée par norethynodrel associée à mestranol: aspects cliniques et tests de laboratoire (rheumatoid arthritis treated with norethynodrel combined with mestranol: clinical aspects and laboratory tests). *Can Med Ass J* 1966;95:350–4.

Dotchev D, Liappis N, Hungerland H. Geschlechtsspezifische unterschiede der serumproteine bei erwachsenen und einfluss der oralen hormonellen kontrazeptiva auf das serumeiweissbild (gender-specific differences in serum proteins of adults and effects of oral hormonal contraceptives on serum protein patterns). *Clin Chim Acta* 1973;44:431–5.

Dutta GP, Kamboj KK. Influence of progesterone and estrogen administration on the recrudescence patterns of Plasmodium knowlesi; infection in female rhesus monkeys (Macaca mulatta) following initial subcurative chloroquine therapy. *Ind J Malariol* 1984;21:79–88.

Dutta GP, Puri SK, Kamboj KK, Srivastava SK, Kamboj VP. Interactions between oral contraceptives and malaria infections in rhesus monkeys. *Bull WHO* 1984;62:931–9.

Dwyer JM, Knox GE, Mangi RJ. Cell mediated immunity in healthy women taking oral contraceptives. *Yale J Biol Med* 1975;48:91–5.

Eidinger D, Garrett TJ. Studies on the regulatory effects of the sex hormones on antibody formation and stem cell differentiation. *J Exp Med* 1972;136:1,098–116.

El Allawy RMM, Nour AM, Said MM, et al. Effect of nutritional status on the interaction between contraceptives and antibilharzial agents. *J Drug Res Egypt* 1977;9:103–18.

El-Boulaqi HA, El-Refaie SA, Bassiouny GA, Amin MA. The relation between trichomonas vaginalis and contraceptive measures. *J Egypt Soc Parasitol* 1984;14:495–9.

Erbach GT, Bahr JM. Effect of chronic or cyclic exposure to estradiol on the humoral immune response and the thymus. *Immunopharmacology* 1988;16:45–51.

European Study Group. Risk factors for male to female transmission of HIV. *Br Med J* 1989;298:411–5.

Fassati P, Motejlova A, Oktabcova M, Spizek J, Fassati M. Immunoglobuliny a hormonalni antikoncepce (immunoglobulins and hormonal contraceptives). *Cesk Gynekol* 1983;48:475–9.

Flynn A. Expression of Ia and the production of interleukin 1 by peritoneal exudate macrophages activated *in vivo* by steroids. *Life Sci* 1986;38:2,455–60.

Fox HS, Bond BL, Parslow TG. Estrogen regulates the IFN-gamma promoter. *J Immunol* 1991;146:4,362–7.

Friedman D, Nettl F, Schreiber AD. Effect of estradiol and steroid analogues on the clearance of immunoglobulin G-coated erythrocytes. *J Clin Invest* 1985;75:162–7.

Gerretsen G, Kremer J, Bleumink E, Nater JP, de Gast GC, The TH. Immune reactivity of women on hormonal contraceptives—phytohemagglutinin and concanavalin-A induced lymphocyte response. *Contraception* 1980;22:25–9.

Gerretsen G, Kremer J, Nater JP, Bleumink E, Gast GC de, The TH. Immune reactivity of women on hormonal contraceptives. *Contraception* 1979;19:83–9.

Gilbert M, Rotstein J, Cunningham C, Ernstrin I, Davidson A, Pincus G. Norethynodrel with mestranol in treatment of RA. *JAMA* 1964;190:235.

Giron DJ, Patterson RR. Effects of steroid hormones on virus-induced diabetes mellitus. *Infect Immun* 1982;37:820–2.

Goedert JJ, Eyster ME, Ragni MV, Biggar RI, Gail MH. Rate of heterosexual HIV transmission and associated risk with HIV-antigen. *Fourth International Conference on AIDS*. Stockholm: 1988;4,019. (abst)

Goldacre MJ, Watt B, Loudon N, Milne LJR, Loudon JDO, Vessey MP. Vaginal microbial flora in normal young women. *Br Med J* 1979;1:1,450–3.

Graff RJ, Lappe MA, Snell GD. The influence of the gonads and adrenal glands on the immune response to skin grafts. *Transplantation* 1969;7:105–11.

Griffiths M, Hindley D. Gonococcal pelvic inflammatory disease, oral contraceptives and cervical mucus. *Genitourin Med* 1985;61:67.

Grossman CJ. Regulation of the immune system by sex steroids. *Endocrine Rev* 1984;5:435–55.

Guerne P-A, Carson DA, Lotz M. IL-6 production by human articular chondrocytes. Modulation of its synthesis by cytokines, growth factors, and hormones in vitro. *J Immunol* 1990;144:499–505.

Guha Mazumder DN, Ghose N, Mitra J, Dutta G, Santra A. Immunological status of women with prolonged oral contraceptives and occurrence of giardiasis. *J Ind Med Assoc* 1990;88:129–31.

Gulshan S, McCruden AB, Stimson WH. Oestrogen receptors in macrophages. *Scand J Immunol* 1990;31:691–7.

Hagen C, Fröland A. Depressed lymphocyte response to P.H.A. in women taking oral contraceptives. *Lancet* 1972;1:1,185.

Hannaford PC, Kay CR, Hirsch S. Oral contraceptives and rheumatoid arthritis: new data from the Royal College of General Practitioners' Oral Contraception Study. *Ann Rheum Dis* 1990;49:744–6.

Hazes JMW, Dijkmans BAC, Vandenbroucke JP, De Vries RRP, Cats A. Reduction of the risk of rheumatoid arthritis among women who take oral contraceptives. *Arthritis Rheum* 1990a;33;173–9.

Hazes JMW, Dijkmans BAC, Vandenbroucke JP, Cats A. Oral contraceptive treatment for rheumatoid arthritis: an open study in 10 female patients. *Br J Rheumatol* 1989;28[Suppl 1]:28–30.

Hazes JMW, Silman AJ, Brand R, Spector TD, Walker DJ, Vandenbroucke JP. Influence of oral contraception on the occurrence of rheumatoid arthritis in female sibs. *Scand J Rheumatol* 1990b;19:306–10.

Hazes JMW, van Zeben D. Oral contraception and its possible protection against rheumatoid arthritis. *Ann Rheum Dis* 1991;50:72–4.

Helgason S, von Schoultz B. Estrogen replacement therapy and the mixed lymphocyte reaction. *Am J Obstet Gynecol* 1981;141:393–7.

Hernandez-Avila M, Liang M, Willet WC, et al. Exogenous sex hormones and the risk of rheumatoid arthritis. *Arthritis Rheum* 1990;33:947–53.

Heywood R, Wadsworth PF. The experimental toxicology of estrogens. *Pharmacol Ther* 1980;8:125–142.

Ho PC, Tang GWK, Fu KH, Fan MC, Lawton JWM. Immunologic studies in patients with premature ovarian failure. *Obstet Gynecol* 1988;71:622–6.

Ho PC, Tang GWK, Lawton JWM. Lymphocyte subsets in patients with oestrogen deficiency. *J Reprod Immunol* 1991;20:85–91.

Holdstock G, Chastenay BF, Krawitt EL. Effects of testosterone, oestradiol and progesterone on immune regulaton. *Clin Exp Immunol* 1982;47:449–56.

Holmdahl R, Carlsten H, Jansson L, Larsson P. Oestrogen is a potent immunomodulator of murine experimental rheumatoid disease. *Br J Rheumatol* 1989;28[Suppl 1]:54–8.

Horne CHW, Howie PW, Weir RJ, Goudie RB. Effect of combined oestrogen-progestogen oral contraceptives on serum levels of alpha2-macroglobulin, transferrin, albumin and IgG. *Lancet* 1970;1:49–50.

Hu S-K, Mitcho YL, Rath NC. Effect of estradiol on interleukin 1 synthesis by macrophages. *Int J Immunopharmacol* 1988;10:247–52.

Huygen K, Palfliet K. Strain variation in interferon gamma production of BCG-sensitized mice challenged with PPD. *Cell Immunol* 1984;85:75–81.

Inman RD, Jovanovic L, Dawood MY, Longcope C. Systemic lupus erythematosus in the male: a genetic and endocrine study. *Arthritis Rheum* 1979;6:624.

Irvine WJ, MacCuish AC, Barnes EW, Urbaniak SJ, Loudon NB. Immunological function in oral contraceptive users. *J Reprod Fertil* 1974;21[Suppl]:33–41.

Jansson L, Mattsson A, Mattsson R, Holmdahl R. Estrogen induced suppression of collagen arthritis V: physiological level of estrogen in DBA/1 mice is therapeutic on established arthritis, suppresses anti-type II collagen T-cell dependent immunity and stimulates polyclonal B-cell activity. *J Autoimmun* 1990;3:257–70.

Joshi UM, Rao SS, Kora SJ, Dikshit SS, Virkar KD. Effect of steroidal contraceptives on antibody formation in the human female. *Contraception* 1971;3:327–33.

Jungers P, Dougados M, Pélissier C, Kuttenn F, Tron F, Lesavre P, et al. Influence of oral contraceptive therapy on the activity of systemic lupus erythematosus. *Arthritis Rheum* 1982;25:618–23.

Kalo-Klein A, Witkin SS. Candida albicans: cellular immune system interactions during different stages of the menstrual cycle. *Am J Obstet Gynecol* 1989;161:1,132–6.

Keisler LW, Kier AB, Walker SE. Effects of prolonged administration of the 19-nor-testosterone derivatives norethindrone and norgestrel to female NZB/W mice: comparison with medroxyprogesterone and ethinyl estradiol. *Autoimmunity* 1991;9:21–32.

Keller AJ, Irvine WJ, Jordan J, Loudon NB. Phytohemagglutinin-induced lymphocyte transformation in oral contraceptive users. *Obstet Gynecol* 1977;49:83–91.

Kenny JF, Gray JA. Sex differences in immunologic response: studies of antibody production by individual spleen cells after stimulus with Escherichia coli antigen. *Pediatr Res* 1971;5;246–55.

Kenny JF, Pangburn PC, Trail G. Effect of estradiol on immune competence: in vivo and in vitro studies. *Infect Immun* 1976;13:448–56.

Kincl FA, Ciaccio LA. Suppression of the immune response by progesterone. *Endocrinol Exp* 1980;14:27–33.

Kinghorn GR, Waugh MA. Oral contraceptive use and prevalence of infection with chlamydia trachomatis in women. *Br J Vener Dis* 1981;57:187–90.

Kita E, Hamuro A, Oku D, et al. Hormonal regulation of soluble immune response suppressor (SIRS): a possible role of SIRS in the maintenance of pregnancy. *Cell Immunol* 1990;130:92–105.

Kittas C, Henry L. Effects of sex hormones on the immune system of guinea pigs and on the development of toxoplasmic lesions in non-lymphoid organs. *Clin Exp Immunol* 1979;36:16–23.

Kjaer SK, Engholm G, Teisen C, Haugaard BJ, Lynge E, Christensen RB, et al. Risk factors for cervical human papilloma virus and herpes simplex virus infections in Greenland and Denmark: a population-based study. *Am J Epidemiol* 1990;131:669–82.

Klipple GL, Cecere FA. Rheumatoid arthritis and pregnancy. *Rheum Dis Clin North Am* 1989;15:213–39.

Koepsell T, Dugowson C, Voigt L, et. al. Preliminary findings from a case-control study of the risk of rheumatoid arthritis in relation to oral contraceptive use. *Br J Rheumatol* 1989;28[Suppl 1]:41.

Kovacs GT, Westcott M, Rusden J, Asche V, King H, Haynes SE, et al. The prevalence of chlamydia trachomatis in a young, sexually-active population. *Med J Aust* 1987;147:550–2.

Kuipers FC. Dimenformon in grote doses ter behandeling van de primair chronische rheumatoïde arthritis (dimenformon in high doses for the treatment of primary chronic rheumatoid arthritis). *Ned Tijdschr Geneesk* 1935;79:5,122–39.

Kvist Poulsen H. Changes in circulating enzyme inhibitors, complement factors, and steroid-dependent proteins during exposure to oral contraceptives and within the normal menstrual cycle. In: *Abstracts XII World Congress of Gynecology and Obstetrics*. Rio de Janeiro: 1988:580–1.

Lahita RG, Bradlow HL, Kunkel HG, Fishman J. Alterations of estrogen metabolism in systemic lupus erythematosus. *Arthritis Rheum* 1979;22:1,195–8.

Lahita RG, Bradlow HL, Kunkel HG, Fishman J. Increased 16alpha-hydroxylation of estradiol in systemic lupus erythematosus. *J Clin Endocrinol Metab* 1981;52:174–8.

Lahita RG, Bucala R, Bradlow HL, Fishman J. Determination of 16alpha-hydroxyestrone by radioimmunoassay in systemic lupus erythematosus. *Arthritis Rheum* 1985;28:1,122–7.

Linos A, Worthington JW, O'Fallon WM, Kurland LT. Case-control study of rheumatoid arthritis and prior use of oral contraceptives. *Lancet* 1983;1:1,299–1,300.

Lockshin MD. Pregnancy does not cause systemic lupus erythematosus to worsen. *Arthritis Rheum* 1989;32:665–70.

Luster MI, Hayes HT, Korach K, Tucker AN, Dean JH, Greenlee WF, Boorman GA. Estrogen immunosuppression is regulated through estrogenic responses in the thymus. *J Immunol* 1984;133:110–6.

Mackowiak PA, Haley ML, Marling-Cason M, Tiemens KM, Luby JP. Effect of human sex hormones on cytomegalovirus growth and Fc receptor expression. *J Lab Clin Med* 1987;110:427–32.

Majumder MSI, Mohiduzzaman M, Ahmad K. Immunocompetence of marginally nourished women on hormonal contraceptives. *Nutr Rep Int* 1987;36:1,285–90.

Maoz H, Kaiser N, Halimi M, et al. The effect of estradiol on human myelomonocytic cells. I. Enhancement of colony formation. *J Reprod Immunol* 1985;7:325–35.

Mathur S, Mathur RS, Dowda H, Williamson HO, Faulk WP, Fudenberg HH. Sex steroid hormones and antibodies to Candida albicans. *Clin Exp Immunol* 1978;33:79–87.

Mati JKG, Sinei SK, Mulandi TN, Ndavi PM, Mbugua S, Mailu CK, et al. Oral contraceptive use and the risk of malaria. *East Afr Med J* 1986;63:382–8.

McCormack WM, Reynolds GH, Cooperative Study Group. Effect of menstrual cycle and method of contraception on recovery of Neisseria gonorrhoea. *JAMA* 1982;247:1,292–4.

McFarland HI, Bigley NJ. Sex-dependent, early cytokine production by NK-like spleen cells following infection with the D variant of encephalomyocarditis virus (EMCV-D). *Viral Immunol* 1989;2:205–14.

Melez KA, Reeves JP, Steinberg AD. Regulation of expression of autoimmunity in NZB × NZW F1 mice by sex hormones. *J Immunopharmacol* 1978–79;1:27–42.

Mintz G, Gutierrez G, Deleré M, Rodriguez E. Contraception with progestogens in systemic lupus erythematosus. *Contraception* 1984;30:29–38.

Mooradian AD, Morley JE, Korenman SG. Biological actions of androgens. *Endocr Rev* 1987;8:1–28.

Mori T, Kobayashi H, Nishimoto H, Suzuki A, Nishimura T, Mori T. Inhibitory effect of progesterone and 20α-hydroxypregn-4-en-3-one on the phytohemagglutinin-induced transformation of human lymphocytes. *Am J Obstet Gynecol* 1977;127:151–7.

Morishima A, Henrich RT. Lymphocyte transformation and oral contraceptives. *Lancet* 1974;2:646.

Musicco M. Oral contraception, IUD, condom use and man to woman sexual transmission of HIV infection. *Sixth international conference on AIDS, vols. 1–3.* San Francisco: University of California; 1990:THC584. (abst).

Neumann F. The physiological action of progesterone and the pharmacological effects of progestogens—a short review. *Postgrad Med J* 1978;54[Suppl 2]:11–24.

Nicol T, Bilbey DLJ, Charles LM, Cordingley JL, Vernon-Roberts B. Oestrogen: the natural stimulant of body defence. *J Endocrinol* 1964;30:277–91.

Nilsson B, Domber MG, von Schoultz B. Effect of estrogen/progestogen combinations on polymorphonuclear leucocyte chemotaxis. *Acta Obstet Gynecol Scand* 1980;59:165–8.

Oriel JD, Partridge BM, Denny MJ, Coleman JL. Genital yeast infections. *Br Med J* 1972;4:761–4.

Paavonen T, Andersson LC, Adlercreutz H. Sex hormone regulation of in vitro immune response. Estradiol enhances human B cell maturation via inhibition of suppressor T cells in pokeweed mitogen-stimulated cultures. *J Exp Med* 1981;154:1,935–45.

Pacifici R, Brown C, Puscheck E, et al. Effect of surgical menopause and estrogen replacement on cytokine release from human blood mononuclear cells. *Proc Natl Acad Sci USA* 1991;88:5,134–8.

Pearce PT, Khalid BAK, Funder JW. Progesterone receptors in rat thymus. *Endocrinology* 1983;113:1,287–91.

Pereira LH, Embil JA, Haase DA, Manley KM. Cytomegalovirus infection among women attending a sexually transmitted disease clinic: association with clinical symptoms and other sexually transmitted diseases. *Am J Epidemiol* 1990;131:683–92.

Persellin RH. The effect of pregnancy on rheumatoid arthritis. *Bull Rheum Dis* 1977;27:922–6.

Petermann B, Brandt M, Elendt D, Malberg K. Wirkung oraler kontrazeptiva auf zirkulierende immunkomplexe (action of oral contraceptives on circulating immune complexes). *Zentralbl Gynäkol* 1982; 104:349–52.

Pillay B, Yap SK. Trichomoniasis-incidence in pill users and associated pap smear abnormalities. *Malays J Pathol* 1979;2:59–62.

Pimstone B. Systemic lupus erythematosus exacerbated by oral contraceptives. *S Afr J Obstet Gynecol* 1966;4:62–3.

Piper JM, Kennedy DL. Oral contraceptives in the United States: trends in content and potency. *Int J Epidemiol* 1987;16:215–21.

Polan ML, Daniele A, Kuo A. Gonadal steroids modulate human monocyte interleukin-1 (IL-1) activity. *Fertil Steril* 1988;49:964–8.

Purtilo DT, Hallgren HM, Yunis EJ. Depressed maternal lymphocyte response to phytohaemagglutinin in human pregnancy. *Lancet* 1972;1:769–71.

Ralston SH, Russell RGG, Gowen M. Estrogen inhibits release of tumor necrosis factor from peripheral blood mononuclear cells in postmenopausal women. *J Bone Min Res* 1990;5:983–8.

Reed BD, Huck W, Zazove P. Differentiation of gardnerella vaginalis, candida albicans, and trichomonas vaginalis infections of the vagina. *J Fam Pract* 1989;28:673–80.

Roubinian JR, Talal N, Greenspan JS, Goodman JR, Siiteri PK. Effects of castration and sex hormones on survival, antinucleic acid antibodies and glomerulonephritis in NZB/NZW F-1 mice. *J Expl Med* 1978;147:1,568–83.

Royal College of General Practitioners. *Oral contraceptives and health.* New York: Pitman Medical; 1974.

Rubin GL, Ory HW, Layde PM. Oral contraceptives and pelvic inflammatory disease. *Am J Obstet Gynecol* 1982;140:630–5.

Sabet El Shammah S, Elwi A, El Hofnawi F, Wasef SA, Mawla NG, Abdallah A. Gestagens and the bilharzial liver. *Asian J Med* 1974;10:56–60.

Sarvetnick N, Fox HS. Interferon-gamma and the sexual dimorphism of autoimmunity. *Mol Biol Med* 1990;7:323–31.

Schlumberger HD. Epidemiology of allergic diseases. *Monographs in Allergy, vol. 21.* Basel; Karger; 1987.

Schreiber AD, Nettl FM, Sanders MC, et al. Effect of endogenous and synthetic sex steroids on the clearance of antibody-coated cells. *J Immunol* 1988;141:2,959–66.

Schuurs AHWM, Verheul HAM. Effects of gender and sex steroids on the immune response. *J Steroid Biochem* 1990;35:157–72.

Schweitzer IL, Weiner JM, McPeak CM, Thursby MW. Oral contraceptives in acute viral hepatitis. *JAMA* 1975;233:979–80.

Sekiya S, Kamiyama M, Takamizawa H. In vivo and in vitro tests of inhibitory effect of progesterone on cell-mediated immunity in rats bearing a syngeneic uterine adenocarcinoma. *JNCI* 1975;54:769–71.

Shaaban MM, Hammad WA, Fathalla MF, Ghaneiman SA, El-Sharkawy MM, Salim TH, et al. Effects of oral contraception on liver function tests and serum proteins in women with active schistosomiasis. *Contraception* 1982;26:75–82.

Shafer MA, Beck A, Blain B, Dole P, Irwin CE, Sweet R, et al. Chlamydia trachomatis: important relationships to race, contraception, lower genital tract infection, and papanicolaou smear. *J Pediatr* 1984;104:141–6.

Shafer MA, Sweet RZ, Ohm-Smith MJ, Shalwitz J, Beck A, Schachter J. Microbiology of the lower genital tract in post-menarchal adolescent girls: differences by sexual activity, contraception and presence of non-specific vaginitis. *J Pediatr* 1985:107:974–81.

Shahani SK, Tezabwala BU. Serum haemolytic complement levels of women using fertility regulating agents. *Ind J Med Res* 1982;76:696–9.

Simonsen JN, Plummer FA, Ngugi EN, Black C, Kreiss JK, Gakynia MN, et al. HIV infection among lower socioeconomic strata prostitutes in Nairobi. *AIDS* 1990;4:139–44.

Spector TD, Hochberg MC. The protective effect of the oral contraceptive pill on rheumatoid arthritis: an overview of the analytic epidemiological studies using meta-analysis. *J Clin Epidemiol* 1990;43: 1,221–30.

Spector TD, Roman E, Silman AJ. The pill, parity and rheumatoid arthritis. *Arthritis Rheum* 1990;33; 782–9.

Spector TD, Brennan P, Harris P, Studd JNN, Silman AJ. Does estrogen replacement therapy protect against rheumatoid arthritis? *J Rheumatol* 1991;18:1473–6.

Staerfelt F, Gundersen TJ, Halsos AM, et al. A survey of genital infections in patients attending a clinic for sexually transmitted diseases. *Scand J Infect Dis* 1983;40[Suppl]:53–7.

Stern R, Fishman J, Brusman H, Kunkel HG. Systemic lupus erythematosus associated with Klinefelter's syndrome. *Arthritis Rheum* 1979;22:1,195–8.

Stock JL, Coderre JA, McDonald B, Rosenwasser LJ. Effects of estrogen in vivo and in vitro on spontaneous interleukin-1 release by monocytes from menopausal women. *J Clin Endocrinol Metab* 1989; 68:364–8.

Stratton JA, Miller RD, Kent DR, Weathersbee PS, Thrupp LD, Richards CA, et al. Effect of oral contraceptives on leukocyte phagocytic activity and plasma levels of prostaglandin E2 and thromboxane B2 in normal menstruating women. *Am J Reprod Immunol Microbiol* 1986;10:47–52.

Sulke AN, Jones DB, Wood PJ. Variation in natural killer activity in peripheral blood during the menstrual cycle. *Br Med J* 1985;290:884–6.

Sullivan DA, Wira CR. Sex hormone and glucocorticoid receptors in the bursa of Fabricius of immature chicks. *J Immunol* 1979;122:2,617–23.

Szekeres-Bartho J, Philibert D, Chaouat G. Progesterone suppression of pregnancy lymphocytes is not mediated by glucocorticoid effect. *Am J Reprod Immunol* 1990;23:42–43.

Tabibzadeh SS, Satyaswaroop PG. Sex steroid receptors in lymphoid cells of human endometrium. *Am J Clin Pathol* 1989;91:656–63.

Tezabwala BU, Hegde UM, Joshi JV, Jaswaney VL, Rao SS. Studies on cell-mediated immunity in women using different fertility regulating methods. *J Clin Lab Immunol* 1983;10:199–202.

Thompson SE, Washington AE. Epidemiology of sexually transmitted Chlamydia trachomatis infections. *Epidemiol Rev* 1983;5:96–123.

Thorogood M, Vessey MP. Trends in use of oral contraceptives in Britain. *Br J Family Planning* 1990; 16:41–53.

Touw JF, Kuipers RKW. The treatment of affections of the joints with progestine. *Acta Medica Scandinavica* 1938;96:501–8.

van Zeben D, Hazes JMW, Vandenbroucke JP, Dijkmans BAC, Cats A. Diminished incidence of severe rheumatoid arthritis associated with oral contraceptive use. *Arthritis Rheum* 1990;33:1,462–5.

Vandenbroucke JP, Hazes JMW, Dijkmans BAC, Cats A. Oral contraceptives and the risk of rheumatoid arthritis: the great transatlantic divide? *Br J Rheumatol* 1989;28(Suppl 1):1–3.

Vandenbroucke JP, Valkenburg HA, Boersma HA, et al. Oral contraceptives and rheumatoid arthritis: further evidence for a preventive effect. *Lancet* 1982;2:839–42.

Vandenbroucke JP, Witteman JCM, Valkenburg HA, et al. Non-contraceptive hormones and rheumatoid arthritis in perimenopausal and postmenopausal women. *JAMA* 1986;255:1299–1303.

Verheul HAM, Schot LPC, Deckers GHJ, Schuurs AHWM. Effects of tibolone, lynestrenol, ethylestrenol and desogestrel on autoimmune disorders in NZB/W mice. *Clin Immunol Immunopathol* 1986a; 38:198–208.

Verheul HAM, Schot LPC, Schuurs AHWM. Therapeutic effects of nandrolone decanoate, tibolone, lynestrenol and ethylestrenol on Sjögren's syndrome-like disorder in NZB/W mice. *Clin Exp Immunol* 1986b;64:243–8.

Verheul HAM, Tittes EV, Kelder J, Schuurs AHWM. Effects of steroids with different endocrine profiles on the development, morphology and function of the bursa of Fabricius in chickens. *J Steroid Biochem* 1986c;25:665–75.

Vessey MP, Villard-Mackintosh L, Yeates D. Oral contraceptives, cigarette smoking and other factors in relation to arthritis. *Contraception* 1987;35:457–64.

Walker SE, McMurray RW, Besch-Williford CL, Keisler DH. Premature death with bladder outlet obstruction and hyperprolactinemia in NZB/W mice treated with ethynyl estradiol (EE) and 17β-estradiol (E2). *Arthritis Rheum* 1991;34[Suppl]:R9.

Washington AE, Gove S, Schachter J, Sweet RL. Oral contraceptives, chlamydia trachomatis infection, and pelvic inflammatory disease. *JAMA* 1985;253:2,246–50.

Weinstein Y, Berkovich Z. Testosterone effect on bone marrow, thymus, and suppressor T cells in the (NZB × NZW)F1 mice: its relevance to autoimmunity. *J Immunol* 1981;126:998–1002.

Weusten JJAM, Blankenstein MA, Gmelig-Meyling FHJ, Schuurman HJ, Kater L, Thijssen JHH. Presence of oestrogen receptors in human blood mononuclear cells and thymocytes. *Acta Endocrinol* 1986;112:409–14.

Willmott FE. Cytomegalovirus in female patients attending a VD clinic. *Br J Vener Dis* 1975;51:278–80.

Willmott FE, Mair HJ. Genital herpes virus infection in women attending a venereal diseases clinic. *Br J Vener Dis* 1978;54:341–3.

Wingrave SJ, Kay CR. Reduction in incidence of rheumatoid arthritis associated with oral contraceptives. *Lancet* 1978;1:569–71.

Wira CR, Sandoe CP. Hormonal regulation of immunoglobulins: influence of estradiol on immuno-globulins A and G in the rat uterus. *Endocrinology* 1980;106:1,020–6.

Wira CR, Sullivan DA. Estradiol and progesterone regulation of immunoglobulin A and G and secretory component in cervicovaginal secretions of the rat. *Biol Reprod* 1985;32:90–5.

Wölner-Hanssen P, Svensson L, Mardh PA, Weström L. Laparoscopic findings and contraceptive use in women with signs and symptoms suggestive of acute salpingitis. *Obstet Gynecol* 1985;66:233–8.

Pharmacology of the Contraceptive Steroids,
edited by Joseph W. Goldzieher.
Raven Press, Ltd., New York © 1994.

27

Teratogenesis and Mutagenesis

Joseph W. Goldzieher

Department of Obstetrics and Gynecology, Baylor College of Medicine,
Houston, Texas 77030

ANIMAL STUDIES

Soon after estrogens became available for biologic investigations, it was found that estrogens were embryocidal in rodents (Hain, 1935) and that the range of dosages administered had to be truncated if liveborn offspring were to be obtained. By the early 1940s extensive studies had been carried out (Greene et al., 1940, 1942) on the intersexuality produced in the offspring of rats and mice given estrogens during gestation. The effects were different in the two species, and with some other steroids even strain differences within a species changed the incidence of anomalies (Fraser and Fainstat, 1951). Teratogenesis from estrogen administration was also reported in guinea pigs and opossums (Greene et al., 1940). Nonsteroidal estrogens such as diethylstilbestrol (DES) produced the same effects, leading to medicolegal controversies that persist today.

The effect of progestins in pregnant rodents varies with the particular compound. Norethynodrel with mestranol induced malformations in rats and rabbits, whereas ethynodiol diacetate/mestranol did not (Saunders and Elton, 1967; Saunders, 1967). Medroxyprogesterone acetate virilized female rat fetuses (Lyster et al., 1959; Suchowsky and Junkmann, 1961), but progesterone itself did not (Revesz et al., 1970). Cyproterone acetate also induced intersexuality in a variety of species (Neumann et al., 1974). In rhesus monkeys, combined oral contraceptives (OCs) may cause abortion during early organogenesis without producing morphological abnormalities in surviving offspring (Prahalada and Hendrickx, 1983). Studies in the baboon during early pregnancy suggest that the embryotoxic and teratogenic effects of medroxyprogesterone acetate may be dose dependent (Tarara, 1984).

Owing to these species differences, which may be due to variations in the metabolism of the compounds involved and their placental transport, as well as the timing and vulnerability of embryological development, a WHO Scientific Group addressing the effect of female sex hormones on fetal development and infant health (WHO, 1981) "placed little weight on animal studies in assessing the potential risks to the human fetus and infant . . . this should not be taken as detracting from or negating the critical importance of animal toxicology and teratological studies in the assessment of drug safety."

HUMAN STUDIES

It is exceedingly difficult to determine if an agent is teratogenic in humans. The effect depends on the specific agent and dose, time during gestation when exposure occurs, and genetic susceptibility of mother and fetus. When used prior to conception (i.e., discontinuation of OCs prior to desired conception), sex steroids may in theory exert effects through their residual endocrine or metabolic impact; this could affect subsequent offspring either by affecting the ova or by changing some important aspect of the maternal endocrine environment. During the first few weeks of fetal life (perhaps 2 weeks), the embryo is relatively resistant to teratogenic agents. A major insult may be lethal; however, if the embryo survives, no organ-specific animalies would occur. Increases or decreases in male/female sex ratio, spontaneous abortion rates, or twinning could occur if early fetal loss rates were selectively altered. By 8 to 10 weeks gestational age, susceptibility is maximum for an organ-specific teratogenic effect. Still later, a teratogen can affect the growth of the fetus or some specific organ, but malformation (except for the brain and gonads) is unlikely to occur.

When women are spacing births, 15% to 35% become pregnant within 2 months of discontinuing OCs. Pharmacokinetic studies of orally administered compounds show rapid clearance; injectable contraceptives may be present for weeks or even months. Residual effects after elimination of the compounds themselves depend on the rate of reversibility of the change (e.g., the half-life of serum proteins whose concentration is affected by contraceptive steroid exposure).

Few studies have distinguished between women who conceive while taking OCs and those who inadvertently begin OC use after conception. Even if contraceptive failures may be as low as 0.3% per year (1% is a more likely figure in the developed world), this rate represents perhaps as many as 160,000 fetuses exposed per year, given current rates of OC use. Supposedly hormone-related events must be examined against a background incidence of about 7% spontaneous birth defects of some kind in the U.S.

Special problems are involved in epidemiological research on OC use (or sex hormones in general) and fetal outcome (WHO, 1981; Polednak, 1985; Bracken, 1990). Prior pregnancy outcomes are important, but rarely investigated or taken into consideration. Ascertaining (let alone dating accurately) the exposure to medications during pregnancy is exceedingly difficult. Records of prescriptions written are no assurance that the OCs were used; the timing of exposure, especially with injectable contraceptives, may be speculation. Recall bias is perhaps the most intractable problem, especially in comparing women who had a child with a birth defect to those who had a normal pregnancy outcome. Klemetti and Saxen (1967), investigating the relationship between congenital malformations and antecedent drug use by the mother, interviewed mothers during and after pregnancy (i.e., prospectively and retrospectively). Only about 25% of the information elicited prospectively was elicited accurately retrospectively, and two thirds of the positive replies elicited retrospectively could not be confirmed. Tilley et al. (1985) interviewed women in the DESAD study. Of the DES-exposed mothers identified through review of their prenatal records, 29% could not remember whether they took DES; an additional 8% said they did not take DES when it was recorded in their charts. In a study of congenital limb reduction deformities and OC use carried out in Australia, the interviews were conducted an average of 4.5 years after the birth of the child (Kricker et al., 1986). It has been emphasized repeatedly that the recall of the mother of a normal child is likely to differ from that of the mother of a child with a birth defect for which she is trying to fix blame. Werler et al. (1989) indicated that recall of OC use around the time of conception is greatly underreported in mothers of healthy newborns compared with mothers of infants with birth defects.

Since there is now a substantial number of prospective studies that avoid this disabling problem of recall bias, no attempt will be made to review or critique the published retrospective case-control studies that, as usual, have been the focus of inordinate attention and concern.

As pointed out by the WHO Scientific Group, there are substantial problems in defining precisely the range of pregnancy outcomes, ascertaining (certain malformations are more common among stillbirths and infants who die soon after birth), and relating the time of exposure to the type of malformation. A noteworthy example of the latter is the incidence of major cardiac malformations reported by Heinonen et al. (1977), who reported a relative risk of 2.3 for sex hormone use during pregnancy. In subsequent litigation, the reluctant authors were required to provide raw data from the Boston Collaborative Perinatal Project. Of the 17 cases classified as hormone users, two took the agent before day 19 (the beginning of the stage of cardiogenesis) and five took it after day 50 (the end of cardiogenesis). Two cases of Down's syndrome and two who took drugs that were not sex hormones at all were also included among the original 17 (Wiseman and Dodds-Smith, 1984).

The problem of confounding is present in virtually all epidemiological research. It is acknowledged that women in developed countries who use OCs are more likely to smoke cigarettes, drink alcohol, and use other medications than women using alternative forms of contraception or no contraception at all. The first two of these confounders are known to be associated with unfavorable pregnancy outcome (Streissguth, 1978; Kline, 1978).

On the basis of general problems with case-control epidemiology (Ibrahim, 1979; Realini and Goldzieher, 1985) and the particular issues described above, further analysis will be limited to prospective studies. A meta-analysis of 12 prospective studies has been carried out by Bracken (1990); it encompasses 6,102 exposed and 83,167 nonexposed women. Three comparison groups were used: 1) women who conceived while using other forms of contraception; 2) women who had used OCs but stopped before conception or the last menstrual period; and 3) women who had never used OCs. Since malformations in spontaneous abortions are often not recorded, the analysis was restricted to stillbirths and live births. For all malformations, the relative risk was almost exactly unity (0.99 with 95% confidence limits of 0.83 and 1.19), regardless of which comparison group was used. Meta-analysis of congenital heart defects (eight prospective studies) yielded a typical relative risk of 1.06 with confidence limits of 0.72 to 1.56. However, this estimate includes the study of Heinonen et al. just analyzed, which contained gross errors of inclusion, and the study of Vessey et al. (1979), which found only a single event in the 38 exposed cases and three events in the 1,767 nonexposed—numbers that do not provide much confidence in the estimate of risk (which, in fact, had confidence limits of 1.61 to 149). Six studies were available for meta-analysis of limb-reduction defects; five of these found zero defects in the exposed mothers, while the sixth found three in 1,448 exposed versus 6 in 4,087 unexposed. The overall risk estimate was 1.04 with confidence limits of 0.30 to 3.55.

In February 1988, the U.S. Food and Drug Administration approved the following labeling: "Extensive epidemiological studies have revealed no increased risk of birth defects in women who have used oral contraceptives prior to pregnancy. Studies also do not suggest a teratogenic effect, particularly insofar as cardiac anomalies and limb reduction defects are concerned when taken inadvertently during early pregnancy."

With respect to long-acting injectables, Pardthaisong and Gray (1991) reported a prospective study of 1,573 pregnancies in which the fetus was exposed to Depoprovera. These consisted of 830 accidental pregnancies during use and 743 infants unknowingly conceived before the first injection was administered. The authors claimed that there was an increased risk of low birth weight (relative risk of 1.9 with confidence limits of 1.4 to 3.2) when conception was estimated to have occurred within 4 weeks of injection. In an invited commentary appended to the paper of Pardthaisong and Gray, Hogue called the comparison group of planned pregnancies "a case of perfect confounding," and pointed out that the authors' claim of a dose relationship was heavily dependent on their ability to establish accurately the time of conception; this also affected the estimate of gestational age and therefore evaluation of the normalcy of the birth weight. The only excess mortality in this study was among those with low birth weight, the cause of which remains necessarily indeterminate.

Six studies summarized by the WHO Scientific Group (1981) indicate that crude rates of stillbirths are consistently lower in pregnancies following OC use; this was also found when subsets controlled for age, parity, and other variables were examined. Both large and small studies have examined the sex ratio of the offspring of previous OC users compared to women who use other or no form of contraception, and no significant difference has been found (WHO, 1981).

MUTAGENESIS

A high proportion of chromosomally abnormal embryos are lost before pregnancy is diagnosed. About 10% of all recognized conceptions have chromosomal anomalies; most of these are lethal early in pregnancy and 90% are lost before the fetus is viable; a further 1% to 2% are lost at or near the time of parturition.

One way by which sex hormone administration could lead to fetal malformations is through effects on chromosome number, changes at a single genetic locus, or cumulative effects on genes at several loci. Evidence of possible effects on lymphocytic chromosomes has been advanced in sporadic reports of chromosome breaks and rearrangements in the blood of women using OCs (reviewed by Briggs and Briggs, 1979) and in the blood of their offspring (Bishun, 1976). Most of these changes have not been statistically significant; the total number of samples surveyed exceeds 20,000 (WHO, 1981). Tests of mutagenicity in bacterial and mammalian cell systems have been negative (Lang and Redman, 1979). It is reasonable to conclude that the possibility of increases in chromosomal abnormalities from OC use is extremely remote.

REFERENCES

Bishun NP. Chromosomes and oral contraceptives. *Proc Roy Soc Med* 1976;69:353–6.

Bracken MB. Oral contraception and congenital malformations in offspring: a review and meta-analysis of the prospective studies. *Obstet Gynecol* 1990;76:552–7.

Briggs MH, Briggs M. Sex hormone exposure during pregnancy and malformations. In: *Advances in steroid Biochem pharmacol, vol. 7*. London: Academic Press; 1979:51–89.

Fraser FC, Fainstat TD. Production of congenital defects in the offspring of pregnant mice treated with cortisone. *Pediatrics* 1951;8:527–33.

Greene RR, Burrill MW, Ivy AC. Experimental intersexuality. The effects of estrogens on the antenatal sexual development of the rat. *Am J Anat* 1940;67:305–44.

Ibrahim MA. *The case-control study: consensus and controversy*. New York: Pergamon Press; 1979:

Hain AM. The physiology of pregnancy in rats: an hormonal investigation into the mechanism of parturition. Effect on the female rat of the antenatal administration of oestrin to the mother. *Quart J Exp Physiol* 1935;25:131.

Heinonen OP, Slone RR, Monson RR, Hook EB, Shapiro S. Cardiovascular birth defects and antenatal exposure to female sex hormones. *N Engl J Med* 1977;296:67–70.

Klemetti A, Saxen L. Prospective vs. retrospective approach in the search for environmental causes of malformations. *Am J Public Health* 1967;57:2,071–5.

Kline J. Smoking: a risk factor for spontaneous abortion. *N Engl J Med* 1978;793–6.

Kricker A, Elliott JW, Forrest JM, McCredie J. Congenital limb reduction deformities and use of oral contraceptives. *Am J Obstet Gynecol* 1986;155:1072–8.

Lang R, Redman U. Non-mutagenicity of some sex hormones in the Ames salmonella/microsome mutagenicity test. *Mutat Res* 1979;67:361–5.

Lyster SC, Lund GH, Dulin WE, Stafford RO. Ability of some progestational steroids to stimulate male accessory glands of reproduction in the rat. *Proc Soc Exp Biol Med* 1959;100:540–3.

Pardthaisong T, Gray RH. In utero exposure to steroid contraceptives and outcome of pregnancy. *Am J Epidemiol* 1991;134:795–803.

Polednak AP. Exogenous female sex hormones and birth defects. *Public Health Rev* 1985;13:89–114.

Prahalada S, Hendrickx AG. Embryotoxicity of norlestrin, a combined synthetic oral contraceptive, in rhesus macaques (macaca mulatta). *Teratol* 1983;27:215–22.

Realini JP, Goldzieher JW. Oral contraceptives and cardiovascular disease: a critique of the epidemiologic studies. *Am J Obstet Gynecol* 1985;152:729–98.

Saunders FJ. Effects of norethynodrel combined with mestranol on the offspring when administered during pregnancy and lactation in rats. *Endocrinol* 1967;80:447–52.

Saunders FJ, Elton RI. Effects of ethynodiol diacetate and mestranol in rats and rabbits, on conception, on the outcome of pregnancy and on the offspring. *Toxicol Appl Pharmacol* 1967;11:229–44.

Simpson JL. Relationship between congenital anomalies and contraception. *Adv Contracept* 1985;1:3–30. Review article.

Streissguth B. Fetal alcohol syndrome: an epidemiologic perspective. *Am J Epidemiol* 1978;107:467–78.

Suchowsky GK, Junkmann K. A study of the virilizing effect of progestogens on the female rat fetus. *Endocrinol* 1961;68:341–9.

Tarara R. The effect of medroxyprogesterone acetate (Depo-provera) on prenatal development in the baboon (papio anubis): a preliminary study. *Teratol* 1984;30:181–5.

Tilley BC, Barnes AB, Bergstralh E, et al. A comparison of pregnancy history recall and medical records. *Am J Epidemiol* 1985;121:269–81.

Vessey M, Meisler L, Flavel R, Yeates D. Outcome of pregnancy in women using different methods of contraception. *Br J Obstet Gynaecol* 1979;86:548–56.

Werler MM, Pober BR, Nelson K, Holmes LB. Reporting accuracy among mothers of malformed and nonmalformed infants. *Am J Epidemiol* 1989;129:415–21.

Wiseman RA, Dodds-Smith IC. Cardiovascular birth defects and antenatal exposure to female sex hormones: a reevaluation of some base data. *Teratol* 1984;30:359–70.

World Health Organization: Report of a WHO Scientific Group: the effect of female sex hormones on fetal development and infant health. *Technical report series no. 657.* Geneva: 1981.

Pharmacology of the Contraceptive Steroids,
edited by Joseph W. Goldzieher.
Raven Press, Ltd., New York © 1994.

28

Drug Interactions

David J. Back and M. L'E. Orme*

*Department of Pharmacology and Therapeutics, University of Liverpool,
Liverpool L69 3BX, United Kingdom*

DRUGS INTERFERING WITH ORAL CONTRACEPTIVE EFFICACY

Anticonvulsant Drugs

A number of anticonvulsant drugs (phenytoin, phenobarbitone, methylphenobarbitone, primidone, carbamazepine, ethosuximide) have been implicated as causing breakthrough bleeding or failure of contraception in women taking OCs (Belaisch et al., 1976; Coulam and Annegers, 1979; Diamond et al., 1985; Gagnaire et al., 1975; Hempel et al., 1973; Janz and Schmidt, 1974; Kenyon, 1972)). Phenytoin appears to be the most commonly reported interacting anticonvulsant, and this is borne out by retrospective data from the United Kingdom Committee on Safety of Medicines (CSM).

Between 1973 and 1984, 43 cases of contraceptive failure in women taking anticonvulsants during OC use were reported to the CSM (Back et al., 1988). Phenytoin accounted for 25 cases and phenobarbitone for 20, with relatively smaller numbers for other anticonvulsants. The CSM monitors adverse drug reactions by means of the yellow card reporting system. However, less than 10% of adverse reactions are actually reported to the CSM (Lumley et al., 1986) the main reasons being that the reaction was too trivial or already well known, or there was uncertainty of causal relationship. If the same degree of under-reporting applies to the OC-drug interactions, then the 43 pregnancies in women concurrently taking anticonvulsant drugs is a very poor estimate of the number that have actually occurred. It should be noted, however, that the reported data tell us nothing of the actual prevalence of the alleged interactions. We do not have good data for unintended pregnancy in women who were: 1) not receiving any other medication, or 2) receiving a drug not implicated in an interaction.

The clinical pharmacokinetic data of this interaction are relatively sparse. In one

---

*We gratefully acknowledge the assistance of many colleagues who have worked in our laboratories and performed many of the studies described in this review.

TABLE 1. *Drugs reported to alter the pharmacokinetics and/or interfere with efficacy of oral contraceptive steroids*

Decreased efficacy	Increased efficacy
Anticonvulsants	Paracetamol
Antibiotics	Vitamin C
Rifampicin	
Griseofulvin	

(See text for critical appraisal.)

study, phenobarbitone 30 mg b.i.d. was given to four young women with epilepsy (Back et al., 1980a). Two of the four women showed a significant fall in steady state EE concentrations when compared to a control cycle, and both had break-through bleeding; however, the other two women showed no change in blood level. Although there was no significant change in the plasma concentration of the accompanying norethindrone, there was a significant increase in sex-hormone-binding globulin (SHBG) capacity. Such an increase effectively reduces the free progestin concentration.

Pharmacokinetic data from other studies (Crawford et al. 1986, 1990) involving single-dose administration of an OC (50 μg EE, 250 μg levonorgestrel) to women before, and 8 and 12 weeks after starting anticonvulsant therapy for tonic/clonic seizures are shown in Fig. 1 and Table 2. In the case of phenytoin, there was a significant decrease in the area under the plasma concentration-time curve (AUC) for both EE and levonorgestrel (LNG) of 49% and 42%, respectively. Similarly, in all patients receiving carbamazepine there was a marked decrease in AUC of both EE (42%) and LNG (40%). The degree of change may well be sufficient to produce contraceptive failure in long-term OC users. In contrast, sodium valproate had no detectable effect on the kinetics of EE or LNG (Table 2). While phenobarbitone, phenytoin, and carbamazepine are known to be enzyme-inducing agents in man, sodium valproate has no enzyme-inducing action. Based on these data, women taking sodium valproate can rely on conventional low-dose OCs for contraceptive control, whereas women receiving phenobarbitone, phenytoin, or carbamazepine might well use a higher dose OC initially for maximum contraceptive protection.

In order to understand the molecular basis of the interaction, it is necessary to examine the mechanism of increased metabolism of OCs, particularly EE. The predominant route of oxidative metabolism of EE_2 is cytochrome P-450-dependent 2-hydroxylation to form the catechol estrogen 2-hydroxy EE. Guengerich (1988) has argued that the specific P-450 isozyme responsible for EE 2-hydroxylation is P4503A4. Evidence for this conclusion included results of studies using enzyme reconstitution, immunoinhibition, correlation of activity, and inhibitors. The hypothesis is that phenobarbitone and other anticonvulsant drugs induce this isozyme, thereby increasing the rate and extent of 2-hydroxylation. Further studies have been performed by Ball et al. (1990). Sixteen human livers were examined for a variety of enzyme activities, including EE 2-hydroxylase. The highest EE 2-hydroxylase activity was found in the liver of a subject who had received phenobarbitone and

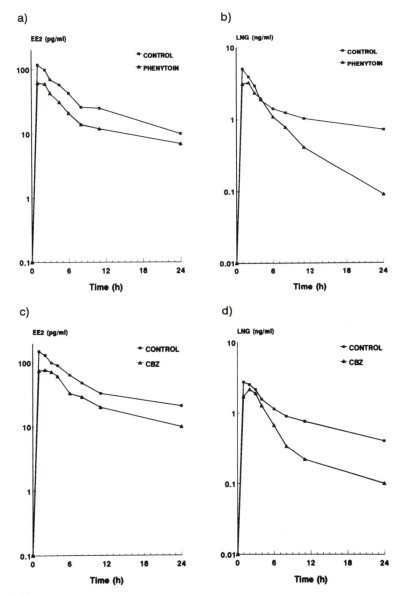

FIG. 1. Plasma concentration-time profiles of ethinylestradiol (EE₂) and levonorgestrel (LNG) in patients taking either phenytoin (a & b) or carbamazepine (CBZ, c & d).

phenytoin for more than 25 years. In other studies, antibodies to rat hepatic cytochrome P450 isozymes raised in rabbits were used to inhibit EE 2-hydroxylase activity of human liver samples. Possible correlations between the proteins recognized by the antibodies by Western blot analysis and 2-hydroxylation rate were determined (Table 3). These experiments show that the 2-hydroxylation of EE cor-

TABLE 2. *Area under the plasma concentration time curve (AUC$_{0-24}$) for ethinyl estradiol and levonorgestrel in patients taking either phenytoin, carbamazepine or sodium valproate*

Group	Daily dose of antiepileptic (mg)	EE$_2$ AUC (pg/ml^{-1}/h) Control	Test	LNG AUC (ng/ml^{-1}/h) Control	Test
Phenytoin (n = 6)	200–300	806 ± 122	411 ± 132*	33.6 ± 19.2	19.5 ± 9.3*
Carbamazepine (n = 4)	300–600	1163 ± 466	672 ± 211*	22.9 ± 9.4	13.8 ± 5.8
Sodium Valproate (n = 6)	400	880 ± 267	977 ± 319	29.1 ± 5.8	29.2 ± 3.8

*$P < 0.05$

relates with CYP3A3/3A4 expression (in agreement with Guengerich, 1988), as well as with CYP2C8 expression. There are no data available on which isozymes are involved in progestin metabolism.

Antibiotics (Excluding Rifampicin)

Broad spectrum antibiotics have been implicated in pill failures. There are a number of case reports (Bacon and Shenfield, 1980; Bainton, 1986; De Sano and Hurley, 1982; Dossetor, 1975), and Back et al. (1988) listed a total of 63 pregnancies reported to the CSM. In this study, the most widely prescribed antibiotics (penicillins and tetracyclines, comprising 74% of all antibiotic prescriptions in England) were implicated in the majority (70%) of pregnancy reports. In a study of pill failures in "reliable" pill takers, documented over a 4-year period (1981–85) in New Zealand by Sparrow (1987), 23% of the 163 cases were stated as being associated with antibiotics. Given these data, it is important to ascertain why clinical pharmacokinetic studies have been singularly unsuccessful in demonstrating any consistent effect of antibiotics on plasma concentrations of contraceptive steroids (see Table 4).

TABLE 3. *Spearman's rank correlations between ethinyl estradiol metabolism and the levels of P450 proteins (as detected by Western blot) in human liver*

P450 protein	Mr (KD)	EE$_2$ 2-hydroxylase
CYP1A2	53.0	0.21
CYP2A6	51.5	0.48
CYP2B6	51.0	0.52
CYP2C9	54.5	0.43
CYP2C8	52.5	0.75*
CYP2D6	51.5	−0.05
CYP2E1	54.5	−0.10
CYP3A3/3A4	52.5	0.78*
CYP4A	51.5	0.10

*$P < 0.05$

TABLE 4. *Clinical pharmacokinetic studies involving antibiotics and oral contraceptives that have failed to show any interaction*

Antibiotic	Number of women	Reference
Ampicillin (500 mg t.i.d. for 7 days)	13	Back et al., 1982c
Ampicillin (250 mg q.i.d. for 16 days)	11	Friedman et al., 1980
Ampicillin (500 mg b.i.d. for 5–7 days)	6	Joshi et al., 1980
Cotrimoxazole (320/1600* mg daily for 7 days)	9	Grimmer et al., 1983
Tetracycline (250 mg b.i.d. for 4 weeks)	5	Orme and Back, 1986
Temafloxacin (600 mg b.i.d. for 7 days)	12	Back et al., 1991a
Clarithromycin (250 mg b.i.d. for 7 days)	10	Back et al., 1991b
Tetracycline (500 mg q.i.d.)	7	Murphy et al., 1991

*Total daily dose of 320 mg trimethoprim 1600 mg sulfamethoxazole

From early studies in pregnant women, the view emerged that antibiotic interference in steroid metabolism was related to an effect on gut microflora (Boehm et al., 1974). There is good evidence that EE can be conjugated with both sulfuric and glucuronic acids, after which it undergoes enterohepatic recirculation. Sulfation occurs primarily in the small intestinal mucosa (Back et al., 1981b; Back et al., 1982b; Rogers et al., 1987a), while conjugation with glucuronic acid occurs mainly in the liver (Helton et al., 1976; Sahlberg et al., 1981). These conjugates are excreted in the bile and thus reach the colon, where they may be hydrolyzed by the bacteria present (principally Clostridia spp., Chapman, 1981) to liberate unchanged EE which can be reabsorbed into the portal circulation. It is difficult to find out how important the recycling of EE is in practical terms. There have been reports in the literature of secondary peaks in plasma concentration time profiles that are presumably due to recycling (Back et al., 1979a; Shenfield and Griffin, 1991), although these peaks do not appear in every or even the majority of subjects.

Oral antibiotics kill off the Clostridia (and other bacteria) responsible for the hydrolytic process. Thus, any conjugates of EE present in the lower part of the gastrointestinal tract are lost in the feces since they are too hydrophilic to be absorbed themselves. In animal studies, the enterohepatic recycling of EE is extensive and clearly diminished by treatment with a variety of antibiotics (Back et al., 1982a). The degree of reduction of recycling can be correlated with the degree of suppression of the gut microflora. However, it has been difficult to duplicate such studies in humans. Thus, ampicillin (Back et al., 1982c; Friedman et al., 1980; Joshi et al., 1980) had no effect on the kinetics of EE in women, even though the ability of fecal microorganisms to hydrolyze steroid conjugates is dramatically reduced (Chapman 1981). Similarly, cotrimoxazole and tetracycline did not cause any reduction of plasma steroid concentrations (Grimmer et al., 1983; Murphy et al., 1991; Orme and Back 1986). Recently, we have failed to show any alteration of OC disposition when women were taking the quinolone antibiotic temafloxacin or the macrolide antibiotic clarithromycin (Back et al., 1991a, 1991b). The only pharmacokinetic study apparently showing a reduction in EE AUC in the presence of an antibiotic is cited by Shenfield and Griffin (1991). In this case, minocycline (100 mg b.i.d.) was given to a woman on a triphasic OC and the AUC was reduced by 70% compared to a control cycle. This individual also had repeated breakthrough bleeding.

Although most studies have failed to show a systematic interaction between antibiotics and OCs, it is nevertheless possible that certain individuals may be at risk of the interaction. Such individuals could be women with a low bioavailability of EE due to extensive steroid metabolism in the gut wall and liver, a large recirculation of EE, and a gut microflora particularly susceptible to the antibiotic being used. For example, if a woman were unable to hydroxylate EE (i.e., was relatively deficient in CYP 3A3/3A4 or CYP2C8 isozymes), she might form EE conjugates to a greater extent and hence have a particularly large enterohepatic recirculation. From an analysis of biliary metabolites, Maggs et al. (1983) identified one woman who was unable to 2-hydroxylate EE.

One objection to some of the reported studies is that the bacteria in the gut develop resistance to antibiotics fairly rapidly, so that if the interaction is looked for after 2 weeks of therapy with the antibiotic it may be missed, since resistance can develop much more rapidly (i.e., over 5 to 6 days; see Leigh et al., 1976). However, several of the studies just mentioned (Back et al., 1982c; Grimmer et al., 1983) looked at the interaction during a 7-day course of the antibiotic starting 3 days after the commencement of the antibiotic therapy—a time when resistance would be unlikely to have developed—and still no interaction was detected.

It is impossible at the present time to evaluate fully the influence of antibiotics on steroid kinetics, and different physicians may well offer different advice.

Rifampicin

Reimers and Jezek (1971) originally reported an interaction between rifampicin and OCs, and this was followed by numerous other reports during the 1970s (reviewed by Orme et al., 1983). Rifampicin is a potent enzyme-inducing agent and, in a clinical pharmacokinetic study in eight patients, EE and norethindrone plasma concentrations were determined both during a course of rifampicin therapy and again 1 month after stopping the antibiotic (Back et al., 1979b, 1980c). There was a reduction in norethindrone AUC from 37.8 to 21.9 ng.ml^{-1}·h (P<0.01), and of EE AUC from 1,749 to 1,015 pg.ml^{-1}·h (P<0.05) during rifampicin. All patients showed evidence of microsomal enzyme induction as judged by an increase in the urinary excretion of 6β-hydroxycortisol and an increased plasma clearance of antipyrine.

There is evidence (Guengerich, 1988; Combalbert et al., 1989) that rifampicin induces CYP3A4, one of the major enzymes involved in EE 2-hydroxylation (as previously discussed); therefore, we can see a molecular basis for the rifampicin—OC interaction.

Griseofulvin

A report by van Dijke and Weber (1984) recorded 20 cases of long-term OC users who experienced intermenstrual bleeding or amenorrhea in the first or second cycle after commencing griseofulvin therapy. Pregnancies were reported in two women. Pregnancy was also reported in the CSM data (Table 3) and in a recent case report by Coté (1990). Although griseofulvin has been shown to modify hepatic enzyme activity in mice (Denk et al. 1977), there is no good evidence of a major inducing effect in humans.

Vitamin C

There are few examples of drugs increasing the therapeutic effect of OCs. Theoretically, any drugs that inhibit the specific enzymes involved in OC metabolism could lead to an elevation of plasma concentration. Thus, if we can find out which drugs are metabolized by CYP3A4 and the other P450 isozymes involved in EE 2-hydroxylation, it may be possible to predict drug interactions with EE. This of course presupposes that with inhibition of one enzyme pathway there is not an increase in turnover of steroid by an alternative pathway.

Vitamin C (ascorbic acid) is occasionally used in high doses and since, like EE, it is metabolized to sulfate conjugates, there is the possibility of transient overload of sulfation in the intestinal wall and/or the liver if vitamin C is coadministered with a combined OC. Two small clinical studies in six and five subjects, respectively (Back et al., 1980b; Back et al., 1981c) seemed to confirm this interaction with EE bioavailability increased by about 50 percent when 1 g of Vitamin C was given a half hour before pill administration. However, the variability of the results was considerable and a much larger group of subjects was necessary to adequately define treatment-related differences. A recent study (Zamah et al., 1993) has reinvestigated the interaction in 37 women using a combined OC for two consecutive cycles. Concomitant daily administration of 1 g Vitamin C taken a half hour before pill intake was randomly assigned to the first or second cycle of OC usage. No effect of Vitamin C was observed on EE AUC_{0-12h} on day 1 or day 15. There was a significantly lower AUC for EE sulfate in the presence of Vitamin C on day 15 but the decline in sulfation was insufficient to alter plasma EE concentrations and is, therefore, unlikely to be of any clinical importance.

Paracetamol

Paracetamol is metabolized primarily by conjugation with sulfuric and glucuronic acid when given in therapeutic doses *in vivo*, but some microsomal oxidation leading to the formation of cysteine and mercapturate conjugates also occurs (Prescott, 1980). Since single-dose paracetamol had been shown to cause partial depletion of inorganic sulfate in man (Levy et al., 1982; Hendrix-Treacey et al., 1986), Rogers et al. (1987a, 1987b) conducted both *in vitro* and *in vivo* studies on the potential for paracetamol to interfere with EE sulfation in the gut wall.

By a technique that involves isolating mucosal sheets from histologically normal ileum and mounting between two chambers (Ussing Chambers), it was shown that paracetamol caused a significant decrease in EE sulfation (Rogers et al., 1987a). This *in vitro* study was followed up by examining the effect of a single dose of paracetamol (1 g) on the plasma concentrations of EE and levonorgestrel in healthy volunteers during the 24-hour period following ingestion of the OC (Rogers et al., 1987b). The AUC of EE was significantly increased following paracetamol administration, with the greatest effect evident in the time period 0 to 3 hours. There was a significant decrease in AUC of EE-sulfate after paracetamol ($7,736 \pm 3,791$ pg·ml^{-1}·h), compared to the control ($13,161 \pm 4,535$ pg·ml^{-1}·h; $P<0.05$). It was concluded that the increase in plasma EE concentrations resulted from a reduction in sulfation of the steroid, substantially in the gut wall, and that this interaction could be of clinical significance in women on OCs who regularly take paracetamol.

Smoking

Polycyclic aromatic hydrocarbons in cigarette smoke are potent inducers of certain cytochrome P450 isozymes (notably CYP1A2) and thereby increase the oxidative metabolism of drugs that are substrates for these enzymes—e.g., antipyrine, propranolol, and theophylline (Vestal et al., 1979; Wood et al., 1979; Jusko et al., 1978; Vestal et al., 1987). In contrast, no effect has been observed on the disposition of other drugs (e.g., diazepam, phenytoin) reviewed by Jusko (1979). With respect to steroid metabolism, Michnovicz et al. (1986) reported a marked increase in estradiol 2-hydroxylation in smokers, with a consequent decrease in circulating E_2 levels. However, Crawford et al. (1981) examined a total of 311 OC users (102 smokers, 209 nonsmokers) and found no significant difference in EE (or levonorgestrel) plasma concentrations, and Kanarkowski et al. (1988) failed to show any significant differences in EE plasma concentration profiles between smokers and nonsmokers. Different P-450 isozymes appear to be involved in the metabolism of E_2 and EE. Ball et al. (1990) have shown that E_2 is metabolised by proteins from the CYP1A (polycyclic aromatic hydrocarbon inducible), CYP2C, and CYP2E gene families, whereas EE is catalyzed by cytochromes from the CYP3A, CYP2C, and CYP2E gene families. Thus, proteins from the CYP1A family appear to play an important role in E_2 metabolism but not in EE disposition. Therefore, from the *in vitro* studies we would not expect EE to be affected by smoking, which is what is found in the pharmacokinetic studies. Little is known as yet about progestin metabolism and smoking from an enzymological perspective.

Adsorbents

Adsorbents such as magnesium trisilicate, aluminium hydroxide, activated charcoal, and kaolin can adsorb a wide variety of substances onto their surface, thereby preventing the absorption of drugs and toxins from the gastrointestinal tract. On theoretical grounds, adsorbents could be expected to interfere with the efficacy of OCs, but there is no firm evidence that this is the case. Joshi et al. (1986) investigated the bioavailability of OCs in women using antacids (magnesium trisilicate + aluminum hydroxide). As judged by peak concentrations and AUCs of EE and LNG, antacid administration had no effect on OC absorption.

Magnesium-containing antacid preparations can induce diarrhea; this raises the question of whether infective or induced diarrhea will lead to a reduced absorption of OCs. Sparrow (1987) and Shenfield (1986) are convinced that diarrhea can induce failure of OC efficacy, and Sparrow records 23 cases of OC failure associated with diarrhea. However, a major consideration is that absorption takes place high in the small bowel, since the bioavailability of OC is not reduced at all in patients with an ileostomy (Grimmer et al., 1986). We know also of a case (Back and Orme, unpublished) of a woman who had resection of all but 30 cm of small bowel and yet showed normal bioavailability of both EE and LNG. So while the case for diarrhea being an important consideration of OC failure is attractive, the pharmacokinetic data are as yet lacking.

Other Drugs

Reports have been published with regard to cases of hepatic cholestasis in women taking the macrolide antibiotic troleandomycin and OCs (Fevery et al., 1983; Haber and Hubens, 1980). Oxidation of troleandomycin by a P450 isozyme produces a derivative (probably a nitroso derivative) that binds tightly to the enzyme and thereby causes inactivation. Guengerich (1988) has indicated that this inhibition is highly selective for CYP3A4 and, since this isozyme is important in EE metabolism, hepatic accumulation of EE is possible. There are in the literature a number of isolated case reports of possible interactions between OCs and a variety of other drugs, including antihistamines and antiasthmatic drugs. However, the evidence for interaction is not convincing from either a clinical or mechanistic viewpoint.

ORAL CONTRACEPTIVES INTERFERING WITH THE METABOLISM OF OTHER DRUGS

There were early indications from animal studies that OCs could inhibit the metabolism of other compounds undergoing oxidative metabolism (Tephly and Mannering, 1968). More recently, Guengerich (1988, 1990) has shown that acetylenic steroids bind covalently to P450 heme after enzymatic oxidation. He demonstrated that both EE_2 and progestogens preincubated with human liver microsomes caused a loss of spectrally detectable cytochrome P-450 and enzyme activity. Similar findings have been published by Back et al. (1991c). These *in vitro* studies provide some mechanistic basis to the numerous literature reports of an inhibitory effect (albeit normally small) of OCs on concurrently administered drugs.

In addition, OCs appear to have the propensity to induce glucuronidation, which will have the opposite pharmacokinetic effect to the inhibitory action on oxidation (Table 5).

TABLE 5. *Drugs for which there is evidence of altered pharmacokinetics in oral contraceptive users*

Increased concentrations	Decreased concentrations
Alprazolam	Acetylsalicylic acid
Antipyrine	Clofibric acid
Caffeine	Morphine
Chlordiazepoxide	Paracetamol
Cyclosporin	Temazepam
Diazepam	
Metoprolol	
Nitrazepam	
Prednisolone	
Theophylline	

Antipyrine

Antipyrine has been widely used as a marker of oxidative drug metabolism in humans. A number of studies have shown inhibition of its metabolism in OC users (Luoma et al., 1987; Teunissen et al., 1982; Pazzucconi et al., 1991). The last of these studies is important because it demonstrated that two modern low-dose OCs produced roughly comparable reductions in antipyrine clearance (Table 6). Clearance to the 4-hydroxy and 3-hydroxymethyl metabolites was most markedly affected.

Benzodiazepines

Oral contraceptives influence the disposition of some benzodiazepines undergoing: 1) oxidation (e.g., chlordiazepoxide; see Roberts et al., 1979, and diazepam; see Abernethy et al., 1982); 2) nitroreduction (e.g., nitrazepam; see Jochemsen et al., 1982); and 3) conjugation (e.g., temazepam; see Stoehr et al., 1984). For benzodiazepines metabolized by oxidative pathways and by nitroreduction, OCs inhibit enzyme activity and reduce metabolic clearance. For example, the elimination half-life of diazepam was significantly longer (69 ± 9 versus 47 ± 4 hours) and the total metabolic clearance significantly less (0.27 ± 0.02 versus 0.45 ± 0.04 ml/min^{-1}/kg^{-1}) in OC users compared to control subjects in the study of Abernethy et al. (1982). Inhibition of the intrinsic clearance of nitrazepam was seen in OC users by Jochemsen et al. (1982). In non-OC users, clearance was 459 ± 40 ml/min^{-1}, whereas in

TABLE 6. *Plasma antipyrine kinetic data obtained in 10 female volunteers before and during administration of two low-dose oral contraceptives*

	Control	EE$_2$ + Gestodene	EE$_2$ + Desogestrel
t½ (h)	11.7 ± 1.0	$15.6 \pm 1.5^{**}$	$17.3 \pm 2.8^{**}$
CL (ml/h^{-1}/kg^{-1})	43.6 ± 4.2	$27.9 \pm 2.6^{**}$	$24.3 \pm 2.4^{**}$
AUC (μg/ml^{-1}/h)	586 ± 62	834 ± 68	$1009 \pm 151^{*}$
Vd (ml/kg^{-1})	680 ± 23	$579 \pm 27^{*}$	$542 \pm 35^{**}$

*P<0.05 versus control
**P<0.01 versus control
(Adapted from Pazzucconi et al. (1991).)

OC users it was 323 ± 30 ml/min^{-1}. It should be noted that, although impaired drug oxidation has been reported for the drugs just outlined, there are others undergoing oxidative metabolism—e.g., bromazepam (Ochs et al., 1987), clotiazepam (Ochs et al., 1984), alprazolam (Scavone et al., 1988)—that show similar pharmacokinetics in both OC users and nonusers.

In contrast to the reduced clearance of some benzodiazepines undergoing oxidative metabolism or nitroreduction, the clearance of temazepam, which is metabolized by glucuronic acid conjugation, is increased by 60% (Stoehr et al., 1984). However, the metabolic clearance of lorazepam, which also undergoes conjugation, remained unaltered in two studies (Stoehr et al., 1984; Abernethy et al., 1983) but increased in another (Patwardhan et al., 1983). Despite the kinetic changes outlined, there is very little evidence that this is an interaction of clinical importance.

Theophylline and Caffeine

The clearance of theophylline and caffeine is reduced by 30% to 40% in OC users (Roberts et al., 1983; Abernethy & Todd, 1985; Rietvald et al., 1984). Studies with human liver microsomes provide evidence of the involvement of two distinct P450 isozymes in the metabolism of theophylline (Robson et al., 1987); at least one of these isozymes must therefore be susceptible to the inhibitory effects of OCs.

Cyclosporin

A potentially important interaction was published as a case report by Deray et al., (1987). A 32-year-old woman was treated with cyclosporin for idiopathic uveitis, her OC use having been stopped 2 months previously. Reintroduction of the OC was associated with increases in plasma concentrations of cyclosporin; aminotransferases, serum bilirubin, and alkaline phosphatase also increased.

Recent *in vitro* studies with human liver have provided evidence that cyclosporin undergoes hydroxylation and N-demethylation, and that CYP3A4 is involved (Kronbach et al., 1988). Again, this same isozyme is at least partially responsible for EE 2-hydroxylation (Guengerich, 1988; Ball et al., 1990).

Analgesic Drugs

Miners et al. (1986) investigated the influence of OCs on salicylic acid and acetylsalicylic acid disposition. Salicylic acid clearance was 41% greater in OC users compared to nonusers due to increases in conjugation pathways (glycine and glucuronic acid). Increased glucuronidation has also been shown for paracetamol (Miners et al., 1983; Mitchell et al., 1983) and was suggested to be the mechanism whereby OCs enhance morphine clearance (Watson et al., 1986).

Corticosteroids

A number of studies have reported changes in prednisolone pharmacokinetics in OC users (Boekenoogen et al., 1983; Meffin et al., 1984; Frey et al., 1984; Legler and Benet, 1986). These alterations (decreased clearance and volume of distribution, and prolonged elimination half-life) result from changes in both protein-binding (which is increased due to increased corticosteroid-binding globulin levels) and unbound clearance (which is decreased, presumably due to inhibition of metabolism). Legler and Benet (1986) have suggested that lower doses of prednisolone should yield clinical efficacy in women taking OCs.

Ethanol

Jones and Jones (1984) found a significantly decreased ethanol elimination rate in women taking OCs compared to nonusers. The implications of this work were that alcohol would be present longer in women taking OCs. However, in another study (Hobbes et al., 1985), no significant effect of OCs on mean peak plasma ethanol concentration, mean time to peak, mean AUC, or mean rate of ethanol disappearance was seen. One surprising finding in this study was that OCs improved tolerance to alcohol, although the reasons were not clear.

Other Drugs

Other isolated reports of OCs influencing the kinetics of concomitantly administered drugs include: 1) an increase in plasma concentrations of metoprolol (Kendall et al., 1982); 2) an increase in plasma clearance of clofibric acid, a drug largely metabolized by glucuronidation (Miners et al., 1984); and 3) a change in the mean metabolic ratio of extensive metabolizers of debrisoquine (Kallio et al., 1988).

INTERACTION BETWEEN PROGESTIN AND ESTROGEN COMPONENTS

In 1989 there was a report that women given a combination of gestodene and EE (75 μg and 30 μg, respectively) showed higher serum levels of EE than women given a combination of desogestrel and EE (150 μg and 30 μg, respectively), despite the fact that the EE dose was the same in both preparations (Jung-Hoffmann and Kuhl, 1989). The difference in EE levels between the treatment groups was observed even after the first oral administration of the two preparations. The authors attributed the difference to a possible inhibitory effect of gestodene on the hepatic cytochrome P-450 system, thereby giving rise to elevated EE levels. However, several subsequent randomized studies in larger populations, including a crossover design and two double-blind studies, contradicted these findings (Table 7).

SUMMARY

Women using OC steroids are likely at some time to receive other drug medication. Over the last 30 years there have been case reports and clinical studies docu-

TABLE 7. *Studies designed to investigate the influence of progestogen (gestodene or desogestrel) on plasma concentrations of ethinyl estradiol*

Study	Type	Length	Finding
JUNG HOFFMAN & KUHL (1989)	Group comparison (n = 22)	12 cycles Multiple blood sampling on 3 days in cycles 1,3,6,12	Significantly higher EE_2 levels during treatment with EE_2/GSD than with EE_2/DG
HUMPEL et al. (1990)	Group comparison (n = 69)	Multiple blood sampling on 1 day in regular OC users	No difference in EE_2 levels between groups
KUHNZ et al. (1990)	Intraindividual crossover (n = 18)	Single dose OC administration Multiple blood sampling	No difference in EE_2 levels between different preparations
DIBBELT et al. (1991)	Group comparison (n = 83)	3 cycles Multiple blood sampling on 3 days in cycles 1,3	No difference in EE_2 levels between groups
ORME et al. (1991)	Intraindividual crossover (n = 10)	Oral and IV administration of EE_2 alone, EE_2 + GSD EE_2 + DG (or 3KDG). Single doses over 3 months	Bioavailability of EE_2 same for each preparation
KUHNZ et al. (1991)	Intraindividual crossover (n = 31)	Administration of each preparation for 3 months Multiple blood sampling on 3 days in cycles 3 and 6	No difference in EE_2 levels between different preparations

menting interactions with OCs. Some of the interactions are of definite therapeutic relevance, whereas others can be discounted as being of no clinical significance. Pharmacological interactions between OCs and other compounds may be of two kinds.

1. Drugs may impair the efficacy of OCs, leading to breakthrough bleeding and/or pregnancy. In a few cases OC activity is enhanced.
2. Oral contraceptives may interfere with the metabolism of other drugs. A number of anticonvulsants (phenobarbitone, phenytoin, carbamazepine) are proven en-

zyme-inducing agents that increase the hepatic concentration of certain cyto-chrome P450 isoenzymes and, in some cases, glucuronyl-transferases.

Since OCs are oxidatively metabolized, hepatic clearance is increased. In contrast, sodium valproate has no enzyme-inducing properties, and thus women on this anticonvulsant can reasonably rely on their low-dose OCs for contraceptive protection. In the past few years the molecular basis of this interaction has emerged, with evidence of specific forms of cytochrome P450 (CYP2C and 3A gene families) being induced by phenobarbitone. Rifampicin, the antituberculous drug, also induces a P450 isozyme that is a product of the CYP3A gene subfamily. This isozyme is one of the major forms involved in ethynyl estradiol (EE) 2-hydroxylation.

Broad-spectrum antibiotics have been implicated in causing pill failure. Although case reports document the interaction and family planning physicians may be convinced that the interaction is real, the problem remains that there is still no firm clinical pharmacokinetic evidence indicating that blood levels of OCs are altered by antibiotics. However, perhaps this should not surprise us given that the incidence of the interaction may be very low. It is our belief that a woman at risk will have a low bioavailability of EE, a large enterohepatic recirculation, and a gut flora particularly susceptible to the antibiotic being used.

Paracetamol gives rise to increased blood concentrations of EE due to competition for sulfation, particularly in the gut wall. However, the interactions are unlikely to be of any real importance. Although on theoretical grounds adsorbents (e.g., magnesium trisilicate, aluminum hydroxide, activated charcoal, kaolin) could be expected to interfere with OC efficacy, there is no firm evidence that this is the case. Similarly, there is no evidence that smoking alters OC pharmacokinetics.

Oral contraceptives are demonstrably able to alter the kinetics of concomitantly administered drugs. The clearance of a number of benzodiazepines undergoing oxidation (chlordiazepoxide, diazepam) and nitro reduction (nitrazepam), theophylline, prednisolone, caffeine, and cyclosporin is reduced in OC users. The clearance of some drugs undergoing glucuronidation (temazepam, salicylic acid, paracetamol, morphine, clofibric acid) is apparently increased.

Finally, despite one early report that the progestin, gestodene, can alter the disposition of EE, a number of subsequent studies has failed to confirm this finding.

The subject of OC drug interactions has been reviewed many times (Back et al. 1981a, 1983; Back and Orme, 1990; Fotherby, 1990; Fraser and Jansen, 1983; Orme, 1982; Orme and Back, 1980; Roberton and Johnson, 1976; Shenfield, 1986; Shenfield and Griffin, 1991; Stockley, 1979; Szoka and Edgren, 1988); the aim of the present review is to give a critical analysis, and where it is known, a mechanistic basis of the interactions.

CONCLUSIONS

There are pharmacokinetic drug interactions with OCs of definite clinical relevance (anticonvulsants, rifampicin) because, in the majority of subjects, the interaction will occur. Data are emerging concerning the cellular/molecular basis for these interactions. However, the interaction of antibiotics and OCs is not as clear; we must await some way of predicting which women may be at risk. Any interaction that causes raised concentrations of EE is of potential importance because of the prevailing concern that high blood levels might correlate with adverse events. To date, there is some evidence that troleandomycin inhibits EE 2-hydroxylation. No firm evidence suggests that the various progestin components of OCs cause differential inhibition of metabolism.

REFERENCES

Abernethy DR, Greenblatt DJ, Divoli M, Arendt R, Ochs HR, et al. Impairment of diazepam metabolism by low-dose estrogen-containing oral-contraceptive steroids. *N Engl J Med* 1982;306:791–2.

Abernethy DR, Greenblatt DJ, Ochs HR, Weyers D, Divoll M, et al. Lorazepam and oxazepam kinetics in women on low-dose oral contraceptives. *Clin Pharmacol Ther* 1983;33:628–32.

Abernethy DR, Todd EL. Impairment of caffeine clearance by chronic use of low-dose estrogen-containing oral contraceptives. *Eur J Clin Pharmacol* 1985;28:425–8.

Back DJ, Bates M, Bowden M, Breckenridge AM, Hall MJ, et al. The interaction of phenobarbital and other anticonvulsants with oral contraceptive steroid therapy. *Contraception* 1988a;22:495–503.

Back DJ, Bates M, Breckenridge AM, Crawford FE, Ellis A, et al. Metabolism by gastrointestinal mucosa-clinical aspects. In: Prescott, Nimmo, eds. *Drug absorption.* Sydney: ADIS Press; 1980b:80–7.

Back DJ, Bates M, Breckenridge AM, Ellis A, MacIver M, et al. The *in vitro* metabolism of ethinyloestradiol, mestranol and levonorgestrel by human jejunal mucosa. *Br J Clin Pharmacol* 1981b;11:275–8.

Back DJ, Breckenridge AM, Crawford FE, Hall JM, MacIver M, et al. The effect of rifampicin on the pharmacokinetics of ethinyloestradiol in women. *Contraception* 1980c;21:135–43.

Back DJ, Breckenridge AM, Crawford FE, MacIver M, Orme ML'E, et al. An investigation of the pharmacokinetics of ethynylestradiol in women using radioimmunoassay. *Contraception* 1979a;20:263–73.

Back DJ, Breckenridge AM, Crawford FE, MacIver M, Orme ML'E, et al. The effect of rifampicin on norethisterone pharmacokinetics. *Eur J Clin Pharmacol* 1979b;15:193–7.

Back DJ, Breckenridge AM, Crawford FE, MacIver M, Orme ML'E, et al. Interindividual variation and drug interactions with hormonal steroid contraceptives. *Drugs* 1981a;21:46–61.

Back DJ, Breckenridge AM, Cross KJ, Orme ML'E, Thomas E. An antibiotic interaction with ethinyloestradiol in the rat and rabbit. *J Steroid Biochem* 1982a;16:407–13.

Back DJ, Breckenridge AM, MacIver M, Orme ML'E, Purba HS, et al. The interaction of ethinyloestradiol with ascorbic acid in man. *Br Med J* 1981c;282:1,516.

Back DJ, Breckenridge AM, MacIver M, Orme ML'E, Purba HS, et al. The gut wall metabolism of ethinyloestradiol and its contribution to the pre-systemic metabolism of ethinyloestradiol in humans. *Br J Clin Pharmacol* 1982b;13:325–30.

Back DJ, Breckenridge AM, MacIver M, Orme ML'E, Rowe PH, et al. The effects of ampicillin on oral contraceptive steroids in women. *Br J Clin Pharmacol* 1982c;14:43–8.

Back DJ, Breckenridge AM, Orme ML'E. Drug interactions with oral contraceptives. *Internat Planned Parenth* Fed 1983;17:1–2.

Back DJ, Grimmer SFM, Orme ML'E, Proudlove C, Mann RD, et al. Evaluation of Committee on Safety of Medicines yellow card reports on oral contraceptive drug interactions with anticonvulsants and antibiotics. *Br J Clin Pharmacol* 1988;25:527–32.

Back DJ, Orme ML'E. Pharmacokinetic drug interactions with oral contraceptives. *Clin Pharmacokin* 1990;18:472–84.

Back DJ, Tjia JF, Martin C, Miller E, Mant T, et al. The lack of interaction between temafloxacin and combined oral contraceptive steroids. *Contraception* 1991a;43:317–24.

Back DJ, Tjia C, Martin C, Miller E, Salmon P, et al. The interaction between clarithromycin and combined oral contraceptive steroids. *J Pharmaceut Med* 1991b;2:81–7.

Bacon JF, Shenfield GM. Pregnancy attributable to interaction between tetracycline and oral contraceptives. *Br Med J* 1980;1:293.

Bainton R. Interaction between antibiotic therapy and contraceptive medication. *Oral Surg* 1986; 61:453–5.

Ball SE, Forrester LM, Wolf CR, Back DJ. Differences in the cytochrome P450 isozymes involved in the 2-hydroxylation of estradiol and 17α-ethinyloestradiol: relative activities of rat and human liver enzymes. *Biochem J* 1990;167:221–6.

Belaisch J, Driguez P, Janaud A. Influence de certains medicaments sur l'action des pilules contraceptifs. *Nouvelle Presse Med* 1976;5:1,645–6.

Boehm FH, Di Pietro DL, Gross DA. The effect of ampicillin administration on urinary estriol and serum estradiol in the normal pregnant patient. *Am J Obstet Gynecol* 1974;119:98–103.

Boekenoogen SJ, Szefler SJ, Jusko WJ. Prednisolone disposition and protein binding in oral contraceptive users. *J Clin Endocrinol Metab* 1983;56:701–9.

Chapman CR. *Absorption and metabolism of steroid prodrugs* [Ph.D. thesis]. University of Liverpool, 1981.

Combalbert J, Fabre I, Febre G, Dalet I, Derancourt J, et al. Metabolism of cyclosporin A. IV. Purification and identification of the rifampicin-inducible human liver cytochrome P450 (cyclosporin A oxidase) as a product of P450IIIA gene subfamily. *Drug Metab Dispos* 1989;17:197–207.

Coté J. Interaction of griseofulvin and oral contraceptives. *J Am Acad Dermatol* 1990;22:124–5.

Coulam CB, Annegers JF. Do anticonvulsants reduce the efficacy of oral contraceptives. *Epilepsia* 1979;20:519–26.

Crawford FE, Back DJ, Orme ML'E, Breckenridge AM. Oral contraceptive steroid plasma concentrations in smokers and nonsmokers. *Br Med J* 1981;182:1,829–30.

Crawford P, Chadwick D, Cleland P, Tjia J, Cowie A, et al. The lack of effect of sodium valproate on the pharmacokinetics of oral contraceptive steroids. *Contraception* 1986;33:51–9.

Crawford P, Chadwick DJ, Martin C, Tjia J, Back DJ, et al. The interaction of phenytoin and carbamazepine with combined oral contraceptives. *Br J Clin Pharmacol* 1990;30:892–6.

Denk H, Eckerstarfer R, Talcott RE, Schenkman JB. Alteration of hepatic microsomal enzymes by griseofulvin treatment in mice. *Biochem Pharmacol* 1977;16:1,125–30.

Deray G, Le Hoang P, Cacoub P, Assogba U, Grippon P, et al. Oral contraceptive interaction with cyclosporin. *Lancet* 1987;1:158–9.

De Sano EA, Hurley SC. Possible interactions of antihistamines and antibiotics with oral contraceptive effectiveness. *Fertil Steril* 1982;37:853–4.

Diamond MP, Greene JW, Thompson JM, Vanttooydonk JE, Wentz A. Interaction of anticonvulsants and oral contraceptives in epileptic adolescents. *Contraception* 1985;31:623–32.

Dibbelt L, Knuppen R, Jutting G, Helmann S, Klipping CO, et al. Group comparison of serum ethinyl estradiol, SHBG and CBG levels in 83 women using two low-dose combination oral contraceptives for three months. *Contraception* 1991;43:1–21.

Dossetor J. Drug interactions with oral contraceptives. *Br Med J* 1975;4:467–8.

Fevery J, Van Steenbergen W, Desmet V. Severe intrahepatic cholestasis due to the combined intake of oral contraceptives and triacetyloleandomycin. *Acta Clin Belg* 1983;38:242–5.

Fotherby K. Interactions with oral contraceptives. *Am J Obstet Gynecol* 1990;163:2,153–9.

Fraser IS, Jansen RPS. Why do inadvertant pregnancies occur in oral contraceptive users. *Contraception* 1983;27:531–51.

Frey BM, Schard HJ, Frey FJ. Pharmacokinetic interaction of contraceptive steroids with prednisone and prednisolone. *Eur J Clin Pharmacol* 1984;26:505–11.

Friedman CI, Huneke AL, Kim MH, Powell J. The effect of ampicillin on oral contraceptive effectiveness. *Obstet Gynecol* 1980;55:33–7.

Gagnaire JC, Tchertchian J, Revol A, Rochet Y. Grossesses sous contraceptifs oraux chex les patients recevant des barbituriques. *Nouvelle Presse Méd* 1975;4:3,008.

Grimmer SFM, Allen WL, Back DJ, Breckenridge AM, Orme ML'E, et al. The effect of cotrimoxazole on oral contraceptive steroids in women. *Contraception* 1983;28:53–9.

Grimmer SFM, Back DJ, Orme ML'E, Cowie A, Gilmore, et al. The bioavailability of ethinyloestradiol and levonorgestrel in patients with an ileostomy. *Contraception* 1986;33:51–9.

Guengerich FP. Oxidation of 17α-ethynylestradiol by human liver cytochrome P-450. *Molec Pharmacol* 1988;33:500–508.

Haber I, Hubens H. Cholestatic jaundice after triacetyloleandomycin and oral contraceptives. *Acta Gastroenterol Belg* 1980;43:475–82.

Helton ED, Williams MC, Goldzieher JW. Human urinary and liver conjugates of 17α-ethynylestradiol. *Steroids* 1976;27:851–67.

Hendrix-Treacey S, Wallace SM, Hindmarsh KW, Wyant GM, Danilkewich A. The effect of acetaminophen administration on its disposition and body stores of sulphate. *Eur J Clin Pharmacol* 1986; 30:273–8.

Hempel Von E, Bohm W, Carol W, Klinger W. Meditamentose enzyminduktion und hormonale kontrazeption. *Zentrabl f Gynakol* 1973;95:1,451–7.

Hobbes J, Boutagy J, Shenfield GM. Interactions between ethanol and oral contraceptive steroids. *Clin Pharmacol Ther* 1985;38:371–80.

Hümpel M, Tauber U, Kuhnz W, Pfeffer M, Brill K, et al. Comparison of serum ethinyl estradiol, sex hormone-binding globulin, corticoid-binding globulin and cortisol levels in women using two low-dose combined oral contraceptives. *Hormone Res* 1990;33:35–9.

Janz D, Schmidt D. Antiepileptic drugs and failure of oral contraceptives. *Lancet* 1974;1:113.

Jochemsen R, Van der Graaff M, Boeijinga JK, Breimer DD. Influence of sex, menstrual cycle and oral contraception on the disposition of nitrazepam. *Br J Clin Pharmacol* 1982;13:319–24.

Jones MK, Jones BM. Ethanol metabolism in women taking oral contraceptives. Alcoholism: *Clin Exper Res* 1984;8:24–8.

Joshi JV, Joshi UM, Sankholi GM, Krishna D, Mandelkar A, et al. A study of interaction of low dose combination oral contraceptive with ampicillin and metronidazole. *Contraception* 1980;22:643–52.

Joshi JV, Sankholi GM, Shar RS, Joshi UM. Antacid does not reduce the bioavailability of oral contraceptive steroids in women. *Internat J Clin Pharmacol Ther Toxicol* 1986;24:192–5.

Jung-Hoffmann C, Kuhl H. Interaction with pharmacokinetics of ethinylestradiol and progestogens contained in oral contraceptives. *Contraception* 1989;40:299–312.

Jusko WJ. Influence of cigarette smoking on drug metabolism in man. *Drug Metab Rev* 1979;9:221–36.

Jusko WJ, Schentag JJ, Clark JH, Gardner M, Yurchak A. Enhanced biotransformation of theophylline in marihuana and tobacco smokers. *Clin Pharmacol Ther* 1978;24:406–10.

Kallio J, Lindberg R, Hulpponen R, Iisalo E. Debrisoquine oxidation in a Finnish population: the effect of oral contraceptives on the metabolic ratio. *Br J Clin Pharmacol* 1988;26:791–5.

Kanarkowski R, Tornatore KM, D'Ambrosio R, Gardner MJ, Jusko WJ. Pharmacokinetics of single and multiple doses of ethinylestradiol and levonorgestrel in relation to smoking. *Clin Pharmacol Ther* 1988;43:23–31.

Kendall MJ, Quaterman CP, Jack DB, Beeley L. Metoprolol pharmacokinetics and the oral contraceptive pill. *Br J Clin Pharmacol* 1982;14:120–2.

Kenyon TE. Unplanned pregnancy in an epileptic. *Br Med J* 1972;1:686–7.

Kronbach T, Fischer V, Meyer UA. Cyclosporine metabolism in human liver: identification of a cytochrome P450III gene family as the major cyclosporine-metabolizing enzyme explains interactions of cyclosporine with other drugs. *Clin Pharmacol Ther* 1988;43:630–5.

Kuhnz W, Back D, Power J, Schutt B, Louton T. Concentration of ethinyl estradiol in the serum of 31 young women following a treatment period of three months with two low-dose oral contraceptives in an intraindividual cross-over design. *Hormone Res* 1991;36:63–69.

Kuhnz W, Hümpel M, Schutt B, Louton T, Steinberg B, et al. Relative bioavailability of ethinyl estradiol from two different oral contraceptive formulations after single oral administration to 18 women in an intraindividual cross-over design. *Hormone Res* 1990;33:40–4.

Legler UF, Benet LZ. Marked alterations in dose-dependent prednisolone kinetics in women taking oral contraceptives. *Clin Pharmacol Ther* 1986;39:425–9.

Leigh DA, Reeves DS, Simmons K, Thomas AL, Wilkinson PJ. Talampicillin: a new derivative of ampicillin. *Br Med J* 1976;2:1,378–80.

Levy G, Galinsky R, Lin JH. Pharmacokinetic consequences and toxicologic implications of endogenous cosubstrate depletion. *Drug Metab Rev* 1982;13:1,009–20.

Lumley CE, Walker SR, Hall GC, Staunton N, Grob PR. The underreporting of adverse drug reactions seen in General Practice. *Pharmaceut Med* 1986;1:205–12.

Luoma PV, Heikkinen JE, Ehnholm C, Ylostalo PR. One year study of effects of an oestrogen-dominant oral contraceptive on serum high-density lipoprotein cholesterol, apolipoproteins AI and AII and hepatic microsomal function. *Eur J Clin Pharmacol* 1987;31:563–7.

Maggs JL, Grimmer SFM, Orme ML'E, Breckenridge AM, Park BK, et al. The biliary and urinary metabolites of ^{3}H-17α-ethinyloestradiol in women. *Xenobiotica* 1983;13:421–31.

Meffin PJ, Wing LMH, Sallustio BC, Brooks PM. Alterations in prednisolone disposition as a result of oral contraceptive use and dose. *Br J Clin Pharmacol* 1984;17:655–64.

Michnovicz JJ, Herschcopf RJ, Naganuma H, Bradlow HL, Fishman J. Increased 2-hydroxylation of estradiol as a possible mechanism for the anti-estrogenic effect of cigarette smoking. *N Engl J Med* 1986;315:1,305–9.

Miners JO, Attwood J, Birkett DJ. Influence of sex and oral contraceptive steroids on paracetamol metabolism. *Br J Clin Pharmacol* 1983;16:503–9.

Miners JO, Grgurinovich N, Whitehead AG, Robson RA, Birkett DJ. Influence of gender and oral contraceptive steroids on the metabolism of salicylic acid and acetylsalicylic acid. *Br J Clin Pharmacol* 1986;22:135–42.

Miners JO, Robson RA, Birkett DJ. Gender and oral contraceptive steroids as determinants of drug glucuronidation: effects on clofibric acid elimination. *Br J Clin Pharmacol* 1984;18:240–3.

Mitchell MC, Hanew T, Meredith CG, Schenker S. Effects of oral contraceptive steroids on acetaminophen metabolism and elimination. *Clin Pharmacol Ther* 1983;34:48–53.

Murphy AA, Zacur HA, Charache P, Burkman RT. The effect of tetracycline on levels of oral contraceptives. *Am J Obstet Gynecol* 1991;164:28–33.

Ochs HR, Greenblatt, DJ, Friedman H, Burstein ES, Locniskar A, et al. Bromazepam pharmacokinetics: influence of age, gender, oral contraceptives, cimetidine and propranolol. *Clin Pharmacol Ther* 1987; 41:562–70.

Ochs HR, Greenblatt DJ, Verburg-Ochs JS, Harmatz JS, Grehl H. Disposition of clotiazepam: influence of age, sex, oral contraceptives, cimetidine, isoniazid and ethanol. *Eur J Clin Pharmacol* 1984;26:55–9.

Orme ML'E. The clinical pharmacology of oral contraceptive steroids. *Br J Clin Pharmacol* 1982;14:31–42.

Orme ML'E, Back DJ. Drug interactions with oral contraceptive steroids. *Pharmacy Internat* 1980;1:38–41.

Orme ML'E, Back DJ. Interactions between oral contraceptive steroids and broad spectrum antibiotics. *Clin Exp Dermat* 1986;11:327–31.

Orme ML'E, Back DJ, Breckenridge AM. Clinical pharmacokinetics of oral contraceptive steroids. *Clin Pharmacokin* 1983;8:95–136.

Orme M, Back DJ, Ward S, Green S. The pharmacokinetics of ethynylestradiol in the presence and absence of gestodene and desogestrel. *Contraception* 1991;43:305–16.

Patwardhan RV, Mitchell MC, Johnson RF, Schenker S. Differential effects of oral contraceptive steroids on the metabolism of benzodiazepines. *Hepatol* 1983;3:248–53.

Pazzucconi F, Malavasi B, Galli G, Franceschini G, Calabresi L, et al. Inhibition of antipyrine metabolism by low-dose contraceptives with gestodene and desogestrel. *Clin Pharmacol Ther* 1991;49:278–84.

Prescott LF. Kinetics and metabolism of paracetamol and phenacetin. *Br J Clin Pharmacol* 1980;10:291S–298S.

Reimers D, Jezek A. Rifampicin und andere antituberkulostatika bei gleichzeitiger oraler kontrazeption. *Prax Pneumol* 1971;25:255–62.

Rietvald EC, Broekman, MMM, Houben JJG, Eskes TKAB, Van Rossum JM. Rapid onset of an increase in caffeine residence time in young women due to oral contraceptive steroids. *Eur J Clin Pharmacol* 1984;26:371–3.

Roberton YR, Johnson ES. Interactions between oral contraceptives and other drugs: a review. *Curr Med Res Opin* 1976;3:647–61.

Roberts RK, Desmond PV, Wilkinson GR, Schenker S. Disposition of chlordiazepoxide: sex differences and effects of oral contraceptives. *Clin Pharmacol Ther* 1979;25:826–31.

Roberts RK, Grice J, McGuffie C, Heilbronn L. Oral contraceptive steroids impair the elimination of theophylline. *J Lab Clin Med* 1983;101:821–5.

Robson RA, Matthews AP, Miners JO, McManus ME, Meyer UA, et al. Characterisation of theophylline metabolism in human liver microsomes. *Br J Clin Pharmacol* 1987;24:293–300.

Rogers SM, Back DJ, Orme ML'E. Intestinal metabolism of ethinyloestradiol and paracetamol *in vitro*: studies using Ussing chambers. *Br J Clinical Pharmacol* 1987a;23:727–34.

Rogers SM, Back DJ, Stevenson PJ, Grimmer SFM, Orme ML'E. Paracetamol interaction with oral contraceptive steroids: increased plasma concentrations of ethinyloestradiol. *Br J Clin Pharmacol* 1987b;23:721–5.

Sahlberg B-L, Axelson M, Collins DJ, Sjovall J. Analysis of isomeric ethynylestradiol glucuronides in urine. *J Chromatog* 1981;217:453–61.

Scavone JM, Greenblatt DJ, Locniskar A, Shader RI. Alprazolam pharmacokinetics in women on low-dose oral contraceptives. *J Clin Pharmacol* 1988;28:454–7.

Shenfield GM. Drug interactions with oral contraceptive preparations. *Med J Austral* 1986;144:205–11.

Shenfield GM, Griffin JM. Clinical pharmacokinetics of contraceptive steroids. An update. *Clin Pharmacokin* 1991;20:15–37.

Sparrow MJ. Pill method failures. *N Zeal Med J* 1987;100:102–5.

Stockley I. Drug interactions: an appraisal of the current situation. *Trends Pharmacol Sci* 1979;1:6.

Stoehr GP, Krobath PD, Juhl RP, Wender DB, Phillips JP, et al. Effect of oral contraceptives on triazolam, temazepam, alprazolam and lorazepam kinetics. *Clin Pharmacol Ther* 1984;36:683–90.

Szoka PR, Edgren RA. Drug interactions with oral contraceptives: compilation and analysis of an adverse experience report database. *Fertil Steril* 1988;49:31–38S.

Tephly TR, Mannering GT. Inhibition of drug metabolism. V. Inhibition of drug metabolism by steroids. *Molec Pharmacol* 1968;4:10–4.

Teunissen MWE, Srivastava AK, Breimer DD. Influence of sex and oral contraceptive steroids on antipyrine metabolite formation. *Clin Pharmacol Ther* 1982;32:240–6.

van Dijke CPH, Weber JCP. Interaction between oral contraceptives and griseofulvin. *Br Med J* 1984;288:1,125–6.

Vestal RE, Cusack BJ, Mercer GD, Dawson GW, Park BK. Aging and drug interactions. I. Effect of cimetidine and smoking on the oxidation of theophylline and cortisol in healthy men. *J Pharmacol Exper Ther* 1987;241:488–500.

Vestal RE, Wood AJJ, Branch RA, Shand DG, Wilkinson GR. Effects of age and cigarette smoking on the disposition of propranolol in man. *Clin Pharmacol Ther* 1979;26:8–15.

Watson KJR, Ghabrial H, Mashford ML, Harman PJ, Breen KJ, et al. The oral contraceptive pill increases morphine clearance but does not increase hepatic blood flow. *Gastroenterology* 1986;90:1,779.

Wood AJJ, Vestel RE, Wilkinson GR, Branch RA, Shand DG. Effects of aging and cigarette smoking on antipyrine and indocyanine green elimination. *Clin Pharmacol Ther* 1979;26:16–20.

Zamah NM, Humpel M. Kuhnz W, et al. Absence of an effect of high vitamin C dosage on the systemic availability of ethynyl estradiol in women using a combination oral contraceptive. *Contraception* 1993; (*in press*).

Zatuchni, GI, Elstein M. What is the relevance of pharmacokinetic and pharmacodynamic data and metabolic studies to OC users? Consensus statement. *Adv Contracept* 1991;7[Suppl 3]:4–5.

Pharmacology of the Contraceptive Steroids,
edited by Joseph W. Goldzieher.
Raven Press, Ltd., New York © 1994.

29

Evaluating Efficacy and Safety

*David A. Edelman and †Joseph W. Goldzieher

*Medical Research Consultants, Madison, New Jersey 07940; †Department of Obstetrics
and Gynecology, Baylor College of Medicine, Houston, Texas 77030*

Establishing the effectiveness and safety of contraceptive drugs is a difficult task for a number of reasons. Quite obviously, the primary purpose of a contraceptive drug is to prevent pregnancy, and a trial should not place women at an unknown or unacceptable risk. Additionally, acceptability needs to be carefully analyzed and evaluated, because adherence to a daily pill-taking regimen will directly affect the risk of pregnancy and the occurrence of side effects, which in turn affects compliance. Since a comprehensive description of the issues and process of evaluating the efficacy and safety of contraceptive steroids would require a book in itself, this chapter is limited to particular issues of the evaluation process.

CONTRACEPTIVE EFFECTIVENESS

In a study on human fertility in 1932, Pearl used an index that was based on the total number of woman-months of exposure (Pearl, 1932). This index, often referred to as the Pearl Index, computes event rates—e.g., pregnancy, as the number of pregnancies divided by the number of woman-months at risk, multiplied by 1,200 to give pregnancies per 100 woman-years. The appeal of this index is its simplicity. Its limitations for the computation of pregnancy rates (or other event rates) include:

1. A disproportionate weight is given by women observed for long periods of time.
2. The index is not suited for estimating pregnancy rates if the risk of pregnancy changes over time or if the character of the population changes with time (i.e., dropouts are not a random sample of the observed population).
3. The rate does not distinguish between the number of women evaluated and the duration of oral contraceptive (OC) use. Thus, 10 users observed for 6 months (total = 60 woman-months of use) is treated the same way as two users observed for 30 months (also a total of 60 woman-months of use).

There are times when it is appropriate to use the Pearl Index for comparing event rates. Where individual published studies have used different methods for computing event rates, the only reasonable procedure for comparing the rates across studies is to compute the Pearl rates. The data necessary for computing a life-table survival rate are usually not available. The Pearl rates should be computed for fixed periods of time such as intervals of 6 months. These rates will give a close estimate of the cumulative gross life-table rate for that time period (Sivin and Schmidt, 1987).

To overcome the limitations of the Pearl Index, survival (life-table) methods should be used. In contraceptive research, these techniques were first used in the 1960s for assessing contraceptive efficacy (Potter, 1969), and they should replace the Pearl Index as an acceptable form of analysis. The life-table method estimates the probability of an event (e.g. pregnancy) during each unit of time, and event rates are expressed as a cumulative rate over a fixed period of time. Standard statistical methods are used to compare the survival distributions, rather than the event rates, at any one point in time.

Since overall pregnancy rates reflect both the intrinsic effectiveness of the method, if used perfectly, and the reliability of the users, it is customary to distinguish between the "theoretical effectiveness" and "use-effectiveness" of OC use (or any other method of contraception).

Theoretical effectiveness is difficult to determine. Putative evidence of ovulation, such as plasma progesterone levels or urinary pregnandiol excretion, indicates the function of a corpus luteum or the absence thereof, but not the release of a viable ovum. Even if an egg is produced and fertilized, no practical test assesses the implantability of the prevailing endometrium. In normal noncontracepting women, very early implantations commonly disintegrate without producing attention-attracting changes in the menstrual cycle; routine monitoring of each cycle of observation with supersensitive β-hCG assays is hardly practicable.

In clinical trials that include relatively few OC users and in which no pregnancies are observed (Goldzieher et al, 1962), the question arises as to what is a reasonable estimate of the pregnancy rate. One approach is to use the upper 95% confidence limit on the observed rate. In Fig. 1, the upper 95% confidence limit for zero pregnancies in 500 to 100,000 cycles of observation is given. However, this approach has some of the same limitations as the Pearl index. If this approach is used to estimate pregnancy rates, the upper 95% confidence values should be obtained for fixed periods of observation, such as successive 6-month periods.

Estimates of the use-effectiveness of OCs vary very widely. In the U.S. for the period 1970–1976, the Guttmacher Institute (Ory et al, 1983) estimated that the percentage of currently married women who became pregnant within the first year of OC use ranged from 2.1% to 4.7%, varying by age group; the highest figure relates to the underage-22 population. Another estimate from this source (Harlap et al, 1991) (in 1991, a time when low-dose OCs were generally used) gave a similar range of 1.9% to 5.0% in the first year of use. In some populations, compliance is so poor that OCs are simply not an acceptable option compared, for example, to injectable contraceptives or surgical sterilization. Jones and Forrest (1992) adjusted

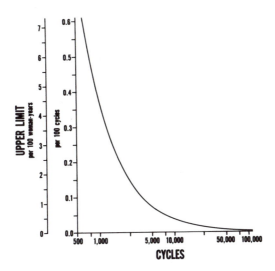

FIG. 1. Upper limit of 95 percent confidence region for "true" incidence rate with zero incidence in a given number of cycles.

for the underreporting of abortion, and calculated even higher failure rates. The long-term implications of failure rates have been discussed by Ross (1989).

An estimate of the sample size required for a cohort study comparing pregnancy rates of two OCs is given in Table 1. The sample sizes were calculated according to the methods of George and Desu (1974) for the comparison of the survival distributions of the two groups of OC users. The calculations are based on the assumption that the subjects are recruited into the study over a 6-month period and followed up for 1 year, and that the only reason for leaving the study is pregnancy. If discontinuations for other reasons were to be taken into account, sample sizes larger than those shown would be required. A simpler approach is to determine sample sizes based on the Pearl Index. This was done by Hines and Goldzieher (1969), who based their calculations on assumed rates of theoretical effectiveness and compli-

TABLE 1. *Sample size requirement for a cohort study of the pregnancy rates of two oral contraceptives*

Alpha	Beta	12-month pregnancy rate per 100 women		Required no. of subjects
		OC #1	OC #2	
0.05	0.20	4.0	2.0	972
		6.0	3.0	855
0.01	0.10	4.0	2.0	1836
		6.0	3.0	1209

TABLE 2. *A study of sample sizes required to differentiate the effectiveness of two oral contraceptives (one (A) twice as effective as the other (B)) in a population which does not take medication with perfect reliability*

Hypothetical pregnancy rate (per 100 w/y)						Calculated number of cycles required for *each* drug	
Due to drug failure		Due to patient failure		Due to patient and drug failure			
A	B			A	B	P = .05	P = .01
0.4	0.8	0.4	(50%)	0.80	1.20	58,000	100,000
0.2	0.4	0.6	(75%)	0.80	1.00	207,000	356,000
0.08	0.16	0.72	(90%)	0.80	0.88	1,210,000	2,080,000
0.04	0.08	0.76	(95%)	0.80	0.84	4,725,000	8,122,000

w/y = women-years

ance (see Table 2). Their calcuations show that to compare two OCs whose theoretical effectiveness rates differ by a factor of two (0.4 and 0.8 per 100 woman-years), and if the pregnancies due to compliance failure are of the same order for both OCs (0.4 per 100 woman-years by the end of the first year), at least 58,000 cycles *with each formulation* are required. This represents an almost impossible task.

Another approach to the evaluation of pregnancy rates is provided by Ketting (1988), who examined the brand of OC used by women who voluntarily terminated a pregnancy and resided in a country where this procedure was legal and available through national health services. A higher-than-expected proportion of the terminated pregnancies was associated with the use of multiphasic formulations, suggesting that these formulations have a smaller margin of error before contraceptive failure occurs. Similar findings were reported by Kovacs et al. (1989) in Australia.

Initial failure rates, both with oral and injectable agents, may be confounded by the presence of a very early, unrecognized pregnancy. With virtually compliance-free methods such as injectables, this complication represents an important component of pregnancies occurring subsequent to the first injection.

Acceptability and compliance are interwoven concepts of great complexity (Benagiano and Shedlin, 1992). In practical terms, compliance is difficult to assess. Even Hippocrates said "[the physician] should keep aware of the fact that patients often lie when they state that they have taken certain medicines . . ." Users' perceptions of prescription drugs in general are seldom based on sound, understandable documentation. Media publicity often generates hysterical outpourings of alleged adverse reactions, which may then be further exploited by vested interests; in a litigious society this becomes a major problem. The documentation that accompanies packages of OCs in the U.S. is generally seen as inadequate, incomprehensible, or both, to the user with a high-school education. The 1984 ACOG survey showed that OC users most commonly get their information regarding OCs from girlfriends and family members, occasionally from sex-education classes, and from other sources. The interaction with health personnel is not seen to be a major source of information. In third-world countries, rumor and misinformation commonly nullify the contraceptive potential of OCs. Thus, acceptability and hence compliance may vary from place to place and time to time, restricting estimates of use-effectiveness to a particular time and locale.

In addition to this background of uninformed or misinformed perceptions, contraceptive agents bear the special burden of opposition of various religious, cultural, or other pro-fertility forces that do not hesitate to exploit reports of adverse reactions or contraceptive failure, and thus diminish acceptability.

SIDE EFFECTS

Phase III clinical trials are the usual procedure for the discovery of common events; rare events require special consideration of sample size. Rare events usually are not discovered until after the agent comes into widespread prescription use. The importance of multicenter trials can hardly be overemphasized; the variability in incidence of subjective and objective symptoms can be startling (Hines and Goldzieher, 1968). Moreover, the incidence of a preexisting complaint such as dysmenorrhea, as well as its response to OC use, can vary widely (Fig. 2). It is well known that the expectations of the candidate population, as well as those of the service delivery personnel, have a profound impact on the results and must be compensated for by appropriate controls.

Women may be questioned directly or indirectly about the occurrence of various side effects and menstrual cycle events. Alternatively, women may be requested to keep a log and record these phenomena on a day-by-day basis. This self-monitoring results in increased observer attention and less loss of useful information due to faulty recall. Whether these biases offset one another is another matter. Presentation and analysis of such data vary greatly in the literature, making comparisons difficult. Rodriguez et al. (1976) and the WHO (Belsey et al., 1991) have suggested standardized formats for the analysis and presentation of data relating to these events.

Placebo-controlled studies can and have been performed repeatedly with OCs; protection against pregnancy can be assured by the simultaneous use of another approved contraceptive modality, such as a vaginal spermicide, or by the use of a population protected against pregnancy by prior tubal ligation. These groups of individuals, however, may have different characteristics from oral or injectable contraceptive acceptors. For example, OC users are more likely to be smokers, and tend to have higher use of other medications. Such confounders need to be taken into account. The importance of placebo controls is evident even for symptoms such as nausea, which is known to occur from oral administration of estrogens. In one double-blind study (Goldzieher et al., 1971, Fig. 3), the incidence of nausea in the placebo cycles ranged around 10%, whereas only two of the five high-dose OCs tested exceeded this level in the first cycle of use.

An anecdotal report typically describes one or more cases of a specific disease, or

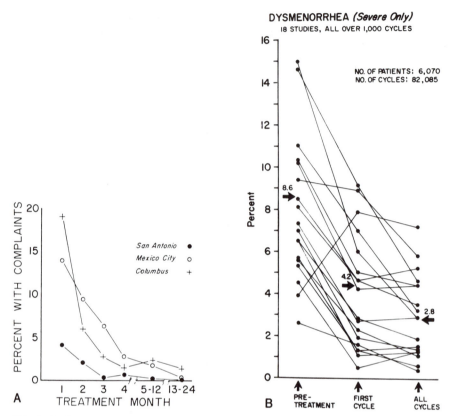

FIG. 2. A. Frequency of complaints by month of use. **B.** Initial incidence and effect of oral contraceptive on dysmenorrhea.

a rare or unusual event. Most such series include too few cases for statistical analysis and should not be used (but frequently are!) to make inferences about what may be expected in larger and diverse populations. Their principal value is to provide an early warning system for potential adverse effects, and to suggest hypotheses that can be tested in other types of study.

In recent years, case-control studies have become a popular method for the study of rare events. Their appeal to researchers often lies in the apparent simplicity of the study design and methods of analysis. A case-control study starts with a group of individuals who have the disease or condition under investigation, and another (more or less matched) group whose individuals are free of the condition. One then determines the frequency of use of the suspected agent (e.g., an OC) in each group, and from the fourfold table (users/nonusers, cases/control) computes the relative risk (RR) of, for example, the risk of disease X among persons exposed to agent Y compared to persons who were not exposed to agent Y. Related to the relative risk is the *attributable risk*, which estimates the proportion of cases of X among OC users

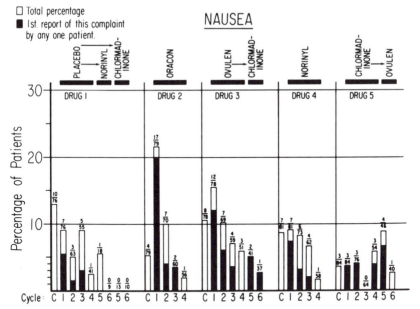

FIG. 3. Incidence of nausea in a placebo-controlled randomized trial of several types of OC. (Numbers on bars indicate number of events/total number of subjects.)

in the general population that is attributable to OC use. Attributable risk is calculated as (RR-1)/RR.

Misuse of case-control studies, which has occurred frequently in the assessment of adverse reactions to OCs (Realini and Goldzieher, 1985) translates into inappropriate interpretation of the data and erroneous conclusions. In the absence of prospective studies, where results may not be forthcoming for years, case-control studies may be the only feasible approach to the evaluation of rare events. However, they are subject to many sources of bias—i.e., systematic flaws (Feinstein, 1977; Ibrahim, 1979; Schlesselman, 1982). Horwitz and Feinstein (1979a, b) have listed 12 methodological principles for case-control study research that, if followed, should minimize the occurrence of many common sources of bias. Unfortunately, most case-control studies in the medical literature fail to adhere to many of these principles. It is therefore not at all surprising that these studies have led to conflicting results. Important examples in the area of investigation of adverse effects of OCs are the British and American case-control studies of cardiovascular hazards attributed to OCs. These studies were confounded by numerous biases (Realini and Goldzieher, 1985), but perhaps most significantly by inattention to the factor of cigarette smoking. When this was taken into consideration, the increased risk of myocardial infarction and other cardiovascular events attributed to OCs disappeared (Croft and Hannaford, 1989; Goldbaum, 1987).

In the case-control studies of deep vein thrombosis, epidemiologists accepted at face value the clinical diagnosis or rationalized its probable accuracy. This occurred

TABLE 3. *Sample size requirements for a case-control study of benign breast disease and long-term oral contraceptive usage*

Relative Risk	P_0	Alpha	Beta	N
0.7	0.2	0.01	0.10	1644
		0.05	0.20	865
	0.4	0.01	0.10	1022
		0.05	0.20	538
0.5	0.2	0.01	0.10	494
		0.05	0.20	260
	0.4	0.01	0.10	288
		0.05	0.20	152

P_0 = estimated proportion of long-term OC users in the control population
Alpha = probability of a type I error
Beta = probability of a type II error
N = number of subjects in the case and control groups
Sample sizes computed using methods given by Schlesselman (1982).

in spite of the fact that available technology (ultrasound, plethysmography, labeled fibrinogen) indicated a false negative diagnostic error of the order of 20% to 50%, and a false positive error that reached 83% when the clinician was aware that the patient was an OC user (for references, see Realini and Goldzieher, 1985).

It is important to consider the sample size required to detect a certain magnitude of the relative risk when a case-control study is to be undertaken. Table 3 illustrates the wide range of sample sizes needed to determine whether long-term OC users are at a reduced risk of benign breast disease. The sample size depends on the probabilities of the type I and type II errors, the magnitude of the relative risk one wants to detect, and the proportion of OC users in the population. There are variables other than OC use *per se* that might affect the risk of benign breast disease (e.g., type of OC, duration of use, age at first use, prior history of benign breast disease, and others). If the study were designed to provide estimates of risk that included these variables, larger samples than those given in Table 3 would be required.

An actual example of the importance of sample size may be found in the study of Mann et al. (1975). Table 4, first half, shows the fourfold data sets for the three age groups. The relative risk for myocardial infarction was 2.8 for the under-40 group and 4.7 for the 40 to 44 age group. Based on this data, as well as apparently confirmatory data provided by the early results of the Royal College prospective study (which also did not correct for smoking), it was recommended that use of OCs be avoided in women aged 40 or over (some used the age of 35 as a cutoff point, for undocumented reasons). These epidemiologists recognized that the data set provided very small numbers for users both in the control and diseased groups, especially in the 40 + age group. They therefore examined the other half of their data for the 40 to 44 age group (only half of the available data had been used for the initial report). The second data set showed a nonsignificant risk of 2.2 (Mann et al., 1976). Unfortunately, the two data sets for the 40 to 44 age group were not combined by the authors, as shown in the Table; if they had been, it would turn out

TABLE 4. British myocardial infarction (MI) studies

		Age < 40		Age 40–44		Age 45–49	
		M.I.	Control	M.I.	Control	M.I.	Control
First half of data	Nonusers	18	49	42	46	44	47
	Users	21	17	8	2	2	0
	Significance	P<.02		P = .05		NS	
	Relative Risk	**2.8**		**4.7**			
Second half of data				36	40		
				10	5		
				NS			
The data combined				78	86		
				18	7		
				P<.05			
				2.8			

that the relative risk for the under-40 and 40-or-over groups was *identical*. In point of fact, neglect of the smoking factor vitiated the entire investigation, but it was nearly 10 years before the FDA removed the age constraint for nonsmokers from the package insert. Undoubtedly, many thousands of women were deprived of access to this contraceptive modality for over a decade because of erroneous inferences from small numbers.

Another example of a problem with case-control studies is illustrated by the issue of hepatomas. To begin with, most of these cases are a consequence of infection with hepatitis B, a sexually transmitted disease whose incidence varies enormously from country to country; virtually all of the early case-control studies ignored this pathophysiology in their investigation of the relationship to OCs. The study of Rooks et al. (1979) showed an astronomical increase in relative risk (up to 503) with increasing years of OC use (see Table 5). The reality, however, is that not one of the large prospective studies in the U.S. and U.K. have reported a single case of hepatoma during the entire duration of these studies.

Prospective studies have their own problems, including selection bias when the contraceptive options are not randomly assigned. Changes in the OC formulations used over time, switching from one formulation to another, and dropouts are just some of the variables that are impossible to control.

Since very few studies include a number of subjects adequate to detect small differences among treatment groups, and since different studies may yield results

TABLE 5. Hepatocellular adenoma and OC use

Duration of use, mos.	Relative risk
0–12	1
13–36	9
37–60	116
61–84	129
Over 85	503

(Rooks et al., 1979)

that apparently are different, how can one best integrate the results of different studies to arrive at a general conclusion about a treatment effect? One approach is through the use of meta-analysis.

The term "meta-analysis" was first used by Glass in 1976 to refer to a method of integrating the findings of different studies. The single most important advantage of meta-analysis (if performed correctly) is that it provides a systematic and quantitative approach for the synthesis of individual study results. For example, Rushton and Jones (1992) identified 27 studies published from 1980 to 1989 that evaluated the risk of breast cancer among OC users. Using meta-analysis methods, they were able to arrive at an overall relative risk estimate for breast cancer in OC users.

An underlying assumption in combining the results from individual studies on, for example, the risk of breast cancer and OC use, is that differences among the studies in their estimates of risk of breast cancer are due to chance alone. Thus, estimates of this risk in the individual studies represent random fluctuations around some true but unknown value. This assumption implies that the results from different studies cannot be pooled without first considering the design, methods of data collection used, subject inclusion and exclusion criteria, and other aspects of the design of the individual studies. Therefore, the prerequisite of any meta-analysis is the development of criteria for the inclusion of individual studies and identification of variables known to affect the risk estimates of the entity to be evaluated. If it appears that the study outcomes are not due to random variation, it may become necessary to perform meta-analyses for certain subgroups of studies and/or make statistical adjustments to the estimates of risk to take into account the effect of important characteristics.

Meta-analysis is a useful tool for providing an objective approach to the assimilation of the results of different studies. However, it is not realistic to expect that a meta-analysis will provide simple statistical answers to complex clinical problems.

REFERENCES

Belsey EM, et al. Menstrual bleeding patterns in untreated women and with long-acting methods of contraception. *Adv Contraception* 1991;7:257–70.

Benagiano G, Shedlin MG. Cultural factors in oral contraceptive compliance. *Adv Contraception* 1992; 8[Suppl]:47–56.

Croft P, Hannaford PC. Risk factors for acute myocardial infarction in women: Evidence from the Royal College of General Practitioners' oral contraceptive studies. *Brit Med J* 1989;298:165.

Feinstein AR. *Clinical Biostatistics*. St. Louis: CV Mosby Co.; 1977:71ff.

Glass GV. Primary, secondary, and meta-analysis of research. *Educ Researcher* 1976;5:3–8.

Goldbaum GM, Kendrick JS, Hogelin GC et al. The relative impact of smoking and oral contraceptive use on women in the United States. *JAMA* 1987;258:1339.

Goldzieher JW, Moses LE, Averkin E, et al. A placebo-controlled double blind crossover investigation of the side effects attributed to oral contraceptives. *Fertil Steril* 1971;22:609–23.

Goldzieher JW, Moses LE, Ellis L. Study of norethindrone in contraception. *JAMA* 1962;180:359–62.

Harlap S, Kost K, Forrest JD. Preventing pregnancy: protecting health. *The Alan Guttmacher Institute* 1991:36–37.

Hines DC, Goldzieher JW. Clinical investigation: a guide to its evaluation. *Am J Obstet Gynecol* 1969;105:450–87.

Hines DC, Goldzieher JW. Large scale study of an oral contraceptive. *Fertil Steril* 1968;19:841–66.

Horwitz RI, Feinstein AR. Case-control study of oral contraceptive pills and endometrial cancer. *Ann Intern Med* 1979a;91:226–7.

Horwitz RI, Feinstein AR. Methodologic standards and contradictory results in case-control research. *Am J Med* 1979b;66:566–74.

Ibrahim MA. *The case control study. Consensus and controversy.* New York: Pergamon Press; 1979: 51ff.

Jones EF, Forrest JD. Contraceptive failure rates based on the 1988 NSFG. *Fam Plann Perspect* 1992; 24:12–9.

Ketting E. The relative reliability of oral contraceptives: findings of an epidemiological study. *Contraception* 1988;37:343.

Kovacs GT, Riddoch G, Duncombe P, et al. Inadvertent pregnancies in oral contraceptive users. *Med J Austral* 1989;150:549–51.

Mann JI, Inman WHW, Thorogood M. Oral contraceptive use in older women and fatal myocardial infarction. *Br Med J* 1976;2:445–7.

Mann JI, Vessey MP, Thorogood D, Doll R. Myocardial infarction in young women with special reference to oral contraceptive practice. *Br Med J* 1975;2:241–5.

Ory HW, Forrest JD, Lincoln R. Making choices. *The Alan Guttmacher Institute* 1983:30.

Pearl R. Contraception and fertility in 2000 women. *Human Biol* 1932;4:363.

Potter RG: Use-effectiveness of intrauterine contraception as a problem in competing risks. In: Freedman RF, Takeshita JY, eds. *Family planning in Taiwan.* Princeton: Princeton University Press; 1969:458.

Realini JP, Goldzieher JW. Oral contraceptives and cardiovascular disease: A critique of the epidemiological studies. *Am J Obst Gynec* 1985;152:729–798.

Rodriguez G, Faundes-Latham A, and Atkinson LE. An approach to the analysis of menstrual patterns in the critical evaluation of contraceptives. *Stud Fam Plann* 1976;7:42–51.

Rooks JB, Ory HW, et al. Epidemiology of hepatocellular adenoma: the role of oral contraceptive use. *JAMA* 1979;242:644.

Ross JA. Contraception: short-term v. long-term failure rates. *Fam Plann Perspect* 1989;21:275–7.

Rushton L, Jones DR. Oral contraceptive use and breast cancer risk: a meta-analysis of variations with age at diagnosis, parity and total duration of oral contraceptive use. *Br J Obstet Gynaecol* 1992;99: 239–46.

Schlesselman JJ. *Case control studies. Design, conduct, analysis.* New York: Oxford University Press; 1982.

Sivin I, Schmidt F. Effectiveness of IUDs. *Contraception* 1987;36:55–84.

Appendix

CHEMICAL NOMENCLATURE: TRIVIAL AND CHEMICAL NAMES

Estrogens

Estradiol cypionate. (17β)-Estra-1,3,5(10)-triene-3,17-diol,17-cyclopentanepropan-
oate.

Estradiol enanthate. (17β)-Estra-1,3,5,(10)-triene-3,17-diol, 17-heptanoate.

Ethynyl estradiol. Ethinyl estradiol; 19-Nor-17α-pregn-1,3,5(10)-trien-20-yne-3,
17-diol.

Ethynyl estradiol methyl ether. Mestranol; 3-Methoxy-19-nor-17α-pregn-1,3,5(10)-
trien-20-yne-17-ol

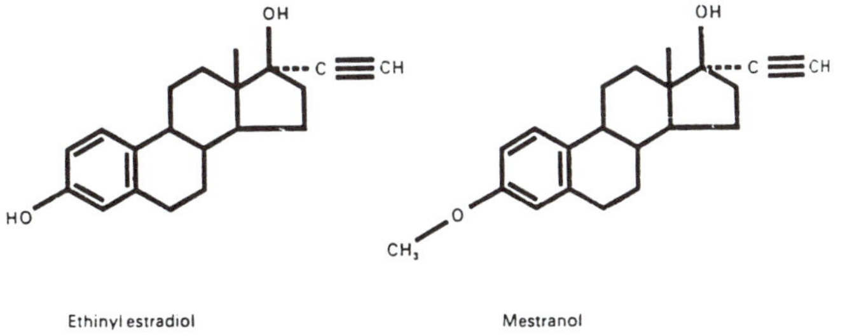

Ethinyl estradiol   Mestranol

FIG. A1. Estrogens.

19-Norprogestins—Norethindrone Group

Ethynodiol diacetate; 19-Norpregn-4-en-20-yne-3β,17-diol diacetate
Lynestrenol; 19-Norpregn-4-en-20-yn-17-ol
Norethindrone,norethisterone; 17-Hydroxy-19-norpregn-4-ene-20-yne-3-one
Norethindrone enanthate; 17-Hydroxy-19-norpregn-4-en-20-yn-3-one enanthate
Norethindrone/norethisterone acetate; 17-Hydroxy-19-norpregn-4-ene-20-yn-3-one
   acetate
Norethynodrel; 17-Ethynyl-19-norpregn-5(10)-en-20-yn-3-one

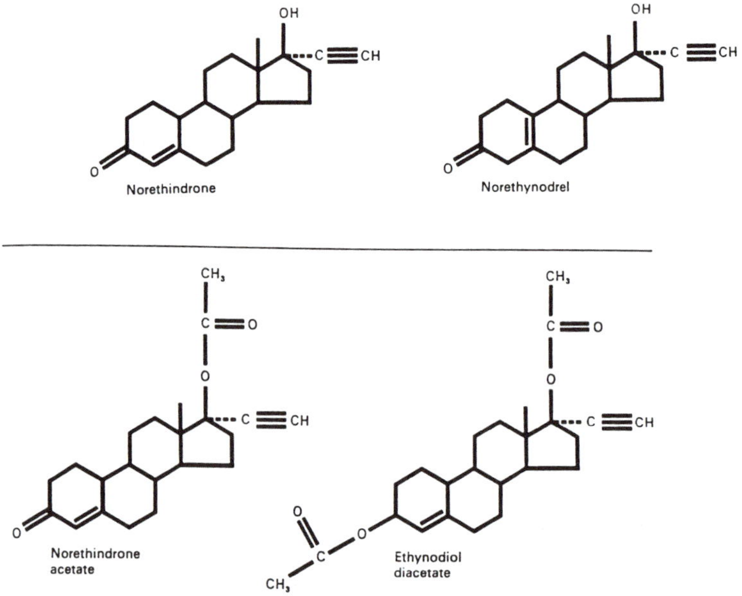

FIG. A2. 19 norprogestins-norethindrone group.

19-Norprogestins—Norgestrel Group*

Desogestrel; (17α)-13-Ethyl-11-methylene-18,19-dinorpregn-4-en-20-yn-17-ol
Gestodene; (17α)-13-Ethyl-17-hydroxy-18,19-dinorpregn-4,15-dien-20-yn-*3*-one
Levonorgestrel;   d(-)-13β-Ethyl-17α-ethynyl-17-hydroxy-18,19-dinorpregn-4-en-3-one
Norgestimate; (17α)-17-Acetyloxy-13-ethyl-18,19-dinorpregn-4-en-20-yn-3-oxime

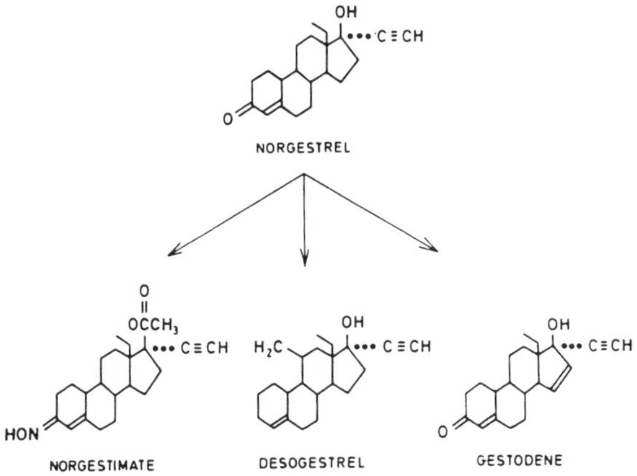

FIG. A3. 19 norprogestins-levonorgestrel group.

* Norgestrel is synthesized chemically, and the final product consists of a racemic mixture that can be resolved into its optically active dextrorotatory (+) and levorotatory (−) enantiomers. On the basis of Reichstein's classification, the absolute stereochemical configuration of (+) norgestrel and (−) norgestrel was designated as *d*-norgestrel and *l*-norgestrel respectively. The *d*- and *l*- prefixes (italicized) assigned to norgestrel refer only to the absolute configuration of a compound. In contrast, the d- and l- prefixes (nonitalicized), which are sometimes used in place of (+) and (−), respectively, refer to a compound's optical rotatory properties. It has been found that naturally occurring steroids generally belong to the *d*-series of Reichstein's classification and are dextrorotatory, on the basis of their absolute stereochemical configuration and optical rotation, respectively. Although some synthetic progestins belong to the same category as the naturally occurring ones, others, such as the biologically active form of norgestrel, belong to the *d*-series but are levorotatory. For this reason, the World Health Organization selected the name *levonorgestrel* for the biologically active enantiomer [*d*-(-)-norgestrel]. The name *norgestrel* for the racemic mixture of the compound [*dl*-(±)-norgestrel] remained the same. Although no name was assigned to the inactive dextrorotatory enantiomer [*l*-(+)-norgestrel], this compound will be referred to as *dextronorgestrel*.

Acetoxyprogestins—Progesterone Group

Chlormadinone acetate; 17-Acetyloxy-6-chloro-pregn-4,6-diene acetate

Cyproterone acetate; 6-Chloro-1,2-dihydro-17-hydroxy-3'H-cyclopropa[1,2] pregn-1,4,6-triene-3,20-dione acetate

Dihydroxyprogesterone acetophenide; (16α)-(R)-16,17-[(1-Phenylethylidine)bis(oxy)]-pregn-4-ene-3,20-dione

Medroxyprogesterone acetate; 17-Hydroxy-6-methyl-pregn-4-ene-3,20-dione acetate

Megestrol acetate; 17-Hydroxy-6-methyl-pregn-4,6-diene-3,20-dione acetate

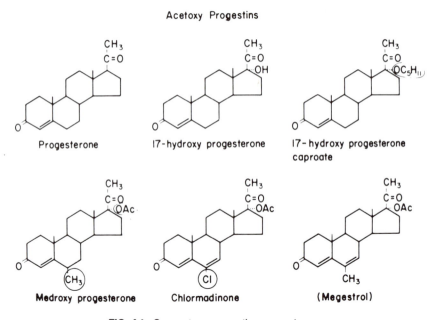

FIG. A4. C_{21}-acetoxy progestins-progesterone group.

Under Investigation

Nomegestrol; 17-hydroxy-6-methyl-19-norpregn-4, 6-diene-3, 20-dione acetate

ST 1435; 17-hydroxy-16-mehtylene-19norpregn-4-ene-3, 20-dione acetate

Subject Index